Sports Injuries

To Sophie and Hildegard

For Butterworth Heinemann

Commissioning Editor: Heidi Allen
Development Editor: Robert Edwards
Project Manager: Ailsa Laing
Design: George Ajayi
Illustrations Manager: Bruce Hogarth
Illustrator: Graeme Chambers

Sports Injuries
Diagnosis and Management

THIRD EDITION

Christopher M Norris MSc CAc MCSP SRP

Director of Norris Associates, Chartered Physiotherapists, Sale, Cheshire, UK

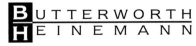

EDINBURGH LONDON NEW YORK OXFORD PHILADELPHIA ST LOUIS SYDNEY TORONTO 2004

BUTTERWORTH-HEINEMANN
An imprint of Elsevier Limited

First published 1993
Second Edition 1998
Third Edition 2004

ISBN 0 7506 5223 3

British Library Cataloguing in Publication Data
A catalogue record for this book is available from the British Library

Library of Congress Cataloging in Publication Data
A catalog record for this book is available from the Library of Congress

Note
Medical knowledge is constantly changing. Standard safety precautions must be
followed, but as new research and clinical experience broaden our knowledge,
changes in treatment and drug therapy may become necessary or appropriate.
Readers are advised to check the most current product information provided by
the manufacturer of each drug to be administered to verify the recommended
dose, the method and duration of administration, and contraindications. It is the
responsibility of the practitioner, relying on experience and knowledge of the
patient, to determine dosages and the best treatment for each individual patient.
Neither the Publisher nor the author assumes any liability for any injury and/or
damage to persons or property arising from this publication.

The Publisher

your source for books,
journals and multimedia
in the health sciences
www.elsevierhealth.com

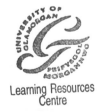

Learning Resources
Centre

12687332

The
Publisher's
policy is to use
**paper manufactured
from sustainable forests**

Printed in China

Contents

Acknowledgements

Models for the photographs were Lindsay Peacock and Helen Doyle, with thanks. Photography by Nina Preece.

Preface

Sports Injuries is a regularly thumbed text in most physio-therapy and sports science libraries. Feedback from students indicated that the practical feel of the book and the varied nature of the treatments, which do not adhere to any particular 'treatment philosophy', were real selling points. For the third edition then, these aspects of the book have been increased with the introduction of specific treatment notes detailing practical techniques, with photographs and accompanying text. Each of these gives pointers to a wide variety of treatment methods, which act as 'snippets' to whet the reader's appetite and encourage them to read further. With over 440 line drawings and 146 photographs, the third edition of *Sports Injuries* is both more visually and more clinically informative.

To make the text even more readable, keypoints and definitions have been included in this edition and the use of two colours has improved the text, making it more appealing to the eye and easier to follow. In addition, the slightly larger format has enabled additional text to be added without making the book too thick and unwieldy.

Material in the book has been updated with new information and references to keep it at the cutting edge of evidence-based practice. Hopefully, by doing this I have also kept *Sports Injuries* as an easy-to-read clinical guide, which will continue to be heavily thumbed by students around the world.

SECTION **1**

Diagnosis

Chapter **1**

Biomechanics of injury

CHAPTER CONTENTS

Human tissue is governed by the laws of mechanics in the same way as other materials. While mechanics is concerned with forces, the effect of these forces on living organisms is the realm of biomechanics. There are two aspects to biomechanics (Dvir, 2000): the study of human performance, and the examination of the way in which biological tissues act when subjected to forces.

Definition

Biomechanics is the study of human motion. It looks at both the mechanics of human performance and the material behaviour of biological tissues.

The association between biological and mechanical aspects of movement has been said to give human motion its sophistication (Williams and Sperryn, 1976). For this reason, the study of biomechanics has a direct application to injury and recovery, and knowledge of this subject is essential for an understanding of the prevention, diagnosis and treatment of sports injuries (LeVeau, 1990).

BIOMECHANICAL PRINCIPLES

Forces

Force is a term used to describe the interaction of an object with its surroundings (Enoka, 1994). It has been defined as the physical action which tends to change the position of a body in space (Stallard, 1984), or the ability to accelerate the object (Dvir, 2000). Consequently, it is an entity which will produce motion, and the study of force and motion is called *kinetics*. The unit of measurement of a force is the newton (N), one newton being the force which would produce an acceleration of $1\,\mathrm{m/s^2}$ when acting on an object with a mass of 1 kg.

The most common forces affecting the human body are those produced by muscles and those occurring as a result of gravity, inertia and contact. There are four important considerations when dealing with forces: the magnitude and direction of the force, and its line and point of application. The combination of magnitude and direction make force a vector quantity (Kent, 1994).

Definition

A *vector* quantity has both magnitude and direction, force and weight being two examples. A *scalar* quantity has magnitude alone, an example being volume or speed.

Forces can therefore be represented graphically by an arrow, the direction of which gives the direction of the force. The arrowhead represents the force's point of application, and the magnitude is given as a value in newtons, or is represented by the length of the arrow. Forces may act in the same line (in series) and are termed linear, or they may act in parallel. In addition, forces of equal magnitude may act opposite to each other to form a force couple. In this case, because the forces are aligned opposite each other no linear displacement occurs, instead a turning force is produced (Fig. 1.1).

The total force acting on a system may be calculated. For forces acting in series, this is simply a matter of subtraction or addition, but when forces act at angles to each other a parallelogram of forces can be constructed to facilitate calculation. Here, the two original or 'component' forces form the adjacent sides of the parallelogram, and the force which represents the two combined (the resultant) is the diagonal of the parallelogram (Fig. 1.2a, b).

This principle (known as the resolution of forces) works equally well in reverse. If one force is known, its two components, acting at 90° to each other, may be determined. Thus when the heel strikes the ground (Fig. 1.2c) two component forces exist causing both shear and compression.

Analysis of human motion is further simplified by using a free body diagram to help visualize the forces acting on the body. A stick figure is used to represent the body isolated from its surroundings. The diagram shows all the external forces acting on the body such as ground resistance and gravity, but not the internal forces such as muscle forces acting across a joint. The forces (input) act on the body in such a way that they produce motion (output).

In Fig. 1.3a, an athlete is running, and we want to calculate the relevant force acting on the body. First, we simplify the action by converting it to a stick figure, to clarify the limb position. Finally (Fig. 1.3b) we show the relevant forces imposed on the athlete's body by the surroundings. In the case of this figure these include air resistance (F_a), the athlete's weight (F_w) and the ground reaction force (F_g).

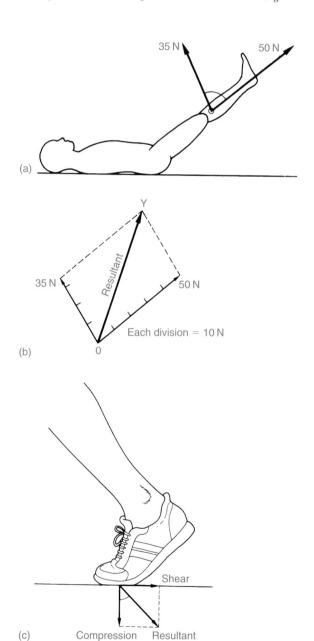

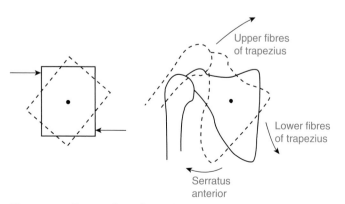

Figure 1.1 Forces of equal magnitude acting in opposite directions produce a turning effect.

Figure 1.2 Parallelogram of forces. The two forces acting parallel to (50 N) and at right angles to (35 N) the lower leg (a) may be resolved into a single force represented by the resultant (b). (c) Components of ground reaction force in a runner.

Newton's laws of motion

Motion, defined as the continual change of relative position of an object in space (Kent, 1994), may be linear, angular or curvilinear. Linear motion occurs in a straight line (for example ice-skating). All parts of the body move the same distance in the same direction and in the same time. Angular (rotatory) motion involves movement of an object about a fixed point (the axis of rotation), so that each part of the object travels in an arc. An example is a dancer pirouetting. Curvilinear motion is the movement of all parts of an object along a curved path (for example a javelin throw). This type of motion has both linear and angular components.

The basic principles of the relationship between force and motion were set down by Newton in 1687 in his classic work *Philosophiae naturalis principia mathematica* ('the mathematical principles of natural philosophy'). These principles are known collectively as the 'laws of motion'.

Newton's first law of motion is the law of inertia. It states that an object remains in its existing state of motion unless acted on by an external force. A stationary object will not begin to move unless acted on by an external unbalanced force, and a body which is moving will keep moving in the same direction and at the same velocity unless it is similarly affected by an external force. Consequently, objects have a resistance to motion change, and this property is called *inertia*.

When a ball is rolling along the ground, it will take more energy to start or stop the ball rolling than it will simply to keep it rolling at the same speed. Similarly, in a vigorous kicking action, inertia will have to be overcome to start the limb moving. If the force required to do this is large enough and rapid enough, muscle damage may occur.

A joint has a certain inertia as a result of its osteological format and the properties of the joint structures. Following immobilization the inertia is likely to be greater because the joint tissues have stiffened and the joint fluid has become more viscous. Gentle, rhythmic swinging exercises are often used to mobilize stiff joints. The continuous motion being more effective than stopping, pausing, and then starting again. In cases of severe weakness after injury, a muscle may be unable to overcome joint inertia to initiate movement. Once the movement has been started by the therapist, the patient's muscles may be strong enough to continue the action – a technique applied in sling suspension.

Definition

Sling suspension is an exercise therapy technique where a patient's limb is held above the treatment couch in canvas slings suspended from a frame by ropes. It can provide free movement without significant resistance.

Heavier objects will be more difficult to start or stop than light objects travelling at the same speed, because heavier things possess more *momentum*. Momentum is the product of an object's mass and its velocity, and is an important consideration during exercise. Rapid, full-range weight training exercises, for example, can be dangerous when muscle fatigue sets in. The combined momentum of the limb and weight may continue movement beyond full physiological joint range to cause tissue damage. Gleim (1984) showed momentum to be a significant factor in injuries to American football players. Taunton, McKenzie and Clement (1988) claimed that the most serious injuries in adolescent football and hockey players occur in the largest athletes, who create larger momentum forces.

Keypoint

Momentum of a limb travelling at speed may continue a movement beyond the normal safe range, causing an injury. This principle is using Newton's first law of motion, that of *Inertia*.

Newton's second law is that of *acceleration*. This law states that the rate of change of momentum of a body takes

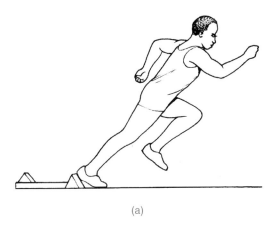

(a)

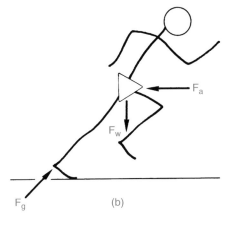

(b)

Figure 1.3   The free body diagram. (a) A sprinter leaving the blocks. (b) Forces due to bodyweight, air resistance and ground reaction.

place in the direction of the force and is proportional to the size of the force and the duration for which it acts.

If a hockey player hits a ball, the force (F) with which the player hits acts for the specific time (t) that the stick is in contact with the ball. The ball has a certain mass (m), and changes its velocity from that at the start (u) to that at the finish of the action (v). We know that momentum is the product of mass and velocity, we know the velocity at the start and at the finish, so the rate of change of this momentum can be obtained by dividing the difference in velocities by time, therefore:

Rate of change of momentum

$$F = \frac{mv - mu}{t}$$

Factorizing this we are left with

$$F = \frac{m(v - u)}{t}$$

since $(v - u)/t$ is the same as change in velocity/t and this is acceleration (a), we are left with the equation $F = ma$.

The amount by which the velocity of an object is increased is dependent both on the magnitude of the force imposed on the object, and the time for which this force acts. This is an important consideration in throwing sports. A greater range of movement will allow a force to be applied on an object for longer, and as a consequence the velocity obtained will be greater. These principles are used in events such as the shot-put and discus throw, where the athlete 'winds up' and spins to apply the greatest force over the greatest time.

Keypoint

In throwing sports an athlete 'winds up' a throw to apply force to the implement (shot, discus, etc.) for a longer period and increase the distance of the throw. In so doing the athlete is applying Newton's second law of motion, that of *acceleration*.

Newton's third law is the law of *reaction*, which states that action and reaction are equal in magnitude but opposite in direction. When a ball is hit with a cricket bat, the player applies a force (action force), and the ball pushes back (reaction force). From Newton's second law we know that:

$$F = \frac{m(v - u)}{t}$$

Suppose the mass of the ball (m) is 0.1 kg, the velocity at the start (u) and finish (v) is 15 m/s and 40 m/s, respectively, and the ball strikes the bat for only 0.05 s (t). Because the initial velocity and the final velocity are in opposite

directions, the difference in velocity is now obtained by summing the two values.

$$F = \frac{0.1(15 - (-40))}{0.05} = 110 \text{ N}$$

When a ball travelling with this force is caught, to avoid injury it is necessary to reduce its momentum. Similarly, when landing from a vertical jump, body momentum must be reduced if injury (a fractured calcaneus) is not to result. The aim in each of these cases is to extend the time taken to dissipate the reaction force (Watkins, 1983). If the cricket ball is stopped with the arms and wrists locked, injury may result from the sudden impact of the force. However, if the arms are extended to meet the ball, and flexed as the ball is brought into the body, the time taken to dissipate the ball's force (deceleration period) is extended and the injury risk reduced.

In the case of landing from a jump, the knees bend to dissipate the reaction force rather than falling directly onto the heels with straight legs.

Keypoint

By extending the time taken to dissipate a reaction force, the injury risk is reduced. This principle applies Newton's third law of motion, that of *reaction*.

Stress and strain

When a force acts on an object, the force, expressed per unit area, is called mechanical stress. Pushing, pulling or twisting are all examples of such forces, but three major categories of stress are important within the context of sports injury. These are tension, compression and shear (Fig. 1.4).

Tension stress is a pulling force. When the ankle is twisted by an inversion injury, the lateral ligament will stretch and tension stress is applied. Similarly, when the spine is flexed, the posterior spinal ligaments are tightened and subjected to a tension stress.

Compression stress is the opposite of tension. It is a pushing force, applied along the length of a tissue. In the upright posture, the menisci of the knee take weight and compression stress is applied. Another example occurs when the quadriceps contract on a bent knee, the patella is pulled against the femur and compression stress is applied to the patellofemoral joint.

Shear stress occurs when opposite forces are applied to a tissue, causing one part of the tissue to slide over another. For example, the sacroiliac joint may encounter shearing stresses with a fall, or a finger may be subluxed by shearing forces when hit by a hard ball.

Both compression and tension stresses occur in line with the tissue fibres, a direction in which the tissues are strongest. Shearing stresses are imposed at an angle to the fibres, making

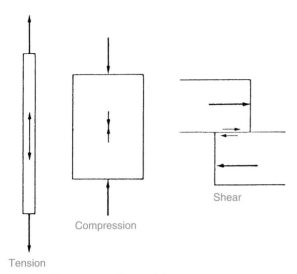

Figure 1.4   Tension, compression and shear stresses.

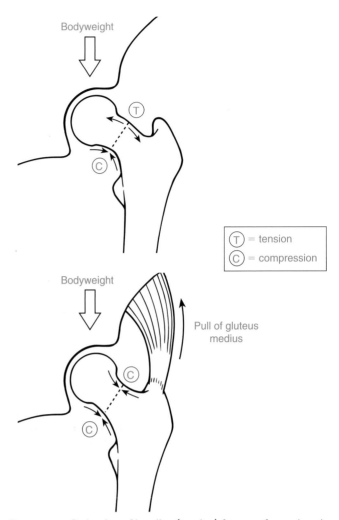

Figure 1.5   Reduction of bending (tension) force on femoral neck by pull of hip abductors.

this type of stress potentially the most dangerous in terms of injury. A fall onto the straight leg, for example, will cause compression stress on the joint structures, especially the cartilage and menisci of the knee. These forces will be largely absorbed, but if severe, compression fracture may occur. During the fall, tension stress will be imposed on the muscles if the joints bend. The elastic capacities of the muscles will now take some of the stress away from the joint. Falling at an angle will again cause some compression and tension, but in addition shearing will take place between the body tissues, and the foot and ground. This type of stress could cause valgus or varus strain at the joint with associated ligament damage or joint subluxation if the force is great.

Bone is structurally better set up to cope with compression forces than with tension forces. Compression forces are withstood by the mineral content of the bone whereas tension forces are resisted only by the collagen fibres within the bone itself. To enable bone to avoid potentially dangerous tension forces, a system is used which is similar to pre-stressing concrete. Pre-stretched steel rods are embedded in a concrete beam before it sets. These rods try to recoil, creating a pulling force a little like a stretched elastic band. The pulling force tends to compress the concrete, and will resist and tension forces imposed on the concrete. As the reinforced concrete beam is subjected to a bending force, one side will compress, and the other will be under tension. The tension force created on the stretched side, however, is resisted by the embedded rods which recoil. This mechanism of pre-stressing is found in the body as muscles are used to unload bone. In the hip joint (Fig. 1.5), the weight of the body acting on the head of the femur causes compression on the lower portion of the femoral neck and tension in the upper portion. This tension force is resisted by the pull of the gluteus medius muscle which pulls on the greater trochanter of the femur generating a compression force within the bone.

> **Keypoint**
>
> Strength and endurance of the gluteus medius muscle is essential in patients with hip pathology, especially that affecting bone, most noticeably osteoporosis.

The relationship between load and deformation

When a stress (load) is applied to a tissue, the tissue will deform, and the deformation is called strain. The relationship between stress and strain is shown graphically by the stress–strain curve (Fig. 1.6). Different materials will each have their own individual curves (Fig. 1.6b), but the general shape of the curves will be the same. The ratio of stress to strain is known as Young's modulus and gives a single figure which represents tissue deformation. A low value represents a flexible substance able to deform easily; rubber has a modulus of 7 and that for cartilage is 24. A high value shows a more brittle substance, bone being 21 000 and glass 70 000.

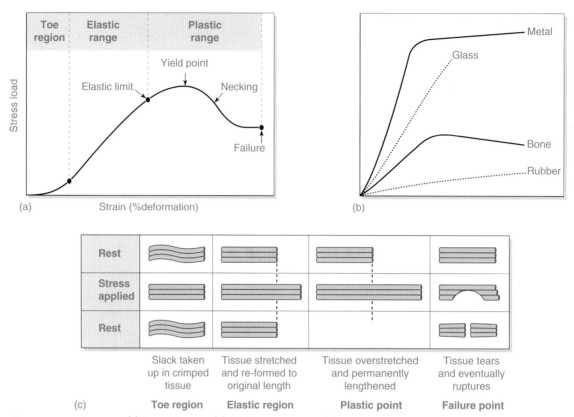

Figure 1.6   The stress–strain curve. (a) General curve. (b) Different materials. (c) Material behaviour.

Definition

Young's modulus (denoted by the letter 'E') is the measure of tissue deformation. It is measured in units of Nm^{-2}. If the value is high, the material distorts very little under load and is said to be 'stiff'.

Initially, the tissue obeys Hooke's law and its deformation is proportional to the force applied to it. As the curve begins (toe region, Fig. 1.6c) deformation occurs with low loading. In the case of a tendon, this initial response is due to straightening out of the 'crimp' in the fibres, which represents 2–4% elongation (Curwin, 1994). This has the effect of protecting the body as most of the movements of daily living occur within this region. As load and deformation increase, a material moves into its *elastic* range, which is represented by the linear portion of the curve. At any point along this part of the line, the material which is put under stress will return to its original size and shape when the stressing force is released.

When the material is stressed beyond the elastic range, it will reach a point at which deformation becomes permanent. At this point, known as the elastic limit, the object will not return to its original form when the force is released. Going past this point, further along the stress–strain curve, the material moves into the *plastic* range. Here, the object will permanently deform, but not rupture. Some materials (including connective tissue) demonstrate both plastic (viscous) and elastic properties combined, and so are termed *viscoelastic*.

The greater the force, the greater the permanent deformation. As the stress imposed on the material increases still further, the yield point (Y) is reached. Now the material continues to deform even though the stress applied to it remains constant, a process known as 'creep'. The stress–strain curve reaches its peak height at this point. As still greater stress is applied to the material, and we move still further along the curve, the material is failing rapidly. Little extra force is required to increase the rate of deformation which is already occurring. This is the necking region. The final load required to produce complete material failure (rupture) is the breaking strength. In the case of a tendon, this occurs when it has elongated 8–10% further than its original length (Butler et al., 1984). The final breaking point represents the tensile strength of the substance, and various values are given in Table 1.1.

The mechanical responses of the connective tissue are due to the complex interaction between the collagen fibres themselves and the protein matrix (ground substance) in which they are contained. The combination of these two materials gives connective tissue a biphasic nature, exhibiting both stress relaxation (a reduction in load over time) and creep (an increase in length under constant loading) (Fig. 1.7). Applying these principles to sport, repeated movement in a constant range of motion such as when

Table 1.1 Tensile strength of biological and non-biological materials

Material	Tensile strength (MNm^{-2})
Rope	82
Nylon thread	1050
Steel	400
Cartilage	3
Skin	10
Tendon	82
Bone	110

From Low and Reed (1996) with permission.

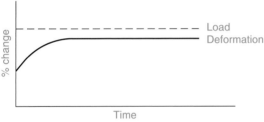

(a) Stress relaxation: load reduces over time

(b) Creep: deformation increases with constant load

Figure 1.7 The biphasic nature of connective tissue.

jogging may lead to stress relaxation and a reduction in loading and therefore resistance to movement. Holding a stretched position (constant load) in sport or daily living will lead to creep and the consequent joint laxity may give a reduction in joint stability.

Factors influencing the stress–strain curve

The stress–strain curve may be influenced by a number of mechanical features of tissue. Of these, we will look at stiffness, creep, fatigue, resilience and toughness.

Structural stiffness occurs when a tissue is less elastic. In this case the initial slope of the stress–strain curve is steeper as less deformation occurs when stress increases. Scar tissue would fall into this category. Scar tissue within a ligament, for example, may be as strong or stronger than the ligament itself, but will not be as elastic and will not therefore respond to stress in the same manner.

Creep occurs when a load (usually small) is imposed on a material over a long time period, causing the material to deform very gradually. Viscoelastic materials demonstrate this property. They deform at a constant rate regardless of the speed with which a force is applied to them. The degree of deformation this time is determined not just by the amount of force applied to a tissue, but also by the duration over which the force is applied. Creep is therefore time dependent. A lesser load applied over a greater time period will produce a larger amount of creep. Creep is related to the viscosity of a tissue, and elevation of temperature will cause corresponding increases in creep. This fact can be used to good effect when stretching tight connective tissue, a warmed tissue which is stretched and held being more pliable than a cold tissue stretched rapidly.

Fatigue is the characteristic of materials to fail before the yield point is reached, when a load is applied repeatedly (cyclically). The larger the load, the fewer repetitions required to produce failure, although a certain minimum load (the endurance limit) must be applied. An example of fatigue through cumulative loading is that of continually bending a wire until it breaks. Fatigue (stress) fractures occur in some athletes who place too much stress on a bone through training. Other things being equal, a heavier athlete is likely to produce fatigue more quickly than a lighter one because the heavier athlete is placing his or her tissues under greater load.

Both resilience and toughness are related to the ability of a material to absorb and release energy. Resilient materials absorb energy well in the elastic range while tough materials do the same in the plastic range. A resilient material will absorb energy and deform, returning to its original shape when the load is released. A tough material will again deform, but will not return to its original shape. Highly resilient materials tend to be bouncy. For example, a rubber ball when dropped will deform, and absorb energy. It will quickly release this stored energy and return to its original shape as it bounces back.

Tough materials will absorb a lot of energy without breaking, but when their failure point is reached, they rupture quickly. Putty is an example here. If something is dropped onto it, it will absorb energy by deforming but will not return to its original shape when released. If subjected to slow tension stress it will stretch, but when stretched quickly it will snap.

Friction and viscosity

When an object rests upon a surface, the force which prevents the object sliding over the other is friction. Friction at rest (a box resting on a sloped surface) is called static friction, while that occurring with movement (when the box slides down the slope) is kinetic friction. Rolling friction occurs when – as the name suggests – an object rolls over a surface rather than sliding over it.

Definition

Friction is a force which resists motion between two contacting surfaces. It is represented by the coefficient of friction (μ), a measure of the roughness between the two surfaces. Surfaces with a coefficient of friction of zero are perfectly smooth.

With kinetic friction, movement is occurring and energy is used. The energy may be released as heat or sound, and causes damage (wearing) to the contacting surfaces. This damage may be reduced by using a lubricant which lowers the coefficient of friction. With rolling friction, damage is lessened and instead the two surfaces deform. The coefficient of several materials is shown in Table 1.2.

Although a surface may appear perfectly smooth to the naked eye, in reality all surfaces are quite rough at a microscopic level. When surfaces are in contact, the peaks of the rough areas (called asperities) are all that is in contact between the two surfaces (Fig. 1.8). The rougher the material, the more the asperities will engage and so the greater the friction produced. Similarly, if the two surfaces are pressed together more firmly, the asperities will be pushed into each other, again increasing the friction. A lubricant placed between the two opposing surfaces will both separate the surfaces and fill in the gaps between the asperities, enabling the surfaces to glide over each other more easily. Lubrication may be provided in a number of ways (Low and Reed, 1996), as shown in Table 1.3.

Viscosity is the property of friction within a fluid, and is defined as the tendency of a fluid to resist motion within itself (Kent, 1994). A fluid with a high viscosity is thick and sticky, like treacle, while a fluid with a low viscosity, such as milk or water, is thin and mobile. When a fluid moves within a container, such as a joint, the fluid in contact with the edge of the container stays fairly static and the next layer of fluid moves over it. The fluid moves layer upon layer, each part moving more easily the further away from the edge of the container it gets. As viscosity is a property which is dependent on the molecules within the fluid moving, heat (which increases molecular movement) reduces viscosity and chilling increases it.

Because viscosity is the resistance to motion within a moving fluid, the more rapid the movement, the more the resistance and the higher the viscosity. When a joint moves, motion is more rapid within mid-range and it is at this point that the resistance to motion due to viscosity is greatest.

Leverage

Types of lever

A lever is simply a device for transmitting (but not creating) force. A typical lever is a rigid bar with one point (the fulcrum or pivot) about which the lever revolves. Two forces are applied to a lever, the effort which tries to move the lever and the resistance which tries to stop movement. The product of the force, and the perpendicular distance between the line of application of the force to the fulcrum, is known as the 'moment' of the force, or torque, and is measured in newton metres (Nm). Torques may be compared between agonist and antagonist muscles (torque ratio), and torque curves may be plotted to show torque generated throughout a range of motion (see Table 1.7, p. 26, Isokinetics).

The distance from the effort to the fulcrum is called the effort arm, and that from the resistance to the fulcrum the resistance arm. The ratio between the effort arm and the

Table 1.2 Coefficient of friction (μ) for various materials

Material	Coefficient of friction
Rubber on concrete	0.7
Dry wood on dry wood	0.3
Bare feet on wooden floor	0.8
Lubricated steel on steel	0.05
Healthy hip joint	0.005
Replacement hip joint	0.10

From Low and Reed (1996), with permission.

Table 1.3 Types of lubrication

Name	Method
Hydrodynamic	As surfaces move they drag lubricant from the periphery to the centre of the joint
Squeeze film	Pressure between the surfaces thins the lubricant and presses it outwards. At the edge of the joint the pressure is less and the lubricant thickens again
Boundary	Some of the lubricant molecules attach to the moving surfaces of the joint
Weeping	Fluid is squeezed into and out of the cartilage in a joint as the surfaces deform
Boosted	Synovial fluid contains water and protein molecules. With loading the water is sqeezed out of the cartilage but the protein remains trapped. The concentration of the lubricant is therefore increased, changing the nature of the lubricant to match the loading conditions

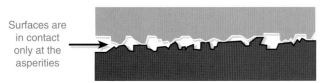

Surfaces are in contact only at the asperities

Figure 1.8 Enlarged cross-section of two surfaces in contact. From Low and Reed (1996), with permission.

resistance arm gives a value for the mechanical advantage. If the effort arm is greater than the resistance arm the mechanical advantage is greater than 1. The mechanical advantage is less than 1 if the resistance arm is the greater of the two.

The relationship between the fulcrum, resistance and effort within a lever system determines the type or 'order' of lever. The first type, or 'first order lever', is one of *balance*. A typical example is a child's see-saw, in which the fulcrum lies between the force and effort. For the lever to balance, the leverage created by the effort must equal that created by the resistance.

With a simple first order lever, a resistance of 6 kg placed 3 m away from the fulcrum gives a torque of 18 Nm ($6 \times 3 = 18$). To balance this out, the effort has to be of the same magnitude. So, the 9 kg weight has only to be placed 2 m from the fulcrum for the lever to balance ($9 \times 2 = 18$). An example of a first-class lever in the body is the skull pivoted on the atlas. The line of gravity of the skull passes anterior to the vertebral column, and to stop the head falling forwards from its own weight, the neck extensors must exert an equivalent balancing force.

In the second order lever, the resistance lies between the fulcrum and the effort. With this type, which is commonly illustrated by a wheelbarrow, the torque produced by the effort is always greater than that produced by the resistance, so the mechanical advantage is also greater than 1. The second order lever is consequently used to produce *power*, but is rarely found in the human body.

The third order lever is the one found most commonly in the body. Here, the resistance arm is the full length of the lever, and the mechanical advantage is always less than 1. The effort is being applied between the fulcrum and resistance. Unlike the second order lever, this does not favour power, but rather *distance* and *speed*. With this type of lever, a contraction of a muscle (the effort) will be magnified and will cause a large movement of the resistance (the limb). In addition, as the distal end of the lever moves a greater distance than the proximal end, the speed of movement of the distal end is greater.

> **Keypoint**
>
> A first order lever works for *balance*, a second order lever for *power* and a third order lever for *speed*.

Leverage and injury

Increased leverage will multiply the effect of a force on body tissue, often making injury more likely (Fig. 1.9). For example, lifting a 10 kg weight is not, in itself, dangerous. However, lifting it at arm's length in a bent-over position with the legs straight will place excessive leverage on the spine, increasing the effect of the weight on the lumbar spine and making injury more likely. As another example, performing a bilateral straight leg raising movement will place excessive strain on the spine, while simply bending the legs will reduce the leverage effect of the legs and so reduce the likelihood of injury.

Some types of athletic equipment may increase the risk of injury by their leverage effects. Running shoes (see p. 295) with flared heels increase the leverage effect on the ankle joints and may, under certain circumstances, predispose the athlete to injury. The face guard on an American football helmet will increase the leverage of neck extension, and a ski will increase leverage forces acting on the tibia.

Centre of gravity

The centre of gravity of an object is the point at which all the weight of the object can be considered to act. This is also the point at which the object would balance. In a symmetrical object such as a ball, the centre of gravity will be at the centre of the object. But, with asymmetrical objects, such as the human body, the centre of gravity will be nearer to the larger and heavier end.

In the human body standing in the anatomical position, the centre of gravity is at the S1–S2 spinal level, but this point will vary as the body position changes.

> **Definition**
>
> Spinal bones (vertebrae) are numbered according to their region, cervical (C), thoracic (T), lumbar (L) and sacral (S). Thus S1 is the first sacral bone and S2 the second, counting from the head downwards.

As the centre of gravity is partially determined by an object's weight, it will shift when something is carried. The centre of gravity of a hiker carrying a heavy rucksack for example, is shifted up and back and would probably lie behind his lower thoracic spine.

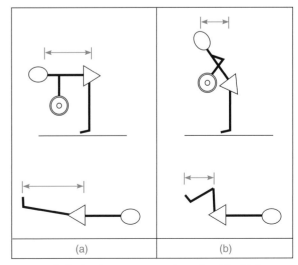

Figure 1.9 Reducing leverage can reduce the risk of injury.
(a) Maximal leverage. (b) Reduced leverage.

By extending the centre of gravity in a line towards the floor, we can calculate the line of gravity, and, importantly, the point at which it passes through an object's base of support.

In order for any object to remain upright, its line of gravity must always pass through its base of support. When the line of gravity moves outside this area, the object will fall over. It follows that an object will be more stable when its line of gravity lies well within its base of support, because it will take a large movement to push the line of gravity to the edge of the supporting base. Take as an example an athlete performing an arm curl exercise with a heavy barbell. In the normal standing position without the barbell the athlete's line of gravity will fall between the feet. However, when the weight is held to the front of the body, the centre of gravity moves forwards, meaning that the line of gravity will now fall nearer to the toes. As the line of gravity is now closer to the edge of the base of support, it will take only a small movement to push it outside the supporting base, and cause the athlete to lose balance.

Keypoint

For an object to remain upright, its line of gravity (L of G) must pass through its base of support. An object whose L of G is well within its base is *more* stable, one where its L of G moves close to the edge of its base is *less* stable.

Stability

During most sports and exercises, an unstable position is a dangerous one, particularly when the body becomes fatigued. An object is more stable when its centre of gravity is lower. Moreover, we say that an object is in stable equilibrium if moving it would cause its centre of gravity to rise. In Fig. 1.10c, the pyramid can either slide sideways, or it would have to be moved onto its side to raise its centre of gravity.

Unstable equilibrium exists when an object's centre of gravity would fall if it were moved (Fig. 1.10b). If the centre of gravity remains the same in all positions, as with a ball, then an object is said to be in neutral equilibrium (Fig. 1.10a).

In addition to the position of the centre of gravity, the size of an object's base of support will also affect its stability. A wide base of support is more stable than a narrow one. Take as an example an ice-skater skating a line. With only the thin blade of the skate on the ice, and the feet close together the base of support is very small. In addition the skater is standing tall, lifting the centre of gravity. The combination of these two features makes the skater quite unstable. However, a judo exponent with feet wide apart has a wide base of support, the knees are bent, lowering the centre of gravity and making the body much more stable.

When moving, the base of support should be widened in the direction of movement. A pulling action such as tug-of-war is therefore safer when a wide stance is taken (increasing the base of support) with one foot in front of the other. Sideways actions, such as lateral flexion of the spine, become more stable and far safer with the feet astride in the frontal plane.

BIOMECHANICS AND KINESIOLOGY OF MUSCLE

Form of muscle

A great number of muscle types exist, but generally speaking muscles may be grouped according to the orientation of their fibres. The fibres may be arranged in parallel, obliquely, or in a spiral fashion, and the arrangement will dictate the power and range of motion that the muscle can produce.

When the fibres are arranged in parallel, the muscle may be strap-like (sartorius) where individual fibres run the whole length of the muscle. The fibres may run between adjacent tendinous intersections which divide the muscle as a whole into sections (rectus abdominis). Alternatively, the fibres may be grouped into discrete bundles producing a fusiform muscle belly which attaches to a tendon (biceps). Another fibre arrangement is the sheet attaching to a broad flat tendon or aponeurosis (internal oblique).

The oblique or 'pennate' grouping sees the muscle fibres attaching to a central tendon. Fibres joining to one side of a tendon only are termed unipennate. When the fibres bind to both sides of a central septum the muscle is bipennate, and when the muscle has several septa it is termed multipennate.

In each case, the muscle fibres can only shorten to half their original length, so the shorter fibres of a pennate muscle will produce less range of motion than the long fibres of a parallel muscle (Fig. 1.16). However, the power of a muscle is determined by the total cross-sectional area of the fibres. With a pennate muscle the total cross-sectional area is much larger than that of a parallel muscle and so the power produced is significantly greater (Fig. 1.17).

The third type of fibre arrangement is the spiralized (Fig. 1.18). Here, the muscle fibres twist as they travel between the two ends of the muscle (pectoralis major, trapezius). As the muscle contracts, the fibres tend to de-rotate and

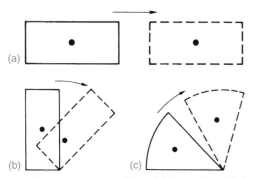

Figure 1.10   Equilibrium and stability. (a) Neutral equilibrium. The centre of gravity remains level as the object is moved. (b) Unstable equilibrium. The centre of gravity moves down as the object is moved. (c) Stable equilibrium. The centre of gravity moves up as the object is moved.

Treatment note 1.1   Mechanical principles of treatment

Mechanical principles may be applied to treatment techniques to increase the effectiveness of treatment and to considerably reduce the stress imposed on the practitioner. From the point of view of injury, excessive stress may be placed on a therapist who is at a mechanical disadvantage compared to the patient. Secondly, if the therapist's body position is poor, stress on the low back may be noticeable and will accumulate over time.

Resisted movements

Where resisted movements are used as part of an objective assessment, therapists must ensure that they place themselves at a mechanical advantage. In elbow flexion, for example (Fig. 1.11), using hand pressure with stronger patients is ineffective. Positioning the therapist's forearm vertically over the patient's forearm increases the mechanical advantage of the therapist and makes the

movement more controlled. Similarly, where trunk lateral flexion is to be resisted, simple hand pressure is ineffective (Fig. 1.12). Placing one hand on the patient's shoulder while the other grips the patient's hand is more effective. In addition, by placing the feet between the patient's feet, the therapist is positioned closer to the axis of rotation of the movement (the patient's sacrum) and so the mechanical advantage is improved.

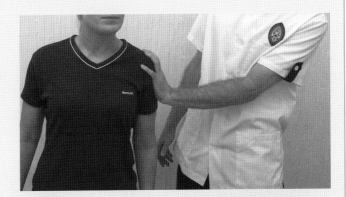

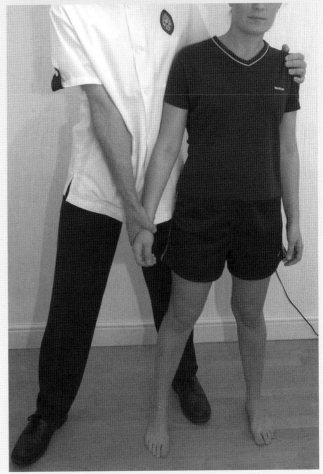

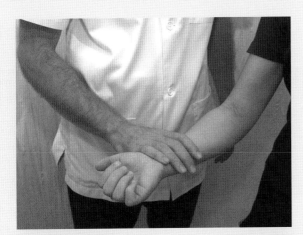

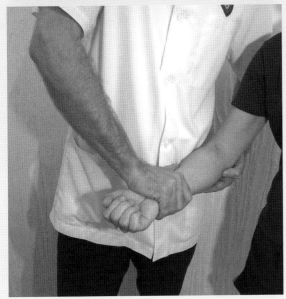

Figure 1.11   Resisted elbow flexion.

Figure 1.12   Resisted trunk side flexion.

Producing power

Many manual therapy techniques require a large amount of force. This is especially the case in sport where a small therapist may be required to treat a very large player (rugby for example). It is essential in these cases that the force for manual therapy is *applied* by the hands but *created* by the therapist's legs and trunk. In a simple effleurage massage technique for example (p. 61), if the hands are used to create the force, the limiting factor is hand and arm strength alone. Taking a walk stance and transferring the weight from one

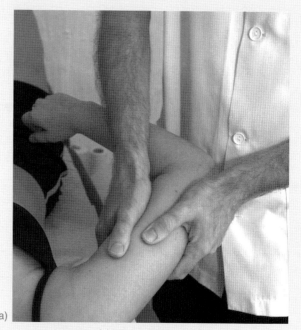

(a)

Figure 1.15   Gripping. (a) Hand alone.

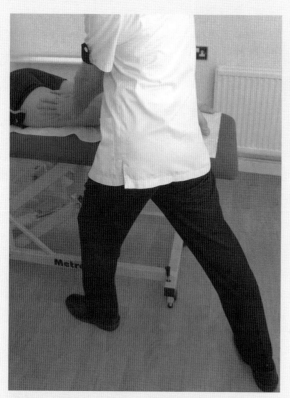

Figure 1.13   Transferring body weight to create power.

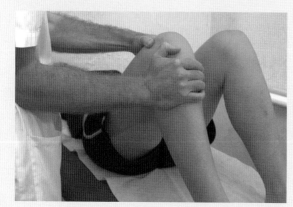

Figure 1.14   Transferring force from the body to the hand.

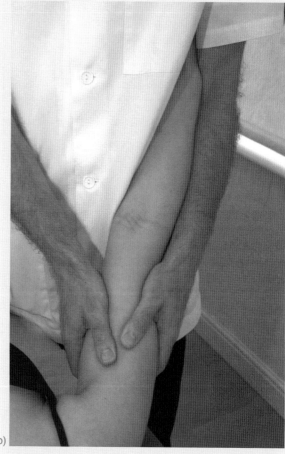

(b)

Figure 1.15   (b) Hand and arm.

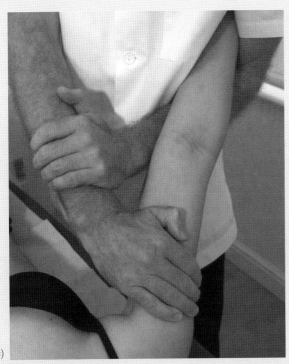

foot to the other allows the therapist to use body sway to create considerable force (Fig. 1.13). Tucking the elbow into the hip (Fig. 1.14) is another technique to transfer the force directly from the body to the hand rather than relying on stability of the shoulder and elbow.

Increasing contact area

The area in contact with the patient has a direct effect on the amount of effort needed from the therapist's hands. Increasing the contact area will proportionally reduce the grip strength required to perform an action. Take a longitudinal distraction (traction) movement for the glenohumeral joint as an example. Gripping the arm and pulling with the arms requires a high degree of grip strength (Fig. 1.15a). Tucking the patient's arm beneath the therapist's arm gives a third area of grip (Fig. 1.15b). Using the same force with three rather than two areas of grip shares the force between the contact areas. Gripping with the whole forearm and locking the patient's arm improves the situation still further (Fig. 1.15c).

(c)

Figure 1.15 (c) Hand, forearm and arm.

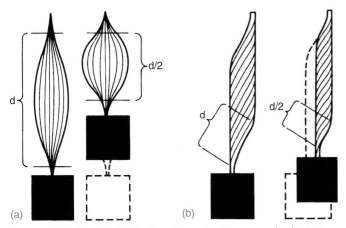

Figure 1.16 Muscle shortening. A muscle fibre can only shorten by half of its original length (d/2), so the range of motion is greater for a parallel arrangement of muscle fibres (a) than for a pennate arrangement (b).

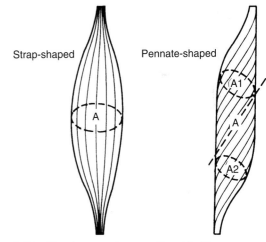

Figure 1.17 Muscle power is proportional to fibre cross-sectional area (A). The total area ($A_1 + A_2$), and so the power, is greater for a pennate-shaped muscle than for a strap-shaped one.

straighten out, imparting a rotation force to the bone on which they attach. In this way, a spiralized muscle not only approximates the bones of the joint over which it acts, but also pulls the bones into the same plane.

Keypoint

A long thin muscle will create a large range of motion, while a short thick muscle will create large amounts of force.

Position of the muscle attachment

The position of the muscle attachment to the bone, and the direction of the muscle, will largely determine its action. Where a muscle attachment is wrapped around the bone, *longitudinal rotation* of the bone will occur (pronator quadratus). Where the distal attachment of the muscle is close to the joint (brachialis), *angular rotation* of the joint is the most prominent movement. If the distal attachment is placed some distance from the joint (brachioradialis) the muscle pull will tend to *approximate* the joint, pulling the joint surfaces together (Fig. 1.19).

Group action of muscles

The properties of muscle contraction are often described for isolated muscle fibres in the laboratory. Functionally, however, muscles do not contract singly, but in a group. The group action of muscles is an important consideration, both with injury and with the process of rehabilitation.

When stimulated, a muscle fibre will develop tension tending to shorten the muscle as a whole. Whether the tension developed is sufficient to cause shortening, or indeed joint movement, will depend on a number of factors. The amount of tension developed, the resistance opposing the muscle, the mechanical leverage system and contraction of neighbouring muscles will all have an effect.

The most effective muscle at producing a particular movement is called the prime mover (agonist). Any muscle which helps to create this same movement but is less effective at doing so is an assistant (secondary) mover. In different situations a muscle may take on both actions. Take as an example a bench-press movement in weight training. If a wide grip is taken, the prime mover will be the pectoral muscles, and an assistant mover will be the triceps. If a narrow grip is taken, pulling the arms in close to the side, the pectorals are shortened and become less effective (length–tension relationship). Now, the triceps becomes the prime mover and the pectorals act as assistant movers.

The muscle which, if it contracted, would tend to oppose the action of the prime mover is the antagonist. Normally through reciprocal innervation (see p. 100), the contraction of the antagonist is reduced. With a co-contraction, however, both prime mover and antagonist may contract. This type of contraction can represent a lack of skill (Wells, 1966) and its reduction has been cited as one way in which strength increases are produced early on in training (Sale, 1988). In actions such as gripping, two joint muscles (see below) are acting, and there may also be a rapid alternation between opposing muscle groups or isometric action to stabilize the joint. The interaction of muscles in co-contraction is complex, and the interested reader is referred to Basmajian and De Luca (1985), and Zehr and Sale (1994) for a full review.

Definition
The muscle responsible for a movement is the prime mover or *agonist*. The muscle which would perform the opposite action is the *antagonist*.

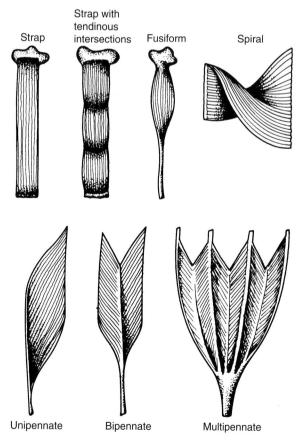

Figure 1.18 Various muscle fibre arrangements. From Williams (1995), with permission.

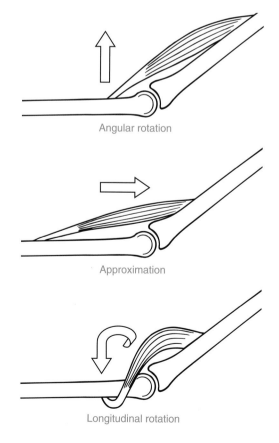

Figure 1.19 Movements determined by muscle attachment.

A muscle acts as a fixator or stabilizer when it anchors or supports a body part to supply a firm base for another muscle (usually the prime mover) to pull on. When a muscle contracts, it will tend to pull both of its ends towards each other. To produce movement at one end only, the bony attachment of one end of the muscle must be stabilized. An example is the contraction of the downwards rotators of the scapula as teres major adducts the humerus. Another situation in which a fixator can act is to resist the pull of gravity to stabilize a body segment. An example of this is a press-up action, in which the abdominal muscles contract to prevent the spine sagging into extension.

A neutralizer is a muscle which contracts to prevent an unwanted action of the prime or assistant mover. Most muscles are capable of several actions, and those not required must be counteracted by activity of a neutralizer. For example, biceps will both flex the elbow and supinate the forearm. If we wish to flex the elbow without forearm rotation, the pronators must neutralize the unwanted supinatory action of the biceps.

Ballistic and reciprocal actions

In rapid actions such as throwing or kicking, the agonist will contract powerfully, but briefly, to move the limb, allowing momentum of the moving limb to maintain the action. EMG studies of this type of action (Zehr and Sale, 1994) have shown a pre-movement silence (depression of the EMG signal) to exist just before initiation of muscle contraction. This silence may potentiate both the force and velocity of the subsequent contraction. At the end of the desired range of motion, the antagonist contracts eccentrically (to a variable degree) to decelerate the limb. Finally, the prime mover works once more to control the final position of the limb. This triphasic muscle action (Fig. 1.20) is known as a ballistic contraction. An overlap may be present between the initial contraction of the prime mover and that of the antagonist in which case a co-contraction occurs. The ballistic action is obviously a highly skilled coordination, and when, with fatigue, the action becomes uncontrolled, injury frequently results.

When an eccentric action immediately precedes a concentric one, a reciprocal contraction occurs, giving a more powerful contraction. LaGasse (1983) demonstrated an 11.4% greater force output from the quadriceps when knee flexion was performed prior to knee extension. Reciprocal contractions occur in most functional movements such as walking and running, and form the basis of power training using plyometrics (p. 109). The stretch incurred by the elastic components of the muscle when working eccentrically is released with the concentric contraction, increasing the force output. In addition the stretch reflex is stimulated in the stretched muscle, facilitating a more powerful contraction through increased recruitment and activation of motor units.

> **Keypoint**
>
> The fast, explosive movements used in sport involve both ballistic and reciprocal actions. These must be retrained to restore full function. To miss out explosive actions in the final period of rehabilitation leaves the athlete open to reinjury.

Two-joint muscles

Most joint complexes contain two-joint or 'biarticular' muscles, and these are frequently the muscles which are torn in sport. Examples in the lower limb are the rectus femoris, hamstrings and gastrocnemius. The important characteristic of these muscles is that they are unable to permit full movement at both joints simultaneously.

When full movement is limited by passive stretch of the muscle, passive insufficiency is present. An example is passive hip extension combined with knee flexion being limited by rectus femoris. When the muscle is unable to shorten sufficiently to produce a full range movement at both joints simultaneously, active insufficiency exists. An example here is the hamstrings flexing the knee and extending the hip.

Because the muscles are not long enough to permit movement at both joints simultaneously, the tension in one muscle is transferred to the other. Using the hip as an example, as the hamstrings contract to extend the hip, tension is transmitted to the rectus femoris enabling it to extend the knee (Wells, 1966). This type of action, involving either extension or flexion at both joints at the same time, is called concurrent movement. The muscle shortens at one end but lengthens at the other, and so maintains its length and conserves tension. When the hip is flexed but the knee extended, the rectus femoris is shortened and rapidly loses tension, while the hamstrings are lengthened and rapidly gain tension, an example of countercurrent movement (Rasch, 1989).

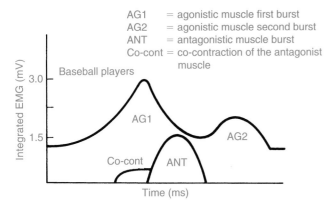

AG1 = agonistic muscle first burst
AG2 = agonistic muscle second burst
ANT = antagonistic muscle burst
Co-cont = co-contraction of the antagonist muscle

Figure 1.20 Triphasic muscle action. Initially the arm is propelled forwards by the agonist muscles (AG1). As the arm reaches its target, the antagonists contract to eccentrically slow the limb (ANT). Some overlap of muscle contraction occurs (Co-cont). Finally the agonist contracts again to finely position the limb (AG2). From McArdle, W.D., Katch, F.I. and Katch, V.L. (1986). *Exercise Physiology: Energy, Nutrition and Human Performance*. Lea and Febiger, Philadelphia. With permission.

Two-joint muscles provide three main advantages to the musculoskeletal system (Enoka, 1994). First, these muscles couple movement at both joints. For example, shoulder and elbow flexion occur together in a feeding pattern, and both actions have a contribution from biceps brachii. Second, the shortening velocity of a two-joint muscle is less than that of a single-joint muscle (van Ingen Schenau, Bobbert and van Soest 1990), contributing to more rapid limb movement. Third, two-joint muscles are said to redistribute muscle force throughout the limb (Toussaint et al., 1992). For example, if hip flexion is performed by iliopsoas, tightness in the hamstrings will tend to flex the knee. This is an appropriate action for the swing phase of gait. Hip extension will tighten rectus femoris tending to extend the knee, an action required during the propulsive gait phase.

> **Keypoint**
>
> When exercising a two-joint muscle, simultaneous movement over both joints will rehearse the complex coordination required for optimal function. Using two separate single-joint actions will still work the full muscle, but coordination will suffer.

Force–velocity relationship

When a muscle is contracting, a relationship exists between the speed of movement it creates and the force which the muscle can develop. The torque generated by the muscle decreases as the velocity of movement increases (Pipes and Wilmore, 1975; Coyle et al., 1981; Burnie and Brodie, 1986). The greatest force being produced at the slowest speeds.

One theory for the force–velocity relationship is that the myosin cross-bridges within the muscle continually move through thermal agitation. The probability of union between the actin and myosin filaments is therefore reduced at higher speeds (Bray et al., 1986), and fewer cross-bridge attachments may occur. In addition, as muscle-shortening speed increases, the rate of cross-bridge cycling increases, but the average force exerted by each cross-bridge is reduced (Enoka, 1994). The speed at which the actin and myosin cross-bridges attach is fairly uniform (a figure known as the rate constant). As force depends on the number of cross-bridges formed, greater speed of contraction means that more filaments slide past each other without binding, and therefore force is reduced. Maximal force is exerted eccentrically (muscle lengthening). As soon as the muscle begins to shorten, force reduces dramatically. When velocity increases to just 10% of maximum, force reduces by 35% (Lieber, 1992).

Length–tension relationship

A further biomechanical relationship exists between the initial length of the muscle and its force production, the so-called length–tension relationship. In the laboratory situation, an isolated muscle can exert its maximal force or tension while in a resting stretched state. If the muscle is shortened or overstretched, less tension can be exerted.

Physiologically, this can be explained in terms of the sliding filament mechanism. In the shortened position, an overlap of the muscle filaments occurs, interfering with cross-bridge coupling. If the muscle is overstretched, the filaments are pulled completely apart, the cross-bridges will not come into contact, and no tension can be developed (Fig. 1.21).

As the relaxed muscle is stretched, however, a passive force due to muscle elasticity is created. This varies between muscles, for example the spinal extensors in man resist a stretching force by purely passive means. Therefore, total force developed by the muscle will be the sum of the active and passive forces.

The length–tension relationship can be used to advantage where two muscles work together to produce a movement as primary and secondary movers. We can emphasize the prime mover by shortening (and therefore 'weakening') the secondary mover. For example, in a sit-up movement with the legs straight both the hip flexors and abdominal muscles are working. However, the hip flexors are generally strong anyway through use in everyday living, so the training effect on these muscles has to be reduced. This is accomplished by bending the knees and hips. The length–tension relationship dictates that the hip flexors will now be able to produce less force.

With a two-joint muscle, the position of the joint at one end of the muscle will help to dictate the potential tension at the other. For example, in the prone lying position the hamstring muscles are shortened at the hip and lengthened at the knee. If this position is used to strengthen the hamstrings, as the knee flexes the hamstrings are further shortened, reducing the tension in the muscle. By flexing the hip, either by using an angled bench (hamstring bench) or by choosing a sitting position, the hamstrings are lengthened at the hip, helping to prevent the muscle shortening as the knee is flexed and so maintaining tension.

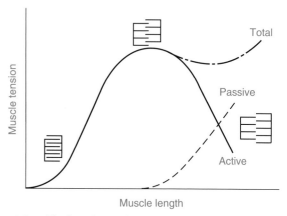

Figure 1.21   The length–tension relationship.

JOINT MECHANICS

Accessory movements

The movements of a joint are of two types, physiological and accessory. Physiological movements are those which the athlete can perform actively, for example flexion and extension of the knee. Accessory movements cannot be produced actively as individual movements, but occur automatically between articulating surfaces of a joint as it moves. Three accessory movements are of particular importance when treating sports injuries: these are roll, slide and spin (Fig. 1.22).

Roll occurs when points at certain intervals on a moving surface contact points at the same intervals on the opposing surface (Hertling and Kessler, 1990). This is similar to a car tyre rolling over the road. If one point on the moving surface stays in contact with a variety of points on the opposing surface, slide is taking place. Spin is a pure rotation around a mechanical axis (Barak, Rosen and Sofer, 1990). Usually when a joint moves, both slide and roll must take place. If roll alone were the only movement, the joint would sublux before any appreciable range had been achieved. If only slide occurred, the edges of the concave aspect of the joint would impinge on the opposing convex lip.

Concave–convex motion

Synovial joints in general consist of both concave and convex surfaces created by the shapes of the bone ends within the joint and their covering cartilage. When a concave surface moves on a convex surface, roll and slide occur in the same direction, the bone sliding towards the direction of movement. When a convex surface moves on a concave surface roll and slide occur in opposite directions, the bone sliding away from the direction of movement. Take as an example knee movement. If the tibia extends on a fixed femur in a leg extension exercise (concave on convex) the joint surface of the tibia rolls and slides forwards in the direction of extension. On the other hand, if the femur extends on a stationary tibia, as with standing up from a chair (convex on concave), the femoral condyles will roll forwards but slide backwards in the opposite direction to the movement. Knowledge of the direction of accessory movements is important when using joint mobilization techniques. For example, if shoulder flexion is limited, although the movement of the humerus is upward, because a convex surface is moving on a concave one, gliding of the joint should be directed downwards (caudally).

> **Keypoint**
>
> When using manual therapy techniques to increase motion or 'mobilize' a joint, apply the concave–convex rule. The accessory movement of a convex joint surface (ball joint of limb) moving on a concave surface (socket) should be in the opposite direction to the physiological movement being regained.

When gliding a joint, the direction of movement is altered with the angle of the joint. The glide direction chosen is called the treatment plane, and is the one in which most translatory motion is possible. In peripheral joints the joint line can be established fairly easily by palpation, and so the treatment plane is determined directly. In the spine, however, the treatment plane is determined by the joint angles of the facets, and is horizontal for C0–C1, angled at 45° between C2 and T12, and almost horizontal for the lumbar area.

Close and loose pack

The two opposing surfaces of a joint do not fit together exactly; they are said to be non-congruent. But, with the joint in one particular position its surfaces will come as close together as they are able, and this is known as 'close pack'. In this position the joint capsule and ligaments twist and pull the joint surfaces together into approximation. The joint space is at a minimum and the concave surface of one bone fits tightly into the convex shape of the other. No further movement is possible in a joint which is close packed, and so this position is avoided when trying to mobilize the joint.

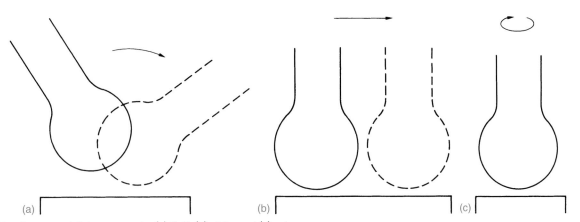

Figure 1.22   Accessory joint movements. (a) Roll, (b) slide, and (c) spin.

Treatment note 1.2   Concept of mobilization and manipulation

Mobilization using accessory movements

Where pain and stiffness limit the normal (physiological) movement of a joint, rather than pressing further into this painful range, *accessory movements* may be used. By increasing the range available to accessory motion, the physiological range may also increase (Maitland, 1986, 1991).

If pain is the dominant factor, this is treated first. When stiffness overshadows pain the aim is to increase the patient's range of motion even though some soreness may be produced during and following treatment. Most patients will present with a combination of pain and stiffness, and when there is doubt as to which is the predominant feature, pain is treated first.

When joint movement is limited, the point of limitation falls short of the anatomical range (that which is available to a joint because of its structure). As the joint is mobilized the point of limitation moves closer to the anatomical range. Within a range of movement four grades of mobilization techniques are used (Table 1.4).

Represented diagrammatically (Fig. 1.23), grades I and II do not reach the end range, and are used when pain is the predominant feature. Grades III and IV are performed to end-range movement and are used when stiffness is the main problem.

A number of techniques may be used. In the knee, for example, lateral movements (Fig. 1.24) and anteroposterior (AP) movements (Fig. 1.25) are useful accessory movements for treatment, while normal bending and straightening (flexion and extension) represent the physiological movements which would be expected to increase as a result of joint mobilization.

Mobilization with movement

With this concept (Mulligan 1999), it is proposed that injury results in not just a reduction in range of motion, but also an alteration in movement throughout the range, or *maltracking*. Three techniques are used. NAGS (natural apophyseal glides) are accessory movements performed in line with the facet plane orientation. SNAGS (sustained natural apophyseal glides) are gliding mobilizations performed as the patient moves (examples are given on pp. 394).

Peripheral joints may also be treated in a similar way using mobilizations with movement (MWM) in an attempt to correct maltracking of the joint. In the case of a hinge joint such as the elbow (Fig. 1.26) the proximal segment is

Table 1.4   Grades of mobilization procedures

Grade I	Small amplitude movement near the starting position of the range
Grade II	Large amplitude movement occupying any free part of the range
Grade III	Large amplitude movement moving into stiffness
Grade IV	Small amplitude movement at the end of range

After Maitland (1986), with permission.

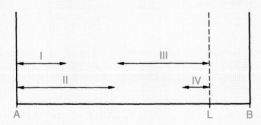

Figure 1.23   Grades of joint mobilization. A, starting point of movement range. B, anatomical limitation of range. L, limitation point due to pain.

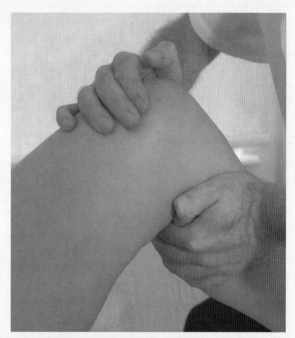

Figure 1.24   Lateral gliding of the knee.

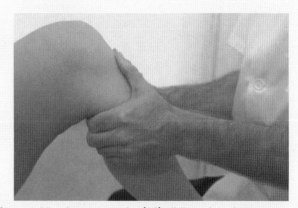

Figure 1.25   Anteroposterior (AP) gliding of the knee.

stabilized while the distal segment is subjected to a gliding (transverse) mobilization by the therapist. The unique feature of this type of mobilization, however, is that the patient then actively performs the previously symptomatic movement.

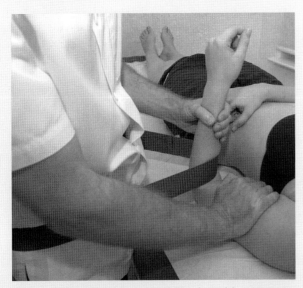

Figure 1.26 Transverse gliding mobilization with movement (MWM) of the elbow.

If pain increases, it indicates that the direction of glide was incorrect and this is reversed and the movement attempted again. Pain reduction should occur; if pain again increases the technique is said to be unsuitable (Wilson, 2001).

Joint manipulation

A manipulation is a high velocity thrust of small amplitude performed at the end-range of motion. The thrust is often accompanied by a pop or click from alteration of gaseous pressure within the synovial fluid when the joint surfaces are tractioned (the suction phenomenon), or a tearing sensation if adhesions are ruptured. Replacing a subluxed joint may also be audible.

Manipulation may be used to stretch out capsular contraction, to rupture joint adhesions, or to move an intra-articular displacement (Cyriax, 1982). Manipulative rupture of adhesions and manipulative reduction is achieved with a high velocity (fast), low amplitude (small) movement. This may be accompanied by traction using some methods. The aim is to perform the technique so quickly that muscle contraction is unable to limit the motion. However, joint manipulation is rarely used where a joint is protected by obvious spasm, as soft tissue techniques to relieve the spasm are normally used first.

Loose pack position is exactly the opposite. As the joint surfaces are released from their close pack position, elastic recoil of the soft tissues surrounding the joint enables its surfaces to move apart, maximizing the joint space. The loose pack position is the resting position often taken up after injury because more joint fluid can accumulate. In loose pack positions joint play is possible. This consists of small accessory movements which give the joint its 'spring'. These are essential to the normal functioning of the joint and play a part in joint nutrition and combined movements.

Definition

In *close pack* the joint surfaces are most congruent with each other. The joint capsule and ligaments are taut and the joint is relatively immobile. In *loose pack* the joint surfaces are non-congruent, the capsule and ligaments lax, and the joint is mobile.

Interestingly many fractures of the upper limb occur with a fall onto the outstretched arm, which is a close packed position, and many ligament sprains occur in loose packed position (Hertling and Kessler, 1990). Examples of close and loose pack positions are given in Table 1.5.

AXES AND PLANES

The human body may, for descriptive purposes, be divided into three planes. The sagittal plane passes through the body from front to back, dividing it into right and left halves. The frontal plane divides the body into anterior and posterior sections, and lies at right angles to the sagittal plane. The transverse plane divides the body into upper and lower portions, and rests at right angles to the other two planes.

Each of the three body planes has an associated axis which passes perpendicularly through it (Fig. 1.27). Movement occurs *in* a plane, but *about* an axis. Abduction and adduction occur in the frontal plane about the anteroposterior axis, flexion and extension occur in a sagittal plane about a transverse axis, and rotations occur in a transverse plane about a vertical axis.

In reality, movements do not occur in one plane, but several. For example, we talk of 'triplane motion' of the subtaloid joint in a runner (see p. 182). This is because a complex series of movements link together to give a motion which occurs in all three planes about an oblique axis.

Table 1.5   Close packed and loose packed positions of selected joints

Joint(s)	Close packed position	Loose packed (resting) position
Facet (spine)	Extension	Midway between flexion and extension
Temporomandibular	Clenched teeth	Mouth slightly open
Glenohumeral	Abduction and external rotation	55° abduction, 30° horizontal abduction, rotated so that the forearm is in the transverse plane
Acromioclavicular	Arm abduction to 30°	Arm resting by side, shoulder girdle in the physiological position
Sternoclavicular	Maximum shoulder elevation	Arm resting by side, shoulder girdle in the physiological position
Ulnohumeral (elbow)	Extension	70° elbow flexion, 10° forearm supination
Radiohumeral	Elbow flexed 90°, forearm supinated 5°	Full extension, full supination
Proximal radioulnar	5° supination	70° elbow flexion, 35° forearm supination
Distal radioulnar	5° supination	10° forearm supination
Radiocarpal (wrist)	Extension with ulnar deviation	Midway between flexion-extension (so that a straight line passes through the radius and third metacarpal) with slight ulnar deviation
First carpometacarpal	Full opposition	Midway between abduction-adduction and flexion-extension
Metacarpophalangeal (fingers)	Full flexion	Slight flexion
Metacarpophalangeal (thumb)	Full opposition	
Interphalangeal	Full extension	Slight flexion
Hip	Full extension, internal rotation and abduction	30° flexion, 30° abduction, and slight external rotation
Knee	Full extension and external rotation of the tibia	25° flexion
Talocrural (ankle)	Maximum dorsiflexion	10° plantarflexion, midway between maximum inversion and eversion
Subtalar	Full supination	Midway between extremes of inversion and eversion
Midtarsal	Full supination	Midway between extremes of range of movement
Tarsometatarsal	Full supination	Midway between extremes of range of movement
Metatarsophalangeal	Full extension	Neutral
Interphalangeal	Full extension	Slight flexion

From Clarkson, H.M. and Gilewich, G.B. (1989) *Musculoskeletal Assessment*. Williams and Wilkins, Baltimore MD. With permission.

BIOMECHANICAL ANALYSIS

Video movement analysis

Analysis of human movement is vital for the prevention and rehabilitation of sports injuries. The most basic analysis may be performed by the clinician simply observing the subject. This type of analysis may be useful, but is limited by the visual memory of the observer. The unassisted human eye sees action at the equivalent of an exposure time of 1/30th of a second (Trew and Everett, 1997). The clinician is therefore unable to follow and retain much of the important detail in even the slowest movement. Although the trained observer may extract considerably more data than the lay person, precise analysis is not possible, even when an action is repeated a number of times.

The situation is improved considerably when an action is recorded on videotape or cine-film to be played back later for accurate analysis. This procedure has previously been complex and expensive, but with the steadily reducing cost and increasing standard of video equipment the task is much easier.

Observing and recording movement

In order accurately to record an action, both the performer of the action and the environment in which the action is performed must be prepared. Subjects should be suitably dressed in shorts or bathing costume to enable accurate location of body segments and joints. Bony reference points or centres of motion are marked on the skin with adhesive tape or reflective markers. The background is cleared, where possible, to allow unobscured vision of the whole movement. The video camera is set up on a stand at a set distance from the subject. The camera should be capable of recording in poor lighting conditions (low lux number), and have a timing/counting facility. If two or more analyses are to be made, the distance between the camera and the subject must remain the same to reduce parallax error. Complex motions are better recorded with two synchronized cameras placed at 90° to each other.

Lighting must be adequate to illuminate the subject in all positions, and where this cannot be controlled (on the field) a low-light camera should be used. Reference points, such

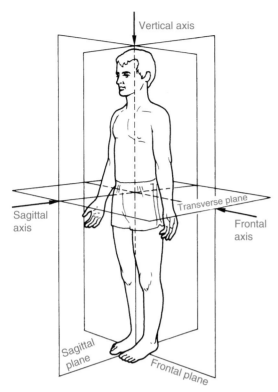

Figure 1.27 Axes and planes of the body.

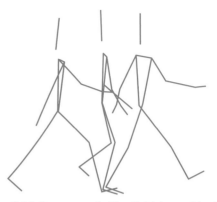

Figure 1.28 Stick figure compiled by digitizing a video image.

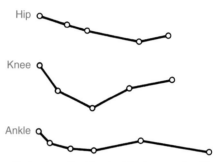

Figure 1.29 Paths described by the hip, knee and ankle reference points. From Williams, J.G. and Davis, M. (1990) KINEMAN: A micro-computer-based digitising system for movement analysis. *Physiotherapy*, **76**(6), 436–440. With permission.

as a measuring stick placed in the field of view, can be useful to give a comparison of distance. Ideally, the whole action should be filmed without moving the camera. To do this the observer must be far enough away from the subject to get a wide field of view.

Analysing movement

The simplest way to analyse a movement is to slow the action down and use an experienced clinical eye. Where the video image is sufficiently clear and reference markers are visible, this is an inexpensive and extremely useful method. The analysis may be taken further, by digitizing the image. Essentially this involves establishing X–Y coordinates of the various marked reference points. The video film is played back on a large flat screen monitor, and the freeze-frame facility used to stop the action at a predetermined point. The relative positions of the various reference points are then recorded. A number of commercially available computer software programs allow the clinician to do this using a digitizing pen. Alternatively, a mouse is used to move the computer cursor to the selected reference point. The software package then records the position of the point in two dimensions. Gradually an image is built which may be used to create a stick figure (Fig. 1.28).

By progressing frame to frame, the limb and centres of rotation for the subject are recorded throughout the movement. Various parameters such as linear and angular displacements and accelerations of the body segments are

then calculated. The overall action is reviewed by analysing the stick figure display, and the paths described by individual reference points (loci) (Fig. 1.29) are studied. In addition, if sufficient joint locations are used, the body's centre of gravity may be determined.

Video analysis still has limitations, particularly with respect to joint rotation and three-dimensional images, though the use of two synchronized cameras reduces this problem. However, with the increasing availability of these systems, they are useful clinical tools for the sports physiotherapist.

Force plates

The force that an athlete exerts on a sports surface may be measured using a force plate. This is essentially a rigid plate set flush into the floor. Beneath the plate, at each corner, sit four transducers capable of recording various components of the ground reaction force (Fig. 1.30). The vertical component (F_z) is a compression force, while the horizontal components (F_y and F_x) are shearing forces. F_y is in line with the long edge of the force plate and is parallel to the direction of travel, whereas F_x is at right angles to the line of travel and parallel to the short edge of the force plate.

In addition to these three fundamental measurements, the force plate will show the moment (turning force) about

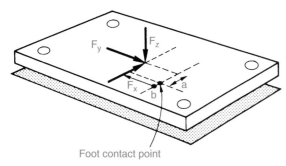

Figure 1.30   Three force components of a force plate a and b represent 'offset' position from centre of force plate.

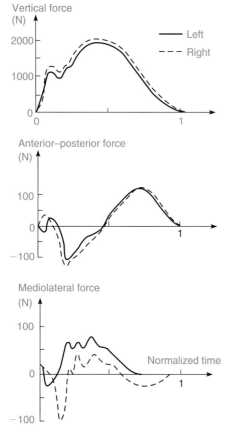

Figure 1.31   Examples of the components of the ground reaction force during running at a speed of 4 m/s (left and right foot). Adapted from Nigg, B.M. (1994) Biomechanics as applied to sports. In *Oxford Textbook of Sports Medicine* (eds M. Harries, C. Williams, W.D. Stanish and L.J. Micheli). Reprinted with permission of Oxford University Press, Oxford.

the central z axis. The position of the line of action of a force is shown by measuring the distance from the force to the centre of the plate, represented by the values a and b.

Using these measurements, ground reaction forces can be plotted for vertical, anterior-posterior, and mediolateral forces (Fig. 1.31). On the time axis, zero represents the point of first contact with the platform (heel strike) and 1 shows the point of last contact (toe off). The vertical force component of running (normal heel–toe gait) has two peaks. The first

Table 1.6   Factors altering an EMG signal

Noise	Artefacts	Distortion
Other muscles contracting, including the heart	False signals caused by EMG machine itself	Uneven amplification of EMG signal
Nearby electrical equipment, power cables, fluorescent lights, and radio waves	Signals from movement of EMG cables (*movement artefacts*)	

From Trew and Everett (1997) with permission.

(vertical impact force peak) occurs from 5 to 30 ms after ground contact and shows the first foot contact with the ground. In barefoot running the peak occurs sooner (5–10 ms), while running in a soft-soled shoe on asphalt gives a slower peak (20–30 ms). In running, impact forces may be as high as four times body weight, while at take off in a jump, forces as high as twelve times body weight may be expected (Nigg, 1994). The second peak (vertical active force peak) is due to movement caused by muscle contraction. This occurs in the middle of the stance phase (100–200 ms after first ground contact). In sprint running, vertical active forces may reach four times body weight (Nigg, 1994).

Electromyography (EMG)

EMG is a useful technique to analyse muscle function, rather than movement itself. When a muscle contracts it produces an electrical change (the muscle action potential or MAP) which lasts for as long 0.25 of a second, and may be from 100 microvolts (μV) to 5 millivolts (mV) (Trew and Everett, 1997). The aim of EMG is to detect this signal and to differentiate it from other electrical signals to ensure that is truly represents muscle contraction. The pure signal is said to be 'clean' and free from noise, artefacts and distortion (Table 1.6).

Electrodes used in EMG may be either surface (usually adhesive) or indwelling (needle). Surface electrodes are more commonly available and easy to use in the clinic environment. They have the disadvantage, however, that the signal must travel from the muscle to the skin, which for a deeper muscle may be some considerable distance. Needle electrodes pick the signal up from directly within the muscle, but the sensation caused by the electrode as the muscle contracts may alter the movement itself.

Surface electrodes are typically silver/silver chloride construction. In *monopolar* placement, one electrode is placed over the muscle being tested and another (the ground electrode) is placed at a distance, usually over a bony prominence, to record a base (zero) value. The difference between the two signals is compared to give an absolute EMG amplitude. With *bipolar* placement both electrodes are placed over the active muscle and the output is the difference between

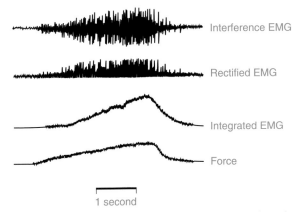

Figure 1.32 EMG signal processing. From Enoka, R.M. (1994) *Neuromechanical Basis of Kinesiology*, 2nd edn. Human Kinetics, Illinois. With permission.

the two signals. The value obtained is therefore one relative to the other but not compared to a base.

An EMG signal can show when a muscle has contracted, but not necessarily how powerfully. The relationship between EMG amplitude and muscle tension development is linear for isometric contraction (Bigland-Ritchie, 1981) but not for isotonic contraction (Lawrence and De Luca, 1983). The unilinear relationship between EMG and force in isotonic contractions is thought to be due to movement of the muscle beneath the electrode which is placed on the skin (Enoka, 1994).

The EMG signal, once amplified, is processed to put it into a more user friendly form. A number of techniques are available for signal processing (Fig. 1.32). Initially the raw signal from a number of muscle action potentials are superimposed (interference EMG). The signal is then compared to zero to give the absolute values of the peaks rather than the values of each peak relative to each other – the peaks are therefore placed against a straight axis (rectified EMG) and then smoothed to give a graph line (integrated EMG) which closely matches the changing muscle force.

ISOKINETIC ASSESSMENT

The use of isokinetic dynamometry is increasing in sports physiotherapy, and the system has both advantages and disadvantages. The system consists of a fixed axis of rotation and a lever driven either hydraulically or electrically. Both systems offer constant angular velocity. Originally hydraulic systems only offered isometric and concentric modes, but electrically powered systems now offer eccentric testing and continuous passive motion (CPM).

Advantages and disadvantages of isokinetic exercise

One of the disadvantages of isokinetics is that dynamometer velocities normally range from 1 to 500 degrees per second (°/s), a speed which is far slower than those obtained in ballistic actions in sport, which may exceed 6000°/s

(Perrin, 1993). In addition, normal muscle contractions do not occur at constant velocities, as offered by a dynamometer. Concentric contractions accelerate, while eccentric actions decelerate a limb. Finally, all human movements are triplane in nature, consisting usually of elements of flexion/extension, abduction/adduction and rotation. Most isokinetic dynamometers will only allow an action in a single plane at any one time. The combination of limited speed, constant speed and single plane motion means that movements on an isokinetic dynamometer cannot be totally functional. In the clinical setting, a number of other factors must by taken into account. The expertise required to perform assessment and exercise accurately and consistently is only acquired with in-depth training. In addition, both the space taken up by the dynamometer and the purchase cost may themselves be limiting factors within a physiotherapy department specializing in sport.

The great advantage of an isokinetic system, used for measurement or training, is the objectivity and reliability that the system has brought to musculoskeletal assessment. Providing the machine is calibrated, and the joint to be measured is accurately positioned and stabilized, reliability is high (Nitschke, 1992). This is especially true when using test velocities lower than 180°/s for the knee (Wilhite, Cohen and Wilhite, 1992). From the point of view of both safety and effectiveness, isokinetic dynamometers score highly. They give continually variable resistance which will match the strength curve of the tested muscle exactly. Because of this, strength testing is not limited to the weakest point in the range of motion, and in addition, testing can accurately identify a weakness at a point within the whole range.

An isokinetic dynamometer can give a number of useful measures to assess muscle function (Table 1.7).

Muscle force

The measurement of torque during maximal concentric contraction is the most common method of isokinetic strength testing. Torque is measured for a single joint movement, the axis of the joint being aligned with that of the dynamometer. In some instances, a rapidly performed movement, such as a throwing action, may exceed the velocity limit of the dynamometer. Equally, extremely strong subjects may produce movements in excess of the torque capacity of the isokinetic apparatus.

When measuring maximum torque, between two and six repetitions are usually performed before a stable measurement is achieved. The maximum torque is normally described as the highest single torque value recorded (Baltzopoulos and Brodie, 1989). However, some authors (Morris et al., 1983; Patton and Duggan, 1987) have used mean values of three or five repetitions respectively, and so the testing methods should always be defined.

The velocity of movement (degrees per second or rads per second) is also recorded, and it must be remembered that torque will reduce as angular velocity increases (Fig. 1.33).

Table 1.7   Parameters measured in isokinetic dynamometry

Torque
The turning effect produced by a force, measured in Newton metres (Nm). Peak torque (PT) is a measure of the force-generating capacity of the muscle and is represented by the highest point on a patient's torque/angle curve. Mean peak torque (MPT) averages this effect over a number of repetitions

Peak torque to weight
Torque expressed per unit of body mass. This measure makes comparisons between patients possible

Time to peak torque
Time to PT measures the ability to produce maximal torque rapidly, and is relevant for ballistic actions. Prolonged time to PT normally represents inefficient recruitment of type II muscle fibres

Torque velocity ratio
The ratio of torque (Nm) to angular velocity (rad/s). Concentric force reduces as velocity increases whereas eccentric force stays constant or may even increase

Work and power
Work is force multiplied by distance, and is represented by the area under the torque curve. Power is work per unit of time, and represents a subject's 'work rate'

Torque ratio
The ratio of agonist to antagonist peak torques expressed as a percentage, for example hamstring to quadriceps (H:Q) ratio

Endurance and fatigue
Endurance is measured as a 'fatigue index'. This gives an indication of type I fibre action.

Torque production and decay
Torque production rate (TPR) is the gradient of the ascending part of the torque curve (from start to peak torque). The torque decay rate (TDR) is the slope of the descending part of the torque curve from peak torque to the end of contraction

Adapted from Urquhart et al. (1995), with permission.

Muscle endurance

Muscular endurance can be assessed using isokinetic dynamometry by computing a fatigue index. Various methods have been used to calculate this index. Probably the most common for knee extension is that described by Thorstensson and Karlson (1976). In this test, subjects perform 50 consecutive knee extensions at 180°/s. The decline in torque over the 50 repetitions is calculated as the percentage difference between the mean torque of the first and last three repetitions.

Patten et al. (1978) used time to muscular exhaustion. Barnes (1981) used the difference (as a percentage value) between the maximum torque and that obtained in the tenth maximal contraction. Norris (1987) used the time to 50% maximal torque, and Baltzopoulos, Eston and McLaren (1988) used the decline in maximum torque over time using a 30-second test period.

Effects of inertia and gravity

Chart recordings of torque from subjects working at high velocities may show an initial high peak known as the 'impact artefact' or 'torque overshoot', followed by oscillations decreasing in amplitude (Fig. 1.34). This occurs in the time from rest to the limb catching up with the preset speed of the dynamometer. During this phase, the limb is accelerating towards the preset speed and is therefore not exercising isokinetically.

The torque overshoot is greater during proximal joint testing owing to the greater limb mass and longer distance between the limb's centre of gravity and the axis of rotation. If the overshoot is interpreted as the peak torque, the subject's muscular capacity will be overestimated (Baltzopoulos and Brodie, 1989).

Signal damping and resistance damping may be used to reduce the effect of torque overload. Signal damping ignores the first part of the torque data, while resistance damping introduces the braking force gradually.

With sagittal and frontal plane movements, the effects of gravity must be considered. With small force outputs, the effect of gravity may obscure results. The dynamometer will only record the force used against its internal resistance. It would normally not show that used to overcome gravity in an upwards movement or the contribution made

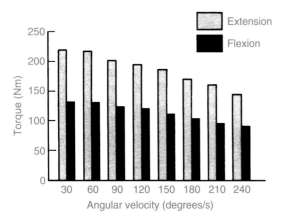

Figure 1.33   The maximum torque at different angular velocities of knee extension and flexion. From Baltzopoulos, V. and Brodie, D.A. (1989) Isokinetic dynamometry. Applications and limitations. *Sports Medicine*, 8(2), 101–116. With permission.

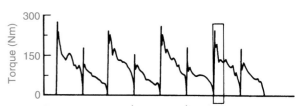

Figure 1.34   Torque overshoot (boxed area) during knee extension-flexion movements. From Baltzopoulos, V. and Brodie, D.A. (1989) Isokinetic dynamometry. Applications and limitations. *Sports Medicine*, 8(2), 101–116. With permission.

by gravity in a downward action. Nelson and Duncan (1983) determined the gravitational torque generated by the limb-lever system when it was allowed to fall passively at various angular positions. From this a correction factor was calculated to be added to the maximum torque registered by the dynamometer. Using this method, results will only be valid if the limb is allowed to fall against the resistance of the dynamometer with the subject's muscles relaxed.

Various computer programs have been produced which correct for gravity and inertial effects. These replace the need for manual data analysis and increase the accuracy of isokinetic dynamometry.

References

Baltzopoulos, V. and Brodie, D.A. (1989) Isokinetic dynamometry. Applications and limitations. *Sports Medicine*, **8**, (2) 101–116

Baltzopoulos, V., Eston, R.G. and McLaren, D. (1988) A comparison of power outputs on the Wingate test and on a test using an isokinetic device. *Ergonomics*, **31**, 1693–1699

Barak, T., Rosen, E.R. and Sofer, R. (1990) Basic concepts of orthopaedic manual therapy. In *Orthopaedic and Sports Physical Therapy* (ed. J.A. Gould), C.V. Mosby, St Louis, pp. 195–211

Barnes, W. (1981) Isokinetic fatigue curves at different contractile velocities. *Physical Therapy*, **60**, 1152–1158

Basmajian, J.V. and De Luca, C.J. (1985) *Muscles Alive*. Williams and Wilkins, Baltimore

Bigland-Ritchie, B. (1981) EMG/force relations and fatigue of human voluntary contractions. In *Exercise and Sport Science Reviews*, **9** (ed. D.I. Miller). Franklin Institute, Philadelphia, pp. 75–117

Bray, J.J., Cragg, P.A., Macknight, A.D.C., Mills, R.G. and Taylor, D.W. (1986) *Lecture Notes on Human Physiology*. Blackwell Scientific, Oxford

Burnie, J. and Brodie, D.A. (1986) Isokinetics in the assessment of rehabilitation: a case report. *Clinical Biomechanics*, **1**, 140–146

Butler, D.L., Grood, E.S., Noyes, F.R., Zernicke, R.G. and Barckett, K. (1984) Effects of structure and strain measurement technique on the material properties of young human tendons and fascia. *Journal of Biomechanics*, **17**, 579–596

Clarkson, H.M. and Gilewich, G.B. (1989) *Musculoskeletal Assessment*. Williams and Wilkins, Baltimore

Coyle, E.F., Feiring, D.C., Rotkis, T.C., Cote, R.U. and Roby, F.B. (1981) Specificity of power improvements through slow and fast isokinetic training. *Journal of Applied Physiology*, **51**, 1437–1442

Curwin, S.L. (1994) The aetiology and treatment of tendinitis. In *Oxford Textbook of Sports Medicine* (eds M. Harries, C. Williams, W.D. Stanish and L.J. Micheli). Oxford University Press, Oxford

Cyriax, J. (1982) *Textbook of Orthopaedic Medicine*, 8th edn. Baillière Tindall, London, vol. 1

Dvir, Z. (2000) *Clinical Biomechanics*. Churchill Livingstone, Edinburgh

Enoka, R.M. (1994) *Neuromechanical Basis of Kinesiology*, 2nd edn. Human Kinetics, Illinois

Gleim, G.W. (1984) The profiling of professional football players. *Clinics in Sports Medicine*, **3**, (1) 185–197

Hertling, D. and Kessler, R.M. (1990) *Management of Common Musculoskeletal Disorders*. J.B. Lippincott, Philadelphia

Kent, M. (1994) *Oxford Dictionary of Sports Science and Medicine*. Oxford University Press, Oxford

LaGasse, P. (1983) Neuromuscular facilitation of muscle tension output by reciprocal muscle work. *Annals of the French-Canadian Association for the Advancement of Science*, **50**, 222

Lawrence, J.H. and De Luca, C.J. (1983) Myoelectric signal versus force relationship in different human muscles. *Journal of Applied Physiology*, **54**, 1653–1659

LeVeau, B.F. (1990) Basic biomechanics in sports and orthopaedic therapy. In *Orthopaedic and Sports Physical Therapy* (ed. J.A. Gould). C.V. Mosby, Philadelphia

Lieber, R.L. (1992) *Skeletal Muscle Structure and Function*. Williams and Wilkins, Baltimore

Low, J. and Reed, A. (1996) *Basic Biomechanics Explained*. Butterworth-Heinemann, Oxford

McArdle, W.D., Katch, F.I. and Katch, V.L. (1986) *Exercise Physiology. Energy, Nutrition, and Human Performance*. Lea and Febiger, Philadelphia

Maitland, G.D. (1986) *Vertebral Manipulation*, 5th edn. Butterworth-Heinemann. Oxford

Maitland, G.D. (1991) *Peripheral Manipulation*, 3rd edn. Butterworth-Heinemann, Oxford

Morris, A., Lussier, K., Bell, G. and Dooley, J. (1983) Hamstring/quadriceps strength ratios in collegiate middle-distance and distance runners. *Physician and Sportsmedicine*, **11**, 71–77

Mulligan, B.M. (1999) *Manual Therapy, Nags, Snags and MWMs*, 5th edn. Plane View Services, Wellington, New Zealand

Nelson, S. and Duncan, P. (1983) Correction of isokinetic torque recordings for the effect of gravity. *Physical Therapy*, **63**, 674–676

Nigg, B.M. (1994) Biomechanics as applied to sports. In *Oxford Textbook of Sports Medicine* (eds M. Harries, C. Williams, W.D. Stanish and L.J. Micheli). Oxford University Press, Oxford

Nitschke, J.E. (1992) Reliability of isokinetic torque measurements: a review of the literature. *Australian Journal of Physiotherapy*, **38**, 125–134

Norris, C.M. (1987) The assessment of a novel physiotherapy technique – combined vacuum and pressure. MSc thesis, University of Liverpool

Patten, W.R., Hinson, M., Arnold, B.R. and Lessard, M.A. (1978) Fatigue curves of isokinetic contractions. *Archives of Physical Medicine and Rehabilitation*, **59**, 507–509

Patton, J. and Duggan, A. (1987) An evaluation of tests of anaerobic power. *Aviation, Space and Environmental Medicine*, **3**, 237–242

Perrin, D.H. (1993) *Isokinetic Exercise and Assessment*. Human Kinetics Publishers, Leeds

Pipes, T.V. and Wilmore, J.H. (1975) Isokinetic vs isotonic strength training in adult men. *Medicine in Science and Sports*, **7**, 262–274

Rasch, P.J. (1989) *Kinesiology and Applied Anatomy*. Lea and Febiger, Philadelphia

Sale, D.G. (1988) Neural adaptation to resistance training. *Medicine and Science in Sports and Exercise*, **20**, (5) 135–145

Stallard, J. (1984) The mechanics of lower limb orthoses. In *Cash's Textbook of Orthopaedics and Rheumatology for Physiotherapists* (ed. P.A. Downie). Faber and Faber, London, pp. 21–42

Taunton, J.E., McKenzie, D.C. and Clement, D.B. (1988) The role of biomechanics in the epidemiology of injuries. *Sports Medicine*, **6**, 107–120

Thorstensson, A. and Karlson, J. (1976) Fatiguability and fibre composition of human skeletal muscle. *Acta Physiologica Scandinavica*, **98**, 318–322

Toussaint, H.M., van Baar, C.E., van Langen, P.P., de Looze, M.P. and van Dieen, J.H. (1992) Coordination of the leg muscles in backlift and leglift. *Journal of Biomechanics*, **25**, 1279–1289

Trew, M. and Everett, T. (1997) *Human Movement*. Churchill Livingstone, Edinburgh

Urquhart, D.S., Garbutt, G., Cova, K., Lennox, C.M.E. and McLatchie, G.R. (1995) Isokinetics: applications in the management of knee soft-tissue injuries. *Sports Exercise and Injury*, **1**, (3) 138–147

van Ingen Schenau, G.J., Bobbert, M.F. and van Soest, A.J. (1990) The unique action of bi-articular muscles in leg extensions. In *Multiple Muscle Systems: Biomechanics and Movement Organisation* (eds J.M. Winters and S.L. Woo). Springer-Verlag, New York

Watkins, J. (1983) *An Introduction to Mechanics of Human Movement.* MTP Press, Lancaster

Wells, K.F. (1966) *Kinesiology.* W.B. Saunders, Philadelphia

Wilhite, M.R., Cohen, E.R. and Wilhite, S.C. (1992) Reliability of concentric and eccentric measurements of quadriceps performance using the Kin-Com dynamometer: the effect of testing order for three different speeds. *Journal of Orthopaedic and Sports Physical Therapy,* **15**, 175–182

Williams, P.L. (1995) *Gray's Anatomy,* 38th edn. Churchill Livingstone, Edinburgh

Williams, J.G. and Davis, M. (1990) KINEMAN: A microcomputer-based video digitising system for movement analysis. *Physiotherapy,* **76**, (6) 436–440

Williams, J.G.P. and Sperryn, P.N. (1976) *Sports Medicine.* Edward Arnold, London

Wilson, E. (2001) The Mulligan concept. *Journal of Bodywork and Movement Therapies,* **5**, (2) 81–89

Zehr, E.P. and Sale, D.G. (1994) Ballistic movement: muscle activation and neuromuscular adaptation. *Canadian Journal of Applied Physiology,* **19**, 363–378

Chapter 2

Healing

The basic processes of soft tissue healing underlie all treatment techniques for sports injuries. We need to know what occurs in the body tissues at each successive stage of healing to be able to select the treatment technique which is most appropriate for that time. A technique aimed at reducing the formation of swelling, for example, would be inappropriate when swelling had stopped forming and adhesions were the problem. Similarly, a manual treatment designed to break up adhesions and mobilize soft tissue would not be helpful when inflammation is still forming and the tissues are highly irritable.

The stages of healing are, to a large extent, purely a convenience of description, since each stage runs into another. Traditionally, the initial tissue response has been described as inflammation, but some authors see inflammation as a response separate to the processes occurring at the time of injury. Van der Meulen (1982) described both in terms of the 'reaction phase', arguing that the classical inflammatory period is preceded by a short (10 minute) period before the inflammatory mechanism is activated. Others (Hunter, 1998), looking at the changes in strength of the healing tissue, have termed the first stage the 'lag phase' because tissue strength does not change. The second stage of healing has been variously called repair, proliferation and regeneration. The tertiary stage has been termed remodelling (Van der Meulen, 1982; Kellett, 1986; Dyson, 1987). The terms injury, inflammation, repair and remodelling will be used in this text.

When describing the stage of healing, the terms acute, subacute and chronic are helpful. The acute stage (up to 48 hours following injury) is the stage of inflammation. The subacute stage, occurring between 14 and 21 days after injury, is the stage of repair. The chronic stage (after 21 days) is the stage of remodelling. The term chronic is also sometimes used to describe self-perpetuating inflammation, where the inflammatory process has restarted due to disruption or persistent

Definition
Treatment must be adapted to the stages of healing, which are injury, inflammation, repair and remodelling.

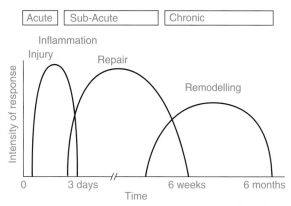

Figure 2.1 Timescale for healing. From Oakes, B.W. (1992) The classification of injuries and mechanisms of injury, repair and healing. In *Textbook of Science and Medicine in Sport* (eds J. Bloomfield, P.A. Fricker and K.D. Fitch). Blackwell Scientific Publications, Melbourne. With permission.

irritation of the healing tissues. The total healing process occurs over a continuum, shown in Fig. 2.1.

INJURY

This stage represents the tissue effects at the time of injury, before the inflammatory process is activated. With tissue damage, chemical and mechanical changes are seen. Local blood vessels are disrupted causing a cessation in oxygen to the cells they perfused. These cells die and their lysosome membranes disintegrate, releasing the hydrolyzing enzymes the lysosomes contained. The release of these enzymes has a two-fold effect. First they begin to break down the dead cells themselves, and secondly, they release histamines and kinins which have an effect on both the live cells nearby and the local blood capillary network.

The disruption of the blood vessels which caused cell death also causes local bleeding (extravasated blood). The red blood cells break down, leaving cellular debris and free haemoglobin. The blood platelets release the enzyme thrombin which changes fibrinogen into fibrin. The fibrin in turn is deposited as a meshwork around the area (a process known as walling off). The dead cells intertwine in the meshwork forming a blood clot. This network contains the damaged area.

The changes occurring at injury are affected by age (Lachman, 1988). Intramuscular bleeding, and therefore haemorrhage formation, are more profuse in individuals over 30 years of age. The amount of bleeding which occurs will be partially dependent on the vascularity of the injured tissues. A fitter individual is likely to have muscle tissue

> **Keypoint**
>
> The tissues of an active athlete are more highly vascularized than those of an inactive subject. The athlete's tissues will therefore bleed more during injury, and bruising will be more noticeable.

which is more highly vascularized, and therefore greater bleeding will occur with muscle injury. In addition, exercise itself will affect gross tissue responses. Muscle blood flow is greatly increased through dilatation of the capillary bed, and again bleeding subsequent to injury will be greater.

INFLAMMATION

The next stage in the healing sequence is that of inflammation. This may last from 10 minutes to several days, depending on the amount of tissue damage which has occurred. The inflammatory response to injury is the same regardless of the nature of the injuring agent or the location of the injury itself (Hettinga, 1990). Various agents can give rise to injury, and Evans (1990a) listed physical, thermal, radiational, electrical and chemical causes.

Inflammation is not simply a feature of soft tissue injuries. It occurs when the body is infected, in immune reactions and when infarction stops blood flowing to an area. Some of the characteristics of the inflammatory response have even been described as excessive (Cyriax, 1982) and better suited to dealing with infection, by preventing bacterial spread, than healing injury (Evans, 1990a).

The cardinal signs of inflammation are heat (*calor*), redness (*rubor*), swelling (*tumor*) and pain (*dolor*). These in turn give rise to the so-called fifth sign of inflammation disturbance of function of the affected tissues (*functio laesa*).

> **Keypoint**
>
> Inflammation is often seen as undesirable. However, inflammation is the first stage of healing and so is a vital step on the road to recovery. The aim should be to prevent excessive inflammation and move the athlete on through the stages of healing towards eventual full function.

Heat and redness

Heat and redness take a number of hours to develop, and are due to the opening of local blood capillaries and the resultant increased blood flow. Chemical and mechanical changes, initiated by injury, are responsible for the changes in blood flow.

Chemically, a number of substances act as mediators in the inflammatory process. The amines, including histamine and 5-hydroxytriptamine (5-HT or serotonin) are released from mast cells, red blood cells and platelets in the damaged capillaries and cause vessel dilatation and increased permeability lasting 10–15 minutes (Lachman, 1988). Kinins (physiologically active polypeptides) cause an increase in vascular permeability and stimulate the contraction of smooth muscle. They are found normally in an inactive state as kininogens. These in turn are activated by the enzyme plasmin, and degraded by kininases.

The initial vasodilatation is maintained by prostaglandins. These are one of the arachidonic acid derivatives, formed from cell membrane phospholipids when cell damage occurs, and released when the kinin system is activated. The drugs aspirin and indometacin act to inhibit this change – hence their use as anti-inflammatory agents in sports injury treatment. The prostaglandins E1 and E2 are two of the substances responsible for pain production, and they will also promote vasodilatation, blood vessel permeability and lymph flow (Oakes, 1992).

> ### Keypoint
>
> Aspirin is one of a group of drugs called non-steroidal anti-inflammatory drugs (NSAIDs). These work by affecting prostaglandins, which are also involved in action of the stomach. For this reason NSAIDs may cause gastric irritation and should not be given to those with a history of peptic ulcers.

The complement system, consisting of a number of serum proteins circulating in an inactive form, is activated and has a direct effect on the cell membrane as well as helping to maintain vasodilatation. Various complement products are involved, and these are activated in sequence. Finally, polymorphs produce leukotrienes, which are themselves derived from arachidonic acid. These help the kinins maintain the vessel permeability.

Blood flow changes also occur through mechanical alterations initiated by injury. Normally, the blood flow in the venules, in particular, is axial. The large blood proteins stay in the centre of the vessel, and the plasmatic stream, which has a lower viscosity, is on the outside in contact with the vessel walls. This configuration reduces peripheral resistance and aids blood flow.

In a damaged capillary, however, fluid is lost and so the axial flow slows. Marginalization occurs as the slower flow rate allows white blood cells to move into the plasmatic zone and adhere to the vessel walls. This, in turn, reduces the lubricating effect of this layer and slows blood flow. The walls themselves become covered with a gelatinous layer (Wilkinson and Lackie, 1979), as endothelium changes occur (Walter and Israel, 1987).

Some 4 hours after injury (Evans, 1980) diapedesis occurs as the white cells pass through the vessel walls into the damaged tissue. The endothelial cells of the vessel contract (Hettinga, 1990), pulling away from each other and leaving gaps through which fluids and blood cells can escape (Fig. 2.2). Various substances, including histamine, kinins and complement factors, have been shown to produce this effect (Fox, Galey and Wayland, 1980; Walter and Israel, 1987).

Swelling

The normal pressure gradients inside and outside the capillary balance the flow of fluid leaving and entering the vessel (Fig. 2.3). The capillary membrane is permeable to water, and so water will be driven out into the interstitial fluid. However, because the tissue fluids usually contain a small

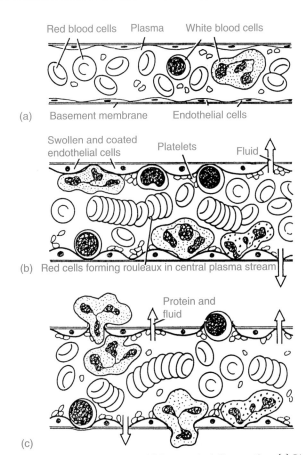

Figure 2.2 Vascular changes which occur in inflammation. (a) Blood vessel starts to dilate. (b) Dilated vessel showing marginalization. (c) White blood cells and fluid pass into tissue. From Evans, D.M.D. (1990a) Inflammation and healing. In *Cash's Textbook of General Medical and Surgical Conditions for Physiotherapists* (ed. P.A. Downie), 2nd edn. Faber and Faber, London. With permission.

amount of protein, and the blood contains a large amount, an osmotic pressure is created which tends to suck water back from the tissue fluid and into the capillary once more. The magnitude of this osmotic pressure is roughly 25 mmHg. At the arteriole end of the capillary the blood pressure (32 mmHg) exceeds the osmotic pressure and so tissue fluid is formed. At the venous end of the capillary the blood pressure has reduced (12 mmHg) and so, because the osmotic pressure now exceeds this value, tissue fluid is reabsorbed back into the capillary.

During inflammation the capillary bed opens and blood flow increases (heat and redness). The larger blood volume causes a parallel increase in blood pressure. Coupled with this, the tissue fluid now contains a large amount of protein, which has poured out from the more permeable blood vessels. This increased protein concentration causes a substantial rise in osmotic pressure, and this, together with the larger blood pressure in the capillary, forces fluid out into the interstitium, causing swelling.

Protein exudation in mild inflammation occurs from the venules only and is probably mediated by histamine (Evans, 1990a). More severe inflammation, as a result of trauma, results in protein exudation from damaged capillaries as well.

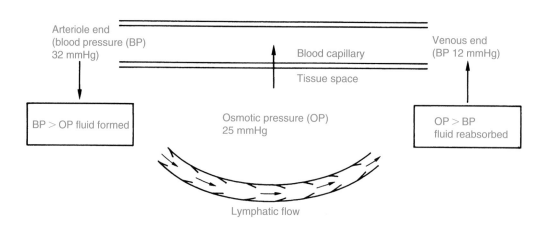

Figure 2.3 Formation and reabsorption of tissue fluid.

During inflammation, lymphatic vessels open up and assist in the removal of excess fluid and protein. The lymph vessels are blind-ending capillaries which have gaps in their endothelial walls enabling protein molecules to move through easily. The lymph vessels lie within the tissue spaces, and have valves preventing the backward movement of fluid. Muscular contraction causes a pumping action on the lymph vessels and the excess tissue fluid is removed to the subclavian veins in the neck.

Pain

Pain is the result of both sensory and emotional experiences, and is associated with tissue damage or the probability that damage will occur. It serves as a warning which may cause us to withdraw from a painful stimulus and so protect an injured body part. Unfortunately, pain often continues long after it has ceased to be a useful form of protection. Associated muscle spasm, atrophy, habitual postures, guarding and psychological factors all combine to make chronic pain almost a disease entity in itself.

Types of pain

Pain may be classified as somatogenic (acute or chronic), neurogenic or psychogenic. Chronic pain may be considered as pain which generally lasts for more than 6 weeks, while acute pain is pain of sudden onset which lasts for less than 6 weeks (Donley and Denegar, 1990).

Definition
Acute pain has a sudden onset and lasts for less than 6 weeks. *Chronic pain* lasts in excess of 6 weeks.

Musculoskeletal pain is not usually well localized – the surface site where the pain is felt rarely correlates directly to injured subcutaneous tissue. Generally, the closer an injured tissue is to the skin surface, the more accurate the athlete can be at localizing it.

Deep pain is normally an aching, ill-defined sensation. It usually radiates in a characteristic fashion, and may be associated with autonomic responses such as sweating, nausea, pallor and lowered blood pressure (Lynch and Kessler, 1990). Pain referral corresponds to segmental pathways, most often dermatomes. The extent of radiation largely depends on the intensity of the stimulus, with pain normally radiating distally, and rarely crossing the mid-line of the body (Cyriax, 1982).

Neurogenic pain is different again. Compression of a nerve root gives rise to ill-defined tingling, especially in the distal part of the dermatome supplied by the nerve. This is a pressure reaction, which quickly disappears when the nerve root is released. Greater pressure causes the tingling to give way to numbness. Compression or tension to the dural sleeve covering the nerve root gives severe pain, generally over the whole dermatome. In contrast, pressure on a nerve trunk usually causes little or no pain, but results in a shower of 'pins and needles' as the nerve compression is released. Pressure applied to a superficial nerve distally gives numbness and some tingling, with the edge of the affected region being well defined (Cyriax, 1982).

Irritability

Irritability may be defined as 'the vigour of activity which causes pain' (Maitland, 1991). It is determined by the degree of pain which the patient experiences, and the time this takes to subside, in relation to the intensity of activity that brought the pain on in the first place. The purpose of assessing irritability is to determine how much activity (joint mobilization, exercise, etc.) may be prescribed without exacerbating the patient's symptoms.

An assessment of irritability may be made at the second treatment session. The amount of movement which the patient was subjected to in the previous session is known, as is the discomfort that he or she feels now. These subjective feelings are then used to determine the intensity of the second treatment session. Similarly, at the beginning of each subsequent treatment session the irritability is again assessed.

Treatment note 2.1   Pain description in examination

During both the subjective examination and the objective examination (see Treatment note 2.4, p. 56) the patient will usually describe pain. Both the type (nature) of pain and its behaviour are important factors in making an accurate clinical diagnosis, and a number of factors should be considered:

- When pain is *decreasing* the condition is generally resolving, while *increasing* pain suggests a worsening condition.
- *Constant* pain which does not change with time, alteration of static posture or activities suggests a non-mechanical condition such as chemical irritation, tumours or visceral lesions (Magee, 2002).
- Where pain *changes* (episodic pain), the therapist should try to determine what activities make the pain worse (exacerbation) and what make it better (remission).
- The therapist should try to determine if the pain is *associated with particular events* (e.g. movements, visceral function), or time of day.
- Pain with sporting activity which *reduces with rest*, in general suggests a mechanical problem, irritating pain sensitive structures.
- *Morning pain* which eases with movement indicates chronic inflammation which takes time to build up and reduces with movement.

The description of pain itself may indicate the structure causing it (Table 2.1) and the behaviour of the pain on physical examination (p. 56) clarifies the picture.

Recording pain

The intensity of pain may be recorded on a visual analogue scale (VAS). The patient is asked to indicate the pain description or number which best represents their pain. Where a 10 cm line is used the distance from the left of the scale to the point marked by the patient may be measured in millimetres and used as a numerical value (Fig. 2.4).

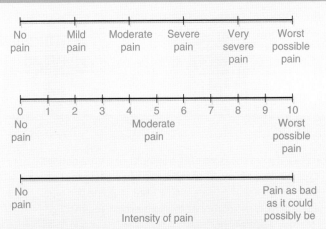

Figure 2.4   Visual analogue scales (VAS) used in pain description. From Petty and Moore (2001) with permission.

Table 2.1   Pain descriptions and related structures

Type of pain	
Cramping , dull, aching, worse with resisted movement	Muscle
Dull, aching, worse with passive movement	Ligament, joint capsule
Sharp, shooting	Nerve root
Sharp, lightning-like, travelling	Nerve
Burning, pressure-like, stinging, with skin changes	Sympathetic nerve
Deep, nagging, poorly localized	Bone
Sharp, severe, unable to take weight	Fracture
Throbbing, diffuse	Vasculature

Source Magee (2002) and Petty and Moore (2001) with permission.

Table 2.2   Red flags in sport examination indicating medical investigation

System/possible pathology	Pain behaviour
Cancer	Persistent night pain Constant (25 hour) pain Unexplained weight loss (e.g. 4–6 kg in 10 days) Loss of appetite Unusual lumps or growths Sudden persistent fatigue Past history of carcinoma
Cardiovascular	Shortness of breath Dizziness Pain or feeling of heaviness in the chest Pulsating sensations in the body Discolouration in the feet Persistent swelling with no history of injury
Gastrointestinal/ genitourinary	Frequent or severe abdominal pain Frequent heartburn or indigestion Frequent nausea or vomiting Change in bladder or bowel habits Unusual menstruation
Neurological	Changes in hearing Frequent or severe headache Problems in swallowing or changes in speech Gait disturbance, or problems with balance/ coordination Drop attacks (fainting) Sudden weakness

Source Magee (2002) and Waddell, G., Feder, G. and Lewis, M. (1997) Systematic reviews of bed rest and advice to stay active for acute law back pain. *British Journal of General Practice*, **47**, 647–652. With permission.

> **Red flags**
>
> It is important for the therapist to appreciate when pain and other symptoms may suggest serious pathology which requires medical investigation – so called 'red flags' (Table 2.2). Where the patient has persistent pain and is generally unwell, the indication is that a pathology other than a musculoskeletal condition exists. In addition, changes in bladder and bowel habits, alteration in vision or gross changes in gait all require further investigation.

> **Keypoint**
>
> Irritability is a measure of the amount of pain a patient experiences as a result of movement (including that of treatment). Irritability should be used to guide the type and intensity of treatment to avoid excessive post-treatment soreness.

> **Keypoint**
>
> Fast pain helps the body avoid tissue damage by provoking a flexor withdrawal reflex. Slow pain enforces inactivity (through muscle spasm) to allow time for healing.

Pain production

Free or 'bare' nerve endings (type IV) respond to painful stimuli and are termed nociceptors (from the Latin *nocere*, to damage). They are largely unresponsive to normal stimuli, but have a low threshold to mechanical and thermal injury, anoxia, and irritation from inflammatory products. Tissues vary in the intensity of pain they will produce when stimulated. The joint capsule and periosteum are the most sensitive to noxious stimuli. Subchondral bone, tendons and ligaments are the next in line in terms of sensitivity, followed by muscle and cortical bone, the synovium and cartilage being largely insensitive.

The pain receptors are supplied by a variety of different nerve fibres. Skin receptors are supplied by thinly myelinated (A delta) fibres which carry 'fast' pain and respond to strong mechanical stimuli and heat above 45°C (Low and Reed, 1990). They give the initial sharp well-localized pain feeling (pinprick). The function of fast pain is to help the body avoid tissue damage and it often provokes a flexor withdrawal reflex.

Impulses from free nerve endings found in deeper body tissues are carried by non-myelinated C fibres. This is 'slow' pain, which tends to be aching and throbbing in nature, and poorly defined. Its onset is not immediate, and the sensation it produces persists after the pain stimulus has gone. The function of slow pain seems to be to enforce inactivity and allow healing to occur and it is therefore often associated with muscle spasm. The C fibres respond to many different types of stimuli and, as such, are said to be 'polymodal'. However, they are most sensitive to chemicals released as a result of tissue damage. Histamine, kinins, prostaglandins E1 and E2, and 5-HT have all been implicated in this type of pain production during inflammation (Walter and Israel, 1987; Lachman 1988).

It can be seen that the pain experienced as a result of sporting injury will usually be either mechanical or chemical in nature. Mechanical pain is the result of forces which deform, or damage the nociceptive nerve endings, and so may be caused by stretching contracted tissue or by fluid pressure. This type of pain is influenced by movement. Chemical pain, on the other hand, results from irritation of the nerve endings, and is less affected by movement or joint position, but will respond to rest.

Articular neurology

In addition to pain receptors (type IV), three other joint receptors are important. Type I receptors are located in the superficial layers of the joint capsule. They are slow adapting, low-threshold mechanoreceptors, which respond to both static and dynamic stimulation. These receptors provide information about the static position of a joint, and contribute to the regulation of muscle tone and movement (kinaesthetic) sense. The type I receptors sense both the speed and direction of movement.

Type II receptors are found mainly in the deeper capsular layers and within fat pads. These are dynamic receptors with a high threshold, and they adapt quickly. They respond to rapid changes of direction of joint movement.

The type III fibres are found in the joint ligaments, and are again high threshold dynamic mechanoreceptors, but are slow adapting. These receptors monitor the direction of movement, and have a 'braking' effect on muscle tone if the joint is moving too quickly or through too great a range of motion. The type IV receptor is the nociceptor described above. Table 2.3 provides a synopsis of the various movement categories to which the receptors respond.

Alteration in the feedback provided by joint receptors is of great importance following sports injury, and is dealt with in the section on proprioceptive training (p. 149).

Pain pathways

Three categories or 'orders' of neurone make up the pain pathways. First order neurones travel from the pain receptors to the spinal cord, second order neurones travel within the cord to the brainstem and third order neurones travel from the brainstem to the higher centres of the cerebral cortex.

Table 2.3 Function of joint receptors

Function	Receptor
Static position	Type I
Speed of movement	Type I
Change in speed	Type II
Direction of movement	Types I and II
Postural muscle tone	Type I
Tone at initiation of movement	Type II
Tone during movement	Type II
Tone during harmful movements	Type III

Adapted from Hertling, D. and Kessler, R.M. (1990) *Management of Common Musculoskeletal Disorders.* JB Lippincott, Philadelphia. With permission.

Keypoint

Type I joint receptors are found in the superficial layers of the joint capsule, type II in the deeper layers. Type III receptors are contained within the joint ligaments themselves.

Seventy percent of the C fibres (slow pain) enter the spine via the dorsal root, while 30% of the fibres enter via the ventral root. The C fibres synapse with second order neurones in the substantia gelatinosa (SG) of the cord and these neurones ascend in the anterolateral funiculus on the opposite side of the cord (Fig. 2.5). From here they travel via the reticular formation to the intralaminar nuclei of the thalamus. The neurones synapse here once more and travel to the prefrontal region of the cerebral cortex. Some of the C fibres travel to the limbic system (cingulate gyrus) and generate emotional responses to pain (described as anxiety, fear and dread). C fibre pain is therefore poorly localized with a large emotional affect (White, 1999).

The A delta fibres (fast pain), on the other hand, synapse in the outer part of the posterior horn of the cord and cross to ascend in the spinothalamic tract to the ventrobasal nuclei in the thalamus, and then to the postcentral gyrus of the cortex.

Fast pain is registered in the parietal lobe and visceral pain in the insular cortex.

With more major injuries both fibres will produce a pain effect. The response to an ankle sprain, for example, will be an intense, well-defined stabbing sensation (A delta) followed by a dull ache accompanied by an emotional response (C fibre).

Clinical note

Acute sports injuries normally give a well-defined stabbing pain followed by a dull ache accompanied by an emotional response.

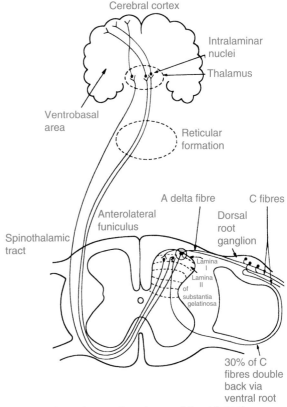

Figure 2.5 Pain pathways. From Low and Reed (1990) with permission.

Pain relief mechanisms

Three concepts of pain control are generally used within physiotherapy:

1. stimulation of ascending fibres to block pain messages (pain gate theory)
2. endogenous opioid formation
3. descending fibre stimulation within the dorsal horn of the spinal cord (descending inhibition).

The pain gate The pain gate theory (Melzack and Wall, 1965) proposed that pain perception was regulated by a 'gate' which could be opened or closed. When stimulated, mechanoreceptors in the skin send impulses via A beta fibres to the posterior horn of the cord. Here, collateral branches are given off. These collaterals affect A delta and C pain fibres in the substantia gelatinosa (SG), reducing their excitability by presynaptic inhibition. Stimulation of A delta fibres by low intensity, high frequency transcutaneous electrical nerve stimulation (TENS) (100–200 Hz) will therefore reduce pain through this gating mechanism (Fig. 2.6).

Endogenous opioids Interneurones within the substantia gelatinosa are able to produce endogenous (made in the body) opioid peptides, which have similar effects to opioids such as morphine, heroin and codeine, which are some of the most powerful analgesics known. These opioids inhibit C fibre cells. Collateral branches of A delta fibres in the posterior horn connect to the interneurones and stimulate them to produce opioids.

The opioids, including enkephalins and endorphins, are produced in various areas of the central nervous system

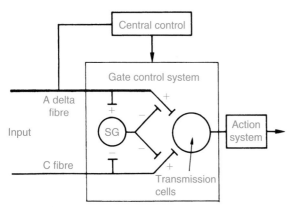

Figure 2.6   The pain gate mechanism. Central control — effects caused by higher centre (brain), action system — pain response. SG, substantia gelatinosa. From Melzack, R. and Wall, P.D. (1965) Pain mechanisms: a new theory. *Science*, **150**, 197. American Association for the Advancement of Science. With permission.

(CNS) including the limbic system and thalamus, pituitary gland, substantia gelatinosa and nerve terminals. These substances inhibit transmission in the A delta and C fibre pathways and so block pain before it reaches sensory levels. Stimulation of the A delta fibres with high intensity low frequency TENS (2–10 Hz) will damp down C fibre activity and reduce pain through this method.

Descending inhibition   Descending inhibition occurs when A delta fibres activate a chain of neurones which travel down the length of the spinal cord. Two separate systems are generally said to be involved (White, 1999), one involving serotonin, the other noradrenaline (norepinephrine). In the first, fibres from the periaqueductal grey matter (PAG) of the midbrain travel to the nucleus raphe magnus and then to the stalked cells in the dorsal horn of the spinal cord. In these cells, serotonin is released, which in turn causes the release of enkephalin to inhibit the cells of the SG. In the second system, the arcuate nucleus of the hypothalamus activates nuclei in the brainstem. Descending fibres in turn release noradrenaline (norepinephrine) into the dorsal horn of the cord to again inhibit the SG. Stimulation at frequencies above 50 Hz may affect this system (De Domenico, 1982).

Treatment note 2.2   Dry needling

Dry needling is an acupuncture technique which involves using a solid (no bore) atraumatic needle inserted into the body tissues. Pain relief has been described through both the pain gate mechanisms and diffuse noxious inhibitory control. In addition, according to Oriental medicine pain can be a result of a blockage and/or stagnation of acupuncture energy (*qi*) and acupuncture is designed to increase the flow of qi energy to stimulate healing and pain relief.

Both painful points (trigger points) and classic acupuncture points may be used. Classic acupuncture points are needled to specific depths described in acupuncture literature (see Norris, 2001). Trigger points may be either needled superficially to a depth of 0.5 cm (Baldry, 1998) or up to 8–10 cm (Gunn, 1996), depending on the mechanism being used. Superficial needling is said to activate A delta nerve fibres responsible for acupuncture pain relief, while deep needling is said to reduce pain but also induce healing through the production of platelet derived growth factor (PDGF) to stimulate new collagen formation (Gunn, 1996).

It should be noted that dry needling carries risks, and requires postgraduate training. Deep needling of the type used in intramuscular stimulation (IMS) in particular is a technique which involves highly specialist training (see Training section at the end of this box).

Technique
Acupuncture needles used for musculoskeletal conditions are of pre-sterilized disposable stainless steel construction and they vary from 0.22 mm to 0.45 mm in diameter and may be up to

4 inches in length. The patient's skin should be cleaned prior to the treatment and the practitioner's hands should be washed and sterilized with an alcohol-based sanitizer before treatment.

The needles are normally inserted using a plastic guide tube which is slightly shorter than the needle (Fig. 2.7). The guide tube is placed on the skin with the needle within it and the needle inserted through the skin surface with a small, brisk tap. Once the needle is inserted the guide tube is removed, and the needle pressed in further to the required depth (Fig. 2.8). Throughout this procedure, sterile practice must be maintained. To guard against infection, each needle is only used once and the shaft of the needle should not be touched.

The needle is often manipulated by rotation, scraping or flicking to increase the sensation felt by the patient – known as sensory propagation along channels or *deqi* in Oriental medicine. The needle may be inserted perpendicular to the skin

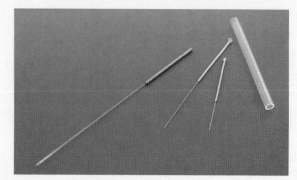

Figure 2.7   Guide tubes and needles.

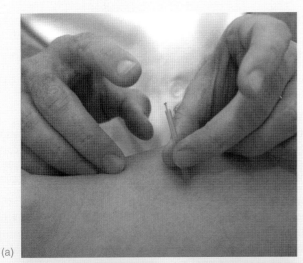

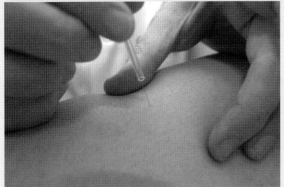

(a)

(b)

Figure 2.8   Use of guide tubes for needle insertion.

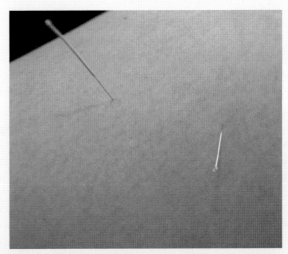

Figure 2.9   Oblique and perpendicular needle insertion.

Precautions and contraindications

Patients who are on anticoagulant therapy and those who have haemophilia should not be treated with dry needling. Diabetic patients should be closely monitored if they are to have needles inserted into hands and feet. Patients with prosthetic or damaged heart valves should be treated with caution. Epileptic patients should not be treated if they have had a fit during the last 3 months. Points on the lower abdomen and the lumbar sacral region should be used with caution during the first trimester of pregnancy. Following needling, it is common for patients to feel drowsy and they should be warned about this.

It is vital that the practitioner using dry needling has a thorough knowledge of underlying anatomy as trauma to body tissues, including the lungs and other organs, has been reported.

Training

Training in dry needling and acupuncture for registered physical therapy practitioners:

Acupuncture Association of Chartered Physiotherapists: www.aacp.uk.com

British Medical Acupuncture Society: www.medical-acupuncture.co.uk

Institute for the Study of Pain (IMS training): www.istop.org

or at oblique and transverse angles (Fig. 2.9). Once the needle is withdrawn the acupuncture point may be pressed with a cotton bud or probe to reduce the likelihood of bruising.

Needles are in general inserted for between 10 and 15 minutes, though shorter insertion techniques may be used to directly stimulate the muscle through intramuscular stimulation (IMS). In addition to muscular treatment, the periosteum of the bone itself may be used as a form of treatment, particularly for joint degeneration. The aim is to strike the periosteum, and the sensation felt is a dull ache rather than the immediate pain of a tissue needle.

Management of inflammation

The effects of acute inflammation can be reduced by slowing the body's response represented by the cardinal signs. Redness and heat are therefore treated by trying to reduce localized bleeding through the use of cold or ice and compression. Swelling is similarly managed by the use of compression to contain local oedema, and gentle movement to assist lymphatic drainage. By reducing the chemical and mechanical effects of the three inflammatory signs above, pain is also reduced.

The amount of rest prescribed during inflammation will depend on the stage of inflammation and the amount of tissue damage.

Chronic inflammation

Inflammation is the beginning phase in the healing process. Ordinarily tissues progress through the healing process sequentially to restore full function. However, in certain cases injuries remain in the inflammatory period, like a computer program that has become stuck in a loop. This is then termed

---

Definition

A *granuloma* is a mass of collagen which occurs in chronic inflammation. It surrounds and isolates foreign material in a wound.

---

chronic inflammation and occurs because macrophages have been unable to completely clear (debride) the area of foreign substances. This material may be dead cells, extracellular blood, or sand or dirt in some cases. Either way, the material is surrounded by collagen to isolate it from the body. This mass of encapsulating scar is called a granuloma.

Chronic inflammation has been shown to have a low concentration of growth factors and a high concentration of protease (Hom, 1995). Adding growth factor to a chronic wound has been shown to improve healing in a number of soft tissues. Platelet derived growth factor has been used to treat ligaments and tendons in general (Evans, 1999) whilst insulin like growth factor (IGF-1) has been used with the achilles tendon (Kurtz, Loebig and Andersen, 1999) and articular cartilage (Nixon, Fortier and Williams, 1999).

REPAIR

Inflammation may continue for 5 days, but with minor trauma it is usually complete by the third day after injury (Evans, 1980). Following this, tissue repair can take place. Repair is by resolution, organization or regeneration, depending on the severity of the injury and the nature of the injured tissues. A minor injury will result in acute inflammation as described above, and the phagocytic cells will clear the area. If there is little tissue damage, the stage of resolution will result in a return to near normal (Lachman, 1988). True resolution rarely occurs with soft tissue injuries, but is more common with inflammatory tissue reactions such as pneumonia.

On the periphery of the injured area, macrophages and polymorphs are active because they can tolerate the low oxygen levels present in the damaged tissue. Cellular division by mitosis is seen in the surrounding capillaries about 12 hours after injury. During the next 3 days capillary buds form and grow towards the lower oxygen concentration of the injured area. These capillaries form loops and blood begins to flow through them. This new capillary rich material is known as granulation tissue. Plasma proteins, cells and fluid pour out of these highly permeable vessels. The gradually increasing oxygen supply to the previously deoxygenated area means phagocytosis can now begin.

New lymphatic vessels bud out from the existing lymphatics, linking to form a renewed lymphatic drainage system. As this process is occurring, fibroblast cells multiply and move towards the injured tissue. By the fifth day after injury they begin to lay down fibrils of collagen, a process requiring adequate amounts of vitamin C.

The individual fibrils form into parallel bundles lying in the direction of stress imposed on the tissue. If no movement

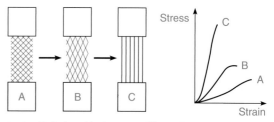

Figure 2.10   Relationship between fibre orientation and stress–strain response. From Oakes, B.W. (1992). The classification of injuries and mechanisms of injury, repair and healing. In *Textbook of Science and Medicine in Sport* (eds J. Bloomfield, P.A. Fricker and K.D. Fitch). Blackwell Scientific Publications, Melbourne. With permission.

occurs to stress the collagen bundles, they are laid down in a haphazard and weaker pattern (Cyriax, 1982). Controlled movement causes the fibrils to align lengthways along the line of stress of the injured structure (Burri, Helbing and Spier, 1973). Variation in longitudinal fibre alignment will determine the stress–strain response of the tissue to loading (Fig. 2.10). Where fibre alignment is parallel to the tissue body, the steep stress–strain curve (C) indicates that less deformation will occur for a given tissue loading. The tissue is therefore 'stronger'.

It becomes clear that external mechanical factors, and not the previous organization of the tissue, dictate the eventual pattern of fibril arrangement (Stearns, 1940). Total rest during this stage of healing is therefore contraindicated in most cases.

Keypoint

External mechanical factors have a positive influence on tissue healing and can dictate the eventual strength of the healing tissues. Long periods of total rest are therefore rarely required when treating sports injuries.

In some tissue full regeneration occurs, damaged cells being replaced by functioning normal tissue. Fractured bone exhibits this property, as do torn ligaments and peripheral nerves providing conditions are suitable (Evans, 1990b).

REMODELLING

The remodelling stage overlaps repair, and may last from 3 weeks to 12 months (Kellett, 1986). During this stage, collagen is modified to increase its functional capacity. Remodelling is characterized by a reduction in the wound size, an increase in scar strength, and an alteration in the direction of the collagen fibres (Van der Meulen, 1982).

Contraction of granulation tissue will occur for as long as the elasticity of the fibres will allow (Van der Meulen, 1982). Fibroblast cells transform into myofibroblasts which then form intercellular bonds. These contain contractile proteins (actomyosin) and behave much like smooth muscle fibres.

Three weeks after injury, the quantity of collagen has stabilized (Van der Meulen, 1982) but the strength of the fibres continues to increase. Strength increases are a result of an expansion in the number of cross-bonds between the cells, and the replacement collagen cells themselves. There is a continuous turnover of collagen, a process influenced by a number of factors, including the age of the patient, the type of tissue injured, the quantity of scar tissue present, the site and direction of the scar and external forces (Van der Meulen, 1982; Frank et al., 1983).

MATCHING TREATMENT TO THE HEALING TIMESCALE

The tensile strength of injured soft tissue will reduce substantially after injury due to mechanical damage to the tissues. By the first postinjury day, tensile strength may have reduced by some 50% . Although healing begins immediately, collagen is not laid down until the fifth postinjury day (Garrett, 1990). The period between injury and the beginning of collagen synthesis has been described as the 'lag phase' (Fig. 2.11). Manual

therapy techniques applied in this period should be aimed at pain resolution and oedema reduction. Only when collagen synthesis begins should therapy aim to prevent adhesions and align collagen fibres in the direction of stress (see p. 64).

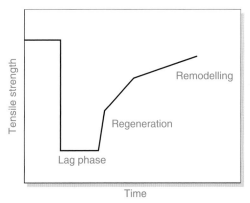

Figure 2.11　Strength of healing tissue following injury. From Hunter (1998) with permission.

Treatment note 2.3　Influencing the mechanical properties of healing tissue

Soft tissue manipulation
The use of deep transverse frictional massage (DTF) has been claimed to assist soft tissue healing. By applying shear and gliding movements to an injured tendon, ligament or muscle, tensile strength of the healing scar may be improved and adhesions reduced. Gentle DTF applied in the acute phase of healing could increase the rate of phagocytosis by inducing agitation of tissue fluid. In the chronic stage of healing the therapeutic movement produced by DTF is said to soften and mobilize adhesions (Kesson and Atkins, 1998). (DTF is covered on pp. 64–68.)

Specific soft tissue mobilization
Specific soft tissue mobilization (SSTM) is a technique pioneered by Hunter (1998). The procedure involves tensioning the tissue using physiological joint movement and accessory joint movement and adding a dynamic soft tissue mobilization. In the acute phase of healing, SSTM is claimed to influence the mechanical properties of healing tissue by altering collagen and ground substance synthesis.

A sustained load of five repetitions of a 30-second hold is used in a treatment session and the patient performs home exercise by self-stretching for three repetitions of a 30-second hold every 3–4 hours. Using the Achilles tendon as an example (Fig. 2.12), the mobility of the tendon is assessed by subjecting it to shearing forces, beginning distally and moving proximally. The aim is to fix the proximal segment of the tendon with the fingers and then move the tendon in the opposite direction with the fingers of the other hand. The shearing motion is moved up the tendon progressively, assessing range and quality of movement.

This same shearing action is used with the tendon on stretch (passive loading) or loaded by mild muscle contraction (dynamic loading).

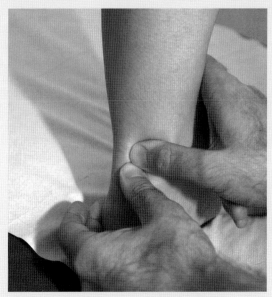

Figure 2.12　Specific soft tissue mobilization (SSTM) of the Achilles.

Eccentric loading
Eccentric loading has been used extensively for rehabilitation of the Achilles tendon. It is claimed that the controlled lengthening of the tendon during eccentric actions increases the tensile strength of the tendon (Stanish, Rubinovich and Curwen, 1986; Kannus 1997) and allows for more storage of elastic energy in the stretch shorten cycle (see p. 8). In addition, eccentric loading may prepare the tendon for rapid unloading. The sudden release of force in this way produces shearing forces within the tendon which could conceivably break up adhesions within the Achilles itself (Curwin, 1994).

INDIVIDUAL TISSUE RESPONSE TO INJURY

In this section we will look at the responses of the individual tissues to injury, and the effects these have upon subsequent rehabilitation. Aspects of tissue structure relevant to sports injury is discussed.

Synovial membrane

The synovium consists of two layers, the intima, or synovial lining, and the subsynovial (subintimal) tissue. The intimal layer is made up of specialized cells known as synoviocytes, arranged in multiple layers. Two types of synoviocytes are present, type A cells, which are phagocytic, and type B cells, which synthesize the hyaluronoprotein of the synovial fluid. The two types are not distinct, however, and appear to be functional stages of the same basic cells (Hettinga, 1990).

The subsynovial tissue lies beneath the intima as a loose network of highly vascular connective tissue. Cells are interspaced with collagen fibres and fatty tissue. The subsynovial tissue itself merges with the periosteum of bone lying within the synovial membrane of the joint. Similar merging occurs with the joint cartilage through a transitional layer of fibrocartilage.

The blood vessels of the joint divide into three branches, one travelling to the epiphysis, the second to the joint capsule and the third to the synovial membrane (Paget and Bullough, 1981). From here the vessels of the subsynovium are of two types. The first is thin walled and adapted for fluid exchange, and the second thick walled and capable of gapping to allow particles, especially nutrients, to pass through.

Once free of the vessels, any material must pass through the synovial interstitium before entering the synovial fluid itself. The passage of this material is by diffusion on the whole, but by active transport for glucose molecules.

The synovium must adapt to movement with normal function of the joint. Rather than stretching, the synovium unfolds to facilitate flexion. The synovium is well lubricated by the same hyaluronate molecules found within the synovial fluid itself, and so the various layers slide over each other. Since the synovium must alter shape within the confines of the joint capsule, the process of synovial adaptation is at its best when the fluid volume of the joint is at a minimum.

Synovial fluid plays a significant role in joint stability. The negative atmospheric pressure within the joint creates a suction effect, which, aided by the surface tension of the synovial fluid, draws the bony surfaces of the joint together.

Response to injury

With minor trauma the synovium is not microscopically disturbed, but will instead suffer a vasomotor reaction (Hettinga, 1990). The synovium will dilate and fluid filtration increases. Protein leaks into the interstitium, changing the osmotic pressure and causing local oedema and joint exudation. This process constitutes a post-traumatic synovitis.

> **Keypoint**
>
> Post-traumatic synovitis initially involves a vasomotor reaction of the synovium rather than actual structural damage.

The slight hyperaemia gives way later to alterations of the intimal layer, the total number of layers increasing threefold. If the trauma does not continue, the protein molecules which were released are cleared by the lymphatics and the osmotic pressures return to normal. If mechanical irritation persists, the intimal layer will continue to thicken. The deep synovial cells now show increased activity and protein synthesis escalates.

Alterations occur in the number of type A and type B synoviocyte cells. The number of type A cells reduces as some of these move into the synovial fluid to become macrophages. The synovial lining becomes filled with fibroblasts, which in turn change into type B cells. Neutrophil cells die, releasing proteolytic enzymes which attack the near joint structures. This process can self-perpetuate the synovitis, even in the absence of further trauma, giving rise to a reactive synovitis.

Onset of symptoms following post-traumatic synovitis usually occurs between 12 and 24 hours after injury and can last for between 1 and 2 weeks. Patients complain mainly of joint tightness, with warmth, erythema and pain being encountered less often. The tightness is due to joint effusion, the increased fluid volume causing the normally negative intra-articular pressure to become positive.

The stability of the joint, no longer created by a negative intra-articular pressure, comes from joint distension instead. This places a traction force on the joint capsule and surrounding ligaments. Pressures are greatest in the effused joint in extremes of flexion and extension, and are reduced at about 30° flexion, this being the resting position taken up by the patient. Haemarthrosis is usually present if swelling occurs within 2 hours of injury, and pain is intense.

> **Keypoint**
>
> If synovitis continues beyond 72 hours the synovium thickens and proteolytic enzymes are released which attack the near joint structures. This process can continue in the absence of further trauma, and represents reactive synovitis.

Surgical removal of the synovial membrane (synovectomy) may be performed in a number of inflammatory joint disorders. With time the synovium will regrow, and the use of continuous passive motion (CPM) may be used to assist this process (Salter, 1990). Without mechanical stimulation synovial membrane will degenerate through the loss of proteoglycan, so movement is vital to its effective healing.

Synovial fluid

Synovial fluid is similar in many ways to blood plasma. The main differences being that synovia does not contain fibrinogen or prothrombin and so is unable to clot. The mucopolysaccharide hyaluronate (hyaluronic acid) secreted by the synoviocytes is contained within the fluid.

The amount of synovial fluid present in a joint is very little – about 0.5–4 ml within large joints such as the knee – and this is spread throughout the joint by structures such as the cartilage, menisci and fat pads.

Synovial fluid is a highly viscous fluid, which becomes more elastic as the rate of joint movement increases. As weight is taken by the joint, synovial fluid is squeezed out from between the opposing joint surfaces. This is resisted by the tenacity of the fluid itself.

As the joint moves, the synovial fluid is pulled in the direction of movement and so a layer of fluid is maintained between the joint surfaces. Any friction produced by movement will therefore occur within the synovial fluid rather than between the joint surfaces. When the joint is statically loaded, however, fluid flows away from the point of maximal load and the joint relies on the articular cartilage to provide lubrication (see below). The synovial fluid provides nutrition for about two-thirds of the articular cartilage bordering the joint space.

Following injury, fluid volume may increase as much as 10 or 20 times, with a decrease in hyaluronate and, with it, fluid viscosity. Pain due to the accumulation of synovial fluid is dependent not on the amount of fluid present, but on the speed with which it forms. Blau (1979) claimed that as much as 100 ml may be extracted from a joint which caused little pain because it took a long time to form, while 15 ml may be exquisitely painful if formed rapidly following trauma.

With injury in which bleeding is not present, the constituents of the synovial fluid remain basically the same. In reactive synovitis, the protein concentration is slightly elevated, and the number of white blood cells increases somewhat from normal values of 100/ml to as much as 300/ml. With post-traumatic synovitis, however, the white cell count is further increased, to as much as 2000/ml.

Haemarthrosis (blood within the joint) causes rapidly developing fluid, which contains fibrinogen. If the synovial membrane is torn, fat can enter the joint from the extrasynovial adipose tissue and will show up in the synovial fluid. The blood from haemarthrosis will mostly stay fluid, and is quickly absorbed by the phagocytic cells to ultimately disappear after several days.

> **Keypoint**
>
> *Synovitis*, an accumulation of synovial fluid alone, forms slowly. *Haemarthrosis*, an accumulation of fluid containing blood, will occur rapidly.

Bone

Types

Bone is essentially a fibrous matrix impregnated by mineral salts (mainly calcium phosphate), and it therefore combines the properties of both elasticity and rigidity. It is a living tissue, which is continually remodelled, and subject to hormonal control.

Two types of bone are generally described, cancellous or spongy bone and compact bone, and important differences exist in both their mechanical properties and methods of healing. Cancellous bone is found at a number of sites, including the bone ends, and is arranged in a system of trabeculae aligned to resist imposed stresses. The shaft of a long bone consists of a ring of compact bone surrounding a hollow cavity. This structure in turn is surrounded by a further layer of compact bone. The bone cavity contains marrow. In infants the bone marrow is red, but this is gradually replaced by yellow bone marrow until, by puberty, only the cancellous bone cavities at the ends of the long bones contain red marrow. With age the bone marrow in these cavities too is replaced, but red bone marrow may still be found in the vertebrae, sternum, and ribs, as well as the proximal ends of the femur and humerus.

The bone is enclosed in a dense membrane called the periosteum, which is absent in the region of the articular cartilage. The periosteum is highly vascular and responsible for the nutrition of the bone cortex which underlies it. The deep layers of periosteum contain bone-forming cells (osteoblasts). These lay down successive layers of bone during growth, and so the periosteum is responsible for alterations in the bone width; in addition these cells play an important part in bone healing. In contrast, the bone cavity is lined by bone-destroying cells (osteoclasts) which erode the inner surface of the bone. A direct blow to the bone which produces bleeding beneath the periosteum will lift it, causing bone deposition by the osteoblasts. This is a common problem over the anterior tibia in footballers and hockey players.

> **Keypoint**
>
> A direct blow to unprotected bone (with a hard ball or boot, for example) may cause bleeding beneath the bone periosteum. Ultimately this may lead to calcification (bone deposits) within the bruised area.

Bone may be further classified into four major types. The long bones are found within the limbs, and consist of a shaft and two enlarged ends. Short bones have a block-like appearance such as those of the carpals, and are mainly cancellous bone. Flat bones are thinner, and consist of two layers of compact bone sandwiching a thin layer of cancellous bone; examples are the skull vaults and the ribs. Finally, irregular bones consist of a thin layer of compact bone surrounded by cancellous bone; examples are the vertebrae.

Definition

Bones may be classified as *long* (limbs), *short* (carpals), *flat* (scapula) and *irregular* (vertebrae).

Development

Skeletal development begins with loosely arranged meso-dermal cells which are mostly converted to hyaline cartilage. Between the seventh and twelfth intrauterine week a primary ossification centre appears within the shaft of the long bone, and spreads towards the bone ends. The centre of the shaft is hollowed out and filled with red bone marrow, and the whole shaft is called a diaphysis. At the end of the bone, secondary centres of ossification appear, usually after birth. Gradually the main part of the cartilage is replaced, leaving only the articular cartilage, and a cartilage plate (growth plate, or physis) between the shaft and end of the bone.

The growth plate is of great importance in paediatric sports medicine. This cartilage layer is responsible for the increase in bone length. As the cartilage grows it becomes thicker, and its upper and lower surfaces are converted to bone. Eventually the cartilage stops growing, but its ossification continues so that the cartilage becomes thinner, until it eventually disappears. At this point the diaphysis and epiphysis are united, and growth in length of the bone is no longer possible. The point at which this occurs may be influenced by a number of factors, including impact stresses (see below).

Intramembranous ossification occurs in the mandible, clavicle, and certain bones of the skull (Palastanga, Field and Soames, 1989). Here, the intermediate stage of cartilage formation is omitted and the bone ossifies directly from connective tissue.

Epiphyseal injury

Two types of epiphysis are found. Pressure epiphyses are found at the end of long bones, and are interarticular. They are subjected to compression stress with weight bearing, and are responsible for changes in bone length. Traction epiphyses (apophyses) occur at the insertion of major muscles. They experience tension stress as the muscles contract, and alter bone shape.

The growth plate itself forms a weak link in the immature skeleton, and shearing or avulsion stresses can cause it to be dislodged. Because the epiphyses are weaker than the major joint structures, injuries which in the adult would cause dislocation or tendon rupture may cause epiphyseal injury in a child.

Five types of injury have been described (Salter and Harris, 1963), as shown in Fig. 2.13. The type I lesion involves horizontal displacement of the growth plate while with the type II lesion the fracture line runs through to the adjacent metaphysis. In the type III and IV fractures the joint surface is involved, so the complication rate is higher (Watson, 1992).

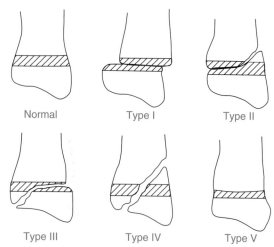

Figure 2.13 Epiphyseal injuries. After Salter and Harris (1963) with permission.

Gentle manipulation under anaesthetic is normally used to realign the epiphysis in the first fracture types. Crush injuries and those through the growth plate may cause more severe problems of growth disturbance. When a fracture crosses the growth plate, bone may fill the gap formed, giving unequal growth. Crush injuries may lead to premature closure of the plate with associated deformities of shortening and altered bony angulation.

Keypoint

If a fracture involves a bone growth plate, bone deformity such as angulation or shortening may result.

Osteochondrosis

Osteochondrosis affects the pressure epiphyses during their growth period, and are the most common overuse injuries seen in children. There is an interference with the epiphyseal blood supply, causing an avascular necrosis to the secondary ossification centre. The bone within the epiphysis softens, dies, and is absorbed (Fig. 2.14). Because the cap of articular cartilage surrounding the epiphysis receives nutrition from the synovial fluid, it remains largely unaffected. The combination of softening bone contained within an intact articular cap leads to flattening of the epiphysis. Gradually the dead bone is replaced by new bone by a process of 'creeping substitution'. Trauma may be one factor which initiates the ischaemic process, either through direct injury or vascular occlusion as a result of traumatic synovitis (Gartland, 1987).

The osteochondroses may be categorized into four groups (Pappas, 1989):

1. Traction osteochondroses (apophysitis) affect the attachments of major tendons, particularly to the knee and heel.

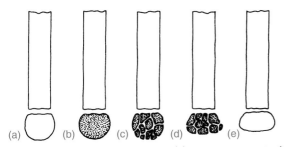

Figure 2.14   Stages of osteochondritis. (a) Normal epiphysis. (b) The bony nucleus undergoes necrosis, loses its normal texture and becomes granular. (c) The bony nucleus becomes fragmented during the process of removal of dead bone. (d) If subjected to pressure the softened epiphysis becomes flattened. (e) Re-ossification with restoration of normal bone texture, but deformity may persist. The whole process takes 2–3 years. From Gartland (1987) with permission.

Table 2.4   The osteochondroses

Classification	Name	Site(s)
Non-articular traction (pulling)	Osgood – Schlatter's Sinding–Larsen – Johannsson's disease Sever's disease	Tibial tubercle Interior pole of patella (quadriceps) Calcaneous (gastrocnemius)
Articular subchondral (crushing)	Perthes' disease Kienböck's disease Köhler's disease Freiberg's disease	Femoral head Lunate (wrist) Navicular (mid-foot) Second metatarsal head
Articular chondral (splitting)	Osteochondritis dissecans	Medical femoral Condyle (knee) Capitellum (elbow) Talar dome (ankle)
Physeal	Scheuermann's disease Blount's disease	Thoracic spine Tibia (proximal)

2. Crushing osteochondroses occur in the hip, wrist, and forefoot.
3. Articular chondral osteochondroses involve splitting of bone near an articular site, with resultant bone fragment formation.
4. Finally, physeal injuries affect the growth plate and result in irregular growth and/or angular deformity.

Any pressure epiphysis may be affected by osteochondrosis, the condition taking the name of the person who first described it in that region. The most common conditions are shown in Table 2.4, and details of these are given in the relevant clinical chapters in Section II of this book.

Healing

Bone healing (see also stress fractures, pp. 260–261) is governed by a number of factors, including the type of tissue which is damaged, the extent of the damage and position of the bony fragments, the amount of movement present at the fracture site as healing progresses, and the blood supply. In a long bone, healing may be divided into five stages, as shown in Figure 2.15 (Crawford-Adams, 1978; Apley and Solomon, 1988). The first stage is that of tissue destruction and haematoma formation. As local blood vessels are torn at the time of injury, blood is released forming a haematoma within and surrounding the fracture site. The bone periosteum and surrounding soft tissues contain the blood, and the periosteum itself is lifted from the bone surface. The deprivation of blood to the bone surfaces immediately adjacent to the fracture line causes these surfaces to die back for up to 2 mm. Some 8 hours after fracture, inflammation and proliferation may be detected as stage two of healing. The deep periosteal cells, and those of the damaged medullary canal, proliferate, and cellular tissue begins to grow forward to meet similar material from the other side of the fracture site and bridge the area. Capillary growth into the region allows the haematoma to be slowly reabsorbed, and the congealed blood itself takes little part in the repair process.

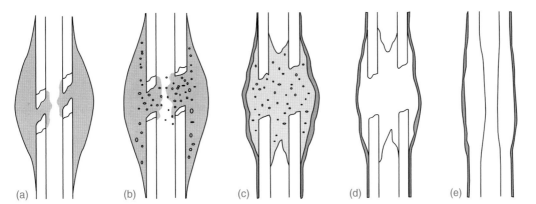

Figure 2.15   Stages of fracture healing. (a) Haematoma. Tissue damage and bleeding occur at the fracture site, the bone ends die back a few millimetres. (b) Inflammation. Inflammatory cells appear in the haematoma. (c) Callus. The cell population changes to osteoblasts and osteoclasts, dead bone is mopped up and woven bone appears in the fracture callus. (d) Consolidation. Woven bone is remodelled to resemble the normal structure (e). From Apley and Solomon (1988) with permission.

The appearance of osteogenic and chondrogenic cells marks the beginning of the third stage of healing. New bone and, in some cases, cartilage are laid down, while osteoclastic cells remove remaining dead bone. The cellular mass which forms is called a callus, and becomes increasingly mineralized into woven bone, uniting the fracture. The callus is larger where there has been much periosteal stripping, when bone displacement is marked, and if the haematoma has been large. The woven bone is transformed into lamellar bone by osteoblasts in the fourth stage of healing.

As the fracture site is bridged by solid bone, the fifth and final stage of healing commences, that of remodelling. A combination of bone reabsorption and formation reshapes the callus, laying down thicker lamellae in areas of high stress and removing excessive bone. The medullary cavity is re-formed.

The rate of healing is dependent on a number of factors. The type of bone is important, cancellous bone healing far more quickly than cortical bone. Also, the fracture type will dictate the speed of healing, with a spiral fracture healing more quickly than a transverse type. If the blood supply has been compromised at the time of injury, or if the fracture has occurred in an area with a poor blood supply, the healing rate will be slower. The age and health of the patient are other determining factors, with fractures in children healing almost twice as fast as those in adults. In general terms, callus may be visible radiographically within 2–3 weeks of injury, with firm fracture union taking about 4–6 weeks for upper limb fractures and 8–12 weeks for those in the lower limb. Full consolidation may take as much as 8 and 16 weeks for upper and lower limb fractures, respectively.

In contrast to long bone, cancellous bone remains fairly immobile when fractured, and heals by 'direct repair' with a minimum of callus formation. The main difference occurs because there is no medullary canal in cancellous bone, and the area of contact between the two injured bone fragments is much greater. Following haematoma formation, new blood vessels and osteogenic cells penetrate the area and meet similar tissue from the opposite bone fragment. The intercellular matrix which is laid down by osteoblasts is calcified into woven bone. This type of healing also occurs when internal fixation is used.

Mechanical properties

Bone responds to mechanical stress in similar ways to other connective tissue, but at a considerably slower rate. Its ability to adapt its structure, size and shape depends on the mechanical stresses placed upon it. When stress is reduced, by prolonged bed rest for example, mineral reabsorption occurs and the bone reduces in strength. Raising stress to an optimal level, by exercise, leads to an increase in bone strength.

In addition to changes in total mineral content, bone varies its strength according to the direction of the imposed stress. At bony attachment sites such as tubercles, alignment of collagen fibres is parallel to the direction of the imposed force. In

> **Keypoint**
>
> As with other tissues in the body, bone responds to mechanical stress by adapting its structure. If stress is reduced (prolonged rest) bone reduces in strength. Raising stress to an optimal level (exercise) leads to an increase in bone strength.

the shaft of a long bone, fibre orientation is along the bone axis, indicating that this part of the bone is designed to resist tension and compression forces. In cancellous bone at the epiphysis, shear stresses are maximal and so fibre alignment is in the direction of the shearing forces.

A number of mechanisms have been proposed to explain how the bone remodels to imposed stress. Bassett (1965) argued that, in theory, mechanical stresses on bone create electrical charges (piezoelectric effect). Areas of compression were said to develop negative charges while those subjected to tensile stress are more positive. The suggestion is that bone deposition by osteoblasts occurs in negatively charged areas, while reabsorption by osteoclasts takes place in regions of positive excitation. Experiments with dogs (Bassett and Pawlick, 1964) have shown that new bone is laid down at an implanted cathode site, although other authors have described bone deposition at both negative and positive sites (Hert and Zalud, 1971) so the effects of polarity are still uncertain.

Electrical fields formed in bone as a result of imposed stresses have been shown to stimulate protein synthesis in frog osteogenic cells (Becker and Murray, 1970), and increased rate of bone formation has been shown as a result of direct current (d.c.) administered through implanted electrodes (Becker, Spadaro and Marino, 1977).

Bone trabeculae subjected to maximum stress will be strengthened by bone deposition, in the direction of the imposed force. Regions of high stress have denser trabeculae, aligned to minimize the bending effect on a bone. Where a bone is subjected to an unbalanced force, which would tend to bend it, remodelling occurs as a result of changes in surface strain (Reigger, 1990). On the convex surface of the bone, osteoclastic activity leads to bone reabsorption, while on the concave surface the reverse occurs and bone deposition is seen. Bone therefore moves towards the concavity which has been induced through loading of the shaft, to minimize the bending effect, a process known as flexural drift. The stress imposed on the bone causes an increase in the calcium concentration found within the interstitial fluid, as a result of changes in bone crystal solubility.

Osteoporosis

Osteoporosis (bone mineral loss) has now reached epidemic proportions in the Western world (Carbon, 1992). The condition involves a progressive decrease in bone mineral density (BMD), due to an imbalance between bone formation and bone reabsorption. Bone mass reaches its peak in the third and fourth decade, and loss occurs normally in both sexes with ageing, but this rate is increased markedly with osteoporosis. Normal bone loss of 3% per decade may increase to as much as 10% per decade for trabecular bone. This leads to a reduction per decade in ultimate stress of 5%, ultimate strain of 9%, and energy absorption of 12% (Behiri and Vashishth 2000).

Osteoporosis may be either *primary*, governed by age and sex, or *secondary* as a result of disease. The most common primary types are postmenopausal osteoporosis and senile osteoporosis.

Definition

Osteoporosis may be either *primary*, governed by sex (postmenopausal) or age (senile), or *secondary* resulting from disease.

The loss of mass makes the bone susceptible to fracture, particularly as a result of microtrauma. Common fracture sites include the distal radius and vertebrae for postmenopausal osteoporosis, and the proximal femur for senile osteoporosis. Fracture of the distal radius presents as a Colles' fracture, while vertebral wedging gives rise to an increased thoracic kyphosis or 'dowager's hump'.

There is a marked increase in the risk of fracture once bone density reduces below a certain level (known as the fracture threshold, Fig. 2.16). The incidence of hip and vertebral fractures rises with age (Fig. 2.17), but the rise in hip fracture incidence in men occurs some 5 years later than that in women (Wolman and Reeve, 1994), an indication of the effect of postmenopausal osteoporosis.

Assessment of osteoporosis

Changes in BMD is the standard objective measure for osteoporosis, but low bone density in itself is asymptomatic. It is only when a fracture occurs or they develop pain or substantial postural changes that individuals seek help. Assessment of BMD may be made by direct examination of X-rays. *Cortical index* measures the thickness of the bone cortex in comparison to the bone shaft. The combined width of the two cortices should be 50% of the total width of the bone at mid-shaft (Apley and Solomon, 1993). *Trabecular index* is a method of assessing bone mass from the radiographic pattern of bone trabeculae in the proximal femur or calcaneus. A more accurate measure of BMD is obtained by *dual energy X-ray absorptiometry* (DXA). The amount of radiation used is relatively small, representing no more than 3% of the natural background radiation in a large city (Lewis, Blake and Fogelman, 1994; Huda and Morin, 1996). Measurement is taken yearly, and only changes greater than 2–3% are significant (Bennell, Khan and McKay, 2000). Results are expressed as BMD in g/cm^2, as a Z score which compares the value to an age matched group, or as a T score which compares the obtained value to a young healthy population. The World Health Organization has classified degrees of BMD loss as shown in Table 2.5.

Subjective assessment includes elements such as family history, fracture status, history of falls, menstrual history, smoking and dietary habits, and exercise status. Objective

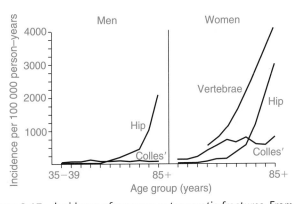

Figure 2.17 Incidence of common osteoporotic fractures. From Wolman, R.L. and Reeve, J. (1994) Exercise and the skeleton. In *Oxford Textbook of Sports Medicine* (eds M. Harries et al.). Reprinted with permission of Oxford University Press, Oxford.

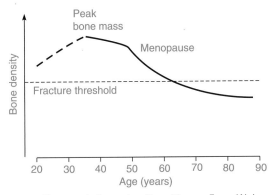

Figure 2.16 Changes in bone density with age. From Wolman, R.L. and Reeve, J. (1994) Exercise and the skeleton. In *Oxford Textbook of Sports Medicine* (eds M. Harries et al.). Reprinted with permission of Oxford University Press, Oxford.

Table 2.5 Classification of osteoporosis

Classification	DXA reading
Normal	>-1
Osteopenia	-1 to -2.5
Osteoporosis	<-2.5
Severe osteoporosis	<-2.5 plus history of fragility fracture

BMD expressed as standard deviations (SD) below the mean of a young adult (T score). World Health Organization (1994) *Assessment of Fracture Risk and its Application to Screening for Osteoporosis. Report of WHO study group.* World Health Organization, Geneva. With permission.

examination is of posture, pain and functional limitation (CSP, 1999; Bennell, Khan and McKay, 2000).

Three main factors are important in the development of osteoporosis: diet, oestrogen level, and physical activity.

Diet

Modern diet can fail to provide an adequate daily intake of calcium. Recommended requirements as high as 1500 mg of calcium and 400 IU of vitamin D have been made for postmenopausal women (MacKinnon, 1988), but many women may consume as little as 300 mg of calcium (McArdle, Katch and Katch, 1986), placing themselves in negative calcium balance. Excess salt or caffeine, and a large intake of meat promote calcium loss in the urine, and an excessive intake of fibre and alcohol can bind calcium in the gut, preventing its absorption (Deakin and Brotherhood, 1992).

Calcium deficiency in animals has been shown to produce osteoporosis (Martin and Houston, 1987), but effects in man are less clear. Studying early postmenopausal women, Nilas, Christiansen and Rodbro (1984) gave a 500 mg calcium supplement over a 2-year period and assessed bone density in the distal radius, while Ettinger, Genant and Cann (1987) gave a 1000 mg supplement and assessed the lumbar vertebrae. Both of these studies failed to show any significant differences between the treatment and non-treatment groups. However, in late postmenopausal women calcium supplementation may be more beneficial (MacKinnon, 1988). However, the effect of calcium supplementation on the incidence of fractures remains unproven (Evans, 1990b)

Adequate calcium is clearly necessary for health, and those individuals who show a deficiency in their calcium intake may need dietary supplementation. Others should receive advice on good diet to enable them to maintain an adequate intake of calcium and vitamin D, remembering that excessive vitamin D intake can be toxic.

Exercise

Weight-bearing exercise creates bone stress and acts as a stimulus for maintaining bone mass. Loss of bone mass has been reported both as a result of prolonged bed rest (Donaldson, Hulley and Vogel, 1970) and following weightlessness (Mazess and Whedon, 1983). Similarly, athletes have been shown to have greater bone density than non-athletes (Nilsson and Westlin, 1977), and tennis players have been shown to have a greater bone density in their dominant arm (Huddleston, Rockwell and Kuland, 1980).

A number of authors have demonstrated the beneficial effects of weight-bearing exercise in slowing bone loss. Smith, Smith and Ensign (1984) assessed the effects of exercise (45 minutes, 3 days per week) on bone loss in postmenopausal women and showed a 1.4% increase in bone mass during the second and third years of their study. Krolner, Toft and Nielsen (1983) studied the effects of exercise

(1 hour, twice per week) on postmenopausal women. They showed a 3.5% increase in bone mineral content of the lumbar spine for the exercising group compared to 2.7% for their control.

High impact exercise which generates a ground reaction force greater than twice body weight is likely to create bone remineralization (Heinonen, Kannus and Sievanen, 1996). Exercise should be performed at least three times per week at intensities beginning with 40–60% maximal oxygen uptake (VO2 max) and progressing to as much as 80% VO2 max, even in the elderly (ACSM, 1998). Strength (weight) training at 70% 1RM has been shown to maintain hip and spine BMD, but programmes must be given progressively, taking clinical history into account. A flowchart to guide exercise prescription is shown in Figure 2.18.

Clearly, regular weight-bearing exercise is important for the prevention and management of osteoporosis. However, the increased risk of fracture in this group means that caution must be shown. Repeated spinal rotation or flexion should be avoided, and high impact activities should be limited at the early stages of treatment, especially where osteoporosis already exists.

> **Keypoint**
>
> Regular weight-bearing exercise slows, and can reverse, bone mineral loss seen in osteoporosis.

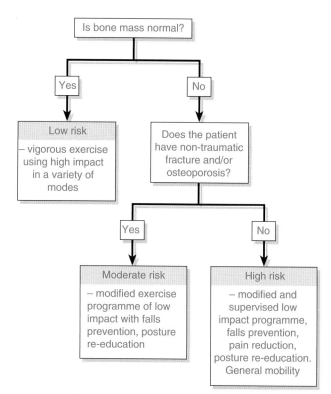

Figure 2.18 Exercise prescription for osteoporosis. Adapted from Bennell, Khan and McKay (2000), with permission.

Hormone replacement therapy

The use of low dosage oestrogen in hormone replacement therapy (HRT) to slow or even halt bone loss in post-menopausal women is widely recommended. HRT is used to make up for the decline in oestrogen levels seen during the menopause. Oestrogen plays an important part in calcium absorption by the body. Secreted by the ovaries and corpus luteum, oestrogen (a steroid hormone) stimulates regeneration of the endometrium, increases mucus output from the cervical glands, and promotes epiphyseal closure and growth of the bones and skeletal muscle.

HRT has been linked with an increased risk of endometrial carcinoma, although the risk is reduced when oestrogen is combined with progesterone (Hedlund and Gallagher, 1988).

Transient osteoporosis

Transient osteoporosis most commonly affects the hip, where it is termed idiopathic transient osteoporosis of the hip (ITOH) (Harrington et al. 2000). It is a relatively rare condition which must be differentiated from both stress fracture and avascular necrosis. The condition was first described in women during late pregnancy (Curtiss and Kincaid, 1959). However, the main group to suffer from this condition are middle-aged (40–70 years) men, who represent over 70% of cases (Lakhanpal, Ginsburg and Luthra, 1987). ITOH is a self-limiting condition which demonstrates bone marrow oedema and slight bone cortex thinning. There is no evidence of the focal subchondral bone defect of the femoral head seen in avascular necrosis (Harrington et al. 2000). Joint fluid is sterile (non-infected) and only mild synovial thickening is present (McCarthy, 1998).

Subjective examination reveals progressive unilateral hip pain referred into the groin and anterior thigh. Pain is exacerbated with weight bearing and eased with rest (contrast with malignancy which gives pain at rest). Typically pain is worse 4–8 weeks after onset, and enforced rest may show disuse atrophy of the quadriceps and gluteal muscles. The joint and greater trochanter may be tender to palpation and the FABRE test positive.

Management is by protected weight-bearing (crutches) and non weight-bearing or partial weight-bearing exercise to pain tolerance (pool/walking/jogging). Non-steroidal anti-inflammatory drugs (NSAIDs) may be of use, and protracted cases have responded to core decompression of the femur (Apel, Vince and Kingston, 1994).

Definition

Core decompression is a surgical procedure which involves taking a plug of bone out of the centre of a bone to reduce pressure.

Articular cartilage

Cartilage is essentially a connective tissue consisting of cells embedded in a matrix permeated by fibres. Two major types are recognized, hyaline cartilage and fibrocartilage. Hyaline cartilage is found over bone ends and is described in more detail below. Fibrocartilage may be either white or yellow. White fibrocartilage is found in areas such as the intervertebral discs and glenoid labrum. Yellow fibrocartilage is found in structures such as the ears and larynx.

Definition

Hyaline cartilage is found in synovial joints, *white fibrocartilage* in the vertebrae and *yellow fibrocartilage* in the ear and larynx.

Articular (hyaline) cartilage is made up of collagen fibres, a protein – polysaccharide complex, and water. Fibres of collagen are embedded in a ground substance of gel-like material. The water content of cartilage is high, between 70 and 80% of its total weight (Bullough, 1981).

Cartilage has no blood vessels, lymphatics or nerve fibres. Nutrition is supplied directly from the synovial fluid, and by diffusion of blood products from the subchondral bone. The tangled structure of cartilage causes it to behave in some ways like a microscopic sieve, filtering out large molecules such as plasma proteins. Fluid movement through the cartilage is by osmosis and diffusion. Movement of the joint increases the rate of diffusion, but in the mature joint there is no transfer across the bone – cartilage interface (Hettinga, 1990).

Intermittent loading creates a pumping effect, squeezing fluid from the cartilage and allowing fresh fluid to be taken up as the load is released. Prolonged loading will gradually press fluid out of the cartilage, without allowing new fluid to be taken up. As much as a 40% reduction in cartilage depth can occur by compression (Hettinga, 1990).

Keypoint

Because cartilage has no direct blood supply, regular movement is vital to supply it with nutrients from the synovial fluid.

The cartilage is arranged in four layers (Fig. 2.19). The collagen fibres of the calcified zone bind the cartilage to the subchondral bone, resisting shear stresses. Within the mid-zone the fibres are randomly oriented. With joint compression, these fibres stretch and will resist the tension forces created within them (Fig. 2.20). This property of elastic deformation (spring) occurs instantly. However, the fluid within the matrix of the cartilage will be compressed. As it does so, proteoglycans within the cartilage will tend to retain water and control its movement through the cartilage matrix. The cartilage will slowly flow away from the compression force, demonstrating the property of creep. When the load is removed, the fluid lost at the time of compression is reabsorbed. These two properties of instant spring and slower creep make cartilage a viscoelastic material.

Cartilage assists joint lubrication by boundary lubrication, and weeping lubrication (see p. 10).

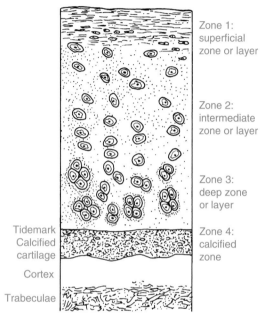

Figure 2.19 Zones in articular cartilage. From Gould (1990) with permission.

Injury

Articular cartilage is to a great extent protected from injury by the elasticity of other joint structures, and the neuromuscular reflexes. Reflex muscular contraction and soft tissue 'give' will largely dampen shock before it reaches the cartilage. However, unexpected loading (such as trauma) which occurs too rapidly to invoke reflex protection will cause injury, but this is more frequently bony fracture rather than damage to the cartilage itself.

If cartilage injury does occur, it is most likely due to slip or shear. Three injury stages have been described (Hettinga, 1990): first, splitting of the cartilage layer at the tidemark between the calcified and uncalcified tissue; secondly, cartilage depression into the subchondral bone; and thirdly, fissuring of the cartilage and underlying bone.

Partial thickness injuries, limited to the articular cartilage alone, heal poorly. The healing which does take place is by proliferation and invasion from soft tissue, and the further away from this tissue the injured area is, the poorer the healing. Full thickness defects, extending through the subchondral bone, heal by superficial tissue bridging the break. Blood vessels grow into the uncalcified cartilage. Osteogenic cells and granulation tissue from the base of the break invade the area, resulting in the formation of fibrous tissue, bony trabeculae and fibrocartilage. There is obvious demarcation of the region into zones, a chondrin-free ring surrounding the uninjured tissue. The healed defect appears as a slightly discoloured roughened area of fibrous tissue.

Figure 2.20 Effects of joint compression on articular cartilage. (a) Compressive loading of the cartilage results in (b) tension stress to the collagenous elements and compression stress to the mucopolysaccharide–water complex. (c) The total response is viscoelastic. The viscous creep with sustained loading is largely the result of a time-dependent squeezing out of fluid. From Hertling, D. and Kessler, R.M. (1990) *Management of Common Musculoskeletal Disorders.* JB Lippincott, Philadelphia. With permission.

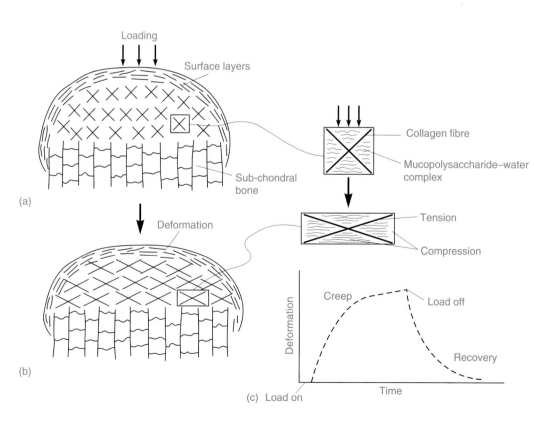

Cartilage repair

Several surgical techniques may be used to aid repair of injury articular cartilage (Table 2.6). The joint surface may be debrided (scraped) and the joint itself washed out (lavaged) to remove fragments of cartilage or subchondral bone. Damaging enzymes produced through cartilage degeneration are also removed. New cartilage cells may be introduced into the damaged area to stimulate healing. Osteochondral grafts of this type may be taken from the patient (autografts) or from cadaveric donors (allografts). A number of tissues have been used for autografts including rib perichondrial cells, periosteum, and chondrocytes themselves. The technique involves two surgical proceedures. First the cells must be removed, then allowed to grow in a laboratory, and finally the cells must be replanted into the damaged cartilage. Allograft techniques can result in high degrees of rejection as a complication (Wroble, 2000) but only involve a single surgical procedure.

Definition
Autografts involve implanting cells or tissue taken from the patient. *Allografts* are taken from a cadaver (dead person).

Drilling, abrasion and microfracture all work by penetrating the subchondral bone and stimulating cell regrowth. The aim is to allow a conduit for clot formation containing mesenchymal stem cells capable of forming repair tissue (Steadman, Rodkey and Singleton, 1997). Unfortunately fibrocartilage rather than renewed hyaline cartilage is produced by these procedures.

Arthritis

The term arthritis tends to be used to describe any chronic inflammatory reaction affecting a joint. However, the term simply means 'joint inflammation', and as such must be qualified by a description of the cause of inflammation. Acute joint injury which causes intracapsular swelling may be termed 'traumatic arthritis'. True osteoarthritis involves cartilage degeneration, initially with little inflammation, so the term osteoarthrosis would seem more appropriate. This condition must be differentiated from inflammatory states affecting multiple joints such as rheumatoid arthritis. The following description is concerned with osteoarthritis (OA) and its connection to sport and exercise.

The initial changes in OA are usually painless and show no swelling. Mild fraying or flaking of superficial collagen fibres within the hyaline cartilage occurs. This happens first at the periphery of the joint in the non-weight-bearing region. Later, damage (fibrillation) is to the deeper cartilage layers in the weight-bearing areas of the joint, extending down to one-third of the cartilage thickness. Small cavities form (blistering) between the cartilage fibres which gradually extend to become vertical clefts. If cartilage fragments break off, they may float free in the joint fluid as loose bodies, giving rise to joint locking and sudden twinges of pain. The presence of a loose body and the by-products of cartilage destruction causes the synovium to inflame, and it is only now that many patients become aware that a problem exists.

Keypoint
Patients usually only become aware that they have arthritis when a joint becomes inflamed and painful. Treatment aimed at reducing pain/inflammation and restoring function will often alleviate the problem, but the structure of the bone remains the same.

Turnover of proteoglycan and collagen within the cartilage ground substance is increased, and the proteoglycan molecules near the fibrillated cartilage are smaller than normal. Mechanically, this altered cartilage is weaker to both compression and tension stresses, but it is still resistant to gliding, and its coefficient of friction remains low (Threlkeld and Currier, 1988). As the cartilage thins the joint space is reduced.

The subchondral bone beneath the fibrillated cartilage becomes shiny and smooth (eburnated). Below the eburnated region the area becomes osteoporotic and local avascular necrosis causes cyst formation where there is complete bone loss. Osteophytes covered with fibrocartilage form at the periphery of the joint, and may protrude into the joint space or more frequently into surrounding soft tissue.

Table 2.6   Management of articular cartilage degeneration

Method	Technique
Debridement	Cartilage layer is removed down to subchondral bone. Results may be poor
Arthroscopic washing	Washing out loose fragments of cartilage/subchondral bone and joint fluid containing degradative enzymes
Drilling, abrasion and microfracture	Work by penetrating the subchondral bone and stimulating cell regrowth. Fibrocartilage rather than renewed hyaline cartilage is produced
Autologous implantation	Transplanting cells of various types into chondral defects. Cells used include rib perichondrial cells, periosteum and chondrocytes
Allograft	Implanting cadaveric cartilage. Rejection is possible

Definition
Two classic signs of osteoarthritis are *eburnation*, where the joint cartilage becomes shiny and smooth, and *osteophytes*, which are bony spurs forming at the edge of the joint.

The synovial membrane becomes thickened and its vascularity increases in line with an inflammatory response (see above). The joint capsule demonstrates small tears filled with fibrous tissue, causing thickening. Contracture usually alters both physiological and accessory movements (see p. 20). For example, when OA affects the knee joint, flexion is often limited and mediolateral stability reduced.

Arthritis secondary to sports injury

The changes which occur in OA, if detected early enough, may be reversible (Hertling and Kessler, 1990). Altered biomechanics of a joint, if corrected, can result in regrowth of fibrocartilage. However, subtle alterations in normal joint mechanics, which may remain long after an injury has 'resolved', may be largely undetectable to a patient or physician. It is not until these changes are well developed and limit physiological joint movement or cause deformity that they become readily apparent. Accessory movements, however, when limited, are detectable to a manipulative physiotherapist at a much earlier stage. It would seem logical therefore to assess and restore accessory movements after joint injury rather than simply full range physiological movement and muscle strength. In this way the onset of OA may be slowed or even avoided.

The use of biomechanical analyses after injury with apparatus such as video playback, isokinetic dynamometry and force plates is helpful to ensure that joint function has been restored.

Arthritis and exercise

Arthritis is often considered a normal ageing process. However, Panush and Brown (1987) cite a study of a population in the age range 70–79 years in which 85% had OA. Importantly, the result indicated that 15% of this age group did not suffer OA, so it seems likely that although ageing is an important factor, other considerations must exist.

Animal studies have failed to show a direct link between exercise and arthritis. Radin, Eyre and Schiller (1979) found no evidence of cartilage deterioration in sheep forced to walk for 4 hours daily on concrete for 12 and 30 months. Videman (1982) found that running did not affect the development of OA in rabbits. Experimentally induced OA was not increased when the animals were forced to run over 2000 metres per week for 14 consecutive weeks.

Studies on runners have also failed to show any significant difference with non-runners. Puranen et al. (1975) found less hip OA in Finnish distance runners than in non-runners of a similar age. Panush et al. (1986) found no greater clinical or radiological evidence of OA in male runners of average age 55 years, and Lane, Oehlert and Block (1998) concluded that runners and non-runners showed similar evidence of hip and knee OA.

Studies have linked OA of particular joints with specific sports. In a review on the subject, Panush and Brown (1987)

cited studies describing OA in the cervical spine and lower extremities of ballet dancers, the upper limb of baseball pitchers, the hands of boxers, cricketers, and downhill skiers, and the ankles and feet of soccer players. Whether these results reflect overuse of the joints involved or altered mechanics following injury to these more frequently used body parts remains uncertain. In general, most authors agree that moderate habitual exercise will maintain joint integrity but sports which subject a joint to repetitive high impact and torsional forces increase the risk of articular degeneration and subsequennt OA development (Eichner, 1999).

It would seem logical that maintaining the normal mobility and strength of a joint throughout life could help maintain the health of the joint structures and perhaps delay the onset of OA. Conversely, high impact loading of an already degenerating joint, such as may occur with running or aerobics on hard unforgiving surfaces, may exacerbate symptoms.

The advice to a patient with OA must be to reduce impact but maintain mobility and strength in a controlled fashion. Athletes must also be made aware of the danger of 'running through the pain' and training with an injury which alters the forces across a joint. Similarly, athletes must be conscious that the cessation of pain following injury does not indicate that full function has returned. Total rehabilitation has only occurred when normal joint mechanics has been restored.

> **Keypoint**
>
> Patients with osteoarthritis should not simply stop exercising. The advice must be to reduce impact but maintain mobility and strength in a controlled fashion.

Arthritis and obesity

Obesity in steadily increasing in the Western world; 55–60% of adults in the USA are overweight (BMI of 25 or more) and 20–25% are clinically obese (BMI 30 or more) (ACSM, 2001). As well as an important effect on cardiovascular health, obesity has an effect on joints. A high percentage of subjects with end-stage hip OA have been shown to be overweight, with a mean BMI of 28.8 (Marks and Allegrante, 2002).

The weight-bearing joints of the lower limb (hip, knee and ankle) are especially at risk from obesity. Obese patients with arthritis of these joints should therefore be helped to lose weight, as this may significantly help the condition.

> **Definition**
>
> Body mass index (BMI) or 'Quetelet index' is a measure of body bulk. BMI is obtained by dividing a person's weight (in kilograms) by their height (in metres) squared. BMI below 20 is considered underweight, 20–25 normal, 25–30 overweight and over 30 obese.

Obese individuals have been shown to be more likely to develop OA in the first place, the increased risk being 4.8 fold in men and 4.0 fold in women. In addition, it has been suggested that obesity increases the risk of the development of bilateral rather than unliteral OA (Felson, 1997).

The joint capsule

The joint capsule is in two parts. The outer part (stratum fibrosum) is fibrous and thickened in areas to form ligaments. The inner layer (stratum synoviale) is loose and highly vascular and blends with the synovial membrane. The capsule consists of parallel fascicles of collagen and some fibrocytes. Blood vessels enter the subchondral bone at the line of capsular attachment and small vessels are found between the individual cartilage fascicles. The nerve supply is very rich, with large fibres giving proprioceptive feedback and small fibres terminating in pain endings.

The capsular response to trauma is an increase in vascularity and eventually the development of fibrous tissue. Cross-linking of collagen fibres occurs, causing a palpable thickening of the capsule. Capsular shrinkage combined with fibrous adhesions will cause loss of movement and occurs particularly after immobilization.

> **Keypoint**
>
> The joint capsule will become thickened and less elastic following trauma and prolonged rest. Ultimately capsular shrinkage will significantly limit movement.

Accumulation of joint fluid through swelling will stretch the capsule and capsular ligaments. The nerve endings situated between the collagen fascicles of the capsule will be stretched, giving rise to mechanical pain. Should the fluid accumulation exceed the elastic limit of the joint capsule, rupture may result.

Joint effusion will stretch portions of the capsule which are normally lax, to facilitate movement. The patient will tend to rest the joint in a position where the joint cavity is of maximum volume (loose pack, see p. 19); in addition, passive movements will be limited in characteristic 'capsular patterns' (Table 2.7).

Ligaments

When a ligament is put under stress, it responds by getting progressively stiffer before later deforming in a regular manner (Amis, 1985). There are two reasons for this. First, the collagen fibres within the ligament are not in line, and so the initial tensile stress is used up by pulling the fibres straight. Secondly, the fibres are not attached to a single point but to an area of bone, and so are of slightly different lengths. When the fibres are stretched, there will be a progressive tightening of the ligament with some fibres becoming taut sooner than others.

Ligaments demonstrate viscoelastic properties. Rapid stretch has been shown to increase stiffness by as much as 20% (Woo, Gomez and Akeson, 1981), and sustained stretch to cause ligament tension to reduce significantly after 2 minutes (Viidik, 1966). The mode of failure also changes with speed, avulsion occurring at slower speeds and ligamentous rupture at higher speeds (Noyes, De Luca and Torvik, 1974).

Clinically, three grades of ligament injuries are recognized (Fowler, 1984). Grade I sprains involve minimal tissue damage with some local tenderness. Swelling is only slight, and function is almost normal. With the grade II sprain, more ligament fibres are injured or the ligament may become partially detached from its bony attachment. Local pain is more intense and movement more limited. Grade III injuries constitute a complete rupture. There is a rapid onset of effusion with considerable pain. The joint is unstable and loss of function is complete. Noyes et al. (1984) argued that this traditional classification, although useful, could be misleading. The grade II injury could refer equally to an injury where only a few ligament fibres are torn, or to a lesion where virtually the total ligament was affected. The grade III injury, they claimed, represented not total rupture, but total loss of function of the ligament, actual continuity of the ligament often being maintained (Table 2.8).

With grades I and II, pain is increased by placing the ligament on stretch. With a grade II injury, some instability may be present, but with a complete rupture instability is always

---

Table 2.7   The capsular patterns

Shoulder – so much limitation of abduction, more than that of lateral rotation, less than that of medial rotation

Elbow – flexion usually more limited than extension, rotations full and painless except in advanced cases

Wrist – equal limitation of flexion and extension, little limitation of deviations

Trapezio-first metacarpal joint – only abduction limited

Sign of the buttock – passive hip flexion more limited and more painful than straight leg raise

Hip – marked limitation of flexion and medial rotation, some limitation of abduction, little or no limitation of adduction and lateral rotation

Knee – gross limitation of flexion, slight limitation of extension

Ankle – more limitation of plantiflexion than of dorsiflexion

Talocalcanean joint – increasing limitations of varus until fixation in valgus

Mid-tarsal joint – limitations of adduction and internal rotation, other movements full

Big toe – gross limitations of extension, slight limitation of flexion

Cervical spine – equal limitation in all directions except for flexion which is usually full

Thoracic spine – limitation of extension, side flexion and rotations, less limitation of flexion

Lumbar spine – marked and equal limitation of side flexions, limitation of flexion and extension

From Cyriax and Cyriax (1983), with permission.

Table 2.8 Ligament injuries

Grade	Signs and symptoms
(I) Mild	Minimal loss of structural integrity No abnormal motion Little or no swelling Localized tenderness Minimal or no bruising
(II) Moderate	Significant structural weakening Some abnormal motion Marked bruising and swelling Often associated with haemarthrosis and joint effusion
(III) Severe	Loss of structural integrity Marked abnormal motion Significant bruising which may track away from area Definite haemarthrosis if capsule remains intact

Adapted from Reid (1992) with permission.

Definition

Grade I ligament injuries are mild, grade II moderate, and grade III severe.

---

present. However, clinically this may be difficult to assess in instances of severe pain and muscle spasm.

Ligamentous viscosity changes with age. The collagen fibres within the ligament enlarge, reducing the water content in the ground substance. Noyes and Grood (1976) showed marked reductions in tensile strength of ligament in the 48–83 year age group when compared with the 16–26 year age group. Noyes et al. (1984) showed three-fold decreases in maximum stress, elastic modulus and strain energy between the ligaments from donors aged 50 years compared to those aged 20 years. The older ligaments failed by bony avulsion rather than ligamentous failure as occurred in the younger tissues. They claimed that ageing produced changes in the ligament/bone systems similar to those found through disuse.

Immobility also has marked effects on ligaments. Laros, Tipton and Cooper (1971) showed strength reductions of 39% after 9 weeks' immobilization, full strength not being regained for 30 weeks. Exercise has been shown to have a beneficial effect on ligament tensile strength (Adams, 1966; Heikkinen and Vuori, 1972; Cabaud et al., 1980). Exercise seems to act as a 'mechanical stimulant', causing increased

Keypoint

Immobilization weakens ligaments, while exercise acts as a mechanical stimulant to cause increased collagen turnover and strengthen the ligament.

collagen turnover within the ligament (Weisman, Pope and Johnson, 1980).

This has important implications for rehabilitation following ligament injury. Wherever possible, complete immobilization should be avoided. While an injured ligament should be protected against excessive external forces which could cause further damage, gentle exercise within the pain-free range should still be encouraged.

The effect of corticosteroids on ligament failure is important, since steroid usage in sport is still popular. Decreases in maximum load of 21% and 39% have been shown 6 and 15 weeks after large dosage cortisone injection (methylprednisolone acetate), with a load reduction remaining for 1 year. In addition, fibrocyte death was seen within the ligament, with delay in reappearance of new fibrocytes for 15 weeks (Noyes et al., 1984).

Muscle

The term 'strain' is generally used to imply a minor injury to any soft tissue structure. However, in this book 'strain' will be confined to injury of muscle while the term 'sprain' will be used for injured joint structures. Strains may be subdivided into acute and chronic types. Acute strains are usually the result of a single violent stretch to a contracting muscle (Fowler, 1984; Keene, 1990), while chronic strains develop over a period of time as a result of repetitive loading.

Definition

Injuries to muscles are termed *strains* while injuries to ligaments and other joint structures are called *sprains*.

Muscle injures may be classified into a variety of types (Table 2.9). At one end of the spectrum is muscle pain, including ischaemia and delayed onset muscle soreness (DOMS) which occurs some time after intense muscle training. These two conditions are covered in Chapter 6. Muscles may be injured through direct trauma (extrinsic injury) or through their own power (intrinsic injury). Extrinsic injury includes contusions (bruising) and tissue damage through laceration such as may occur through an open impaling injury or compound fracture, where the fractured bone pierces muscle and skin.

Contusions are common in contact sports such as rugby, where a quadriceps contusion or 'dead leg' is a common site. Bruising may be greater than for grade (I) or grade (II) injuries, and the amount of blood released into the tissues makes possible scarring or calcification a concern. Contusions, as with grade (III) injuries, may be classified as intermuscular, where the blood is released from the muscle and spreads downwards (tracking). Tracking disperses the blood, facilitating healing and minimizing the risk of scarring. The tense muscle resolves fairly quickly, allowing an earlier recovery of range of motion. Blood appears in distal parts of

Table 2.9 Muscle injuries

Grade	Signs and symptoms
Exercise induced muscle soreness	Muscle pain during training (ischaemia) or aching occurring 24–48 hours after intense unaccustomed activity (delayed onset muscle soreness – DOMS)
Contusion	Pain and marked bruising tracking distally. Failure to increase range of motion suggests blood clot is trapped (intramuscular haematoma)
(I) Mild strain	Small number of muscle fibres torn, giving minimal bleeding. Pain and spasm well localized. Muscle function normal, but endurance may be reduced
(II) Moderate strain	Larger number of muscle fibres injured, but muscle fascia remains intact. Bleeding contained causing an increase in intramuscular pressure. Palpation reveals definite mass and considerable pain. Contractility and extensibility of muscle reduced.
(III) Severe strain	Greater area of muscle affected, with muscle fascia partially torn. Bleeding more profuse, and blood may track distally. Function severely impaired
(IV) Rupture/avulsion	

Sources Fowler, J.A. (1984) Soft tissue injuries and sports injuries. In *Cash's Textbook of Orthopaedics and Rheumatology for Physiotherapists* (ed. P.A. Downie). Faber and Faber, London. With permission. Keene (1990) and Reid (1992).

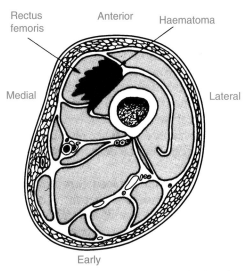

Figure 2.21 An intermuscular haematoma affecting the rectus femoris. From Fowler, J.A. (1984) Soft tissue injuries and sports injuries. In *Cash's Textbook of Orthopaedics and Rheumatology for Physiotherapists* (ed. P.A. Downie). Faber and Faber, London. With permission.

the limb. With an intramuscular haematoma, blood is trapped within the muscle septum, giving a palpable mass. The inflammatory response is generally greater (Reid, 1992) and the risk of scarring and myositis ossificans must be considered. Range of motion remains restricted, and this is one of the most important early clinical signs.

> **Clinical note**
>
> Following a muscle contusion, if range of motion remains restricted, intramuscular haematoma must be suspected.

Three grades are used to describe actual muscle strains, while a complete rupture is sometimes described as a grade four sprain (Fowler, 1984). The grade (I) (mild) strain is a contusion in which there is tearing of a small number of muscle fibres with the fascia remaining intact. Bleeding is minimal, with pain and spasm being localized. Muscle function is normal, but endurance may be reduced.

Grade (II) (moderate) strains result from more severe trauma. A larger number of muscle fibres are injured, and injury occurs over a greater area. The fascia still remains intact so bleeding is contained within the muscle (intramus-

cular haematoma) but with considerably less accumulation of blood than with a contusion. The contained bleeding will cause an increase in intramuscular pressure, which in turn will compress the bleeding points and stop further haemorrhage (Williams and Sperryn, 1976). A definite palpable mass is evident with this injury, and pain to palpation is considerable. Function of the muscle is impaired, with contractility and extensibility being greatly reduced.

With grade (III) (severe) strains, a larger area of muscle is affected. The muscle fascia is partially torn, and more than one muscle may be involved. Bleeding is more profuse, and spread over a larger area, as the haemorrhage is no longer contained by the muscle sheath. The torn fascia releases the blood to form an intermuscular haematoma (Fig. 2.21), and blood may track distally.

The grade (IV) injury is a complete rupture or avulsion. The muscle ends contract and a definite gap is apparent. In some cases a snapping sound may be heard at the time of injury. Bleeding and swelling are considerable, and active contraction of the muscle is not possible. Avulsion injuries may occur at a number of specific sites (Table 2.10). High contraction forces cause the bony muscle attachment to separate, pulling a small plug of bone off. A muscle will fail at its weakest point, and this is normally the middle of the muscle belly or the musculotendinous junction. However, in the adolescent, the unclosed growth plate is weak, making avulsions more common in the 14–17 age group, although as the ischial apophysis does not close until later, ischial avulsions are seen up to the age of 25 (Toomey, 1995).

The site of the injury is especially important with regard to the treatment regimen chosen. Muscle-tendon injuries can be to the muscle belly itself, the musculotendinous (MT) junction or the teno-osseous (TO) junction. Garrett (1990) showed that both passive stretching, and stretching a

Table 2.10   Common sites for avulsion injuries

Site	Muscle
Anterior superior iliac spine (ASIS)	Sartorius
Anterior inferior iliac spine (AIIS)	Rectus femoris
Iliac crest	External oblique
Ischial tuberosity	Hamstrings
Olecranon process	Triceps
Patella	Quadriceps tendon
Lesser trochanter	Iliopsoas

pre-contracted isolated rabbit muscle consistently caused failure at the MT junction, a small (0.1–1 mm) amount of muscle tissue being left attached to the tendon.

Garrett (1990) also showed that pre-contracted muscles absorbed 100% more energy than passively stretched muscle fibre, and used these results to emphasize the importance of muscles as energy absorbers. He argued that conditions which interfere with a muscle's contractile ability, such as fatigue or muscle weakness, might diminish the energy absorbing ability of the muscle and possibly predispose to injury.

Cyriax (1982) claimed that muscle belly injuries would respond to therapeutic exercise. Muscle contraction causes broadening of the fibres and, he claimed, would reduce intramuscular scarring. Injury at the MT or TO junctions would not respond to exercise as no muscle broadening occurs at these points. Cyriax argued that passive therapy, such as transverse frictional massage or injection, was more appropriate to these sites.

Myositis ossificans traumatica

Myositis ossificans traumatica (MOT) is soft tissue ossification of muscle resulting in the formation of non-neoplasmic bone (Booth and Westers, 1989). It usually occurs in the proximal limb muscles, and is seen most commonly following contusion of the quadriceps femoris musculature (Jackson, 1975), although other regions include the elbow flexors and hip abductors.

Several aetiological theories have been suggested (Booth and Westers, 1989). Calcification of a muscle haematoma can occur following fibrosis, or intramuscular bone formation may result from periosteal detachment. Rupture of the periosteum may lead to the proliferation of osteoblasts and their escape into the surrounding muscle. Intramuscular connective tissue may undergo metaplasia into bone, and Urist et al. (1978) demonstrated that certain skeletal muscle cells, known as inducible osteogenic precursor cells (IOPC), have the capability of differentiating into osteoblasts. Certain individuals have been shown to have a predisposition to the condition (Rothwell, 1982).

Clinically, the patient presents with severe post-traumatic pain and limitation of movement. There is local swelling and erythema, with the area being warm and tender to palpation.

Keypoint

Myositis is most common after quadriceps haematoma (dead leg). The classic sign is reduction in movement range over time.

Tenderness usually becomes more pronounced with time, and tissue signs do not respond to conservative management. The factor which should alert the practitioner to the possibility of MOT is a reduction in movement range over time. Normally, an increasing range would be expected as a condition resolves. Radiological evidence of ossification is usually seen within 2 months following injury, and other investigations, including computed tomography (Vas et al., 1981) and ultrasound scanning (Kramer et al., 1979), have been used.

Management of MOT is aimed at lessening any disability rather than affecting the bone mass. Initially, the soft tissue response to trauma, especially bleeding, is limited by the use of such regimens as rest, ice, compression and elevation (RICE). Rehabilitation is slower than with a normal muscle haematoma, isometric exercises being used 7–14 days following injury, but active exercises (within the pain-free range) are not used until 2–4 weeks after injury (Booth and Westers, 1989).

Tendons

A variety of conditions may affect tendons, the most common in sport being tenosynovitis, tendinitis and tenovaginitis. Tendinitis is an inflammation and scarring of the tendon which can occur in varying degrees. Scarring may interfere with tendon function and/or cause persistent local inflammation. Tenosynovitis is a lesion to the gliding surfaces of the outside of the tendon and the inside of its sheath, but not the sheath itself (Fowler, 1984). The lesion is usually as a result of overuse or compression (Williams and Sperryn, 1976). Pathological features are similar to those seen in rheumatoid arthritis (Williams and Sperryn, 1976), including an increase in the number of lining cells of the sheath, together with proliferation of local blood vessels, oedema and cellular changes. As the roughened surfaces of the sheath move against each other pain and crepitus occur. The same condition occurring to tendons which do not have a true sheath is termed peritendonitis. Here, the paratenon thickens, and shows fibrinoid degeneration and dense fibrous adhesions (Snook, 1972). Local oedema is evident, sometimes with palpable crepitus, and pain may disappear with activity (Williams and Sperryn, 1976).

Tenovaginitis occurs when the tendon sheath is chronically inflamed and thickens. It is the fibrous wall of the tendon sheath rather than the synovial lining which is affected. Common sites include the flexor sheaths of the fingers or thumb. When the sheaths of extensor pollicis brevis and abductor pollicis longus are affected, de Quervain's syndrome is present.

Nerves

The nervous system can be affected by injury through both internal (intraneural) and external (extraneural) means. Intraneural pathology has an effect on the elasticity of the neural system (Slater, Butleter and Shacklock, 1994). When tension is taken up at one point in the nervous system, this is transferred further along, a little like pulling on a rope. Altered mechanics may be accompanied by changes in physiology. Altered microcirculation and axonal transport may occur through compression (Lundborg, 1988), with nerve swelling occurring both proximal and distal to a compression force. (MacKinnon, Dellon and Hudson, 1984).

Definition

Axonal transport is active movement of chemical substances through the cell fluid (axoplasm) of a nerve.

The nervous system consumes 20% of the oxygen used by the body. This is supplied to the nerves through the vasa nervorum, a network of extraneural and intraneural vessels.

Nerve injury may occur along a number of sites (Fig. 2.22) where nerve movement is restricted. Typically, injury is either through trauma or through overuse conditions caused by friction, compression or stretch which cause adverse neural tension (ANT). If sustained, compression may lead to deterioration of the neurone.

Box 2.37   Definition

Adverse neural tension (ANT) is an abnormal physiological or mechanical response from neural structures caused by alteration in their movement or stretch capability (Butler, 1991).

The two major issues affecting nerves in sport injury management are vascular factors and mechanical factors. An alteration in pressure to the blood vessels supplying the nerves of as little as 20 mmHg will affect nerves, and at pressures of 80 mmHg the nerve blood flow is cut off completely (Rydevik, Lundborg and Bagge, 1981). With increasing pressure, the nerve will initially become hypoxic, leading to local venous stasis. If maintained, oedema will form due to alteration in osmotic pressure (see p. 32). With time, the blood capillaries will deteriorate and fibrosis will set in. Eventually

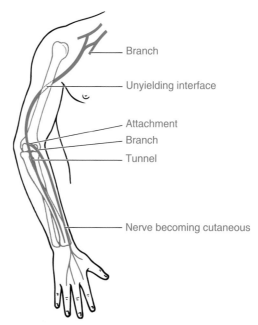

Figure 2.22   Sites of restricted movement in a nerve. From Butler (1991) with permission.

the condition becomes chronic, with scar tissue formation, and the nerve becomes a tough fibrous cord (Butler, 1991).

Mild pressure or friction can lead to oedema of the epineurium, and tearing of the epineurium itself is common in ankle injury (Nitz, Dobner and Kersey, 1985). In such injuries the intraneural and extraneural blood vessels may also rupture. Mechanical damage can again lead to fibrosis with increased stiffness and reduced elasticity occurring in the damaged nerve (Beel, Groswald and Luttges, 1984). The mechanical change in the nerve will alter tension in the whole nervous system as the structures are continuous. Further, the combination of mechanical change and vascular alteration will alter the firing pattern of the nerve and the transport system within the nerve itself (axonal transport). This type of alteration can cause changes further along the nerve creating a *double crush syndrome*. In these cases a condition such as carpal tunnel syndrome can give rise to altered neural mechanics and eventual pathology in the neck (Upton and McComas, 1973), or carpal tunnel syndrome on the other side of the body (Hurst, Weissberg and Carroll, 1985).

Skin

Skin wounds may be divided into two categories: open and closed. Closed wounds occur when there is no penetration of the epidermis, and open wounds are those where the epidermis has been pierced. Closed wounds encompass contusions, abrasions and friction burns, such as those caused by gravel. Open wounds in sport include cuts such as lacerations and puncture wounds.

A contusion or bruise involves a direct blow to the skin surface. Bleeding occurs from torn blood vessels into the skin and subcutaneous tissues, forming a bruise or ecchymosis.

The size of the bruise is dependent on the vascularity of the affected tissue as well as the size of the blood vessels damaged and the laxity of the surrounding tissues. Normally, bruising requires conservative management, but conditions such as retrobulbar haemorrhage (behind the eyeball) and scrotal haematoma may require surgical evacuation (Ray and Soutar, 1993). Following contusion, released blood will clot and degrade, producing superficial colour changes.

An abrasion or graze occurs through a glancing injury or repeated microtrauma to the skin surface. The skin surface breaks through, but the damage is not full thickness. The condition may be complicated by ingrained tattooing where embedded particles remain beneath the surface. The material may become covered by epithelium, giving a visible and hypertrophic scar. An abrasion of this type should be treated as early as possible after the injury by vigorous scrubbing with a stiff nail brush and an antiseptic wash to remove the embedded dirt.

Clinical note

An abrasion from a fall onto a grit surface runs the risk of *ingrained tattooing*. The wound must be thoroughly scrubbed with an antiseptic wash to remove all dirt, before being dressed.

Extensive areas of skin may be affected during an abrasion, and intense pain usually occurs as raw nerve endings are exposed. Bleeding may be widespread, but healing is rapid unless infection ensues. Extensive debriding injuries involving large areas of skin loss (for example from a motor-cycle accident) may require grafting.

A laceration is a full thickness skin injury which exposes the subcutaneous tissue. A force sufficient to break the skin in this way will also give considerable associated deep tissue damage. In addition the edge of the skin break will be uneven and surrounded by a contusion. Clean lacerations may require stitching but heal well; jagged injuries involving skin tearing may leave more scarring.

Pressure or friction may cause an abrasion where the skin surface is removed, or a blister, where the epidermal surface skin layer is detached from the underlying tissue. The gap between the two layers is filled with lymph, exposing nerve endings to fluid pressure, so causing pain. When pressure or friction is applied progressively, the epidermal skin layer may adapt to form a thickened callus (Williams, 1979).

Healing of an incised wound such as a cut, where the wound edges are in apposition, occurs by *first intention*. If the wound edges are separated and more major skin damage has occurred (or if infection has intervened), then healing is by *second intention* (Evans, 1990a).

With healing by first intention, slight haemorrhage occurs and the cut is filled with a blood clot on the first day. By the second and third day the clot has become organized and epithelial cells from the two sides of the cut have joined. This single layer of covering multiplies to form stratified squamous epithelium – normal epidermis. Fibroblasts lay down collagen in the granulation tissue and a band of scar tissue is formed by 2 weeks after the injury.

Healing by second intention takes longer as the spread of epithelial cells over the larger area takes time. The large amount of granulation tissue results in more extensive scarring and likely contracture.

Treatment note 2.4   Principles of physical examination

Physical examination is conducted after a full subjective examination (see Treatment note 2.1), and aims to determine the structure(s) which are responsible for producing the patient's symptoms (Petty and Moore, 2001). The examination consists of a number of stages within the whole framework of clinical diagnosis (Table 2.11) and some or all of the elements will be used on each patient.

Observation and inspection
1. The patient should be observed in general before the individual body part is focused on more closely. Postural characteristics, gait and facial expression can be important pointers in both static and dynamic situations. Simple tasks such as walking into the treatment room and undressing can hold valuable clues. Formal posture assessment is covered on pages 137–140, and gait analyis is discussed on pages 183–185.
2. Inspection of the affected body part must identify any deformity such as alteration in joint or spinal alignment as well as skin colour changes including redness (indicating inflammation) and any rashes or skin injury. Swelling indicates an inflammatory response, and the speed with which it formed is important (see p. 31). Other abnormalities such as soft/hard bumps, ganglia and nodules should also be noted and may require medical investigation. Muscle contour is important as it may indicate wasting, spasm or imbalance.

Palpation
1. General palpation of the area looks at temperature, swelling, and synovial thickening before individual structures are identified through examination of surface anatomy. Increased temperature (heat) indicates inflammation as before, and a cold clammy skin feeling suggests autonomic disturbance. The firmness (condition) and mobility of the soft tissues should be determined as well as the general presence of swelling. The production of muscle spasm suggests pain and/or trigger point activation (p. 147).

Table 2.11 Clincal examination

Element	Detail
Observation	Face
	Gait
	Posture
History (subjective examination)	Age, occupation, activities
	Site and spread
	Onset and duration
	Symptoms and behaviour
	Past medial history (PMH)
	Other joint involvement
	Drug history (medication)(DH)
Inspection	Deformity (bony?)
	Colour changes
	Muscle wasting
	Swelling
Palpation	Temperature
	Swelling
	Synovial thickening
Active movements	Range/movement pattern
	Pain/symptoms
	Power
	Willingness
Resisted movements	Pain/symptoms
	Power
Passive movements	Pain/symptoms
	Range and quality
	End-feel

After Kesson and Atkins (1998) with permission.

2. The unaffected side of the body should be palpated first to establish a baseline for comparison with the affected body part. Superficial palpation should precede deep palpation so that important findings are not obliterated – in general, 'harder pressure feels less'.

Movements

1. Active movements may be used to assess willingness to move, and then resisted movements look at the production of pain (or symptoms) and power graded to normal values and assessed in comparison to the uninjured side.
2. Passive movements determine pain, range, and end-feel (Table 2.12) as well as the presence of a capsular pattern (Table 2.7, p. 51). They are used to examine non-contractile (inert) structures.

Table 2.12 End-feel

Type	Example
Normal	
Hard	Bone to bone approximation – elbow extension
Soft	Soft tissue approximation – elbow flexion
Elastic	Tissue stretch – lateral rotation of the shoulder joint
Abnormal	
Hard	Bony degeneration – osteoarthritis (OA)
Springy	Mechanical joint displacement – loose body, meniscal tear
Spasm	Involuntary muscle spasm – irritable joint
Empty	Patient stops movement – anticipation of pain/instability

From Cyriax (1982), Kesson and Atkins (1998) with permission.

References

Adams, A. (1966) Effect of exercise upon ligament strength. *Research Quarterly*, **37**, 163–176

American College of Sports Medicine (ACSM) (1998) Position stand on exercise and physical activity for older adults. *Medicine and Science for Sports and Exercise*, **30**, 992–1008

American College of Sports Medicine (ACSM) (2001) Intervention strategies for weight loss and prevention of weight regain for adults. *Medicine and Science for Sports and Exercise*, **33**, 2145–2156

Amis, A.A. (1985) Biomechanics of ligaments. In *Ligament Injuries and their Treatment* (ed. D.H.R. Jenkins). Chapman and Hall, London

Apel, D.M., Vince, K.G. and Kingston, S. (1994) Transient osteoporosis of the hip: a role for core decompression? *Orthopedics* **17**, (7) 629–632

Apley, A.G. and Solomon, L. (1988) *Concise System of Orthopaedics and Fractures.* Butterworth-Heinemann, Oxford

Apley, A.G. and Solomon, L (1993) *Apley's system of orthopaedics and fractures*, 7th edn. Butterworth Heinemann, Oxford

Baldry, P.E. (1998) Trigger point acupuncture. In *Medical Acupuncture* (eds J. Filshie and A. White). Churchill Livingstone, Edinburgh

Bassett, C.A.L. (1965) Electrical effects in bone. *Scientific American*, **213**, (4) 18

Bassett, C.A.L. and Pawlick, R.J. (1964) Effects of electric currents on bone in vivo. *Nature*, **204**, 652

Becker, R.O. and Murray, D.G. (1970) The electrical control system regulating fracture healing in amphibians. *Clinical Orthopaedics and Related Research*, **73**, 169

Becker, R.O., Spadaro, J.A. and Marino, A.A. (1977) Clinical experience with low intensity direct current stimulation of bone growth. *Clinical Orthopaedics and Related Research*, **124**, 75–83

Beel, J.A., Groswald, D.E. and Luttges, M.W (1984) Alterations in the mechanical properties of peripheral nerve following crush injury. *Journal of Biomechanics* **17**, 185–193

Behiri, J. and Vashishth, D. (2000) Biomechanics of bone. In *Clinical Biomechanics* (ed. Z. Dvir). Churchill Livingstone, Edinburgh

Bennell, K., Khan, K. and McKay, H. (2000) The role of physiotherapy in the prevention and treatment of osteoporosis. *Manual Therapy*, **5**, (4) 198–213

Blau, S.P. (1979) The synovial fluid. *Orthopaedic Clinics of North America*, 10, 21–35

Booth, D.W. and Westers, B.M. (1989) The management of athletes with myositis ossificans traumatica. *Canadian Journal of Sports Science*, **14**, (1) 10–16

Bullough, P.G. (1981) Cartilage. In *Scientific Foundations of Orthopaedics and Traumatology* (eds R. Owen, J. Goodfellow and P. Bullough). Heinemann Medical, Oxford

Burri, C., Helbing, G. and Spier, W. (1973) Rehabilitation of knee ligament injuries. In *The Knee.* Springer, New York

Butler, D.S. (1991) *Mobilisation of the Nervous System*. Churchill Livingstone, Edinburgh

Cabaud, H.E., Chatty, A., Gildengorin, V. and Feltman, R.J. (1980) Exercise effects on the strength of the anterior cruciate ligament. *American Journal of Sports Medicine*, **8**, 79–86

Carbon, R.J. (1992) The female athlete. In *Textbook of Science and Medicine in Sport* (eds J. Bloomfield, P.A. Fricker and K.D. Fitch). Blackwell Scientific Publications, Melbourne

Chartered Society of Physiotherapy (CSP) (1999). *Physiotherapy Guidelines for the Management of Osteoporosis*. Chartered Society of Physiotherapy, London

Crawford-Adams, J. (1978) *Outline of Fractures*. Churchill Livingstone, London

Curtiss, P.H. and Kincaid, W.E. (1959) Transitory demineralization of the hip in pregnancy: a report of three cases. *Journal of Bone and Joint Surgery (Am)*, **41**, 1327–1333

Curwin, S.L. (1994) The aetiology and treatment of tendinitis. In: *Oxford Textbook of Sports Medicine* (eds M. Harries et al.). Oxford Medical Publications, Oxford

Cyriax, J. (1982) *Textbook of Orthopaedic Medicine*, 8th edn. Baillière Tindall, London, vol. 1

Cyriax, J.H. and Cyriax, P.J. (1983) *Illustrated Manual of Orthopaedic Medicine*. Butterworths, London

De Domenico, G. (1982) Pain relief with interferential therapy. *Australian Journal of Physiotherapy*, **28**, (3) 14–18

Deakin, V. and Brotherhood, J.R. (1992) Nutrition and energy sources. In *Textbook of Science and Medicine in Sport* (eds J. Bloomfield, P.A. Fricker and K. D. Fitch). Blackwell Scientific Publications, Melbourne

Donaldson, C.L., Hulley, S.B. and Vogel, J.M (1970) Effects of prolonged bed rest on bone mineral. *Metabolism*, **19**, 1071–1084

Donley, P.B. and Denegar, C. (1990) Pain and mechanisms of pain relief. In *Therapeutic Modalities in Sports Medicine* (ed. W.E. Prentice). Times Mirror/Mosby College Publishing, Philadelphia

Dyson, M. (1987) Mechanisms involved in therapeutic ultrasound. *Physiotherapy*, **73**, (3) 116–120

Eichner, E.R. (1999) Comment. *Yearbook of Sports Medicine*. Mosby, St Louis, pp. 365–366

Ettinger, B., Genant, H.K. and Cann, C.E. (1987) Postmenopausal bone loss is prevented by low dosage estrogen with calcium. *Annals of Internal Medicine*, **106**, 40–45

Evans, P. (1980) The healing process at cellular level: a review. *Physiotherapy*, **66**, (8) 256–259

Evans, D.M.D. (1990a) Inflammation and healing. In *Cash's Textbook of General Medical and Surgical Conditions for Physiotherapists* (ed. P.A. Downie), 2nd edn. Faber and Faber, London

Evans, R.A. (1990b) Calcium and osteoporosis. *Medical Journal of America*, **152**, 431–433

Evans, C.H. (1999) Cytokines and the role they play in the healing of ligaments and tendons. *Sports Medicine* **28**, 71–76

Felson, D.T. (1997) Understanding the relationship between bodyweight and osteoarthritis. *Clinical Rheumatology*, **11**, 671–681

Fowler, J.A. (1984) Soft tissue injuries and sports injuries. In *Cash's Textbook of Orthopaedics and Rheumatology for Physiotherapists* (ed. P.A. Downie). Faber and Faber, London

Fox, J., Galey, F. and Wayland, H. (1980) Action of histamine on the mesenteric microvasculature. *Microvascular Research*, **19**, 108–126

Frank, G., Woo, S.L., Amiel, O., Harwood, F., Gomez, M. and Akeson, W. (1983) Medial collateral ligament healing: a multidisiplinary assessment in rabbits. *American Journal of Sports Medicine*, **11**, 379–389

Garrett, W.E. (1990) Muscle strain injuries: clinical and basic aspects. *Medicine and Science in Sports and Exercise*, **22**, 436–443

Gartland, J.J. (1987) *Fundamentals of Orthopaedics*, 4th edn. W.B. Saunders, Philadelphia

Gould, J.A. (ed.) (1990) *Orthopaedic and Sports Physical Therapy*, 2nd edn. C.V. Mosby, St Louis

Gunn, C.C. (1996) *Treatment of Chronic Pain*, 2nd edn. Churchill Livingstone, Edinburgh

Harrington, S., Smith, J., Thompson, J. and Laskowski, E. (2000) Idiopathic transient osteoporosis. *Physician and Sportsmedicine*, **28**, (4) 1–9

Hedlund, L.R. and Gallagher, J.C. (1988) Estrogen therapy for postmenopausal osteoporosis: current considerations of the menopause. *Annals of Clinical and Laboratory Science*, **15**, 219–228

Heikkinen, E. and Vuori, I. (1972) Effect of physical activity on the metabolism of collagen in aged mice. *Acta Physiologica Scandinavica*, **84**, 543–549

Heinonen, A., Kannus, P. and Sievanen, H. (1996) Randomised controlled trial of effect of high impact exercise on selected risk factors for osteoporotic fractures. *Lancet*, **348**, 1343–1347

Hert, J. and Zalud, J. (1971) Reaction of bone to mechanical stimuli. (VI). Bioelectrical theory of functional adaptation of bone. *Acta Chirurgicae Orthopaedicae et Traumatologicae Cechoslovaca*, **38**, 280

Hertling, D. and Kessler, R.M. (1990) *Management of Common Musculoskeletal Disorders*. J.B. Lippincott, Philadelphia

Hettinga, D.L. (1990) Inflammatory response of synovial joint structures. In *Orthopaedic and Sports Physical Therapy*, 2nd edn (ed. J.A. Gould). C.V. Mosby, St Louis, pp. 87–117

Hom, D.B. (1995). Growth factors in wound healing. *Otolaryngologic Clinics of North America*, 28, 933–953

Huda, W. and Morin, R.L. (1996) Patient doses in bone mineral dosimetry. *British Journal of Radiology*, **69**, 422–425

Huddleston, A.L., Rockwell, D. and Kuland, D.N. (1980) Bone mass in lifetime tennis athletes. *Journal of the American Medical Association*, **244**, 1107–1109

Hunter, G. (1998). Specific soft tissue mobilization in the management of soft tissue dysfunction. *Manual Therapy*, **3**, (1) 2–11

Hurst, L.C., Weissberg, D. and Carroll, R.E. (1985) The relationship of double crush to carpal tunnel syndrome. *Journal of Hand Surgery*, **10B**, 202–204

Jackson, D.W. (1975) Managing myositis ossificans traumatica. *Physician and Sports Medicine*, **October**, 56–61

Kannus, P (1997) Tendon pathology. *Sports Exercise and Injury*, **3**, 62–75

Keene, J.S. (1990) Ligament and muscle tendon unit injuries. In *Orthopaedic and Sports Physical Therapy*, 2nd edn (ed. J.A. Gould). C.V. Mosby, St Louis

Kellett, J. (1986) Acute soft tissue injuries: a review of the literature. *Medicine and Science in Sports and Exercise*, **18**, (5) 489–500

Kesson, M. and Atkins, E (1998) *Orthopaedic Medicine*. Butterworth-Heinemann, Oxford

Kramer, F.L., Kurtz, A.B., Rubin, C. and Goldberg, B.B. (1979) Ultrasound appearance of myositis ossificans. *Skeletal Radiology*, **4**, 19–20

Krolner, B., Toft, B. and Nielsen, S. (1983) Physical exercise as a prophylaxis against involutional bone loss: a controlled trial. *Clinical Science*, **64**, 541–546

Kurtz, C.A., Loebig, T.G. and Anderson, D.D. (1999) Insulin like growth factor 1 accelerates functional recovery from achilles tendon injury in a rat model. *American Journal of Sports Medicine*, **27**, 363–369

Lachman, S. (1988) *Soft Tissue Injuries in Sport*. Blackwell, Oxford

Lakhanpal, S., Ginsburg, W.W. and Luthra, H.S. (1987) Transient regional osteoporosis: a study of 56 cases and review of the literature. *Annals of Internal Medicine*, **106**, (3) 444–450

Lane, N.E., Oehlert, J.W., Bloch, D.A. and Freis, J.F. (1998) The relationship of running to osteoarthritis of the knee and hip and bone mineral density of the lumbar spine: a 9 year longitudinal study. *Journal of Rheumatology*, **25**, 334–341

Laros, G.S, Tipton, C.M. and Cooper, R.R. (1971) Influence of physical activity on ligament insertions in the knees of dogs. *Journal of Bone and Joint Surgery*, **53A**, 275–286

Lewis, M.K., Blake, G.M. and Fogelman, I (1994) Patient dose in dual X-ray absorptiometry. *Osteoporosis International*, **4**, 11–15

Lewis, T. and Grant, R.T. (1924) Vascular reactions of the skin to injury. *Heart*, **11**, 209–265

Low, J. and Reed, A. (1990) *Electrotherapy Explained: Principles and Practice*. Butterworth-Heinemann, Oxford

Lundborg, G. (1988) *Nerve Injury and Repair*, Churchill Livingstone, Edinburgh

Lynch, M.K. and Kessler, R.M. (1990) Pain. In *Management of Common Musculoskeletal Disorders*, 2nd edn (eds D. Hertling and R.M. Kessler). J.B. Lippincott, Philadelphia

McArdle, W.D., Katch, F.I. and Katch, V.L. (1986) *Exercise Physiology: Energy, Nutrition, and Human Performance*, 2nd edn, Lea and Febiger, Philadelphia

McCarthy, E.F. (1998) The pathology of transient regional osteoporosis. *Iowa Orthopedic Journal*, **18**, 35–42

MacKinnon, J.L. (1988) Osteoporosis: a review. *Physical Therapy*, **68**, (10) 1533–1540

MacKinnon, S.E, Dellon, A.L. and Hudson, A.R. (1984) Chronic nerve compression: an experimental model in the rat. *Annals of Plastic Surgery*, **13**, 112–120

Magee, D.J. (2002) *Orthopedic Physical Assessment*, 4th edn. Saunders, Philadelphia

Maitland, G.D. (1991) *Peripheral Manipulation*, 3rd edn. Butterworth-Heinemann, Oxford

Marks, R. and Allegrante, J.P (2002) Body mass indices in patients with disabling hip osteoarthritis. *Arthritis Research*, **4**, (2) 112–116

Martin, A.D. and Houston, C.S. (1987) Osteoporosis, calcium and physical activity. *Canadian Medical Association Journal*, **136**, 587–593

Mazess, R.B. and Whedon, G.D. (1983). Immobilization and bone. *Calcified Tissue International*, **35**, 265–267

Melzack, R. and Wall, P.D. (1965) Pain mechanisms: a new theory. *Science*, **150**, 971

Nilas, L., Christiansen, C. and Rodbro, P. (1984) Calcium supplementation and post-menopausal bone loss. *British Medical Journal*, **289**, 1103–1106

Nilsson, B.E. and Westlin, N.E. (1977) Bone density in athletes. *Clinical Orthopaedics and Related Research*, **77**, 179–182

Nitz, A.J., Dobner, J.J. and Kersey, D. (1985) Nerve injury and grade II and III ankle sprains. *American Journal of Sports Medicine*, **13**, 177–182

Nixon, A.J., Fortier, L.A. and Williams, J. (1999) Enhanced repair of extensive articular defects by insulin like growth factor 1 laden fibrin composites. *Journal of Orthopaedic Research*, **17**, 475–487

Norris, C.M. (2001) *Acupuncture: Treatment of Musculoskeletal Conditions*. Butterworth-Heinemann, Oxford

Noyes, F.R., De Luca, J.L. and Torvik, P.J. (1974) Biomechanics of anterior cruciate ligament failure: an analysis of strain-rate sensitivity and mechanisms in primates. *Journal of Bone and Joint Surgery*, **56A**, 236–253

Noyes, F.R. and Grood, M.J. (1976) The strength of the anterior cruciate ligament in humans and rhesus monkeys: age-related and species-related changes. *Journal of Bone and Joint Surgery*, **58A**, 1074–1082

Noyes, F.R., Kelly, C.S., Grood, E.S. and Butler, D.L. (1984) Advances in the understanding of knee ligament injury, repair and rehabilitation. *Medicine and Science in Sports and Exercise*, **16**, (5) 427–443

Oakes, B.W. (1992) The classification of injuries and mechanisms of injury, repair and healing. In *Textbook of Science and Medicine in Sport* (eds J. Bloomfield, P.A. Fricker and K.D. Fitch). Blackwell Scientific Publications, Melbourne

Paget, S. and Bullough, P.G. (1981) Synovium and synovial fluid. In *Scientific Foundations of Orthopaedics and Traumatology* (eds R. Owen, J. Goodfellow and P. Bullough). Heinemann Medical, Oxford

Palastanga, N., Field, D. and Soames, R. (1989) *Anatomy and Human Movement*. Heinemann Medical, Oxford

Panush, R.S. and Brown, D.G. (1987) Exercise and arthritis. *Sports Medicine*, **4**, 54–64

Panush, R.S., Schmidt, C., Caldwell, J., Edwards, N.L. and Longley, S. (1986) Is running associated with degenerative joint disease? *Journal of the American Medical Association*, **255**, 1150–1154

Pappas, A.M. (1989) Osteochondroses: diseases of growth centers. *Physician and Sports Medicine*, **17**, 51–62

Petty, N.J. and Moore, A.P. (2001) *Neuromusculoskeletal Examination and Assessment*, 2nd edn. Churchill Livingstone, Edinburgh

Puranen, J., Ala-Ketola, L., Peltokalleo, P. and Saarela, J. (1975) Running and primary osteoarthritis of the hip. *British Medical Journal*, **1**, 424–425

Radin, E.L., Eyre, D. and Schiller, A.L. (1979) Effect of prolonged walking on concrete on the joints of sheep. Abstract. *Arthritis and Rheumatism*, **22**, 649

Ray, A.K. and Soutar, D.S. (1993) Skin injuries and would healing. In *The Soft Tissues* (eds G. R. McLatchie and C.M. Lennox). Churchill Livingstone, Edinburgh

Reid, D.C. (1992) *Sports Injury Assessment and Rehabilitation*. Churchill Livingstone, Edinburgh

Reigger, C.L. (1990) Mechanical properties of bone. In *Orthopaedic and Sports Physical Therapy*, 2nd edn (ed. J. A. Gould). C.V. Mosby, St Louis, pp. 3–47

Rothwell, A.G. (1982) Quadriceps haematoma: a prospective study. *Clinical Orthopaedics and Related Research*, **171**, 97–103

Rydevik, B., Lundborg, G. and Bagge, U. (1981) Effects of graded compression on intraneural blood flow. *Journal of Hand Surgery*, **6**, 3–12

Salter, R.B. (1990) The biological concept of continuous passive motion of synovial joints. In *Articular Cartilage and Knee Joint Function* (ed. J.W. Wing). Raven Press, New York

Salter, R.B. and Harris, W.R. (1963) Injuries involving the epiphyseal plate. *Journal of Bone and Joint Surgery*, **45A**, 587

Slater, H., Butleter, D.S. and Shacklock, M.O. (1994) The dynamic central nervous system: examination and assessment using tension tests. In Boyling et al (eds) *Grieve's Modern Manual Therapy*, 2nd edn (ed. J. Boyling, N. Palastanga). Churchill Livingstone, Edinburgh

Smith, E.L., Smith, P.E. and Ensign, C.J. (1984) Bone involutional decrease in exercising middle-aged women. *Calcified Tissue International*, **36**, 129–138

Snook, G.A. (1972) Tenosynovitis in long distance runners. *Medicine and Science in Sports and Exercise*, **4**, 166

Stanish, W.D., Rubinovich, R.M. and Curwin, S. (1986) Eccentric exercise in chronic tendinitis. *Clinical Orthopaedics*, **208**, 65–68

Steadman, J., Rodkey, W. and Singleton, S. (1997) Microfracture technique for full-thickness chondral defects. *Operative Techniques in Orthopaedics*, **7**, (4) 300–304

Stearns, M.L. (1940) Studies on development of connective tissue in transparent chambers in rabbit's ear. *American Journal of Anatomy*, **67**, 55

Threlkeld, A.J. and Currier, D.P. (1988) Osteoarthritis: effects on synovial joint tissues. *Physical Therapy*, **68**, (3) 364–370

Toomey, M. (1995) The pelvis, hip and thigh. In *Sports Physiotherapy* (eds M. Zaluaga et al.). Churchill Livingstone, Edinburgh

Upton, A.R. and McComas, A.J. (1973) The double crush in nerve entrapment syndromes. *Lancet*, **2**, 359–362

Urist, M.R., Nakagawa, M., Nakata, N. and Nogami, H. (1978) Experimental myositis ossificans: cartilage and bone formation in muscle in response to a diffusible bone matrix derived morphogen. *Archives of Pathology and Laboratory Medicine*, **102**, 312–316

Van der Meulen, J.C.H. (1982) Present state of knowledge on processes of healing in collagen structures. *International Journal of Sports Medicine*, **3**, 4–8

Vas, W., Cockshott, W.P., Martin, R.F., Pai, N.K. and Walker, I. (1981) Myositis ossificans in haemophilia. *Skeletal Radiology*, **7**, 27–31

Videman, T. (1982) The effect of running on the osteoarthritic joint: an experimental matched pair study with rabbits. *Rheumatology and Rehabilitation*, **21**, 1–8

Viidik, A. (1966) Biomechanics and functional adaptation of tendons and joint ligament. In *Studies on the Anatomy and Function of Bone and Joints* (ed. F.G. Evans). Springer, Berlin

Waddell, G., Feder, G. and Lewis, M. (1997) Systematic reviews of bed rest and advice to stay active for acute low back pain. *British Journal of General Practice*, **47**, 647–652

Walter, J.B. and Israel, M.S. (1987) *General Pathology*, 6th edn. Churchill Livingstone, London

Watson, A.S. (1992) Children in sport. In *Textbook of Science and Medicine in Sport* (eds J. Bloomfield, P.A. Fricker and K.D. Fitch). Blackwell Scientific Publications, Melbourne

Weisman, G., Pope, M.H. and Johnson, R.J. (1980) Cyclic loading in knee ligament injuries. *American Journal of Sports Medicine*, **8**, 24–30

White, A. (1999) Neurophysiology of acupuncture analgesia. In *Acupuncture: A Scientific Appraisal* (eds E. Ernst and A. White). Butterworth-Heinemann, Oxford

Wilkinson, P.C. and Lackie, J.M. (1979) The adhesion, migration and chemotaxis of leucocytes in inflammation. *Current Topics in Pathology*, **68**, 47–88

Williams, J.G.P. (1979) *Injuries in Sport*, Bayer (UK), Haywards Heath, England

Williams, J.G.P. and Sperryn, P.N. (1976) *Sports Medicine*. Edward Arnold, London

Wolman, R.L. and Reeve, J. (1994) Exercise and the skeleton. In *Oxford Textbook of Sports Medicine* (eds M. Harries et al.). Oxford University Press, Oxford

Woo, S.L.Y., Gomez, M.A. and Akeson, W.H. (1981) The time and history-dependent viscoelastic properties of the canine medial collateral ligament. *Journal of Biomechanical Engineering*, **103**, 293–298

World Health Organization (WHO) (1994) Assessment of Fracture Risk and its Application to Screening for Osteoporosis. Report of WHO study group. World Health Organization, Geneva

Wroble, R.R. (2000). Articular cartilage injury and autologous chondrocyte implantation – which patients might benefit? *Physician and Sportsmedicine*, **28**, (11) 43–49

Chapter 3

Sports massage

Massage is one of the original core skills of physiotherapy (Copestake, 1917), which unfortunately fell from popularity because of the belief that it was 'unscientific'. Thankfully, massage is making a re-emergence in the more fashionable guise of 'sports massage', both within physiotherapy and through the development of specialist massage therapists. Various massage procedures are used within sport and most influence the tissues by stretching or compression, resulting in both reflex and mechanical effects. The classical massage procedures are outlined in Table 3.1.

MASSAGE TECHNIQUES

Effleurage

Two types of effleurage are used (Fig. 3.1). The first is a superficial stroking movement designed to produce a sensory reaction, either of relaxation (slow stroking) or stimulation (fast stroking). The second is a deep action aimed at assisting lymphatic and venous drainage. The tissue manipulation starts distally and proceeds proximally in the direction of the heart, for example, 'knee to groin' or 'elbow to axilla'. The proximal portion of the limb is treated first to clear lymphatic and venous congestion. This will allow the tissue fluids mobilized by the distal massage to move against less restriction.

Table 3.1 Massage procedures

Effleurage
Unidirectional stroking movement travelling proximally

Petrissage
Soft tissue compression including kneading, picking up, wringing, rolling and shaking

Frictions
Small, deep circular or transverse movements at specific anatomical sites

Tapotement
Percussive actions including clapping, hacking, beating, tapping, shaking and vibration

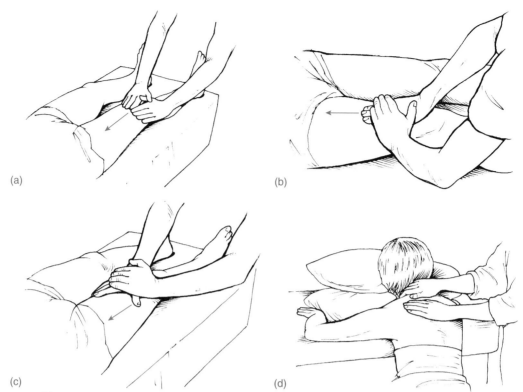

Figure 3.1 Effleurage. (a) Both hands cover the surface of the limb. (b) Reinforced hand for deeper pressure. (c) Thumb web used to contour limb. (d) Superficial stroking — the flat hands or fingertips are pulled towards the therapist.

> **Keypoint**
>
> Where deep stroking (effeurage) is used to assist lymphatic flow, the massage direction is from *distal to proximal*, towards the heart.

The therapist uses the hands either together or separately with one supporting the other to create more force. Skin contact is maintained throughout the action, and as they move, the hands change shape to contour the limb. The whole of the hand, and not just the leading edge should apply the pressure, to avoid sticking or jerking.

The force for the movement should come from overall body motion and not simply arm strength. The therapist adopts a stance with one foot in front of the other (walk standing) and transfers his or her weight from the rear to the front foot. The arms and hands transmit, rather than create, the force. At the beginning of the action the elbows will be bent, and at the end, full reach is achieved by straightening the arms. At this end-point a slight overpressure is applied and the movement pauses before being repeated.

> **Keypoint**
>
> The hands are used to *transmit* force created by the legs and trunk. The hands should not create force themselves.

Some therapists prefer to maintain skin contact with a light stroking action as the hand is returned to the starting position. The advantage of this technique is that the movement is continuous, but the disadvantage is that sometimes the light pressure can be uncomfortable to a ticklish subject.

A light effleurage movement may be used to begin massage, to spread oil and acclimatize the athlete to massage and assist in relaxation. In addition, the lightness of the touch helps the practitioner to feel altered areas of tissue tension which may be focused on later. As effleurage proceeds, the depth of the movement can increase, developing the superficial stroking action into deep longitudinal pressure.

Petrissage

Various petrissage movements are used (Fig. 3.2). In each case the hands maintain contact with the skin and do not glide over the skin surface except when progressing from one area to another. *Kneading* is a circular motion carried out by compressing the tissues against underlying structures. This may be performed with the flat of the hand, the heel of the hand, or the pads of the fingers and thumbs. The choice of contact area is dependent on the size of the body part being treated and the depth of the manipulation being carried out. Pressure is applied on the upward part of the circle, and released on the downward portion. At this point the hand is moved, lightly brushing over the skin surface to maintain contact.

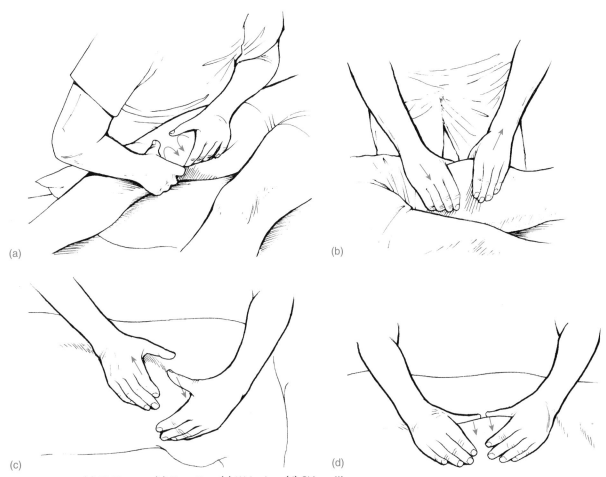

Figure 3.2 Petrissage. (a) Picking up. (b) Kneading. (c) Wringing. (d) Skin rolling.

Picking up is performed by compressing, then lifting and squeezing the tissues. The therapist's thumb and thenar eminence work against the medial two or three fingers to compress rather than pinch. The web between the thumb and first finger stays in contact with the skin so that the whole lateral portion of the hand surrounds the athlete's tissues. The action is more normally performed alternately, enabling the therapist's hands to recover between tissue compressions.

In a *wringing* movement, both hands pick the tissues up (see above), and then work against each other, pulling and pushing the tissues before they are released. The hands progress by gently 'walking' them up and down the body of the muscle. With large muscles, the fingertips face each other and the elbows are apart to create power through the transmission of body sway. The whole of the hand grips the tissues in this case. For smaller muscles, the grip is confined to the thumb and fingers alone. Now, the fingers face forwards and the elbows are held in, the movement coming from the elbows and wrists only.

With *rolling*, the skin is lifted away from the underlying tissues, and rolled between the thumbs and fingers of both hands. The technique is usually used on large body areas which have flat expanses of skin, for example the back,

abdomen and thigh. The flat of the hands are placed on the skin at a distance to the therapist. The hands are pulled towards the therapist to gather the skin up. As the skin bunches up, the thumbs press forwards and adduct to present their combined inner surfaces as a flat surface against the skin roll. Along the length of the spine, continuous skin rolling may be used. Again, the fingers feed the skin towards the approaching thumbs, but this time the fingers 'walk' along the skin surface to allow a continuous movement. The heels of the hands must be kept down on the skin surface to avoid the thumb tips 'digging in' as the hands move forwards.

> **Keypoint**
>
> When gripping the tissues for rolling and wringing, the flat surface of the fingers is used rather than the tips. This avoids the fingers 'digging in' painfully.

Muscle shaking is used within sports physiotherapy to reduce muscle tone and relax a muscle. This is useful following strenuous activity for example, or where muscle spasm is present due to pain. In addition, hypertonity due

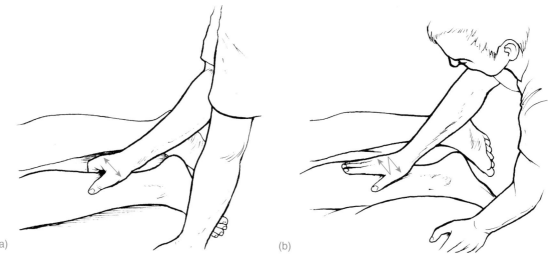

(a)

(b)

Figure 3.3   Vibration and shaking. (a) Vibration — applied locally. (b) Muscle shaking — flat of hand moves whole muscle belly.

to postural changes may be usefully reduced using shaking prior to proprioceptive neuromuscular facilitation (PNF) stretching procedures. The terms 'shaking' and 'vibration' are often used to describe very similar techniques. From the point of view of this book, shaking affects the whole of a structure (ribcage, limb or muscle) while vibration affects only part of the structure, having a more local effect (Fig. 3.3).

For shaking, the flat of the hand is used with slight pressure lightly gripping the muscle belly. As muscle resistance to palpation reduces, deeper pressure is used. Using shaking on a dependent muscle, for example the calf or hamstrings in crook lying, has the advantage that gravity pulls the muscle away from the bone, thus broadening the muscle. The practitioner has to exert less pressure therefore, to achieve a similar effect. *Vibration* differs from muscle shaking in that it is used locally with only the fingertips (singly or reinforced) transmitting the force. The effect is deeper and more focused than shaking with the force directed into, rather than along, the muscle. It is stimulatory in nature and may be used over trigger points, for example.

Frictional massage

With frictions, only the therapist's fingers or thumbs are used to give an accurate, deep, soft tissue manipulation (Fig. 3.4). The fingers should be held locked but not hyperextended. With small areas, the first and second fingers are used overlapping as one unit. Larger areas may require the use of all of the fingertips of one hand reinforced by the other hand. The friction may either be circular or transverse.

Circular frictions are normally used to break up thickened oedema, particularly around a joint. Three or four circular actions are used, gradually increasing in depth depending on patient tolerance. Pressure is released and the hand moved to another position before the friction is resumed.

Table 3.2   Aims of deep transverse frictions (DTF)

Produce therapeutic movement
Induce traumatic hyperaemia in chronic lesions
Give pain relief
Improve function

Deep transverse frictions

Deep transverse frictional massage (DTF) is a specific manipulation technique pioneered by Cyriax (1941). The aim of the technique (Table 3.2) is to move the tissues with a view to improving function, and to induce hyperaemia and pain relief (Kesson and Atkins, 1998). DTF involves a transverse sweeping movement of the connective tissues which aims to discourage cross-link formation between collagen fibres. By applying shear and gliding movements in this way, tensile strength of the healing scar may be improved and adhesions reduced. Gentle DTF applied in the acute phase of healing could increase the rate of phagocytosis by inducing agitation of tissue fluid. In the chronic stage of healing, the therapeutic movement produced by DTF is said to soften and mobilize adhesions (Kesson and Atkins, 1998) in preparation for later tissue mobilization.

Hyperaemia may be produced by DTF in the underlying tissues. Clinically, a red, raised area is seen on the skin as the technique is applied, and it is assumed that the same increase in regional blood flow occurs in the underlying tissues (Winter, 1968). The potential increase in the inflammatory response is required in chronic lesions but not in acute lesion. For this reason DTF, if used in the acute phase of injury, must be gentle and given over a shorter period to avoid hyperaemia production.

The pain reduction seen with DTF may result from the massage acting as a noxious stimulus (counter-irritant)

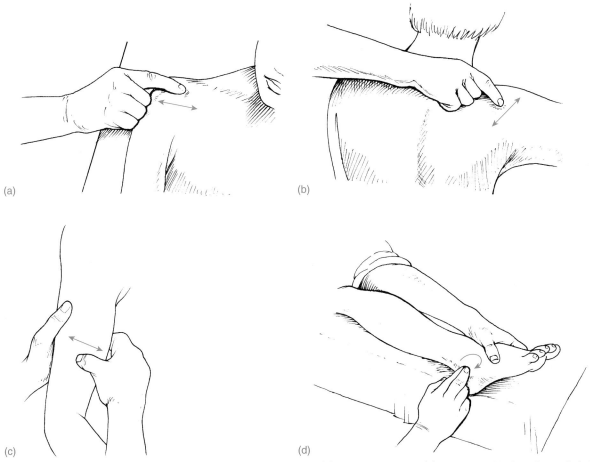

Figure 3.4   Frictional massage. (a) Deep transverse friction – single finger. (b) Reinforced finger. (c) Transverse friction of muscle belly. (d) Circular friction to break up oedema.

Treatment note 3.1   Saving your hands

Massage and manual therapy are powerful techniques; however, by their very nature they can cause considerable stress to the therapist's hands. One study has shown that manual therapists are 3.5 times more likely to develop pain in the wrists and hands compared to non-manual therapists (Bork et al., 1996). Another study showed that therapists who used manual therapy were 7.7 times more likely to develop thumb pain and 4.0 times more likely to report wrist pain. Clearly this is an 'at risk' area and anything which can be done to reduce this risk is important.

Hyperextending finger joints

Many people have hyperextending finger joints (Fig. 3.5), meaning that, as they place pressure with the pad of their finger or thumb, the terminal digit is unstable and the joint extends further than normal, stressing both the ligaments and the muscles in the finger. In order to prevent this, both deep transverse frictional massage (p. 64) and joint

mobilization techniques should be carried out with other parts of the hand.

Mobilization procedures can be carried out using the pisiform bone of the hand (Fig. 3.6). This small bone has approximately the same area as the thumb, and pressure can be placed through the straight wrist and carpel bones directly on to the pisiform itself. Where this area is too large, a plunger (Fig. 3.7) can be used. These come with a variety of different sized heads to correspond to different treatment areas.

For transverse frictional massage, the elbow may be used on large joints (Fig. 3.8). Because the elbow has a tendency to slip, it should be supported using the web of the finger and thumb of the opposite hand. Where direct digital pressure is needed over a period of time, for example deactivating trigger points deep within a muscle, a 'knobber' is useful (Fig. 3.9). This is a plastic device with a variety of different shaped balls on the end which can be used for greater or lesser pressure. These can be easily held in the

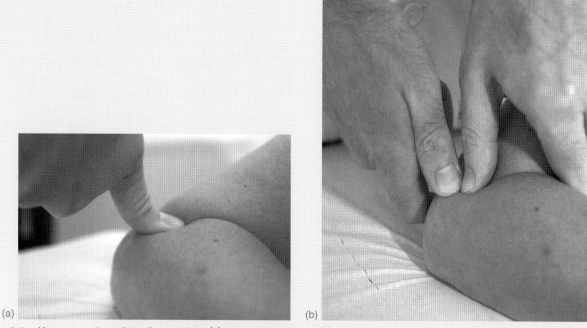

Figure 3.5   Hyperextension of the finger joints. (a) Hyperextended and (b) corrected.

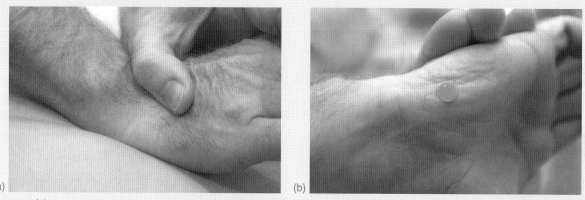

Figure 3.6   (a) Use of pisiform bone to transmit pressure. (b) Contact area on pisiform.

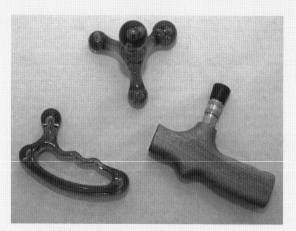

Figure 3.7   Various plungers used in massage.

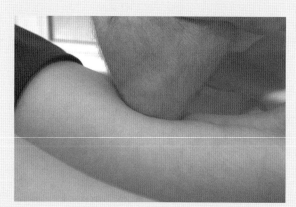

Figure 3.8   Use of the elbow for deep transverse frictions (DTF).

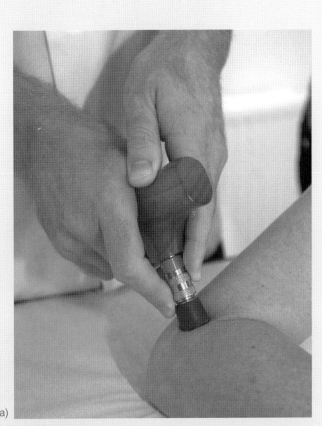

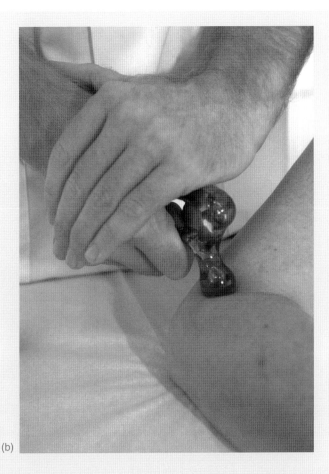

(a)

(b)

Figure 3.9   Using a plunger.

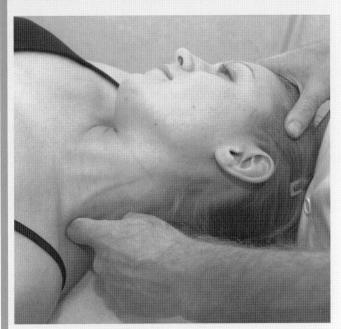

Figure 3.10   Use of knuckles for direct pressure.

hand to provide direct pressure to the trigger point. As an alternative, either a single knuckle or two knuckles may be used to provide greater or lesser pressure (Fig. 3.10).

Strain on the flexed wrist

Tendons around the wrist can become inflamed if the wrist is held in a flexed or adducted position for a long time. Where joint distraction movements are used (Fig. 3.11) it is important to pull through a straight angle of the wrist with the carpals and radius and ulna in line rather than flexed. This will ensure that the tendon sheath is not stretched and therefore compressed against the tendon itself. In addition, when using the thumb for manual therapy, again it is important that the wrist is in its neutral position and you avoid stretching the thumb tendons over the radial styloid.

As a general guide, the practitioner's elbow should be kept tucked into the side of the body, the wrist should be in line with the radius and ulna, and the finger tendons should be as relaxed as possible. In addition, exercises to warm up the hands and fingers should be performed before starting clinic sessions, aiming to take the wrist and finger joints to their full range of motion in each direction, maintaining the stretch position for 20–30 seconds.

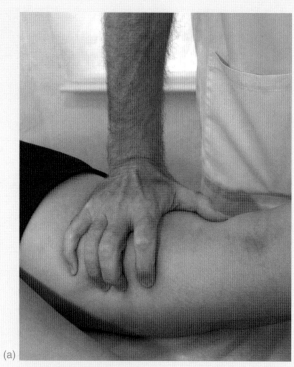 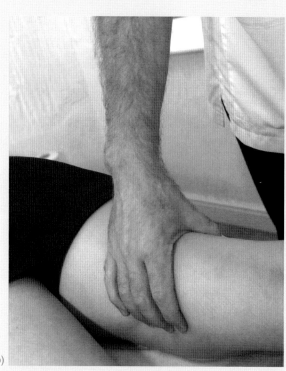

Figure 3.11   Avoiding stress on the wrist and hand. (a) Poor wrist and hand alignment. (b) Corrected.

through mechanoreceptor activity. This would explain why DTF used aggressively gives better pain reduction than DTF given lightly, as the more aggressive approach will cause greater mechanoreceptor stimulation, which has been shown to increase pain suppression (Bowsher, 1988). Pain relief seen clinically is often fairly long-lasting, and a study by de Bruijn (1984) showed pain relief for up to 48 hours following DTF of 5 minutes maximum.

Restoration of function is often the most striking effect of DTF. On reassessment, range of motion is usually significantly increased and muscle contraction more easily performed. Kelly (1997) confirmed this in a study looking at 46 subjects who showed an increase in force of muscle contraction and an increased range of dorsiflexion after DTF of the gastrocnemius muscle.

DTF technique

DTF is performed with the skin of the patient and the finger(s) of the therapist acting as a single unit. A number of hand positions may be used to maximize the force applied to the tissues but minimize the stress imposed on the practitioner's hands (Fig. 3.12). The action demands great anatomical accuracy and must be of sufficient depth and sweep to affect the desired tissues. The point at which the DTF is applied corresponds to the lesion in the tissues rather than the painful point, as pain is often referred away from the original site of injury.

> **Keypoint**
>
> With DTF the practitioner's fingers and the patient's skin move as one unit. The fingers must not glide over the skin surface.

Tendons are generally frictioned in a stretched position, with the lesion often lying at the teno-osseous junction. Tendons in a sheath are again placed on stretch with the aim of rolling the sheath around the tendon as the DTF is given. Muscles are treated in relaxed inner range, to facilitate broadening and separation of the muscle fibres in an imitation of normal function. Ligaments are placed under slight stretch to allow the practitioner's fingers access to the lesion.

Transverse frictions to the Achilles tendon are shown on page 264, to the shoulder tendons on page 386, and to the elbow on page 415.

Tapotement

The percussive movements may be used to stimulate, or for evacuation of a hollow cavity. Percussion for evacuation, such as that used in chest physiotherapy, is not within the context of this book.

For stimulating tapotement the hands are relaxed, and follow each other in a succession of alternating movements.

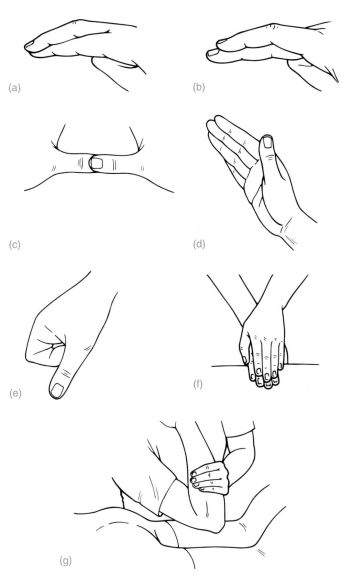

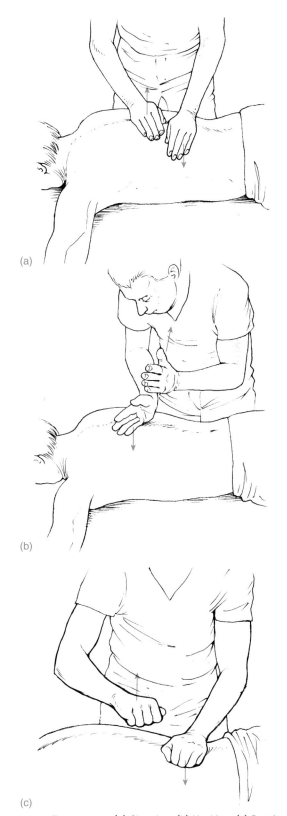

Figure 3.12 Hand positions for deep transverse frictions (DTF). Modified from Kesson and Atkins (1998). (a) Single finger. (b) Reinforced finger. (c) Reinforced thumb. (d) Knife edge of the hand. (e) Single knuckle. (f) Reinforced finger pads. (g) Elbow.

With clapping, the wrists are flail and the cupped hand strikes the body creating a hollow (rather than slapping) sound. Hacking involves striking the skin with either the ulnar border of the hand (severe) or the back of the tips of the fingers by using a pronation/supination movement of the forearm (mild). Beating or pounding is performed with the ulnar border of the semi-closed fist and tapping with the fingertips. The percussion techniques are used over bulky muscle areas but must avoid bony areas (spine of the scapula, patella) as these will be painful if struck (Fig. 3.13).

Figure 3.13 Tapotement. (a) Clapping. (b) Hacking. (c) Beating.

Massage medium

Massage can require both slip (lubrication) and grip (friction), depending on the particular technique being performed. Grip media include talc or corn starch, while lubricants may be oils, creams or lotions. Where one technique progresses onto another, practitioners may often find themselves wanting

Table 3.3 Function of media used in massage

Lubricant (slip)	Friction medium (grip)
Reduces friction on the skin	Massage technique can be more deeply applied
Protects skin from abrasion	
Protects hairy skin from being pulled	Skin and hand move as one unit
Some oils (e.g. wheatgerm) may be nutrient to the skin	Tissue more accurately manipulated
Enhances gliding techniques	Powder will absorb perspiration
Perfumed oil may have a beneficial psychological effect on the patient	
Essential oils have a medicinal effect	

Sources Holey and Cook (1997) and Kesson and Atkins (1998) with permission.

one medium while using another. The functions of grip and slip media are shown in Table 3.3. It must be noted, when using oil, that patients may be allergic to nuts and suffer anaphylactic shock. Peanuts are the most common nut allergen with approximately 1 in 500 of the population affected (Demain, 1996). Traditionally used arachis oil is derived from peanuts, and oils such as almond are obviously nut based.

Clinical note

Anaphylactic shock can present as respiratory distress, hypotension, oedema, rash, tachycardia, pale clammy skin and sometimes convulsions and cyanosis. It can be life-threatening if oedema affects the larynx as airflow is obstructed.

Vegetable oils are absorbed into the skin, whereas mineral oils remain on the skin surface to create a 'sheen' or skin gloss. Vegetable oils may therefore be used as carriers for essential oils and can have a nutrient effect on the skin. Mineral oils, because they remain on the skin surface, maintain their lubrication properties and last longer. Some vegetable oils may be thick and viscous, feeling tacky to the touch. In addition, vegetable oils have a shorter shelf-life and will go rancid (oxidize) when exposed to the air.

PRACTICAL APPLICATION OF TECHNIQUES

The lower limb

Posterior thigh

Massage to the posterior aspect of the leg begins with the athlete lying prone with the knee slightly flexed to take the stretch off the popliteal structures. The shin is supported by a rolled towel. A towel is placed over both legs, and folded

back to reveal the leg to be massaged. The towel covers the leg again to maintain body heat once leg massage has finished, and the other leg is uncovered and massaged in turn. Where swelling is the main concern, the massage procedures begin in the upper leg to clear the lymphatic vessels here before fluid is pushed into them by lower leg massage. Effleurage begins the movement. A skin inspection is carried out. Cuts are either protected by waterproof taping, or the practitioner must wear protective gloves. Where a skin lesion is large, massage should not proceed directly over the area. A small amount of gel or cream is placed on the practitioner's hand and warmed, through friction, before application.

Where increased muscle tone is detected, muscle shaking is used to aid relaxation. The palm may be placed across the fibres of the muscle with the shaking movement perpendicular to the leg (transverse shaking). Alternatively, with a smaller limb, the hand may grip the muscle belly with the fingers parallel to the muscle fibres (longitudinal shaking). The palm contact for the shaking procedure causes the whole muscle to vibrate, and the effect is general. Where a more local effect is required, the fingertips are used, rather than the palm, in a 'claw hand' contact for local vibration. The action is now directed downwards into the depth of the muscle rather than along its length.

The effleurage stroke begins over the popliteal fossa and proceeds up the centre of the thigh to the buttock crease. The second stroke is medial, and the third stroke is lateral, both ending at the buttock crease.

Petrissage strokes begin with palmar kneading, one hand reinforcing the other, and is carried out over the bulky middle area of the hamstrings. Picking up is used over the length of the muscle, with wringing and rolling used over the muscle bellies. In each case, the tissue manipulation begins just above the popliteal fossa and proceeds centrally, medially and laterally, the number of 'muscle strips' depending on the size of the athlete's leg.

Local massage to the adductors may be given with the athlete supine and the hip flexed, abducted and externally rotated. The knee then rests on a folded pillow or the therapist's pelvic rim, with the far hand stabilizing the knee. Alternatively, half crook side lying may be chosen (Fig. 3.14). The near hand begins the massage with effleurage and shaking, moving from the medial epicondyle of the knee to the groin. Palmar kneading and picking up are used, followed by deep effleurage along the length of the adductor fibres using the thumb pad. Transverse frictions, if required, may be given by altering the hand so that the dominant hand lies perpendicular to the thigh. Flicking, using the ulnar borders of the hands in a rapid alternating action, is the most appropriate percussion technique. Hacking can be painful due to the fusiform nature of the muscle, while clapping tends to be better carried out with the athlete in side lying (see below). The massage finishes with effleurage, and the athlete's position lends itself well to the use of passive stretching techniques, including contract–relax (see p. 102) for the short adductors. An alternative starting position, which allows the

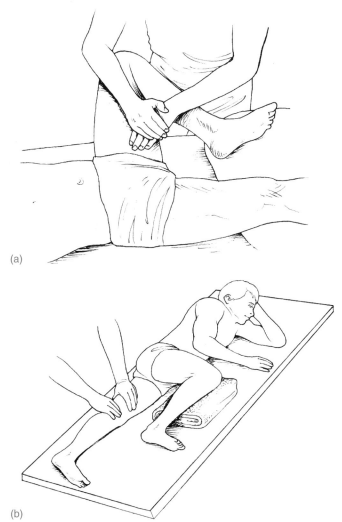

(a)

(b)

Figure 3.14 Treating the adductors. (a) Thigh rests on therapist's pelvis. (b) Bent upper leg rests on rolled towel.

application of more pressure, is half crook side lying with the affected leg extended on the couch. The unaffected leg lies forwards with the hip and knee flexed and the knee supported on a pillow to prevent pelvic and spinal rotation.

Calf and Achilles

The calf area is treated after the posterior thigh in cases of general massage where swelling is the major concern. The shin is supported on a folded towel, or the leg being treated may be hooked over the other leg. Effleurage and muscle shaking are used to begin the treatment. Superficial strokes are applied longitudinally from Achilles to knee with the hands working side by side or one hand resting over the other, depending on limb size. The stroking movement is localized by using the thumb pads placed side by side, with the movement directed along the muscle fibres (Fig. 3.15). Kneading is given to the muscle bellies only, with picking up and muscle rolling being especially useful in cases of consolidated oedema. Circular frictions are applied along each

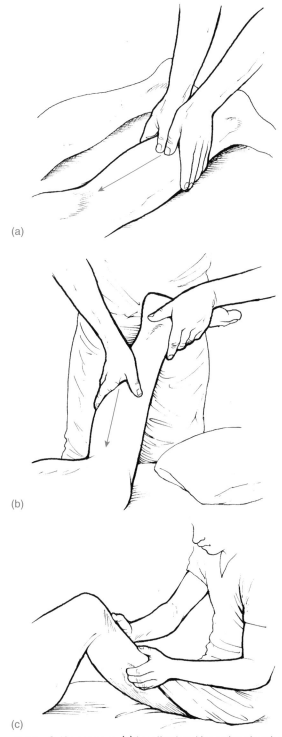

(a)

(b)

(c)

Figure 3.15 Calf treatment. (a) Localized stoking using thumb pads. (b) Effleurage using thumb web. (c) Massage of the peronei.

side of the Achilles tendon. This may be applied with one finger supporting the other or using a light pinch grip massaging both sides of the Achilles at once.

An alternative starting position is with the knee held flexed by the therapist's hand while the other hand supplies the effleurage stroke, with the web of the hand. The calf is then massaged in two or three sections, depending on size. Where more pressure must be exerted, crook lying is the position of choice. The therapist sits on the couch and supports the athlete's foot against his or her thigh. Effleurage is given with one cupped hand over the other. The therapist can lean back to exert more pressure. Local stroking is then applied with the fingertips rather than the thumbs. In the crook lying position, the edge of tibialis posterior and the peronei may be massaged using either the fingertips or the thumb, with the rest of the fingers stabilizing the hand.

Anterior thigh

Massage to the anterior thigh proceeds in a similar order to that of the posterior thigh. Less direct pressure is used due to the reduced muscle bulk, and percussion movements are rarely used. Finger kneading may be used effectively around the patella especially over the suprapatellar pouch in the case of local pooling of oedema within this area. Kneading is probably the most useful procedure over the quadriceps because of the ease with which the muscle bellies are picked up.

Shin

Massage is only applied to the peronei over the lateral aspect of the shin due to the lack of muscle over the medial tibia. The size of the lateral compartment dictates that the whole hand cannot be used. Effleurage is applied with the thumbs held side by side or with the fingers, with the thumb stabilizing the hand. Alternatively, the hypothenar eminence may be used in larger subjects.

The back

Lower back

The subject is in the prone lying position with a rolled towel beneath the shins to flex the knees and take the stretch off the sciatic nerve. If the lordosis is very deep, some subjects find it more comfortable to have a folded towel placed beneath the abdomen. Massage to the back may be given in any direction, and the practitioner does not need to work 'distal to proximal', as with the limbs. The massage begins with effleurage from the posterior iliac crest to the scapula (Fig. 3.16). The fingers follow the line of the erector spinae muscle fibres and cover the back in two or three sections, depending on the athlete's size. Lateral effleurage (lateralizing) then follows, from the spine around the trunk to the abdomen. Kneading with the palms and heels of the hands begins at the inferior angles of the scapulae and works down towards the sacrum with alternating pressure movements of the hands. The line follows the line of the erector spinae. Both kneading and picking up may be used over the quadratus lumborum. Transverse kneading may be used across the erector spinae with the fingertips pulling towards the therapist and the sides of the thumbs pushing away. Local finger

stroking is used with the thumbs pressing together, and finger kneading is performed with the pads of the fingers along the length of the erector spinae, across the posterior rim of the pelvis, and along the posterior aspect of the lower ribs. Skin rolling is used from the ilium to the scapula and transversely around the circumference of the lower trunk.

Fascial stretching may be used to good effect in the lower spine. The forearms are crossed and the hands are placed flat over the back. The practitioner leans forwards and down exerting pressure and pressing the hands apart to impart and stretch on the lumbar fascia. The hand must not slide over the skin surface as this will cause painful friction: the skin and hand move as one unit.

The lower back massage finishes with effleurage and light finger stroking movements to aid relaxation.

Upper back

When applying upper back massage, the therapist stands at the couch side and later changes position to the head of the couch facing caudally (Fig. 3.17). Effleurage begins over the trapezius in a diamond shape, from the inferior angle of the scapula to the occiput, out to the acromion and down to the inferior angle once more. Kneading with the heel of the hand is used from the occiput to lower scapula. Petrissage is especially useful over the middle fibres of trapezius, with ringing and rolling both appropriate techniques. Kneading, using the pads of the fingers, is useful along the length of the cervical extensors and to the rhomboids and levator scapulae. If the shoulder is internally rotated (hand behind the back), the medial border of the scapula can be lifted from the ribcage and the side of the therapist's hand can be used to massage beneath the undersurface of the scapula (serratus anterior and subscapularis muscles). Hacking, clapping and flicking actions are used over the middle trapezius fibres only, the superficial bony surfaces making these techniques inappropriate over the scapula and upper spines.

The therapist then transfers to the head of the couch. Kneading and pressure techniques to the middle fibres of trapezius are more effective from this position. In addition, finger kneading and friction may be carried out to the occiput. Where massage is required to the upper cervical and sub-occipital regions only, the athlete may be positioned supine, lying with the head supported on a folded towel. The therapist sits at the head end of the couch and uses finger kneading and friction to the sub-occipital tissues. From this position, passive stretching techniques for the upper trapezius and levator scapulae may then be carried out.

The upper limb

Shoulder and upper arm

Arm and shoulder massage may be carried out in either sitting or supine positions (Fig. 3.18). When sitting, the athlete's arm is supported on a small table, or if lying, the arm

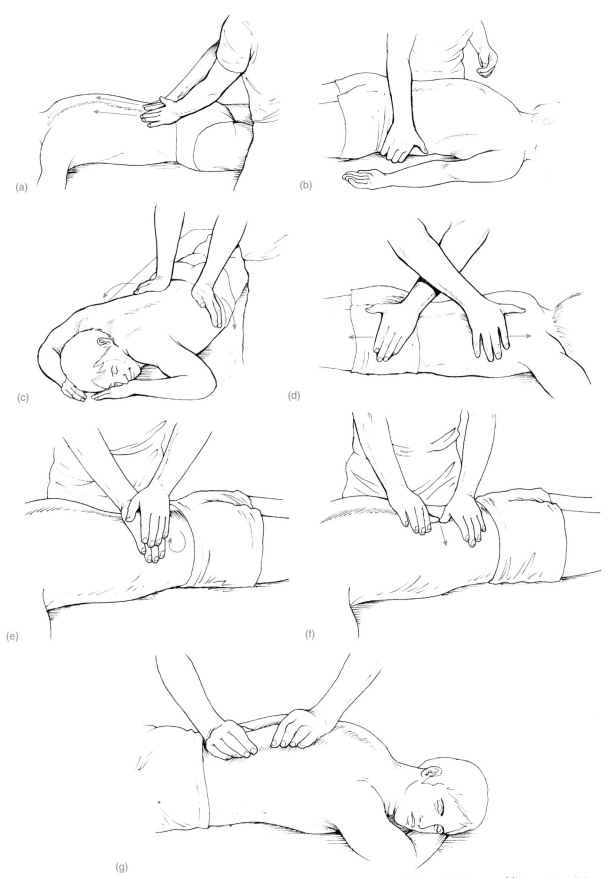

Figure 3.16   Lower back massage. (a) Effleurage following the line of the erector spinae. (b) Lateral effleurage. (c) Deep lateralizing.
(d) Fascial stretch. (e) Kneading. (f) Transverse kneading. (g) Skin rolling.

Figure 3.17 Upper back massage. (a,b) For upper back massage the therapist stands at the couch side and later changes to the head end. (c) Kneading the middle fibres of trapezius. (d) With the shoulder internally rotated the medial border of the scapula is lifted. (e) Massage to the upper trapezius. (f) Suboccipital techniques.

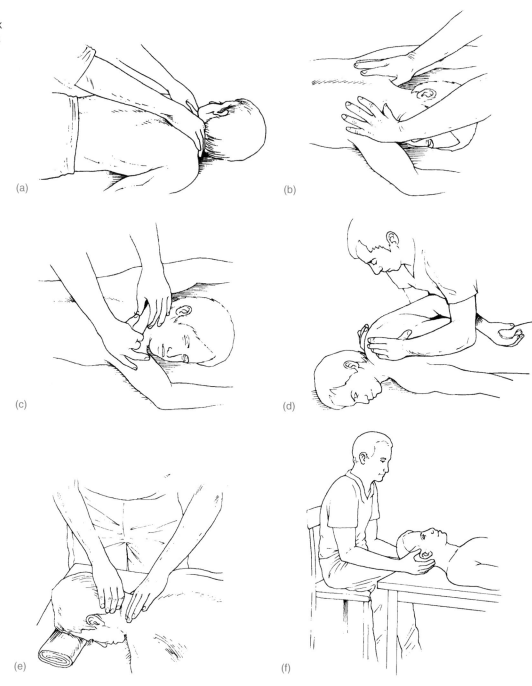

is supported on a pillow or folded towel. Alternatively, the arm may be usefully supported across the therapist's leg (covered by a folded towel) for certain upper arm and shoulder procedures. The treatment begins with effleurage, the therapist holding the athlete's hand for limb stability. The therapist anchors the athlete's near hand. The palm of the therapist's far hand rests over the extensor aspect of the athlete's hand to begin the effleurage stroke. The movement begins distally, with the therapist's far hand moving from the athlete's fifth finger along the ulnar aspect of the forearm, across the under edge of the upper arm to end at the axilla. For the second stroke, the athlete's forearm is moved

into mid-pronation. The action begins at the back of the athlete's hand and covers the radial side of the forearm and side of the upper arm, to again end at the axilla. For the flexor aspect of the arm, the therapist changes hands so that the near hand carries out the massage stroke. The movement begins at the thumb, and glides along the radial side of the forearm and anterior aspect of the upper arm to the axilla. The next stroke begins over the athlete's palm, and proceeds over the flexor aspect of the forearm and inner edge of the upper arm to the axilla. The last effleurage stroke begins on the flexor aspect of the fifth finger and moves across the inner edge of the forearm and upper arm to the inner axilla.

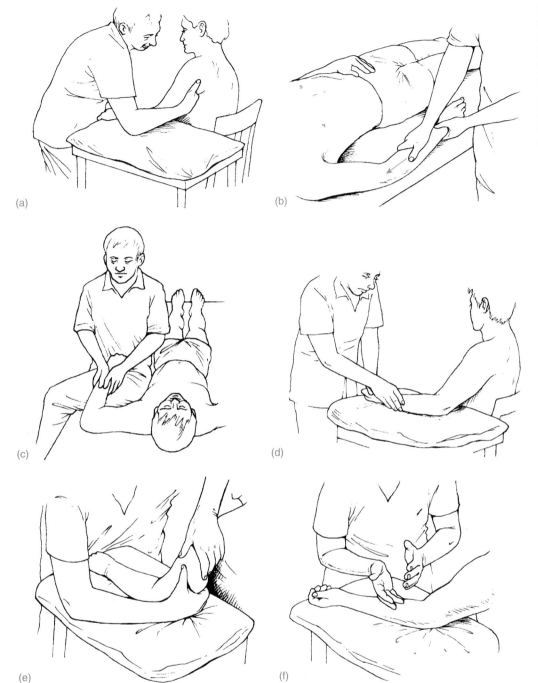

Figure 3.18 Massage of the shoulder and upper arm. (a) Arm supported on table in sitting. (b) Supine lying. (c) Using the therapist's leg for support. (d) Effleurage using the thumb web. (e) Wringing the triceps. (f) Hacking the flexor aspect of the forearm.

(a)

(b)

(c)

(d)

(e)

(f)

Muscle shaking is performed using the same single-handed grip as effleurage. The deltoid and triceps are shaken using the outer hand, while the biceps is shaken using the inner hand. In each case the other hand holds the athlete's hand to stabilize the arm.

Kneading begins with the hands placed on the anterior and posterior aspects of the deltoid. The hands press together, compressing the shoulder, and work alternately in circular motions. The alternate movement continues down the length of the upper arm with the hands gripping biceps and triceps, and moving around the arm slightly to cover the flexor and extensor aspects of the forearm. Each hand

moves along the skin only as the compression pressure is released. Thumb kneading may be used for the forearm, with the thumbs lying side by side. The pressure is transmitted with the length of the distal phalanx rather than the tip ('along' rather than 'in').

Picking up and muscle rolling may be performed single-handed or with both hands alternately. The single-handed action maintains the grip on the athlete's hand (or elbow in the case of shoulder treatment) for stability. The therapist's outer hand is used for procedures on the posterior deltoid, triceps and forearm extensors, the inner hand for the anterior deltoid, biceps and forearm flexors. Double-handed actions are used for the middle fibres of the deltoid following on from kneading for the upper fibres of trapezius (see above). The thumb and finger grip must avoid placing pressure over the acromion.

Wringing is used over the bellies of the biceps and triceps. In the case of the biceps, the therapist stands in front of the athlete with the hands over the anterior position of the arm and the fingers placed medially. For the triceps, the hands cup the posterior portion of the arm, again with the fingers medially placed. The wringing action is carried out using the cupped hands in opposition. The forearm flexors are wrung using the thumb pads in opposition to the pads of the index and ring fingers.

Percussion techniques are performed first on the flexor aspect of the whole arm with the forearm supinated, and then on the extensor aspect with the forearm pronated. For the extensor aspect the therapist stands level with the athlete's waist and faces the head. With the athlete's forearm pronated, the action works from the posterior axilla and posterior deltoid across the triceps and then to the forearm extensors. For the flexor aspect, the therapist changes position to stand above the athlete's arm facing the feet. The athlete's forearm is supinated and the action begins at the medial axilla, and works down the front of the deltoid, over the biceps and across the forearm flexors. The therapist must take care to avoid contact with bony prominences and superficial tendons at the shoulder and elbow.

Foot massage

Foot massage (Fig. 3.19) may be used following an injury where swelling and scar tissue are present. In addition, foot massage is particularly beneficial as an aid to relaxation. Reflexology is a specialized form of foot massage not covered in this book.

Foot massage is often combined with passive joint movement (physiological and accessory), because the joints of the foot often become stiff through the use of constricting footwear. The reader is referred to Maitland (1991) and Kaltenborn (1989) for details of the techniques.

Effleurage is given by starting with the therapist's hands cupping the athlete's foot, with the fingers resting medially. Initially, both hands move from the toes to the ankle. As the action becomes firmer, one hand remains stationary to support the foot while the other carries out the massage stroke. General kneading is carried out with one hand holding the toes and the other imparting pressure through the hypothenar eminence. More specific finger kneading and circular frictions are used for the interossei. Firm digital pressure is used over the sole of the foot with the thumb pads or single knuckle. Light percussion techniques (finger tapping) are used only over the medial longitudinal arch with the foot supported in slight plantarflexion. A stretching action is used for the metatarsals. The hands surround the foot, with the thumbs on the plantar surface and the fingertips coming together on the dorsal surface. The action is to press the thumbs into the plantar surface of the metatarsal heads and pull the neighbouring metatarsal bones down with the fingers. Slow passive movements are then used to fully stretch the tissues. Each toe is tractioned in turn, and flexion, extension, abduction and adduction are used for each of the metatarsal phalangeal (MTP) joints. Circular frictions and finger kneading are used around the malleoli, and to each side of the Achilles tendon.

EFFECTS OF MASSAGE

Effects of massage are achieved through mechanical, physiological and psychological processes, and the interrelation between these three. Compression and squeezing will improve venous and lymphatic drainage, visible when superficial vessels are massaged (Hollis, 1987). Interstitial pressure is increased and fluid absorbtion aided. Fresh blood will enter the area. The superficial skin response to vigorous massage is an axon reflex. Redness results (flare) through dilatation of skin arterioles and slight swelling (wheal) occurs through increased permeability of the capillary wall, allowing tissue fluid to escape into the surrounding area. The deep response to vigorous massage, however, can be a reduction in blood flow, if muscle tone is increased and blood flow through the muscle reduces as a consequence.

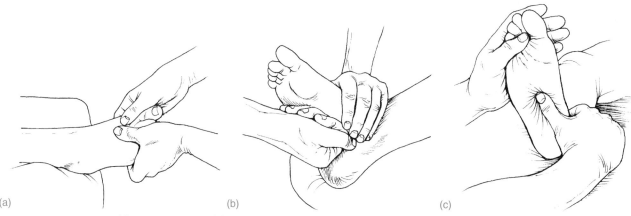

Figure 3.19   Foot massage. (a) Finger kneading. (b) Plantar kneading using the knuckles. (c) Deep digital pressure of the sole.

Treatment note 3.2 Trigger points

Trigger points (myofascial trigger points) are highly sensitive local areas which often lie within a tight band of the muscle fibres. In general, trigger points (TrP) can cause pain in a muscle at rest, or, particularly, when a muscle is placed on stretch. Because the TrP is painful when the muscle is placed on stretch, it prevents the muscle from lengthening and so can alter body alignment (see Muscle imbalance, Ch. 6).

TrPs are painful to palpation and often appear as nodules or tight bands within the muscle itself. Sudden pressure or flicking the fingers across the band can cause the muscle to jump, a reaction known as the 'twitch response' or 'jump sign'.

Some trigger points lie over traditional acupuncture points, while others are simply within the muscle.

A TrP may either be *active* or *latent*. A latent TrP does not cause pain at rest, but only when it is palpated. Although not painful, the muscle that the TrP is associated with can still be shortened and restrict movement. An active TrP causes both pain and tenderness at rest or when the muscle is stretched during daily activities. Palpation of an active TrP causes pain and referral of the pain in a pattern which mimics the patient's main symptoms.

TrPs may be located within the belly of a muscle (*central TrP*) or at the muscle attachment (*attachment TrP*). In the case of the latter, a TrP may be found at both the teno-osseous and musculotendinous junctions where the muscle attaches to bone, tendon or aponeurosis (sheet of tendon).

A number of theories have been proposed for TrP activation, including damage to the muscle sarcolemma resulting in an alteration to the muscle contraction threshold, local muscle ischaemia, and an alteration in the release of acetylcholine from the motor end plate.

Massage treatment of trigger points (TrPs)

TrPs may be treated through a number of mechanisms (see Table 6.5, p. 147), including several massage techniques, dry needling and stretching.

Ischaemic compression

In this technique, pressure is applied slowly and progressively to the TrP (sudden pressure can stimulate the TrP). The pressure is maintained until the tenderness to palpation has reduced and the end-feel of the tissue changes from a hard elastic recoil to a softer resistance. As this occurs, a slow continuous stretch may be placed on the muscle to lengthen it.

Ischaemic compression relies on heavy pressure from the practitioner and either the thumbs or supportive finger (see Treatment note 3.1 may be used, or several mechanical devices are available (Fig. 3.20).

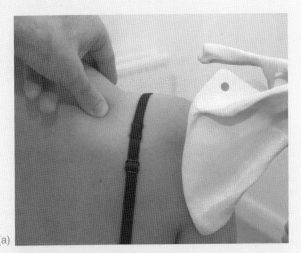

(a)

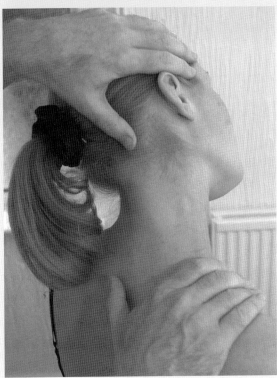

(b)

Figure 3.20   Ischaemic pressure and muscle stripping.

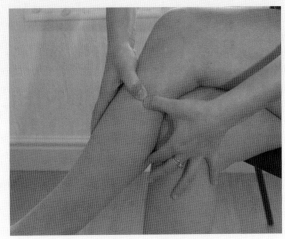

Figure 3.21   Self-treatment using the hands.

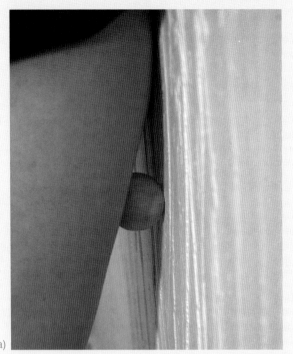
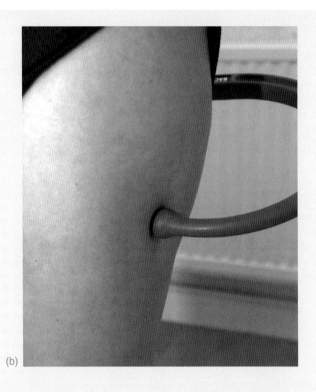

(a)
(b)

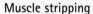
Figure 3.22   Self-treatment using pressure from a ball or plunger.

Muscle stripping

This is a deep stroking massage applied with minimal lubrication to the skin to prevent friction only. Firm pressure is used along the length of the taut band at a rate of approximately 2–3 cm every 3 seconds. The direction should be distal to proximal, creating a 'milking movement' and causing a reflex hyperaemia that returns the muscle site to its normal condition.

Self techniques

Athletes may be taught to compress TrPs using a small rubber ball (squash ball or tennis ball) or their fingers. Fingers can provide direct pressure (Fig. 3.21), while the athlete may lean on the ball with the ball paced between themselves and the floor or wall (Fig. 3.22).

Deep stroking and kneading of the calf for a 10-minute period has been shown to increase blood volume for 40 minutes (Bell, 1964), and blood pressure has been shown to reduce following back massage (Barr and Taslitz, 1970). Intradermal dye injections have been used to show lymph flow improvements with massage (McMaster, 1937), and massage has been shown to be significantly better at improving lymph flow compared to electrical stimulation and passive movements (Ladd, Kottke and Blanchard, 1952).

A decrease in the viscosity of both blood and plasma has been shown following a 20-minute whole body massage (Ernst et al., 1987). Studies of muscle tone using the Hoffman (H) reflex, have shown a decrease in H reflex amplitude during, but not following, massage (Morelli, Seabourn and Sullivan, 1990; Sullivan et al., 1991).

Short-term pain relief, particularly through friction massage, is thought to be brought about by the closure of the pain gate and stimulation of endogenous opioids (Cyriax, 1980). In contrast, gentler techniques do not appear to give this response. No significant change has been shown in beta endorphin or beta lipotrophin levels on pain-free subjects using effleurage and petrissage of the back over a 30-minute period (Day, Mason and Chesrown, 1987).

Massage has been found superior to relaxation therapy in the treatment of fibromyalgia (Sunshine et al., 1996). Two 30-minute massage periods were given weekly over a 5-week period and the significant changes included an increased number of sleep hours and a reduction in substance P, pain rating and number of tender points.

One of the greatest benefits from massage seems to be psychological, with increased feelings of wellbeing and decreased arousal levels (Longworth, 1982; Hemmings, 2001). Massage has been shown to improve mood state in a group of amateur boxers during intensive training (Hemmings, 2000) and perceived recovery following athletic training and competitive performance (Hemmings et al., 2000). Pre-competition sports massage has been shown to produce a positive response, with athletes able to cope better with physical exertion (Harmer, 1991).

Tissues are mobilized as they are moved over each other, and adhesions stretched with more forceful actions. Massage has been shown to aid recuperation from muscle fatigue (Balke, Anthony and Wyatt, 1989), and is commonly used both before and after exercise with this in view. Sports massage has been shown to be effective at reducing delayed onset muscle soreness (DOMS) when it is applied within 2 hours of eccentric exercise (Smith et al., 1994). Creatine kinase (CK) levels were reduced, and a slight increase in both neutrophil emigration and cortisol levels was noted. Stimulatory massage, however, may have the reverse effect. CK and lactate dehydrogenase (LDH) have been shown to increase significantly following vigorous whole body massage, possibly illustrating mechanical trauma to the muscles, with resultant increased cell membrane activity (Arkko, Pakarinen and Kari-Koskinen, 1983). Tissue damage of this type has been used to argue the case for rigorous training for therapists applying massage to athletes (Callaghan, 1993).

Stimulatory mechanical massage has been shown to be ineffective at increasing blood flow and aiding recovery (Carafelli et al., 1990). This type of massage can cause muscle contraction through the initiation of a tonic vibration reflex, and will therefore reduce blood perfusion through the muscle.

References

Arkko, P.J., Pakarinen, A.J. and Kari-Koskinen, O. (1983) Effects of whole body massage on serum protein and hormone concentrations, enzyme activities and haematological parameters. *International Journal of Sports Medicine*, **4**, 265–267

Balke, B., Anthony, J. and Wyatt, F. (1989) The effects of massage treatment on exercise fatigue. *Clinical Sports Medicine*, **1**, 189–196

Barr, J.S. and Taslitz, N. (1970) Influence of back massage on autonomic functions. *Physical Therapy*, **50**, 1679–1691

Bell, A.J. (1964) Massage and the physiotherapist. *Physiotherapy*, **50**, 406–408

Bork, B., Cook, T.M., Rosecrance, J. and Engelhardt, K. (1996) Work related musculoskeletal disorders among physical therapists. *Physical Therapy*, **76**, 827–835

Bowsher, D. (1988) Modulation of nociceptive input. In *Pain Management by Physiotherapy*, 2nd edn (eds P.E. Wells, V. Frampton, and D. Bowsher). Butterworth-Heinemann, Oxford

Callaghan, M.J. (1993) The role of massage in the management of the athlete: a review. *British Journal of Sports Medicine*, **27**, (1) 28–33

Carafelli, E., Sim, J., Carolan, B. and Libesman, J. (1990) Vibratory massage and short term recovery from muscular fatigue. *International Journal of Sports Medicine*, **11**, 474–478

Copestake, B.M.G. (1917) *The Theory and Practice of Massage and Medical Gymnastics*. H.K. Lewis, London

Cromie, J., Robertson, V. and Best, M. (2000) Work related musculoskeletal disorders in physical therapists. *Physical Therapy*, **80**, (4) 336–351

Cyriax, J. (1941) *Massage, Manipulation and Local Anaesthesia*. Hamilton, London

Cyriax, J. (1980) *Textbook of Orthopaedic Medicine*, 10th edn. Baillière Tindall, London

Day, J.A., Mason, R.R. and Chesrown, S.E. (1987) Effect of massage on serum level of B-endorphin and B-lipotrophin in healthy adults. *Physical Therapy*, **67**, 926–930

de Bruijn, R. (1984) Deep transverse friction: its analgesic effect. *International Journal of Sports Medicine*, **5**, 35–36

Demain, S. (1996) Departmental danger of death. *Physiotherapy*, **82**, (1) 71

Ernst, E., Matrai, A., Magyarosy, I., Liebermeister, R.G.A., Eck, M. and Breu, M.C. (1987) Massages cause changes in blood fluidity. *Physiotherapy*, **73**, 43–45

Harmer, P.A. (1991) The effect of pre-performance massage on stride frequency in sprinters. *Athletic Training. Journal of the National Athletic Training Association of America*, **26**, 55–59

Hemmings, B. (2000) Sports massage and psychological regeneration. *British Journal of Therapy and Rehabilitation*, **7**, 425–429

Hemmings, B., Smith, M., Graydon, J. and Dyson, R. (2000) The effects of massage on physiological restoration, perceived recovery and repeated sports performance. *British Journal of Sports Medicine*, **34**, 109–115

Hemmings, B.J. (2001) Physiological, psychological and performance effects of massage therapy in sport: a review of the literature. *Physical Therapy in Sport*, **2**, (4) 165–170

Holey, E.A. and Cook, E.M. (1997) *Therapeutic Massage*. Butterworth-Heinemann, Oxford

Hollis, M. (1987) *Massage for Therapists*. Blackwell Scientific Publications, Oxford

Kaltenborn, F.M. (1989) *Manual Mobilization of the Extremity Joints*. Olaf Norlis Bokhandel, Norway

Kelly, E. (1997) The effects of deep transverse frictional massage to the gastrocnemius muscle. *Journal of Orthopaedic Medicine*, **19**, 3–9

Kesson, M. and Atkins, E. (1998) *Orthopaedic Medicine*. Butterworth-Heinemann, Oxford

Ladd, M.P., Kottke, F.J. and Blanchard, R.S. (1952) Studies of the effect of massage on the flow of lymph from the foreleg of the dog. *Archives of Physical Medicine and Rehabilitation*, **33**, (8) 971–973

Longworth, J. (1982) Psychophysiological effects of slow stroke back massage in normotensive females. *Advances in Nursing Science*, **July**, 44–61

Maitland, G.D. (1991) *Peripheral Manipulation*, 3rd edn. Butterworth-Heinemann, Oxford

McMaster, P.D. (1937) Changes in the cutaneous lymphatics of human beings and in the lymph flow under normal and pathological conditions. *Journal of Experimental Medicine*, **65**, 347

Morelli, M., Seabourn, D.E. and Sullivan, J. (1990) Changes in H-reflex amplitude during massage of triceps surae in healthy subjects. *Journal of Orthopaedics and Sports Physical Therapy*, **12**, 55–59

Smith, L.L., Keating, M.N., Holbert, D. et al. (1994) The effects of athletic massage on delayed onset muscle soreness, creatine kinase, and neutrophil count: a preliminary report. *Journal of Orthopaedics and Sports Physical Therapy*, **19**, 93–99

Sullivan, S.J., Williams, L.R.T., Seabourne, D.E. and Morelli, M. (1991) Effects of massage on alpha motoneuron excitability. *Physical Therapy*, **71**, 555–560

Sunshine, W., Field, T., Schanberg, S. et al. (1996). Massage therapy and transcutaneous electrical stimulation effects on fibromyalgia. *Journal of Clinical Rheumatology*, **2**, 18–22

Winter, B. (1968) Transverse frictions. *South African Journal of Physiotherapy*, **24**, 5–7

Chapter **4**

Taping in sport

CHAPTER CONTENTS

Strapping or taping is used extensively in the prevention and treatment of sports injuries, and this chapter looks at the more common taping methods. The aim is to set out some fundamental principles of both tape application and the mechanisms by which taping achieves its effect. Where appropriate, specific strapping techniques are described in Section II of this book.

TAPING MATERIALS

Various forms of tape are available, either elastic or inelastic. In general, elastic tape is used with injured contractile tissue to provide a graded resistance or compression. Inelastic tape is more often used with non-contractile tissue injuries, to take the place of a ligament in reinforcing a joint. Zinc oxide tape is the most common inelastic type. It is air permeable, allowing the skin to breathe and some moisture to escape through the tape. The tape is backed with a strong adhesive which may be a hypoallergenic formation. The tape strength is largely dependent on the number of individual threads per inch, a value known as the thread count (Lutz et al., 1993). The higher quality tapes generally have a higher thread count and are therefore stronger and less affected by body heat and moisture. The edge of zinc oxide taping may be serrated to make tearing off strips of tape during application easier.

Definition
The thread count of a tape refers to the number of threads per inch. Higher thread counts give stronger tapes.

The elastic tapes may be either adhesive backed or adherent. Adhesive elastic tapes will normally stretch both longitudinally and transversely. Typically, this type of tape will recoil to 125% of its original length when initially stretched lengthways (Austin, Gwynn-Brett and Marshall, 1994). However, multiple stretching will cause the tape to fatigue. Rather than tensile strength, elastic tape has good compression qualities and will pull on the skin if applied pre-stretched.

Table 4.1 Taping supplies

Taping and padding materials
Zinc oxide tape (various sizes)
Elastic tape (various sizes)
Cohesive tape (various)
Waterproof tape
Felt and foam padding (various thicknesses)
Underwrap
Tubular elasticated bandage (various sizes)
Blister protectors
Cotton gauze squares (sterile and non-sterile)
Sterile plasters (various sizes)
Paraffin gauze

Skin care preparations
Adhesive spray
Adhesive remover
Antiseptic solution and ointment
Moisturizing skin cream
Skin toughener spray
Petroleum jelly

Instruments/apparatus
Razor and soap
Tape cutters, bandage scissors, sharp/blunt scissors
Cotton wool, cotton-tipped applicators
Surgical gloves

From Norris (1994), with permission.

Adherent or cohesive tapes are normally impregnated with latex, enabling them to stick to themselves rather than to the wearer's skin. This feature makes the cohesive tapes reusable to a certain extent, giving cost savings. Most tapes are water-repellent to some degree, but the latex coated cohesive tapes may also be water-resistant, enabling an athlete to bathe with them on and so maintain fitness by exercising in water.

Beneath the tape, padding materials are used to protect the skin or bony prominences and to fill in superficial anatomical cavities. The padding may be either foam or fibre based. Polyester urethane foam underwrap is used to prevent tape adhering to the skin and to provide a more even compression. Fibre padding such as orthopaedic felt, or its synthetic equivalent, is used where thicker packing is required. These have the advantage that they may be cut and shaped. A variety of taping supplies are listed in Table 4.1.

Splinting or bracing materials vary from thermoplastic materials used to support unstable joints to anatomical braces used to immobilize a joint, especially after surgery. In addition, a variety of elasticated stockinets and purpose-designed braces are available for most major joints. Elasticated braces may be shaped to accommodate the contours of the joint. For example, knee sleeves may be open to reduce compression over the patellar area, while ankle braces are shaped to contour the foot and lower shin. These braces offer compression to prevent pooling of oedema and heighten confidence in a body part through proprioceptive enhancement.

Braces may be made of neoprene where the additional advantage of heat retention is useful. Metal or plastic stays are often built into braces to make them more robust.

APPLICATION

Skin preparation

The limb is generally positioned with the injured structure, or part to be protected, in a shortened position. For example, the lateral ligament of the ankle is strapped with the joint held everted and dorsiflexed. Where a general limitation of all movements is required at a joint, the functional mid-range position is chosen.

The contact between the skin and strapping should be as firm as possible to prevent excessive movement which may lead to skin abrasion. Anything that reduces this skin contact will result in a loss of adhesiveness. Substances which are secreted or excreted from the skin, such as the hydrolipid film, dead epidermal cells and sweat, will stick to the tape rather than allowing direct skin contact. Clean and dry skin is therefore a requirement for good adhesion.

Some athletes will have hypersensitivity to components within the strapping and may show severe allergic reactions. Chemical skin reactions are more likely with strong zinc oxide adhesive than with hypoallergenic preparations based on polyacrylate. Where this type of adhesive still causes irritation, cohesive strapping is chosen. Mechanical irritation can result if the drag of the strapping exceeds the elastic properties of the skin, or if the strapping starts to slip and 'burn' the skin.

Before tape is applied, the body area and skin condition is inspected. Sensation and circulation of the skin should be assessed before and after tape application. Minor scratches and abrasions can be protected by petroleum jelly or paraffin gauze, while larger areas should be covered by a sterile dressing. It must be remembered, however, that in cases of a large wound, first aid is required and not simply taping.

The skin is lightly shaved or the hair flattened down and an underwrap applied. Skin preparation products such as tincture of benzoin or adhesive spray can be useful where strapping fixation is poor. The use of underwrap does allow the strapping to be applied onto non-shaved skin, but the cutaneous stimulation is likely to be less than with direct skin application. This may make underwrap better where mechanical rather than functional strapping is used. Superficial skin damage occurs more commonly over areas of soft skin, such as within the popliteal and cubital fossae. In addition, taping over unprotected bony prominences can lead to pressure points if the tape is applied too tightly. This is common over the base of the fifth metatarsal with fore-foot taping for example.

Tape application

Tape may be either cut or torn prior to application. To cut tape, it should be loosely folded over the lower blade of the scissors with the non-adhesive face inwards (Fig. 4.1a).

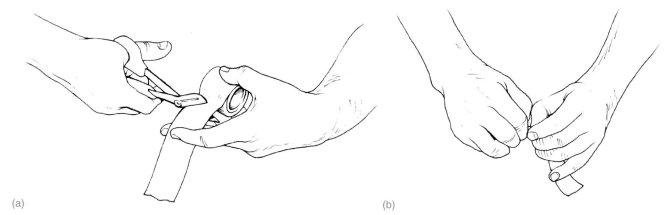

Figure 4.1   Tape may be either cut or torn prior to application.

If the adhesive face is directed outwards, the tape will stick to the scissors and jam between the blades. When tearing tape, speed rather than strength is the deciding factor. The tape should be stretched over the tips of the thumbs with the non-adhesive face inwards. The thumbs should be held together, and one hand twisted against the other with the aim of rapidly breaking the tape edge (Fig. 4.1b). The faster the action, the less strength required.

In many circumstances, the strapping is applied along the line of the tissue fibres, so knowledge of the underlying anatomy is obviously important. The aim is to reduce the movement which stresses the injured tissues, but allow a near normal range of motion in other directions.

Tape may either be applied in a number of individual strips or as a continuous roll. Application in strips has the advantage of accuracy both in terms of the underlying anatomy and the tension applied to the individual strips. It can, however, be slow. Continuous application, while being considerably quicker, uses more tape and can make tension difficult to control.

Where strapping is applied in layers, the overlap between successive pieces is normally half the width of the tape. This ensures that the tape layers do not part with movement of the body (Adams, 1985). Gapping of the tape can trap skin between the tape layers, causing skin damage. The tape should be applied smoothly and moulded to the anatomical contours of the body part. Creases should be avoided as these will create pressure spots. Tape is secured to the skin via anchoring strips (Fig. 4.2a). These are either elastic or inelastic strips applied directly to the skin without traction. Care must be taken not to compress the skin as the anchor tape is surrounding the limb and can easily impair the circulation. From the anchors, reins or stirrups may be attached, under traction. A rein travels between two anchor strips (Fig. 4.2b), while a stirrup is a U-shaped loop which passes beneath a body part, for example under the heel and up either side of the shin (Fig. 4.2c). The reins or stirrups are applied along the length of anatomical structures or to pull a joint into a particular position. They relieve stress from ligaments or perform the actions which a muscle would

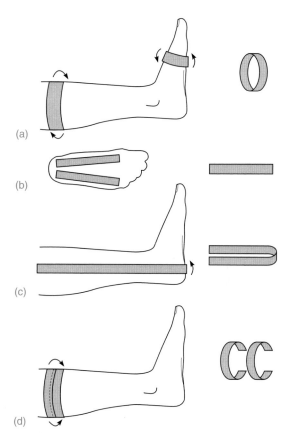

Figure 4.2   (a) Anchor, (b) reins, (c) stirrup and (d) fixing strips. From Norris (1994) with permission.

perform were it to contract. Care must be taken to avoid tape slippage which can lead to a friction burn of the skin.

> **Keypoint**
>
> Take care to avoid tape slippage, as this can lead to a friction burn of the skin.

The reins are therefore attached to the anchor strips or skin by secure fixing strips. These run at 90° to the reins and attach in a semicircular fashion, not surrounding the limb (Fig. 4.2d). Once the main skeleton of the taping has been formed, the components are supported by casting strips to hold the reins in place and perform a firm cover for the tape. An additional protective layer may be provided by a piece of elasticated stockinet placed over the whole taping. A glossary of terms used when taping is shown in Table 4.2.

The aim of functional taping is not to immobilize the limb completely. Instead, movement which stresses the injured tissues is reduced, while a near normal range of motion is allowed in other directions. This allows the athlete to continue with modified and reduced intensity training while protecting those tissues damaged during the original injury. In addition, the tape may be used to re-educate movement giving the athlete feedback (see below). To achieve this, the limb is positioned with the injured structure to be protected in a shortened position. For example, the lateral ligament of the ankle is strapped with the joint held everted and dorsiflexed. Where a general limitation of all movements is required at a joint, the functional mid-range position is chosen.

Aftercare and tape removal

The athlete must be observed for 2 or 3 minutes after taping application to ensure against circulatory complications. The finger- or toenail of the treated limb should be firmly pressed and released to ensure that colour returns readily, demonstrating that an adequate blood flow is reaching the nail bed. However, even with correctly applied strapping complications may occur later, so the athlete must be warned to remove the strapping immediately in the presence of skin discoloration in the fingers or toes, increasing swelling, increasing pain or numbness/tingling. Both passive and active joint movements are performed to ensure that the tape limits the range of motion correctly, and that it stays on.

The strapping is removed by lifting the end and pressing the skin down to form a tunnel. A tape cutter or bandage scissors are then used (lubricate the tip of the cutter) to cut the tape. The tape should be pulled back on itself and the skin pressed down at the same time to avoid too much skin traction. Residual adhesive should be cleaned from the skin. Frequent tape removal and re-application will increase skin irritation, as will tape slippage which can lead to a skin burn. Each time the tape is taken off, some of the protective corneum is stripped, so the skin must be protected with a moisturising cream over the treated area.

TAPING MECHANISMS

Taping appears to achieve its effects by both mechanical and functional mechanisms (Table 4.3). Mechanically, the range of motion at the joint is reduced by taping and the force required to displace the joint is increased. Radiographic studies of static talar tilt and anterior displacement, for example, have shown significant movement reductions with ankle taping (Larsen, 1984; Vaes et al., 1985). Electrogoniometry has also been used to demonstrate reduced inversion/eversion and plantarflexion during active exercise with the ankle taped (Laughman et al., 1980; Fumich et al., 1981). The limitation to movement is quickly reduced as the tape degrades with body heat and moisture. Forty percent of the supportive strength of ankle tape is lost after just 10 minutes of vigorous exercise (Rarick et al., 1962). In addition, the typical tensile strength of zinc oxide tape is considerably less than the tensile strength of the anterior talofibular ligament, for example (Andreasson and Edberg, 1983; Attarian, McCrackin et al., 1985), meaning that multiple layer application is required to secure the joint effectively. Although the mechanical stabilizing effect of tape is reduced following exercise, taping has been shown to reduce the incidence of ankle injuries (Garrick and Requa, 1973; Ekstrand, Gillquist and Liljedahl, 1983). Clearly, another mechanism must be working to aid joint stability.

Table 4.2   Glossary of taping terms

Anchor	The first tape strips applied to the skin, for the attachment of additional tape
Butterfly	Tape strips applied from a single fixed point and fanning out
Buttress	Material used to support or limit movement
Casting strips	Tape placed over reins to hold them firm
Continuous taping	A single length of tape wound around a structure repeatedly
Fixing strip	Tape used to make reins secure
Lock	Inelastic tape which secures an anatomical structure
Padding	Foam or fibre-based material used to protect bony prominences or fill superficial cavities
Rein	A strip of tape travelling between two anchor points
Skin toughener	Skin preparation products such as tincture of benzoin or spray adhesive
Stirrup	A U-shaped loop of tape
Strip taping	Applying a number of individual strips of tape
Underwrap	Thin polyester urethane foam placed beneath tape to protect the skin

From Norris (1994), with permission.

Table 4.3   Effects of taping

Category	Effect
Mechanical	Range of motion at the taped joint reduced
	Force required to displace the taped joint increased.
Functional	Reflex stimulation of skin
	Learning process due to skin drag
	Enhanced proprioception
	Alteration of underlying muscle contraction

The additional mechanism may be an enhancement in functional stabilization of a joint through skin stimulation. Two mechanisms seem to act here: first, direct reflex stimulation, and second, a learning process. Activation of a cutaneous reflex response is a familiar occurrence, and is demonstrated in both the abdominal reflex and the flexor withdrawal response. Cutaneous stimulation causes muscle contraction within the region of the stimulant. It is possible that the stimulation of adhesive tape, and particularly the drag caused by the tape on the skin with movement, will initiate this response, as cutaneous receptors can stimulate proprioceptive reflexes (Darton, Lippold and Shahani, 1985). Peroneal reaction time has been shown to shorten with taping application (Karlsson and Andreasson, 1992) and the peroneus brevis has been shown to function for a longer period at the end of the swing phase of gait (Glick, Gordon and Nishimoto, 1976). In addition, during single leg standing, peroneal muscle activity has been shown to be significantly greater in taped than in non-taped ankles (Loos and Boelens, 1984).

Ankle proprioception has been shown to be enhanced by taping (Robbins, Waked and Rappel, 1995). Using a series of angled blocks, subjects were asked to estimate perceived slope direction and amplitude. Absolute foot position error was 4.11° for subjects wearing athletic footwear, 3.13° for those wearing taping and athletic footwear and 1.96° for barefoot athletes. When compared to the barefoot condition, untaped subjects wearing athletic footwear were 107.5% worse and taped subjects were 58.1% worse. This study demonstrated not just the ability of taping to enhance proprioception, but also the detrimental effect of athletic footwear on proprioception (see p. 294).

The use of taping on the patella has been shown to change the vastus medialis obliquus (VMO) timing in subjects with patellofemoral pain (Gilleard, McConnell and Parsons, 1998). With taping applied to reduce pain by 50% (see p. 219), a step-up movement was performed; VMO activity occurred earlier in the movement while vastus lateralis (VL) activity remained unchanged. During a step-down action (eccentric control of the quadriceps) VMO activity occurred earlier and VL activity was delayed, showing that taping affected muscle contraction timing.

The other way cutaneous stimulation seems to work is by reminding the athlete not to perform an unwanted action. Skin drag is uncomfortable, and can be used to great effect to correct faulty technique through feedback. In this situation, the athlete learns to adjust muscle control to prevent the skin drag (McLean, 1989). A good example is the avoidance of repeated flexion of the lumbar spine. Strips of pre-stretched elastic adhesive tape placed either side of the spine will drag on the skin as the person flexes, reminding them to avoid this action.

This cutaneous stimulation of underlying protective mechanisms may be used in other regions. For example, it is unlikely that a mechanical strapping could immobilize the hamstrings sufficiently to prevent tearing while still allowing unhindered function. However, elastic adhesive tape applied pre-stretched along the length of the muscle may remind the athlete not to overstretch and could therefore be useful in the subacute phase of injury to this body part.

USES

Strapping in sport is normally used either to prevent injury or to promote the safe use of an injured body part, and may be used at any stage of healing. Its use in the acute phase of an injury must be treated with caution. Although its protective function is useful, accumulation of swelling and the need for regular inspection of the body part usually make the use of compression bandages or inflatable splints more appropriate. The aim of taping in the subacute phase of injury is to support the injured structure, by reducing the range of motion of actions which place stress on the damaged tissues. The use of functional taping should allow near normal movements in ranges other than those which stress the injury.

The great majority of publications describe strapping to the ankle, with particular reference to the lateral ligament, perhaps because this is one of the most commonly injured areas in sport. Reduction in the rate of ankle injuries following strapping application has been shown by a number of authors. Studying a population of 2562 college basketball players, Garrick and Requa (1973) showed an injury rate for non-strapped ankles of 32.8 sprains per 1000 players. This reduced dramatically to 14.7/1000 when a basketweave strapping with heel-lock was used. When the effect of strapping was studied on players who had previous ankle sprains, the injury rate reduced from 27.7/1000 to 16.4/1000. Ekstrand, Gillquist and Liljedahl (1983) taped half the previously injured, or unstable, ankles of Swedish football players. After a 6-month period, those taped had no lateral ligament injuries to the ankle, but those without taping had suffered nine ligament injuries.

Some therapists believe that restricting movement at one joint by the use of taping may throw stress on other joints in the limb, although the evidence for this is inconclusive. Ankle taping has been shown to cause the heel to lift sooner in the stance phase of barefoot walking. In non-taped athletes, heel lift has been shown to occur at 71.5% of the stance phase, but at 67.1% in those athletes who wore ankle taping (Carmines, Nunley and McElhaney, 1988). This alteration of the biomechanics may adversely affect the metatarsophalangeal joints (particularly the first) increasing forefoot stress. This could make turf toe a contraindication to ankle taping. Neither Glick, Gordon and Nishimoto (1976) nor Garrick and Requa (1973) found any increase in knee injuries as a result of ankle taping in their subjects.

TAPING EXAMPLES

Three procedures will be used as illustrative examples here: first, the use of reins to support the plantarfascia; secondly, the use of proprioceptive taping to reduce lumbar flexion in low back pain; and thirdly, the use of padding and anatomical taping in the treatment of a lateral ligament sprain to the ankle.

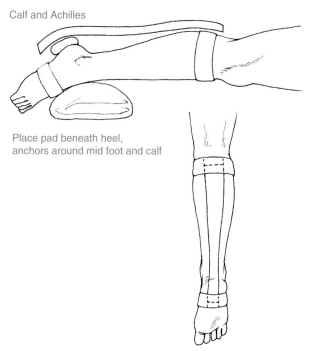

Calf and Achilles

Place pad beneath heel, anchors around mid foot and calf

Figure 4.3   Calf and Achilles. Place elastic anchors around the mid-foot and calf, and a felt heel raise below the heel. Tape with the athlete prone and the foot plantarflexed. Three reins run between the foot and calf to maintain the plantarflexed position.

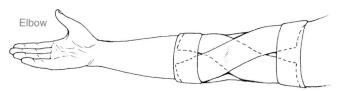

Elbow

Figure 4.4   Elbow. Begin with the arm slightly flexed. Place elastic anchors around the forearm and upper arm. Reins cross the elbow to maintain flexion. Apply several layers as required.

Use of check reins

The plantarfascia is taped with the foot in its neutral position as plantarflexion places the structure on stretch (see p. 285). The skin is sprayed with skin preparation to improve tape adhesion.

> **Keypoint**
>
> Spray adhesive or a skin prep can be used to improve tape adhesion. Wash dirt from the skin first and dry thoroughly.

Anchor strips of 5-cm zinc oxide tape are placed across the plantar aspect of the forefoot, covering the first and fifth metatarsal heads. The strip runs to the dorsal surface of the first and fifth metatarsals but does not encircle the foot. A second anchor is placed around the calcaneum and a third below the heel pad to cover the whole of the heel. Three strips of zinc oxide tape are then used as reins from the heel,

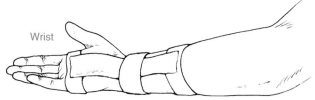

Wrist

Figure 4.5   Wrist. Begin with the wrist slightly flexed. Place anchors around the hand and mid-forearm. Reins link the two anchors on the palmar surface of the forearm. The taping may be reinforced by fixing strips around the wrist.

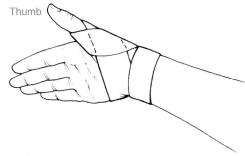

Thumb

Figure 4.6   Thumb. Hold the thumb slightly flexed and adducted to protect against an overextension injury. Using 2-cm zinc oxide tape, loop around the wrist (loosely) and then continue a figure-of-eight around the thumb and back onto the wrist.

fanning out towards the forefoot. When the patient weight bears, the taping should prevent the foot from flattening completely, and take the stretch off the plantarfascia.

Fixing strips may be used, and placed at 90° to the reins. Each strip starts and finishes at the edge of the dorsum of the foot.

Proprioceptive taping for postural re-education

In cases of lumbar pain, where a large component of the condition is due to stress accumulation through repeated bending, proprioceptive taping is used to remind the patient not to flex the lumbar spine, but to move at the hips instead (see p. 88). The patient lies prone, and two strips of adhesive fleece net taping are placed over the erector spinae at each side of the spine, with the skin relaxed, from the crest of the ilium to the lower thoracic region.

> **Clinical note**
>
> Adhesive fleece net taping is used to protect the skin from zinc oxide tape adhesive. Fleece net taping will allow some skin breathing and reduce moisture build-up.

On top of this, two 5-cm strips of zinc oxide tape are placed to stretch the skin. The tape is adhered to the lower thoracic region and then gently pulled caudally to traction the skin. Only slight skin bunching should be noticed. Once the tape has set, it will restrict lumbar flexion by pulling on the skin,

Ankle (strip taping)

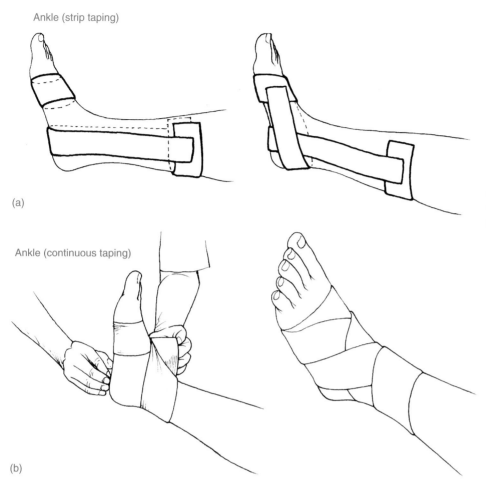

(a)

Ankle (continuous taping)

(b)

Figure 4.7 Ankle. (a) Strip taping. Place elastic reins around the forefoot and mid-calf. Place the first stirrup from the calf rein and beneath the heel. Place a second stirrup from the forefoot rein around the calcaneum. Alternate stirrups, building up a 'basket-weave' taping. (b) Continuous taping. Evert and dorsiflex the foot (for an inversion injury). Begin the taping on the outer edge of the foot. Take it across the dorsum of the foot and beneath the sole, pulling the foot into eversion. Loop around the lower shin forming a figure-of-eight. Leave the heel free to enable the athlete to wear a shoe.

Medial aspect of knee

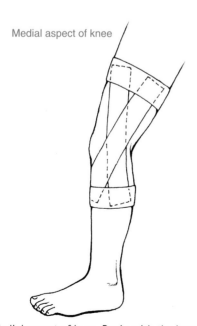

Figure 4.8 Medial aspect of knee. Begin with the knee slightly flexed. Place elastic anchors around the upper calf and lower thigh. Join these with several layers of overlapping zinc oxide taping, crossing on the joint line.

and encourage the patient to perform the 'hip hinge' action when bending (Fig. 4.10).

Anatomical taping with padding

Padding and anatomical taping are used to support the ankle after tearing of the anterior talofibular ligament. Underwrap is wound around the foot and ankle from the metatarsal heads to a point 20 cm above the malleoli. Plantarflexion and inversion are the movements which must be limited to reduce stress on the healing ligament. To achieve this a felt or foam rubber wedge is placed beneath the calcaneum with the larger side placed laterally to evert the rearfoot. A felt horse-shoe is placed beneath and to the sides of the lateral malleolus to avoid oedematous pooling and to create an automassage effect when walking. Two strips of 5-cm zinc oxide tape are used as heel locks. These are adhered medially and pulled laterally to force the ankle joint into eversion.

A figure of eight is then used to lock the ankle and 5-cm elastic tape is used (continuous) to add compression. The tape begins over the tubercle of the fifth metatarsal and is pulled over the dorsum of the foot and around the forefoot forcing the foot into eversion. As the tape emerges laterally, once more it is pulled tightly over the medial malleolus to

Figure 4.9   Thigh. (a) Place elastic tape around the thigh to compress the area. (b) Reinforce with zinc oxide reins lengthways, to provide resistance to overstretch.

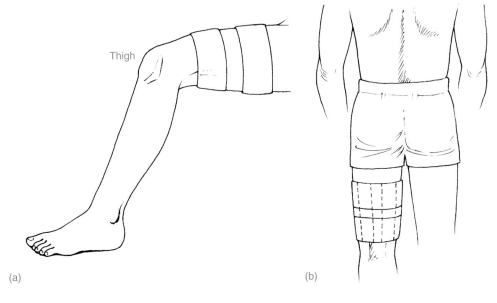

Thigh

(a)   (b)

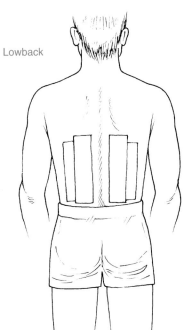

Lowback

Figure 4.10   Low back. Begin with the spine in lordosis. Place overlapping strips of zinc oxide taping either side of the spine, to provide skin feedback to flexion.

Table 4.4   Taping procedures illustrated in this book

Procedure	Page number
Patella	219
Patella fat pad	251
Turf toe	282
Plantarfascia	285
Heel pad	285
Metatarsal	286
Acromioclavicular joint	381
Proprioception for shoulder	395

pull the foot into dorsiflexion. The tape winds behind the calcaneum and then across the dorsum of the foot overlapping the first piece of taping by one-half. Tension is placed on the tape to pull the foot into dorsiflexion once more and the tape passes over the Achilles to finish on the dorsum of the foot. Here, the edge of the tape is held down by a small piece of 5-cm zinc oxide tape. Gaps or 'windows' between the tape should be avoided to guard against blister formation. Table 4.4 lists the taping procedures used in the clinical chapters of this book, while Figures 4.3–4.10 illustrate some common taping techniques used in sport.

References

Adams, I. (1985) *Strapping in Sport.* Johnson and Johnson Wound Care, Baillière Tindall, London

Andreasson, G. and Edberg, B. (1983) Rheological properties of medical tape used to prevent athletic injuries. *Textile Research Journal*, **53**, 225–230

Attarian, D.E., McCrackin, H.J., Devito, D.P., McElhaney, J.H. and Garrett, W.E. (1985) Biomechanical characteristics of human ankle ligaments. *Foot and Ankle*, **6**, 54–58

Austin, K.A., Gwynn-Brett, K.A. and Marshall, S.C. (1994) *Illustrated Guide to Taping Techniques*, Mosby Year Book/Wolfe Medical, London

Carmines, D.V., Nunley, J.A. and McElhaney, J.H. (1988) Effects of ankle taping on the motion and loading pattern of the foot for walking subjects. *Journal of Orthopaedic Research*, **6**, 223–229

Darton, K., Lippold, O.C.J. and Shahani, M. (1985) Long latency spinal reflexes in humans. *Journal of Neurophysiology*, **53**, 1604–1608

Ekstrand, J., Gillquist, J. and Liljedahl, S. (1983) Prevention of soccer injuries. *American Journal of Sports Medicine*, **11**, 116–120

Fumich, R.M., Ellison, A.E., Geurin, G.J. and Grace, P.D. (1981) The measured effect of taping on combined foot and ankle motion before and after exercise. *American Journal of Sports Medicine*, **9**, 165–170

Garrick, J.G. and Requa, R.K. (1973) Role of external support in the prevention of ankle sprains. *Medicine and Science in Sports and Exercise*, **5**, 200–203

Gilleard, W., McConnell, J. and Parsons, D. (1998) The effect of patellar taping on the onset of vastus medialis obliquus and vastus lateralis muscle activity in persons with patellofemoral pain. *Physical Therapy*, **78**, 25–32

Glick, J.M., Gordon, R.B. and Nishimoto, D. (1976) The prevention and treatment of ankle injuries. *American Journal of Sports Medicine*, **4**, 13–14

Karlsson, J. and Andreasson, G.O. (1992) The effect of external ankle support in chronic lateral ankle joint instability: an electro-myographic study. *American Journal of Sports Medicine*, **20**, (3) 257–261

Larsen, E. (1984) Taping the ankle for chronic instability. *Acta Orthopaedica Scandinavica*, **55**, 551–553

Laughman, R.K., Carr, T.A., Chao, E.Y., Youdas, J.W. and Sim, F. (1980) Three dimensional kinematics of the taped ankle before and after exercise. *American Journal of Sports Medicine*, **8**, 425–431

Loos, T. and Boelens, P. (1984) The effect of ankle tape on lower limb muscle activity. *International Journal of Sports Medicine*, **5**, (Suppl.) 45–46

Lutz, G.E., Barnes, R.P., Wickiewicz, T.L. and Renstrom, P.A.F.H. (1993) Prophylactic athletic taping. In *Sports Injuries* (Volume IV of the encyclopaedia of sports medicine) (ed. P.A.F.H. Renstrom), Blackwell Scientific, Oxford

McLean, D.A. (1989) Use of adhesive strapping in sport. *British Journal of Sports Medicine*, **23**, (3) 147–149

Norris, C.M. (1994) Taping: components, application and mechanisms. *Sports Exercise and Injury*, **1**, 14–17

Rarick, G.L., Bigley, G., Karst, R. and Malina, R.M. (1962) The measurable support of the ankle joint by conventional methods of taping. *Journal of Bone and Joint Surgery*, **44A**, 1183–1190

Robbins, S., Waked, E. and Rappel, R. (1995) Ankle taping improves proprioception before and after exercise in young men. *British Journal of Sports Medicine*, **29**, (4) 242–247

Vaes, P., De Boeck, H., Handelberg, F. and Opdecam, P. (1985) Comparative radiologic study of the influence of ankle joint bandages on ankle stability. *American Journal of Sports Medicine*, **13**, (1) 46–50

Chapter 5

Physical training and injury

CHAPTER CONTENTS

PRINCIPLES OF TRAINING

Supercompensation

In any form of training the body is exposed to a workload or physical stress of a *type*, *intensity*, *duration* and *frequency* sufficient to cause physical change. To achieve a training effect, the body must be *overloaded*, that is, exposed to a physical stress which is greater than that encountered in everyday living. The response to this training stress is catabolism, the breakdown of metabolic fuels or tissues. Following the catabolic response, the tissues react by adapting and becoming better suited to coping with the imposed stress, this adaptation is known as anabolism, and involves tissue growth (Astrand and Rodahl, 1986). With training, the anabolic effect is excessive, causing the tissues to grow stronger, a process called *supercompensation*.

The process of adaptation to an imposed demand (stress) is succinctly described by the general adaptation syndrome or GAS (Seyle, 1956). Initially there is an *alarm reaction* or 'shock' This may last for several weeks, and during this time an athlete's performance will be impaired, leading to stiffness. Over time, the body adapts to the stress and the athlete enters the *resistance* phase which is the process of 'supercompensation', enabling the body to more effectively cope with stress at that imposed level. However, if the stress imposed on the body is too great, or if an athlete fails to allow a sufficient recovery period for the body to adapt, the *exhaustion* phase may be reached. The body becomes stiff and sore again and the athlete quickly loses motivation. Boredom sets in – 'overtraining' has occurred. Lack of adequate rest, poor diet and too little sleep to allow recovery can all lead to exhaustion.

> **Keypoint**
>
> Failure to allow sufficient recovery following a training session can lead to overtraining and exhaustion.

Progressive exercise

As fitness improves, the *intensity* of the load which is required to produce a training effect will increase. Adaptation to the load occurs, and so further improvement will only occur if the training intensity is increased. Physical activity in itself is therefore not synonymous with physical training. A training effect will only occur if an activity is sufficiently demanding.

In addition to a minimum intensity, the training load must be continued for a certain *duration*. High intensity training which is too brief may not allow time for the physical adaptations required by the body. The frequency of training – that is, how often it is carried out – is also important. Training is a stimulus which causes an anabolic adaptation. This adaptation will take time, and so adequate recovery must be allowed between training sessions for the body tissues to modify themselves. The type of training will dictate the type of tissue adaptation which occurs, a principle known as specificity (McCafferty and Horvath, 1977) (see below).

Training effects are not permanent. The motor system adapts to the level (overload) and type (specificity) of stress that is imposed on it. If the stress is removed, and training ceases, the motor system will again adapt to the new, now lower, level of stress, and *detraining* will occur. This transient nature of training adaptation is known as the *reversibility principle* (Thorstensson, 1977; Enoka, 1994).

Definition
The *reversibility principle* describes the gradual loss of training effects when the training overload is reduced, a process referred to as *detraining*.

When training for aerobic (cardiopulmonary) fitness or stamina, exercise intensity may be assessed by measuring heart rate or maximal oxygen uptake (VO_2 max). The American College of Sports Medicine (1978) recommended the quantity and quality of exercise required to develop and maintain aerobic fitness and body composition. A training frequency of 3–5 days per week is required, at an intensity of 60–90% of the maximum heart rate reserve, or 50–85% VO_2 max. This should be carried out for a duration of 15–60 minutes, and be continuous or rhythmical in nature. These recommendations were later updated to include the provision of resistance training, flexibility, and weight loss (ACSM, 1990, 2002). For strength gains, one set of 8–12 repetitions was recommended, with 8–10 exercises for the major muscles groups, for 2 days per week. A balanced flexibility programme should include both static and dynamic range of motion exercise to work the major muscle/tendon groups. Each stretch should be held for at least 10–30 seconds, and four repetitions should be used for each group two to three times per week. To achieve significant weight loss, 4½ hours of moderate exercise with an energy expenditure of at least 2000 calories per week is recommended. To achieve this, either continuous or accumulative exercise

Table 5.1 Recommended quantity and quality of exercise to gain a training effect

Type	Recommendation
Cardiovascular	3–5 days/week 50–85% VO_2 max 15–60 minutes Continuous and rhythmical in nature
Muscular strength	One set of 8–12 repetitions 8–10 exercises for the major muscles groups 2 days per week
Flexibility	Static and dynamic stretching to work major muscle/tendon groups Each repetition held for 10–30 seconds 4 repetitions for each group 2–3 times per week
Weight loss	4½ hours exercise/week, expending 2000 calories in total Continuous or accumulative exercise Intensity of 55–69% maximal heart rate Accumulated daily duration 30–40 minutes

Source ACSM (1978, 2002). American College of Sports Medicine (ACSM) (1978) The recommended quantity and quality of exercise for developing and maintaining fitness in healthy adults. *Medicine and Science in Sports and Exercise*, **10**, vii–x.
ACSM (2002) Progression model in resistance training for healthy adults. *Medicine and Science in Sports and Exercise*, **34**, 364–380. With permission.

may be used at an exercise intensity of 55–69% maximal heart rate. Accumulated daily duration should be 30–40 minutes per day (Table 5.1).

FITNESS

Physical fitness has been defined as a set of attributes that relate to the ability of people to perform physical activity (McArdle et al., 1991), or the ability of a person to function efficiently and effectively to enjoy leisure, to be healthy, to resist hypokinetic disease, and to cope with emergency situations (Kent, 1994).

Fitness can be thought of as a continuum from optimal fitness at one side through average fitness to complete lack of fitness and death (Fig. 5.1). The exact components of fitness required to make an individual optimally efficient and effective will be determined largely by the physical activity to be performed.

Fitness may be subdivided into two types: task (performance)-related fitness is that required for sport and within occupational activities; health-related fitness includes components which are associated with some aspect of health. Physical training will improve fitness, but may not always enhance health. Extreme development of any one of the fitness components, in isolation, will upset the delicate balance between the components, and may actually be detrimental to health. For example, excessive development of flexibility will lead to hyperflexibility and, when strength

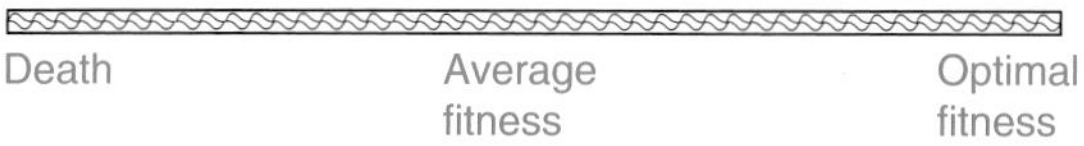

Figure 5.1   The fitness continuum.

Table 5.2   'S' factors of fitness

Factor	Concept
Stamina	Cardiopulmonary and local muscle endurance
Suppleness	Passive and active flexibility
Strength	Isometric, isotonic (concentric and eccentric) isokinetic strength
Speed	Speed (rate of movement) and power (rate of doing work)
Skill	Motor skill
Specificity	Overload must match tissue adaptation required
Spirit	Psychological aspects of injury, including illness behaviour

lags behind, instability. Excessive development of strength may reduce range of motion, leaving an athlete 'muscle bound'. Favouring some muscles to the detriment of others will often lead to a change in the equilibrium point (resting position) of a joint.

Fitness components

The fitness components may be conveniently defined as 'S' factors (Table 5.2). The term 'stamina' is used to encompass both cardiopulmonary and local muscle endurance. Cardiopulmonary endurance is associated with a reduced risk of coronary heart disease (Ashton and Davies, 1986), and local muscle endurance is a factor in any sustained activity, especially joint stability. Suppleness (flexibility) and strength (see below) are concerned with the health of the musculoskeletal system, to maintain both range of movement and joint integrity. Speed (rate of movement) and power (rate of doing work) are both needed in later stage rehabilitation as part of proprioceptive training (see p. 147). Skill training is important, not just for sports specific actions, but for the skill of individual movement such as scapulohumeral rhythm or gait re-education, for example. The principles of skill training and their relevance to rehabilitation are discussed on page 149.

The term 'specificity' refers to the SAID principle, that is 'specific adaptation to imposed demands'. The change taking place in the body of an athlete (adaptation) as a result of training (the imposed demand) will be determined by the type of training which is used, and will be specific to it.

Specificity applies to strength and power development, but also to the energy systems used while exercising. A particular cardiopulmonary training programme will cause specific training adaptations. Aerobic fitness developed on a cycle ergometer, for example, will differ slightly from that obtained while running.

It is important, therefore, that training matches as accurately as possible the action which the athlete will use in a sport in terms of joint range, muscle work, energy system and skill.

The term 'spirit' covers the psychological effects of exercise as discussed below.

> **Keypoint**
>
> *Specificity* of training means that exercise must match, as accurately as possible, the actions which an athlete will use in sport.

PSYCHOLOGICAL EFFECTS OF EXERCISE

Exercise and self-concept

Several psychological characteristics have also been shown to change as a result of participation in a regular exercise programme. Enhancement of self-confidence, self-esteem and body image are seen, and reductions in anxiety, depression, stress and tension have been demonstrated.

> **Definition**
>
> *Self-esteem* is the degree to which individuals feel good (positive) about themselves. *Body image* is the perception of one's own body and general physical dimensions.

Enhanced well-being

Athletes often claim that exercise makes them 'feel good', and the 'runners' high' is a widely reported phenomenon. Reductions in stress and anxiety have been reported, lasting for between 2 and 5 hours after the cessation of training (Morgan, 1985), and decreased depression has been demonstrated as a result of 6–20 week exercise programmes (Greist et al., 1979). In addition, altered states of consciousness have been described following distance running (Mandell, 1979). Weight training programmes have been shown to enhance self-concept in both male (Dishman and Gettman, 1981; Tucker, 1982) and female (Brown and Harrison, 1986) athletes. Three theories exist to explain these phenomena: the distraction hypothesis, and the production of monoamines and endorphins.

How exercise makes an athlete feel better

The distraction hypothesis proposes that participation in vigorous exercise distracts the athlete from stress. Comparison between exercise, meditation and distraction show similar reductions in state anxiety, but the effect resulting from exercise appears to last longer (Morgan, 1985).

Depression is also affected by exercise. Reductions in the monoamine chemicals noradrenaline (norepinephrine) and serotonin (5-HT) are associated with depressed states in humans, and these same chemicals have been shown to increase in rats subjected to chronic exercise (Brown et al., 1979). Increases in the release of endorphins and enkephalins, or slowing of the dissociation rates of these chemicals has also been proposed (Pert and Bowie, 1979). By measuring plasma levels of these chemicals or using opiate antagonists to neutralize them, researchers have demonstrated some association between exercise and endorphins (Farrell et al., 1983).

Exercise addiction

Exercise addiction, or exercise dependence, is the physiological or psychological dependence on regular exercise, usually distance running but other forms of exercise such as body-building may also show this trend. Athletes who are addicted to exercise show symptoms of withdrawal and show uncontrollable craving for a particular exercise type at the expense of other training.

Definition
Exercise addiction is physical or psychological dependence on regular exercise of a single type. Athletes show uncontrollable craving and symptoms of withdrawal when the exercise is not practised.

The experience of exercise for an athlete, and the way in which this fits into the rest of his or her life, is one factor which determines whether or not an exercise becomes addictive (Crossman, Jamieson and Henderson, 1987). An individual's need for exercise can be either positive or negative. *Positive addiction* exists when an athlete receives some psychological or physical benefit from an activity, and is able to control the activity.

The *negatively addicted* athlete is controlled by the activity and will experience severe negative effects (withdrawal) with a missed exercise bout. Such athletes often engage in an activity at the expense of their health or at the expense of other factors, such as relationships and career prospects. The negatively addicted athlete may be failing to gain approval from significant others and may harbour feelings of inadequacy or unattractiveness. This type of athlete often exercises alone or in isolation from the group. They experience feelings of enhanced self-concept and even euphoria during exercise. Importantly, such individuals are more likely to ignore pain or injury and work through this to complete a workout. In the same vein, they tend to be anxious if a workout is missed and almost appear to suffer 'withdrawal symptoms' (Table 5.3).

WARM-UP

Many athletes conscientiously warm up in the belief that they will protect themselves against injury, and enhance

Table 5.3 Characteristics of exercise addiction

The athlete may:

1 Perform several bouts of exercise per week for up to an hour at a time
2 Experience a high degree of positive effect after exercising
3 Exercise alone or isolate themselves when in a group
4 Be highly satisfied and less self-critical when exercising than at any other time
5 Experience a state of euphoria when exercising
6 Be more depressed/anxious/angry after missing a workout
7 Tend to ignore physical discomfort/injury in order to complete exercise regime

Adapted from Glasser, W. (1976) *Positive Addiction.* Reprinted by permission of HarperCollins Publishers Inc. and Anshel, M.H. (1991) A psycho-behavioral analysis of addicted versus non-addicted male and female exercisers. *Journal of Sport Behavior*, 14(2), 145–154. With permission.

their sporting performance. While neither of these beliefs have been conclusively proven, there is mounting evidence in the literature to suggest that both may contain elements of truth. This section does not attempt to be a full review of the subject, but will draw on some of the many studies concerning warm-up to illustrate important points.

Warm-up types

Warm-up may be either *passive*, involving an external heat source, or *active*, involving body heat. An active warm-up, in turn, may be *general*, using the whole body, or *specific*, working only those body parts to be used in competition, and studies have shown improvements from each (Table 5.4).

Many external heat sources are suitable for a passive warm-up. Common types used by athletes include hot baths or showers and saunas. Clinically, physiotherapists use a number of modalities including hot packs, whirlpool baths and electrotherapy (short-wave diathermy in particular). Benefits are claimed to result from the increase in tissue temperature, and physical performance has been improved using this type of warm-up.

With a passive warm-up, no significant active body movement is used, and little energy is expended. Subsequent physical work will not therefore be impaired due to depletion of energy stores. This type of warm-up can be useful clinically, when active movement is either not desirable or not possible.

General warm-ups are the type most commonly used in sport. The overall body temperature is raised by active exercise, increasing the temperature of the deep muscles and body core. Specific warm-up involves movements which are to be used in actual competition, but at a reduced intensity. Rehearsal of body movement takes place, and the specific tissues directly involved in the activity are heated. This type of warm-up would seem especially appropriate for events requiring highly skilled and coordinated actions.

Table 5.4 Some historical studies on efficiency of warm-up

Reference	Warm up type	Result
Carlile (1956)	Passive	Improvements in swimming times after hot showers (8 minutes at 40°C)
Davies and Young (1983)	Passive	Warmed the triceps surae muscles using hot water baths. Showed increases in peak power output with cycling and jumping tasks
Sargeant (1987)	Passive	Water baths. Showed increases in peak force and power of 11% after heating, and reductions of up to 21% after cooling
Richards (1968)	Active – general	Stool stepping before vertical jump task. 1- and 2-min warm-ups improved performance by 23%. 4 min had no effect. 6 min warm-up reduced performance by 27%
DeVries (1959)	Active – specific	Compared passive (hot showers and massage), active (calisthenics) and specific (swimming) warm-up prior to swimming task. Significant improvement only after specific warm-up

---

Definition

A *passive* warm-up increases tissue temperature by using an external heat source. An *active* warm-up uses body heat produced during exercise, and may be *general*, using the whole body, or *specific*, working body parts to be used in competition.

Effects of warm-up

A warm-up achieves its effect through physiological, psychological and biomechanical methods. Physiological effects are largely due to increases in tissue temperature, while psychological effects are mainly due to practice. Biomechanical effects are achieved by alterations in the tissue response to mechanical strain.

Cardiovascular changes

The change from a relaxed resting state to a higher training level should be gradual, to avoid suddenly stressing the cardiovascular system. Equally, to stop training quickly, and reduce cardiac output too rapidly, can compromise venous return.

A warm-up of sufficient intensity will cause an alteration in regional blood flow. When resting, only 15–20% of the total blood flow goes to the skeletal muscles, but after about 10 minutes of general exercise this figure is increased to 70–75% (Renstrom and Kannus, 1992). During a warm-up, blood flow is increased to active muscles and reduced to visceral tissues earlier than would occur without a warm-up. Increased blood flow causes the delivery of nutrients and removal of metabolic wastes to be enhanced.

Barnard et al. (1973) examined the effects of sudden strenuous exercise on men with no symptoms of cardiac problems. Each subject ran vigorously on a treadmill for 10–15 seconds without a warm-up. In 70% of these subjects, abnormal changes were seen on an ECG trace, indicative of subendocardial ischaemia. These changes were reduced, or even abolished, when a warm-up was performed before activity. Similarly, the effect of sudden onset exercise on blood pressure was improved. Average systolic blood pressures of 168 mmHg were seen without warm-up and these reduced to 140 mmHg when warm-up preceded exercise.

One of the reasons for these changes is that the adaptation of the coronary blood flow to strenuous exercise is not instantaneous. The cardiac output is unable to increase quickly enough to meet the demands of sudden high intensity work (Astrand and Rodahl, 1986), and a warm-up gives the cardiovascular system time to respond.

Keypoint

A warm-up reduces the stress on the cardiovascular system by allowing the adaptation of coronary blood flow to occur more gradually.

Tissue temperature

The ability to perform physical work is improved by elevated temperature (Bergh and Ekblom, 1979a). Warm-up prior to maximal exercise will enable the adaptations necessary for these changes, to occur sooner.

Oxygen dissociation from haemoglobin is more rapid and complete, and oxygen release from myoglobin is greater at higher temperatures (Astrand and Rodahl, 1986). The critical level of various metabolic processes is lowered, causing an acceleration in metabolic rate and a more efficient usage of substrates. Muscle contraction is more rapid and forceful (Bergh, 1980). The sensitivity of nerve receptors and speed of transmission of nervous impulses are both increased as temperature rises (Astrand and Rodahl, 1986). This more rapid transmission of kinaesthetic signals is particularly important when complex highly skilled movements are used. These temperature-dependent changes are summarized in Table 5.5.

The increased tissue temperature created by a warm-up will alter the force-velocity curve of a muscle (see p. 18). The effect is to shift the curve to the right by 12% for each 1°C increase in temperature (Enoka, 1994). The change in contraction velocity (maximal velocity of shortening) results in an increase in peak power output of the muscle (Fig. 5.2).

Large temperature changes have been shown to affect maximal isometric force. Cooling the hand muscles to 15°C reduced maximum isometric force by 30% (Ranatunga, Sharpe

Table 5.5 Warm-up mechanisms

Improvement	Mechanism
Muscle work	Faster muscle contraction and relaxation speeds
Economy of movement	Lowered viscous resistance within muscle
Oxygen delivery and usage	Haemaglobin releases oxygen more easily as tissue temperature rises
Nerve conduction	Increased temperature accelerates metabolic rate within nerve. Specific warm-up rehearses motor pattern
Blood perfusion	Local vascular bed dilated

Source McArdle, W.D., Katch, F.I. and Katch, V.L. (2001) *Exercise Physiology, Energy, Nutrition and Human Performance*, 5th edn. Lea and Febiger, Philadelphia. With permission.

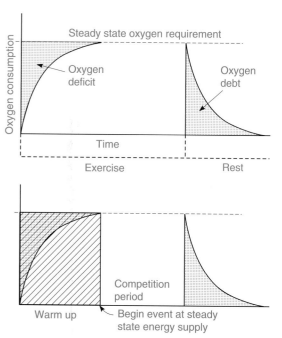

Figure 5.3 The effect of warm-up on oxygen deficit.

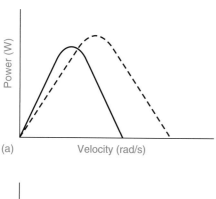

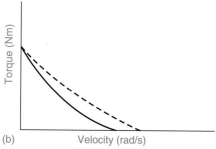

Figure 5.2 Effect of tissue temperature increase due to warm-up. (a) Peak power is increased demonstrated by increased height obtained on vertical jump test. (b) Maximum velocity of shortening increased and torque–velocity curve shifts to the right. Adapted from Enoka, R.M. (1994) *Neuromechanical Basis of Kinesiology*, 2nd edn. Human Kinetics, Illinois. With permission.

and Turnbull, 1987), while warming the quadriceps changed maximal isometric torque from 262 Nm at 30.4°C to 312 Nm at 38.5°C, an increase of 2.4%/1°C (Bergh and Ekblom, 1979b).

Mobilization hypothesis

In the initial period of intense exercise, high amounts of energy are required immediately. The anaerobic reserves are quickly used up, and the aerobic system has not yet become fully functional. The difference between the energy needed and that which can be supplied is known as the *oxygen deficit*, and represents stored energy and the build up of

metabolic wastes (Fig. 5.3). When exercise stops, the body continues to provide energy aerobically to replenish the energy stores and metabolize waste products which have accumulated. This, in turn, creates the *oxygen debt*.

Gutin and Stewart (1971) argued that a function of warm-up was to mobilize the body's cardiovascular system to reach a steady state. As warm-up was stopped, a brief rest period before competition allowed the oxygen debt to be repaid, without letting the cardiovascular system return to normal levels. When competition commenced, the oxygen deficit would be smaller, and some anaerobic energy would be available to the athlete at the end of exercise.

Gutin et al. (1976) asked subjects to pedal a cycle ergometer at an intensity sufficient to produce a heart rate of 140 b.p.m., a rate which they claimed equated with a 50–60% VO2 max. The subjects' performance in a subsequent exercise task was significantly better than a control group who did not undertake a warm-up, a result possibly due to the mechanism described above.

A rest period is essential after the warm-up, to allow the oxygen debt to be repaid. But, following rest, the body must be kept warm to maintain the warm-up effects until the athlete competes. As an illustration, Andzel and Gutin (1976) used bench stepping both as a warm-up and exercise task. A 30- or 60-second rest after the warm-up resulted in improved performance, but when no rest period followed the warm-up, performance remained unchanged.

How long should a warm-up last, and what intensity of exercise should be used? A number of papers have addressed these questions. Andzel (1982) compared warm-up periods at an intensity sufficient to produce a heart rate of 120 and 140 b.p.m., followed by a 30-second rest period. Performance was significantly better with the 140 b.p.m. group. Richards (1968)

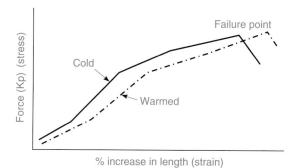

Figure 5.4   The effect of warm-up on tissue failure. After Safran, M.R. et al. (1988) The role of warmup in muscular injury prevention. *American Journal of Sports Medicine*, **16**(2), 123–129. With permission.

argued that while some warm-ups would enhance performance, others could interfere with performance if fatigue set in. By varying the length of stool stepping, she concluded that a 1- or 2-minute warm-up was superior to a 4- or 6-minute period in her study. Bonner (1974) saw similar effects by altering warm-up periods with a static cycle task. Where performance was reduced in these examples, the workload was obviously too high. Sargeant and Dolan (1987) compared warm-up periods with changing intensity assessed by percentage of VO_2 max, and concluded that a 39% VO_2 max intensity was superior to a warm-up at 56% VO_2 max.

Unfortunately there are no hard and fast rules to guide the athlete in terms of warm-up duration and intensity, but, generally, once the heart rate has reached about 140 b.p.m., this should be sustained for 2–3 minutes. This workload should be sufficient to induce light sweating, and is appropriate for the cardiopulmonary part of the warm-up. Obviously, the time taken to achieve this heart rate will depend on exercise intensity and fitness level, so the total warm-up period will be considerably longer.

> **Keypoint**
>
> A warm-up should be of sufficient intensity to induce mild sweating.

Biomechanical effects

Safran et al. (1988) showed that a greater force and length of stretch was required to tear isometrically preconditioned muscles (Fig. 5.4). They claimed that the rise in temperature occurring during the warm-up period could alter the viscosity of the connective tissue within the muscle, and that isometric contractions caused a stretch at the musculotendinous junction. LaBan (1962) showed a 1.5% increase in the length of a stretched tendon following a temperature increase to 42.5°C. Warren, Lehmann and Koblanski (1971) demonstrated increases of 5.8% in length and 58% in force to failure for tendons heated to 45°C.

Shellock and Prentice (1985) argued that muscle elasticity is dependent on blood saturation. They claimed that cold muscles with lower blood saturation levels were therefore more susceptible to injury. Fluids exhibit higher viscosity with lower temperatures, and so joint inertia will be greater when the synovial fluid of a joint is colder.

Changes have also been noted in structural stiffness of muscle following warm-up and exercise. Immediately following activity, muscle stiffness is increased, but can be significantly reduced by stretching. The increase in stiffness is thought to result from thixotropy (Enoka, 1994), the property exhibited by materials whereby they become more fluid when disturbed (shaken). Within muscle, stable bonds are formed between actin and myosin filaments. The bonds are increased following activity, but disengaged by stretching. This has important implications for both warm-up and cool-down. Warm-up will help minimize general muscle stiffness, while cool-down will reduce the actin and myosin bonding which remains following exercise (see also DOMS, p. 116).

Proprioception has been shown to improve as a result of warm-up (Bartlett and Warren, 2002). Joint position appreciation (see p. 148) is more sensitive in the knee after a warm-up, demonstrating that joints seem to accommodate to increased ligamentous laxity which results from a reduction in stiffness due to exercise. The method through which this occurs is thought to be an increase in the sensitivity of the proprioceptive mechanisms around the knee.

Psychological effects

Psychological aspects of warm-up fall broadly into two categories: first, there are psychological effects of a physical warm-up which will be dealt with below; secondly, aspects of sports psychology, such as visualization and imagery, which are dealt within the section on sports psychology related to injury.

Two psychological factors are important in the context of warm-up; these are *rehearsal* and *arousal*.

Rehearsal   Rehearsal will only take place when an athlete performs a specific warm-up, with actions relevant to the sport to be performed in competition. During the warm-up, the athlete is re-familiarizing him- or herself with the skilled movements required by a sport. Confidence is improved, and the athlete may be more relaxed following this practice.

When an athlete is performing a skilled task, a period of rest followed by resumption of the same task may result in impaired performance. This phenomenon is called *warm-up decrement* (WUD), and is well documented (Adams, 1961; Schmidt, 1982).

> **Definition**
>
> *Warm-up decrement* is the gradual loss of the effects of the warm-up in the period between the warm up and competition.

A number of explanations have been suggested to account for WUD. At a basic level it is seen as simply forgetting an aspect of the motor skill. Nacson and Schmidt (1971) suggested that WUD results from a loss of *'activity set'*. They claimed that a number of variables such as arousal level and attention had to be adjusted (tuned) to a specific task. With practice, the adjustments reach an optimal level, which is reduced with rest. They showed that WUD could be reduced if, during the rest period, a completely different movement was practised. This second movement could not contribute to the memory of the first task, but did require a similar activity set to the original skill.

So far, we have dealt with skills which were practised during the warm-up period to improve subsequent sporting performance. Where one type of training has a direct effect on another, a *transfer effect* is taking place.

Definition

A *transfer effect* is the interaction between two similar forms of training. An *activity set* is a group of variables which are adjusted or 'tuned' to a specific physical task.

When the practice of one task improves the performance of another, *positive transfer* is occurring. However, if during a warm-up skills are practised which are different to those needed for competition, they may interfere with the learning process and *negative transfer* can occur. Here, performance suffers because a slightly different skill, with a different activity set, is remembered. An example would be practising tennis strokes with a racquet of different weight and size to that of the one used in competition.

Arousal   The second psychological effect of warm-up is that of *arousal*. The relationship between level of arousal and performance, is demonstrated by the inverted-U hypothesis (Fig. 5.5). In a plot of arousal level against performance, initially increased arousal correlates initially with improved performance. But, as arousal continues to increase, an optimal level is reached. Above this point, further arousal is detrimental to performance.

The point of optimum arousal is related to the psychological profile of the athlete and the complexity of the task to be performed. Activities which require fine muscular control

(such as archery) or involve important decision-making (such as wicket-keeping) generally require lower arousal levels. Where actions involve gross muscular actions without fine control and without complex decision-making (power-lifting, for example) a higher level of arousal is generally required.

The function of warm-up, therefore, must be to psychologically prepare the athlete, and place him or her at the level of arousal appropriate to the task to be undertaken. A highly motivated (aroused) athlete may need to be relaxed prior to a complex activity. Conversely, a poorly motivated athlete due to compete in a strength event may need to be 'psyched up' to an increased arousal level.

Keypoint

A warm-up should *psychologically prepare* an athlete, and place him or her at a level of arousal appropriate to the task to be performed.

Warm-up technique

The intensity and duration of the warm-up period will depend on both the type of activity to be undertaken and the athlete's fitness. A fitter athlete competing at a high level will take longer to warm-up as the body's thermoregulatory system will be more efficient.

During cold weather it will take longer for the body's core temperature to increase, and so the warm-up should be longer or more vigorous. A warm-up should generally be of sufficient intensity and duration to raise the body's core temperature by 1–2°C, recognized by the onset of mild sweating. The warm-up effects may persist for 45–80 minutes, the time variation being dependent on the rate of heat loss (DeVries ,1980).

Practically, the warm up may be divided into three parts: *pulse raising, mobility,* and *rehearsal* (Norris, 2002).

Pulse raising

The pulse raising (cardiovascular, or 'CV') portion of a warm-up should induce mild sweating, and is best performed wearing a full track suit or other insulating clothing. This will retain body heat and maintains the benefits of the warm-up until competition. Gentle jogging, light aerobics, or using CV machines in a gym are all pulse raising activities.

Mobility

Mobility exercises should be performed that are sufficient to take the joints through their full range of motion, the exact range being determined by the movements to be used during sport. The aim is to ensure that the movements used in sport will not overstretch the tissues. A distinction must be made here between *maintenance stretching* and *developmental stretching*. Maintenance stretches are used prior to a sport to take the tissues to their maximum comfortable range. For developmental stretching, exercises are used which aim to

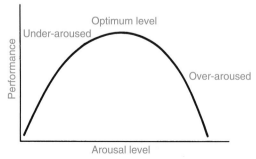

Figure 5.5   Relationship between arousal and performance.

increase this range of motion, and so a thorough warm up is performed first. Maintenance stretches therefore form part of a warm-up, while developmental stretches are practised in a separate stretching session.

Rehearsal

To rehearse complex actions in a warm-up, movements may either be performed at a lower intensity level, or split up into their subcomponents. For example, in weight training, the first set of an exercise can be carried out with a light resistance, or even an unweighted bar or stick. In hurdling, the leg action may be practised slowly and to lower levels, gradually increasing in both speed and height until the normal hurdling action has been achieved.

Only when the individual can perform the movement correctly has the rehearsal portion of the warm-up achieved its aim.

WARM-DOWN

On cessation of exercise it is important to reverse the processes which occurred during the warm-up. The heart is no longer helped by the rhythmic contraction and relaxation of the leg muscles. Consequently, to stop intense exercise immediately will increase the demand on the cardiovascular system, causing the heart rate to rise. Metabolic waste products formed during exercise, such as lactic acid, will no longer be carried away from the working area with so much vigour. Instead they will remain in the area, causing pain. This is thought to be one possible cause of delayed onset muscle fatigue (Byrnes and Clarkson, 1985). Flushing the area with fresh blood by performing a gentle warm-down can reduce this effect.

FLEXIBILITY TRAINING

Flexibility is the range of motion possible at a specific joint or series of articulations, or the amount (amplitude) of joint movement and the general absence of stiffness (Cureton, 1941; Reilly, 1981).

Two types of flexibility are generally recognized, *static* and *dynamic*. Static (or extent) flexibility refers to the amount of movement obtained by passively moving a limb to a maximum degree. Dynamic flexibility is concerned with the amount of active movement possible as a result of muscle contraction. The concern here is not so much the degree of movement present as the ease with which it is obtained. This type of flexibility is probably more important in speed events (Hardy and Jones, 1986).

> ### Definition
>
> *Static flexibility* is the amount of movement obtained by passively moving a limb. *Dynamic flexibility* is the active movement possible as a result of muscle contraction.

Dynamic flexibility must not be confused with agility, which can be defined as the ability to rapidly change the direction of either the whole body or individual body parts without loss of balance (Borms, 1984).

Effects of flexibility training

Flexibility training is generally thought to achieve effects in two broad areas, those of performance enhancement and injury prevention, and these two areas will be addressed here.

Improved performance

To achieve maximal performance, a limb must be able to move through a non-restricted range of motion (Shellock and Prentice, 1985). In sprinting, for example, lack of adequate dynamic flexibility could result in a reduced stride length with possible reductions in sprinting speed. In addition, greater resistance to movement through increased joint inertia and muscle stiffness at the end of movement range is more energy consuming.

Good flexibility is associated with good sporting performance in all activities where a maximal amplitude of movement is required to achieve the best technical effects. Similarly, a limited range of movement can reduce work efficiency in these situations (Borms, 1984). In addition, if flexibility is increased, force may be applied over an increased distance (Reilly, 1981), thus facilitating acceleration of an implement.

Injury prevention

A variety of authors have argued that flexibility may condition tissues to have greater tensile strength and elasticity (Cureton, 1941), leading to injury prevention (Holt, Travis and Okita, 1970) and a reduction in soft tissue pain (DeVries, 1962). This has led some to suggest that the type of training programmes undertaken could affect the number of injuries suffered (Ekstrand et al., 1983). There is some evidence to support this stand. Netball players, who had not warmed up have been shown to have an increased risk of injury (Hopper, 1986), while warming up and stretching have been shown to be important factors in the prevention of hamstring injuries in Australian football (Seward and Patrick, 1992). In a study of army recruits, Hartig and Henderson (1999) showed the effect of hamstring stretching over a 13-week period on overuse injuries. Using 298 subjects, they showed an incidence rate of 29.1% for the control (non-stretching) group and 16.7% for the stretching group.

Muscle stiffness has been shown to reduce as a result of stretching (McNair and Stanley, 1996). Using five repetitions of a static stretch and holding each repetition for 30 seconds, stiffness was reduced to the same degree as with a warm-up for 10 minutes at 60% HR max. Static stretching has also been shown to improve muscle compliance and enhance muscle force development (Rosenbaum and Henning, 1995) as well as reduce the passive resistance offered by a muscle. This latter effect has been shown to return to pre-stretching levels within 1 hour (Magnusson, Simonsen and Kjaer, 1996). These biomechanical changes affecting muscle stiffness could lead to an injury prevention effect of stretching.

Although individual studies indicate the possibility of an injury prevention effect of stretching, taken as a whole the research does not support this. Herbert and Gabriel (2002) summarised the information gained from five studies and concluded that there was no evidence that stretching either before or after exercise protects against muscle soreness or risk of injury. In a later study Weldon and Hill (2003) conducted a review of seven papers and decided that no definitive conclusions could be made concerning the value of stretching, due to the poor quality of the available studies.

Tightness occurs in muscle groups in set patterns, with the biarticular muscles (mobilizers, see p. 122) showing a greater tendency to shorten. For example, of the hip extensors, it is the hamstrings (biarticular) rather than the gluteals (uniarticular) which commonly show tightness and injury through tearing. Tightness of the muscle may pull a joint out of alignment, altering the equilibrium point of the joint and predisposing to joint injury. Further details of this type of change or 'muscle imbalance' is given on pages 122–137.

Flexibility training and muscle power output

Muscle power depends not just on muscle contraction, but on a combination of active contraction, muscle reflex activity and elastic recoil of the non-contractile elements associated with a muscle (pp. 109–111). We have seen that one effect of flexibility training is to reduce muscle stiffness. This in turn could have a direct effect on power development by changing the elastic forces created by the rebounding muscle.

Kokkonen et al. (1998) tested subjects with a one repetition maximum (1RM) lift, and found the subject's lifting ability to be reduced by 7–8% following static stretching. Using a footplate to stretch and measure strength output from the soleus muscle Fowles et al. (2000) used 13 maximal passive stretches over a ½-hour period, holding each stretch for over 2 minutes. Again they measured maximal muscle contraction and found that strength in the stretching group reduced by 28% immediately after stretching, reducing to 12% after 30 minutes and 9% after 60 minutes. Using a leg extension exercise Behm et al. (2001) used 20 minutes of static stretching, with each repetition held for 45 seconds. These authors found a 12% decline in maximal leg strength, confirming the results of the previous studies.

A number of mechanisms may be responsible for this stretch-induced decline in strength output. EMG measurement has revealed a 20% decline in quadriceps activity after stretching (Behm et al., 2001). Muscle activation (using interpolated twitch) has also been shown to decrease by 13% (Fowles et al., 2000).

In addition to alteration in muscle stiffness and electrical changes to the muscle, microscopic damage similar to that seen following eccentric activity also seems to occur. Creatine kinase (CK) levels have been shown to increase by

---

Definition

Interpolated twitch (IT) is a method of electrically stimulating a muscle to create a muscle twitch which can then be measured. *Creatine kinase* (CK) is a chemical produced in a muscle following intense eccentric actions. It is created by the breakdown of damaged muscle cells.

---

over 60% following intense stretching (Smith et al., 1993), confirming this.

Muscle reflexes

A number of structures can limit joint range of motion (Table 5.6) and the ability of muscle to relax and allow a stretch to occur is one of the most important in sport. For this reason, three muscle reflexes are important when using flexibility training, the *stretch reflex*, *autogenic inhibition*, and *reciprocal innervation* (Table 5.7).

When a muscle is stretched, elongation is detected by the muscle spindle afferent nerve fibres. These receptors send

Table 5.6   Factors limiting range of motion at a joint

Osteological design of joint
Joint degeneration (osteophytes)
Cartilage and cartilaginous joint structures
Muscle tone (active)
Muscle elasticity (passive)
Ligament
Fascia
Tendon passing over the joint
Nerve length (passive)
Nerve activation (active)
Skin, scarring and subcutaneous tissue
Soft tissue contact
Joint fluid viscosity (ease of movement) and quantity (movement range)
Consolidated oedema, fibrous tissue

Table 5.7   Muscle reflexes and stretching

Stretch reflex	
Responds to:	
— change in velocity (phasic) (e.g. knee jerk reflex)	Facilitatory (↑ tone)
— change in length (postural) (e.g. body sway)	
Autogenic inhibition (the reverse stretch reflex)	
— Golgi tendon organ (GTO) measures tension	Inhibitory (↓ tone)
Reciprocal innervation	
— Agonist contracts, antagonist relaxes to allow movement	Inhibitory (↓ tone)

impulses to the dorsal roots of the spinal cord, and a reflex is caused which contracts the extrafusal fibres of the same muscle, in opposition to the original stretching force. The reflex is therefore facilitatory. The stretch imposed may be either sudden (as in a knee jerk reflex), where the muscle responds to a change in velocity, or prolonged (as with postural sway), where the muscle measures the change in length.

In addition to the muscle spindle, the Golgi tendon organ (GTO) in the muscle tendon will also register stretch. Both these receptors are affected by changes in muscle length, but the GTO is also receptive to changes in muscle tension (Bray et al., 1986).

When a muscle is stretched, there is a corresponding stretch of the muscle spindle. But, if the stretch lasts for longer than 6 seconds, the GTO registers not only the change of length of the muscle, but also the alteration in tension in the muscle tendon. The GTO will then cause a reflex relaxation of the muscle, a process known as autogenic inhibition or the reverse stretch reflex. This has a protective function, causing the muscle to relax and allowing it to stretch before it is damaged. It is therefore inhibitory.

Stretching which involves short jerking movements will tighten the muscle through the stretch reflex, while movements lasting for longer than 6 seconds will allow the muscle to relax again through stimulation of the GTO, which will override the stretch reflex. If the tension of the muscle to be stretched is increased through isometric contraction, once relaxed the muscle tone will reduce below normal resting levels, enabling a greater stretch to be applied. The stretch reflex (H reflex) has been shown to be suppressed for 10 seconds following isometric contraction of this type (Moore and Kukulka, 1991), giving a 10-second period during which stretching may be applied.

> **Definition**
>
> The *H reflex* (Hoffman reflex) is an artificially induced equivalent of the stretch reflex produced in a laboratory by stimulating a muscle with a single electric shock.

When a muscle is tensed, a reflex relaxation of the antagonist will occur, a process known as *reciprocal innervation*. If, for example, the biceps muscle contracts to flex the elbow, its antagonist, the triceps, must relax to allow the movement to occur. This reflex is modified in *co-contraction*, where both the agonist and antagonist muscles contract simultaneously (Levine and Kabat, 1952). Co-contraction functions to increase joint stiffness and contributes to stability and accuracy of rapid movements (Enoka, 1994).

Most coaches, athletes and therapists would recognize that regular stretching can increase range of motion. One of the methods by which this occurs may be neural plasticity at spinal level (Alter, 1996). Experiments with monkeys (Wolpaw, Lee and Carp, 1991) have shown that the H reflex can be modified as a result of using EMG biofeedback. The magnitude of the H reflex can be increased, reduced or altered completely, and following surgical transection of the spinal cord these changes remain, indicating that the plasticity is occurring at spinal level rather than through brain influence. It may be possible that the threshold of the stretch reflex in man can be altered through a process of desensitization (habituation) so that the reflex threshold is higher (less likely to occur). This would modify the muscle's resistance to stretching and thereby increase available range of motion. Neuronal activity has been shown to reduce with both static and ballistic stretching (Vujnovich and Dawson, 1994).

> **Definition**
>
> *Habituation* (desensitization) is a learning process which results in the reduction of a response or sensation. It occurs in the presence of continual stimulation with a constant stimulus.

Techniques of flexibility

Five methods of stretching are generally recognized: static, ballistic, active, and two proprioceptive neuromuscular facilitation (PNF) techniques (Table 5.8).

Static stretching

During static stretching, a muscle is stretched to the point of discomfort and held there for an extended period. As the muscle is held, the athlete will feel a reduction in the pain stimulus from sharp acute pain to a more dull diffuse sensation. If the static stretch is held by the therapist, the end-feel of the muscle resistance will change from a strong (firm) elastic feel to a more yielding feel. Static stretches should be held for a prolonged period. A 30-second hold has been shown to be more effective than a 15-second hold, with no greater benefit seen when the holding time is extended to 60 seconds (Bandy and Irion, 1994). Four or five repetitions should be

Table 5.8 Summary of stretching techniques

1 Ballistic – rapid jerking actions at end of range to force the tissues to stretch
2 Static stretching (SS) – slowly and passively stretching the muscle to full range, and maintaining this stretched position with continual tension
3 Active stretch – contract the agonist muscle to full inner range to impart a stretch on the antagonist
4 contract-relax (CR) – isometrically contracting the stretched muscle, and then relaxing and passively stretching the muscle still further. This action is usually performed by a partner
5 Contract-relax-agonist-contract (CRAC) – the same as CR except that during the final stages of the stretching phase, the muscle opposite the one being stretched is contracted

performed, as no further benefit is seen when the number of repetitions is increased from this (Taylor et al., 1990).

> **Keypoint**
>
> Optimal static stretching is achieved by holding the stretch for 30 seconds and performing 4–5 repetitions of this movement.

Ballistic stretching

Ballistic stretching involves taking the limb to its end of movement range, and adding repetitive bouncing movements. There is a suggestion that injury may result from abrupt stretching of this type (Etnyre and Lee, 1987) and so the technique has become less popular. Although this may be true for vigorous ballistic stretches which are uncontrolled, adding small stretches to the end of range gained by static stretching (pulsing) has been shown to reduce neurone excitability further than static stretching alone (Vujnovich and Dawson, 1994). To perform ballistic stretching more safely, firstly it should be given after static stretching, and secondly it should be given progressively in terms of both velocity of stretch and range of motion. Such a stretching session would begin with a warm-up and then move to static stretching (5 reps, each held for 30 seconds) this would then progress to 3–5 reps of end range

> **Keypoint**
>
> Ballistic stretching must only be used as a *progression* on static stretching. Short range high velocity movements are used at end range (pulsing) to further increase flexibility. The movements must remain controlled throughout.

pulsing (high velocity, short range). This would then progress to longer range movements at slow velocity, and finally to long range movements at steadily increasing velocity.

Active stretching

Active stretching involves pulling a limb into full inner range so that the antagonist muscle is stretched passively while the agonist is strengthened. This type of stretch is important when correcting muscle imbalance (see p. 126). The inner range contraction is used to shorten a lengthened (lax) muscle, while the shortened muscle is stretched using a functionally relevant movement.

When stretching a biarticular muscle, full inner range contraction is not possible at both ends simultaneously and so the opposing muscle cannot be fully stretched. For example, the hamstrings cannot pull the hip to full inner range extension and the knee to full inner range flexion at the same time, as they are activity insufficient (p. 17). This means that the rectus femoris muscle will in turn not be fully stretched. Passive range of motion will therefore be greater than active range of motion for a biarticular muscle. One of the aims of stretching, however, should be to reduce this difference to a minimum, giving the athlete active control over a greater range of motion (Fig. 5.6), as this may reduce the likelihood of injury (Lashville, 1983). In addition, although passive range of motion is greater than active, the active range normally more closely resembles the movements used in sport and so is more specific.

One of the main advantages of active stretching in the early period of rehabilitation is the control that the athlete has where pain is present. As one muscle is being tightened to stretch another, the athlete is in control of the movement throughout. This may give the athlete the confidence to stretch into ranges which they would not normally be prepared to enter in the presence of pain.

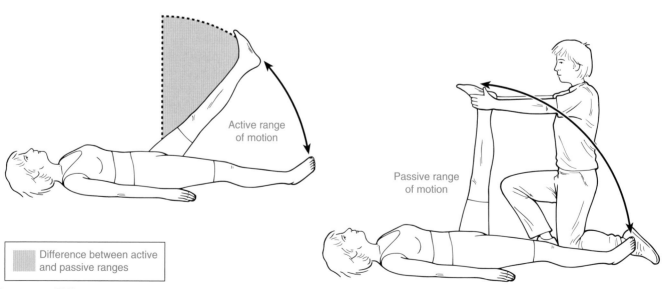

Figure 5.6   Difference between active and passive ranges of motion.

Treatment note 5.1 Passive stretching

There are several passive stretching techniques which are useful in the clinic situation. The therapist applies these on the patient initially without the patient taking an active part in the procedure. Once full passive range has been obtained through a hold-relax technique, contract-relax and CRAC procedures may be used with the same exercise (see p. 102).

Hamstrings

Straight leg raising may be performed with the patient's leg resting on the therapist's shoulder. The leg is held with one hand to stop it slipping and the other hand keeps the knee locked. The therapist takes up a walk standing position with the weight on the back leg to begin (Fig. 5.7); as the stretch is put on, the therapist shifts the weight onto the front leg by lunging forward. In this way the therapist protects his or her back and avoids moving into a flexed position of the trunk.

To emphasize the upper portion of the hamstrings (ischial origin), the patient's knee is flexed by 20° by altering the hand position. The whole leg is pressed into hip flexion, maintaining the slightly flexed knee position (Fig. 5.8).

Rectus femoris

The rectus femoris is stretched in a side lying position (Fig. 5.9). The affected leg is uppermost and the patient bends the underneath knee and holds onto this, to guard against anterior pelvic tilt and hyperextension of the lumbar spine as the stretch is put on. The therapist flexes the knee and holds this flexed position using pressure of his/her abdomen. The femur is then pulled back into extension using hand pressure over the knee and pelvis. Where the upper portion of the rectus is to be targeted, knee flexion is released slightly to allow for a greater extension stretch at the hip. It should be remembered that only 15° of extension is available at the hip before anterior pelvic tilt begins. Further extension range will therefore affect the lumbar spine rather than impose a greater stretch on the rectus.

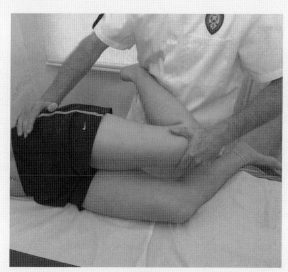
Figure 5.9 Rectus femoris stretch.

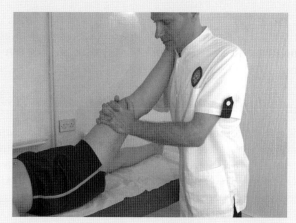
Figure 5.7 Hamstring stretch using straight leg raise (SLR).

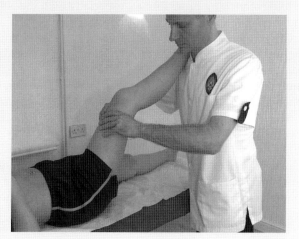
Figure 5.8 Emphasizing the upper portion of the hamstrings.

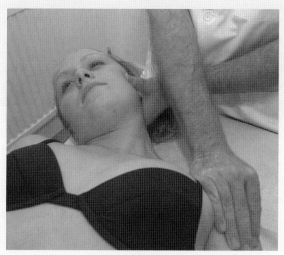
Figure 5.10 Upper trapezius stretch.

Upper trapezius

The upper trapezius is frequently overactive and may develop painful trigger points. The stretch is performed in supine lying to allow the therapist to use massage techniques over the muscle belly if required.

For the right trapezius (Fig. 5.10), begin by elevating the right shoulder to relax the trapezius. Laterally flex the neck to the left and maintain this position using pressure with the right hand. Impart the stretch by pressing down on the right shoulder with the left hand. An X grip of this type is easier for the therapist to apply, while pressing on the shoulder rather than the neck is more comfortable for the patient. The stretch may be varied by using neck flexion with the patient's head on a block or rolled towel.

When using massage techniques with the muscle on stretch, the neck and shoulder position may be maintained by using the left forearm as a 'strut' between the two structures. The right hand is then free to apply the massage technique.

Keypoint

With active stretching the aim is to match the range of motion available using a passive stretch.

PNF stretching

PNF (proprioceptive neuromuscular facilitation) techniques have been adopted by the sporting world from neurological physiotherapy treatments. These techniques use alternating contractions and relaxations of muscles and capitalize on the various muscle reflexes to achieve a greater level of relaxation during the stretch.

Two PNF techniques are used in sport, contract-relax (CR) and contract-relax-agonist-contract (CRAC). The CR technique involves lengthening a muscle until a comfortable stretch is felt. From this position, the muscle is isometrically contracted, and held for a set period. The muscle is relaxed, and then taken to a new lengthened position until the full stretch is again felt by the subject. The rationale behind the CR method is that the contracted muscle will relax as a result of autogenic inhibition, as the GTO fires to inhibit tension. Some authors argue that a maximal isometric contraction is needed to initiate relaxation through the GTO mechanism (Janda, 1992). Others recommend the use of minimal isometric contractions (Lewit, 1991) which seem more appropriate in situations where pain is present.

With the CRAC method, the muscle is stretched as above, but in the final stages of the stretch, the opposing muscle groups are isometrically contracted as the stretch is applied, to make use of reciprocal inhibition of the agonist and reduce its tension. PNF stretches have been shown to be more effective than static or ballistic movements (Holt, Travis and Okita, 1970; Cornelius and Hinson, 1980; Holt and Smith, 1983; Etnyre and Abraham, 1986), with CRAC methods generally being better than CR.

There are two major disadvantages to PNF techniques. First, the extra tension developed in the muscle results in greater pain, and this in turn may reduce user compliance, an important consideration in early rehabilitation. Secondly, as PNF involves isometric contractions, the user must be discouraged from holding the breath and using a valsalva manoeuvre. The raised intra-abdominal and intra-thoracic pressure which occurs with this technique can lead initially to a reduction in venous blood flow to the heart and a decreased cardiac output. On expiration, increases in blood pressure in excess of 200 mmHg have been recorded (Alter, 1996).

Keypoint

When using PNF stretching athletes must not hold their breath during the isometric phase of the movement. They should breathe normally throughout the motion range.

A number of stretching exercise positions are shown in Appendix 2. The reader is referred to Norris (1999) and Norris (1996) for further examples.

Factors affecting flexibility

The amount of movement present at a joint during a stretch (amplitude) is affected by internal (body) and external (environmental) factors (see Table 5.6). Internal factors include the bony contours of the joint. These will differ between individuals, and in certain pathologies such a arthritis, movement will decrease as bone formation changes. These factors cannot readily be affected by flexibility training but must be taken into consideration when prescribing stretching programmes, especially with the elderly and during rehabilitation.

Other internal factors include volume of surrounding tissue, an obese individual frequently being less flexible than a lean one. Muscle tissue, tendons, and joint capsules are other internal factors which may result in movement limitation. Jones and Wright (1982) indicated that 47% of mid-range stiffness is due to the joint capsule, 41% due to muscle fascial sheaths, 10% due to the tendon, and 2% due to the skin. Other factors include cartilage and viscosity of joint fluid (Holland, 1968). Muscle tension will limit range of motion, providing *active resistance*. When a muscle is relaxed, the connective tissue framework of the muscle rather than the myofibrillar elements will provide a *passive resistance*.

Temperature is one external factor which affects flexibility (see p. 95). An increase in tissue temperature can result in both a reduction in synovial fluid viscosity and increased soft tissue extensibility. At a temperature of approximately 40°C a thermal transition of collagen occurs, allowing a greater plastic deformation when stretched (Rigby, 1964). Elastic (recoverable) deformation of connective tissue is favoured by high force, short duration stretching with tissue at normal body temperature or slightly cooled, while plastic deformation (permanent lengthening) is greater with lower force, longer duration stretching at elevated temperatures. If the tissue is then allowed to cool in this stretched position, results may be better (Sapega et al., 1981).

Individual variations in body structure can have apparent effects on flexibility. Individuals with long slender limbs are likely to be more flexible than shorter individuals with thicker musculature. However, good flexibility in one joint does not guarantee similar attributes in other joints, because flexibility has been shown to be joint specific (Harris, 1969).

In general, flexibility decreases with age (Harris, 1969), although between individuals this trend is very much dependent on activity levels and other lifestyle factors (Borms, 1984). A general belief is that girls are more flexible than boys, but it is not clear whether this is due to body structure or social and environmental influences (Goldberg, Saranitia and Witman, 1980).

Therapeutic stretching

When stretching is used as a manual therapy to mobilize a joint after injury or surgery, the various techniques will be combined. If muscle spasm is the limiting factor, ice may be used to limit the pain and this may be combined with PNF stretching (cryostretch procedures). However, to stretch connective tissue effectively, higher than normal temperatures are required, so heat is the modality of choice, where muscle spasm does not limit movement.

The ability of the heat source to reach the tissue to be stretched must be considered, and this will largely depend on the tissue depth and vascularity. In superficial tissues and joints superficial heat (heat lamp, hot pack, hot water soak) will have a beneficial effect on tissue extensibilty. The deeper tissues will not be heated directly. However, muscle spasm may reduce as a result of pain relief. Deeper heating (microwave, shortwave diathermy, ultrasound) may have a direct heating effect on deeper tissues, enabling some of the temperature dependent effects on tissue to be achieved (Sapega et al., 1981).

After heating, passive stretching may be applied by the therapist, or, where long term stretch is to be used, pulley systems and weights can apply the passive stretch. This especially useful for an immobile joint where adhesions limit movement.

STRENGTH TRAINING

Strength is the ability to overcome a resistance; it is the maximum tension which a muscle can produce (McArdle, Katch and Katch, 2001). Strength is usually measured as the torque exerted in a single maximal isometric contraction of unrestricted duration (Enoka, 1994). However, clinically it is important to define the type of strength by prefacing the term with the category of muscle contraction which was used. We should therefore talk of isometric or isotonic strength, rather than simply strength alone.

Adaptation to resistance training

Muscular contraction involves a combination of physiological and neurological processes, and consequently adaptations to resistance training are both *myogenic* (structural) and *neurogenic* (seen on EMG only) in nature (Table 5.9).

Table 5.9 Physiological adaptations to resistance training

Variable	Response
Muscles fibres	
• Number	?
• Size	Increase
• Type	?
• Strength	Increase
Capillary density	
• Bodybuilders	No change
• Powerlifters	Decrease
Mitochondria	
• Volume	Decrease
• Density	Decrease
Twitch contraction time	Decrease
Enzymes	
• Creatine phosphoskinase	Increase
• Myokinase	Increase
• Phosphofructokinase	Increase
• Carbohydrate metabolism	Increase
Basal metabolism	Increase
Intramuscular fuel stores	
• ATP	Increase
• Phosphocreatine (PC)	Increase
• Glycogen	Increase
• Triglyceride	?
VO$_2$ max	
• Circuit weight training	Increase
• Heavy resistance training	No change
Connective tissue	
• Ligament strength	Increase
• Tendon strength	Increase
Body composition	
• % fat	Decrease
• Lean body mass	Increase
Bone	
• Mineral content/density	Increase
• Cross-sectional area	No change

Source McArdle, W.D., Katch, F.I. and Katch, V.L. (2002) *Exercise Physiology*, 5th edn. Lippincott, Williams and Wilkins, Philadelphia. With permission.

Myogenic changes

Hypertrophy   One of the most noticeable myogenic adaptations to resistance exercise is increased muscle size through muscle growth or *hypertrophy*. Increased cross-sectional area has been found to result from an increase in size of individual muscle fibres. Hypertrophied muscle fibres may have 30% greater diameter and 45% more nuclei (McArdle, Katch and Katch, 2001). The increase in size occurs in both type I (slow twitch) and type II (fast twitch) fibres. Selective hypertrophy can occur, causing just the type I or just the type II fibres to increase in size, the ratio between the two fibre types remaining the same. In normal adults the ratio is about 1:1 or 2:1, but in competitive bodybuilders ratios as high as 6:1 have been found, compared to 0:1 in sprinters (Astrand and Rodahl, 1986). In addition, heavy resistance training has been shown to increase the proportion of type IIA (fast oxidative glycolytic) fibres (Bandy, Lovelace-Chandler and McKitrick-Bandy, 1990).

In addition to the increase in fibre size, which occurs with hypertrophy, connective tissue proliferation is also seen (McArdle, Katch and Katch, 2001). Thickening of the muscle's connective tissue support, and that of the musculotendinous junction, may reduce the risk of soft tissue trauma.

Endurance training has long been known to increase the number of mitochondria and the capillary density (number per square millimetre of tissue). However, resistance training is thought to lead to hypertrophy without a significant increase in the number of capillaries (Astrand and Rodahl, 1986). As the number of capillaries stays the same but the size of the muscle tissue increases, the capillary density is reduced. Each capillary must now supply a greater fibre area with oxygen and nutrients, a factor which may account for the relatively poor aerobic capacity of athletes who train solely for strength.

Alterations in muscle energy stores have been reported following resistance training programmes. Increased intramuscular stores of adenosine triphosphate (ATP) and creatine phosphate (CP) have been reported (MacDougall et al., 1977). Similarly, increases in two of the enzymes of anaerobic glycolysis (phosphofructokinase and lactate dehydrogenase) have been reported (Costill et al., 1979). Increases in phosphogen stores and the enzymes of anaerobic glycolysis could be expected to prolong the maintenance of a maximal muscle contraction (Bandy, Lovelace-Chandler and McKitrick-Bandy, 1990).

Hypertrophy in seniors   Weight training was once thought of as the preserve of the young. However, research now shows that muscle training effects are significant in seniors as well. Increases of muscle volume of 26%, peak torque of 46% and 28.6% in total work output have been reported following resistance training programmes for healthy men with an average age of 67 years (Roman, 1993; Yarasheski, 1993; Sipala and Suominen, 1995). In even older subjects (Fiatarone, 1994) a 10-week resistance programme on 63 women and 37 men showed average strength increases of 113% and increase in cross-sectional area of 2.7%. Perhaps of more importance were the improvements in functional ability which these physiological changes achieved, with significant improvements in gait velocity (11.8%) and stair climbing speed (28.4%).

Hyperplasia   The possibility of muscle fibre splitting (*hyperplasia*) in humans has always been a contentious subject. A greater number of muscle fibres is seen in competitive bodybuilders, but this is thought to be a congenital feature of the more successful athletes (Bandy, Lovelace-Chandler and McKitrick-Bandy, 1990). New muscle fibres may develop from *satellite cells*. These cells lie between the sarcolemma and the basal lamina of the muscle fibre at the end of the muscle. They are normally dormant, but become active in the case of muscle injury, and when stimulated they proliferate. With high intensity muscle training, satellite cell activation may occur to replace cells damaged by training. There may be no significant gain in fibre number therefore. *Longitudinal splitting* may occur where a large muscle fibre splits into two daughter cells (a process known as lateral budding) (Gonyea et al., 1986). In mammals, hyperplasia through satellite cell proliferation and longitudinal splitting does occur, but only where hypertrophy is not the main system of muscle growth (McArdle, Katch and Katch, 2001). In humans, most authors agree that the increase in cross-sectional area following resistance training is the result of hypertrophy rather than hyperplasia.

Neurogenic changes

Significant strength gains may be made at the beginning of a strength training programme without noticeable changes in muscle size. The increase in strength is thought to be the result of more efficient activation of the motor units (Astrand and Rodahl, 1986). As Sale (1988) stated, 'strength has been said to be determined not only by the quantity and quality of the involved muscle mass, but also by the extent to which the muscle mass has been activated.'

Increased EMG activity occurs during maximal muscle contraction following a resistance training programme, indicating an increased recruitment of motor units and a greater firing rate (Bandy, Lovelace-Chandler and McKitrick-Bandy, 1990). For a muscle to produce its greatest force, all of the motor units it contains must be recruited. Normally, high threshold motor units are only recruited in periods of extreme need, with the smaller motor units being recruited first. The small slow oxidative (SO) fibres are

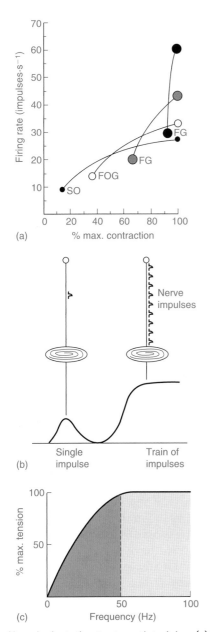

(a)

(b)

(c)

Figure 5.11 Neural adaptation to strength training. (a) The size of motor unit recruitment. The small slow twitch oxidative (SO) motor units are recruited at low force levels. The largest high threshold fast twitch glycolytic (FG) are not recruited until 90% maximal force is obtained. Between these two extremes are the lower threshold FG units and the fast twitch oxidative glycolytic (FOG). For each line, the low point shows the recruitment threshold and the high point shows the maximum firing rate obtained with maximum contraction force. (b) Effect of firing rate on muscle force. A single impulse from the axon to the muscle creates a twitch contraction giving a low force output. A high frequency train of impulses (high firing rate) creates a longer tetanic contraction, giving a force which is ten times greater. (c) Force–frequency curve. At low frequencies small increases in frequency give very large increases in force. At high frequencies the reverse is true, and doubling the frequency from 50 Hz to 100 Hz gives virtually no corresponding increase in force. From Sale, D.G. (1992) Neural adaptation to strength training. In *Strength and Power in Sport* (ed. P.V. Komi). IOC Medical Publication, Blackwell Scientific, Oxford. With permission.

recruited at low force levels, while the fast glycolytic (FG) fibre may not be recruited until 90% of maximum force production is reached. Between these two extremes, lower threshold FG and fast oxidative glycolytic (FOG) fibres are recruited (Fig. 5.11a).

In addition to enhanced recruitment, an increase in firing rate (frequency) of motor units is also seen. A single nerve impulse will cause an isolated twitch response, while a number of impulses are required to produce a sustained contraction (Fig. 5.11b). The greater the excitation of a motoneurone, the greater the firing rate of the motor unit in impulses per second (Hz). Motor units fire at rates of between 10 and 60 Hz, with large increases in force seen for small increases in frequency at the lower end of the spectrum. At the higher end (Fig. 5.11c), increasing the frequency of motor unit excitation has little effect on force production.

With strength training, a subject may gain the ability to recruit the large motor units more easily and so increase the muscle force production. In addition, the firing rate of the motor units utilized in a contraction may be enhanced with training.

Motor unit synchronization (groups of motor units being activated together) has been shown to be greater in strength athletes than control subjects, and is likely to increase as a result of a resistance training programme. This change is more likely to increase the rate of force development rather than peak force itself (Sale, 1988).

Evidence for neural adaptation following strength training comes from EMG studies which show increased activation of prime movers, as a result of improved skill and coordination. For example, during plyometric exercise (see p. 109) the high stretch load can result in a period of inhibition at the start of the eccentric phase while the trained individual shows facilitation, possibly as an adaptation of reflex response (Sale, 1992).

Activation of the prime mover may be limited by insufficient motivation, or inhibition. During new strength tasks, excessive co-contraction may occur to stabilize and protect the moving joints. Simultaneous contraction of the antagonist will reduce the force output of the agonist through reciprocal inhibition. Training could reduce the co-contraction and allow greater activation of the agonist muscle group resulting in a greater force output (Sale, 1988). Such inhibition may explain the phenomenon of bilateral deficit (Sale, 1992). In a weight-training exercise which requires the simultaneous use of both limbs (for example, the squat, leg press or arm pressing movements), the total force which a subject can produce is often considerably less than the sum of the force of the individual limbs acting alone. In contrast to this inhibitory interlimb effect, cross-education represents an overflow of chronic changes from the working muscle to the non-working muscle. This is commonly seen in rehabilitation where an injured muscle may be enhanced by working its uninjured counterpart. Both bilateral deficit and cross-education represent neural adaptation as there are often no significant morphological changes.

Increases in load may occur in resistance training without substantial elevations in strength. Rutherford (1988) cited an example of subjects training on a leg extension exercise. Improvements of 200% in load lifted were accompanied by strength increases of only 11%. He argued that increased coordination of muscles used as 'fixators' in the leg extension movement could account for the improved weight training ability.

Whatever the exact mechanisms involved, it seems clear that neural adaptation is largely responsible for the initial strength gains following a resistance training programme. Gains made later on are more likely to result from muscle hypertrophy. In addition, neural adaptation is likely to be one of the factors leading to specificity of strength training.

Specificity of strength training

Maximum force production from a muscle is, then, the result of a blend of myogenic and neurogenic adaptations which are specific to a particular movement pattern. Improvements in contractile properties such as maximum force, velocity of shortening and rate of tension development can vary with the type of contraction used in training. Training a muscle to perform in a particular movement is not simply a question of overloading it against a resistance. For example, strengthening the leg muscles with a squatting exercise will not increase the performance on a leg extension movement to the same degree as training the same muscles on a leg extension bench. To strengthen a muscle for a specific movement, an exercise must mimic the movement as closely as possible. Similarly, strength gains resulting from isometric training will be specific to the joint angle at which the training was carried out.

Training a muscle at a specific velocity will result in strength gains at speeds close to, or less than, the training velocity (Rutherford, 1988), a phenomenon known as *velocity specificity*. One explanation of this principle is that before training, subjects are unable to produce maximal contractions at all velocities, and through practice they learn to fully activate their prime movers only at the velocities used during training.

Another possibility is preferential hypertrophy of one fibre type. There is little evidence for transformation of one fibre type to another, except following electrical stimulation. Preferential hypertrophy of type II fibres does occur, but at both fast and slow velocities, so the neural explanation seems more likely.

Muscle work

Muscle contractions may be categorized into two types, static (isometric) where the limb segments do not move, and dynamic (isotonic) where movement does occur. The term isotonic (same tension) is confusing, however, because as the limb segments move, leverage forces change and the muscle tension varies continually.

Dynamic contractions may be subdivided into either concentric (muscle shortening) or eccentric (muscle lengthening). Isokinetic contractions are dynamic (and may be concentric or eccentric), but the speed of contraction is held constant by continually varying the resistance. Isokinetic systems do not permit acceleration, the speed being held constant. Isoacceleration (Westing, Seger and Thorstensson, 1991) involves a subject working against a preset acceleration (concentric) or deceleration (eccentric).

The term 'isotonic' has come to be used to describe a concentric or eccentric contraction performed using free weights or a machine which offers a fixed resistance, and this convention is adhered to in this book for clarity.

During concentric contractions, alterations in leverage of the limb throughout the movement mean that the resistance imposed can be no greater than the weakest part of the muscle force curve. If the resistance exceeds the weakest point, the movement is not completed, and the subject reaches a 'sticking point'. The force generated with concentric exercise cannot therefore be maximal throughout the range.

Eccentric training

During an eccentric contraction the muscle is lengthening under active tension. Eccentric contractions are frequently used to resist gravity, the muscles being used as a 'brake'. Tensions developed during eccentric contractions are greater than those of concentric or isometric contractions, leading some authors to argue that the training effect is superior (Darden, 1975).

Greater strength increases have been demonstrated using eccentric training in comparison with concentric activity. Subjects working eccentrically for six repetitions at 120% of the concentric 1 RM have been shown to produce equivalent strength gains to those performing 10 repetitions at 80% of 1 RM (Johnson et al., 1976). However, the amount of muscle soreness (DOMS) encountered with pure eccentric work makes it more appropriate to start a training period with concentric contractions and progress to eccentric contractions in the final stages. In addition, training specificity and safety considerations make eccentric training in isolation less desirable.

Lengthening a muscle immediately before a concentric action will increase the force output of the muscle, a process known as *pre-loading*. Vertical height attained in a single leg and a two leg squat is significantly increased with pre-loading (Fig 5.12) (Enoka 1994). The pre-load effect occurs because it takes time for the chemical processes involved in muscle contraction to come on line. Actin and myosin coupling is not immediate but is 'ramped up' as the muscle is stimulated. By beginning a jump with the muscle partially contracted, this period is taken up (Jaric, Gavrilovic and Ivancevic, 1985).

Another method of producing power during eccentric action is the *stretch–shorten cycle*. Here, the muscle to be worked is first stretched, and the total power produced

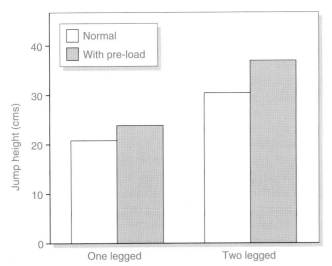

Figure 5.12   Effect of pre-loading on vertical jump height. From Enoka, R.M. (1994) *Neuromechanical Basis of Kinesiology*, 2nd edn. Human Kinetics, Illinois. With permission.

consists of contractile force and elastic recoil of the inert muscle structures.

Definition

Pre-loading a muscle consists of contracting it not from rest, but from a partially contracted state. The *stretch–shorten cycle* contracts the muscle from a previously stretched position.

Plyometrics

Rapid eccentric contraction used immediately before an explosive concentric action (stretch–shorten cycle) forms the basis of plyometric training. This type of training was first used in Eastern block countries in the development of speed (Verhoshanski and Chornonson, 1967). The movements involve a pre-stretch of a muscle, followed by a rapid contraction, causing the athlete to move in the opposite direction. Effects are achieved in both the contractile and inert structures of the muscle.

The rapid stretch of the muscle stimulates a stretch reflex, which in turn generates greater tension within the lengthening muscle fibres. In addition to increased tension, the release of stored energy within the elastic components of the muscle makes the concentric contraction greater than it would be in isolation. Increased tension will in turn stimulate Golgi tendon organ (GTO) activity, inhibiting excitation of the contracting muscle. Desensitization of the GTO has been suggested as a possible mechanism by which plyometrics allows greater force production (Bosco and Komi, 1979).

The use of muscle contraction involving acceleration in the concentric phase and deceleration in the eccentric phase more closely matches the normal function seen in sport, and

---

Table 5.10   Proposed neuromuscular adaptations to plyometric training

Increased inhibition of antagonist muscles
Better co-contraction of synergistic muscles
Inhibition of neural protective mechanisms
Increased motor neuron excitability

Source Potteiger, J.A. (1999) Muscle power and fiber characteristics following 8 weeks of plyometric training. *Journal of Strength and Conditioning Research*, 13(3), 275–279. With permission.

---

therefore has advantages in terms of training specificity. However, the rapid movements involved are not suitable in early stage training as they can be relatively uncontrolled.

Several neuromuscular adaptations have been proposed for the effect of plyometric exercise (Table 5.10), and exercise of this type has been shown to significantly increase peak power output (Potteiger, 1999). Comparing plyometric exercises with their non-power equivalents demonstrates the advantages of this training. A plyometric jump compared to a deep knee bend action used 22% less energy, produced 9% more work and was 40% more efficient (Lees and Graham-Smith, 1996), while a rebound bench press compared to a standard lift gives 30% more work, allowing the athlete to lift 5.4% greater weight.

Practical considerations of plyometric training

Plyometric exercise is only effective when the concentric contraction occurs immediately following the pre-stretch cycle. If there is a pause in activity, some of the benefits are lost as elastic energy is wasted, and the effect of the stretch reflex is altered (Voight and Draovitch, 1991). The ability to recover the stored elastic energy within the tissues depends on the time period between concentric and eccentric activity, known as the coupling time. The stored elastic energy of the leg extensor muscles has a half life of 4 s (Lees and Graham-Smith, 1996), and the coupling time in plyometric exercise has been measured at average periods of 23 ms. Providing the coupling time remains at these levels, nearly all the stored elastic energy can be utilized.

Injury considerations in plyometrics

This type of training is intense, and should only be used after a thorough warm-up, and usually at the end of an exercise programme. To perform plyometrics, the athlete needs a good strength base, and his proprioceptive activity should be tested using single leg standing and single leg half squats (eyes closed, position maintained for 30 seconds) before training commences. Any loss in proprioception may cause the athlete to fall as fatigue sets in. Safety considerations, including proper clothing and footwear and a firm non-slip sports surface, are essential.

Compression forces present in plyometrics have the potential for injury. Spinal shrinkage has been measured at 1.75 mm after 25 repetitions of a drop jump from a height of 1.0 m so this type of exercise is not suitable for individuals with a history of low back pain of discal origin. In normal walking, deceleration forces have been measured at 3 g (three times earth's normal gravity), while in a drop jump from a height of 0.4 m the deceleration has been measured at 23 g (Lees and Graham-Smith, 1996). This type of force acting on the lower limb makes plyometrics unsuitable for those with a history of arthritis in the joints of the lower limb or spine.

Keypoint

Plyometrics is an advanced, intense form of exercise, not suitable for the beginner. *Safety considerations* are essential throughout.

Three types of exercises are normally used: in-place, short response, and long-response (Table 5.11). In-place activities include such things as standing jumps, drop jumps and hopping. Short-response actions are those such as the standing broad jump, the standing triple jump and box jumps. Long response movements include bounding, hopping and repeated hurdle jumps.

Although plyometric activity is primarily used for lower limb training, is does have an important place for the upper limb and trunk. Overhead throwing actions using a medicine ball, and throwing and catching from a bent-knee sit-up position are examples of this.

Resistance may be added to increase the overload on the working muscles as the plyometric activity is used. Vertical jumps may be performed using light dumb-bells, or a squat/leg press machine, and horizontal movements (lateral jumps, side hops) can be overloaded using an elastic cord.

Plyometrics has its use in late stage rehabilitation, and functional pre-competitive testing following injury. The adaptations produced by this type of activity within a previously injured muscle are likely to make it more capable of withstanding explosive effort, as encountered in sprinting and jumping activities, for example. This, in turn, may reduce the risk of re-injury. Using heavy resistance exercise in late stage rehabilitation of the injured athlete may allow the limb to regain lost strength, but without plyometric activity it is likely that the limb could still break down in the competitive situation, because the strength activity does not match the speed and power of the action to be used on the field of play.

Resistance training methods

Exercise progression

As with exercise in general, strength training requires a muscle to be 'overloaded' or worked at a resistance greater than that normally encountered. This may be achieved in a number of ways, the most common of which in the context of sports injuries is weight training.

To increase the overload placed on a muscle, and progress the exercise, a number of methods may be employed, as listed below:

1. Resistance
2. Leverage
3. Isolation
4. Gravity
5. Sets/repetitions
6. Rest interval
7. Frequency of training
8. Speed of movement
9. Range of motion
10. Duration of exercise
11. Type of muscle work
12. Group action of muscles
13. Starting length of muscle
14. Momentum/inertia.

Increasing the resistance, exercise duration, and frequency will make the exercise harder, as will reducing the rest interval. Altering the effect of gravity, by inclining or declining a bench, will affect the point of maximal leverage. Changing the length of the lever arm will also alter the resistance, for example arm abduction performed in the standing position will be harder with a weight bag in the hand than with one fastened to the elbow.

Table 5.11   Plyometric exercises

Exercise type	Movement	Description
In-place	• Standing jumps	Jumping and landing on the same spot, to emphasize the vertical component of the jump
	• Drop jumps	Use gravity and body weight to increase resistance and emphasize eccentric component of movement
	• Hopping	Straight, zig-zag, or rotatory hopping on the same spot
Short response	• Standing broad jump	Emphasizes horizontal component of jump
	• Standing triple jump	Combines several jumps and hops over a distance
	• Box jumps	Jump over an object to emphasize both vertical and horizontal component of jump
Long response	• Bounding	Greater horizontal range than others. Single/double/alternate legs
	• Hopping	Repeated combinations of straight/zig-zag/rotatory hopping
	• Repeated hurdle jumps	Horizontal and vertical jump component for endurance

The relationship between length–tension and force–velocity (see p. 18) means that altering the starting length of a muscle or the speed of movement will change the overload. For example, when performing a sit-up exercise the hip flexors and abdominal flexors will work. By bending the hips, the work of the hip flexors will be reduced, increasing the overload of the abdominal flexors.

As the speed of movement increases, the force output from the muscle is reduced. In addition, more rapid actions have more momentum and are therefore harder to stop (a safety consideration) and are performed with ballistic muscle actions.

The type of muscle work (isometric or isotonic) and the function of the muscle (agonist/fixator, etc.) can be used to great effect, as can the range of movement. Initial rehabilitation exercises, where range of movement is limited, tend to be isometric in nature, progressing to isotonic and increasing the range of motion. The motor skill involved with group muscle action makes it vital that a muscle is not simply worked as a prime mover, but as a fixator and synergist as well.

The combination of repetitions (number of complete executions of an exercise) and sets (number of repetitions grouped together) in weight training is the subject of considerable debate. In general, low numbers of repetitions have been traditionally used to increase strength, while higher numbers have been favoured for endurance. Medium numbers of repetitions are usually referred to as 'power' training, although it is unlikely that this would be effective unless the speed of the movement were increased.

A number of combinations of sets and repetitions have been developed, the most widely used probably being that of DeLorme and Watkins (1948).

Weight training programmes

DeLorme and Watkins

This method requires the user to first discover the maximum weight which can be lifted for the 10 repetition maximum (10 RM). The programme then consists of three sets of 10 repetitions at percentages of this maximal value, as follows:

1. 1st set, 10 repetitions at 50% of 10 RM
2. 2nd set, 10 repetitions at 75% of 10 RM
3. 3rd set, 10 repetitions at 100% of 10RM.

Strength gains were assessed using a 1RM (single repetition maximum) each week, and gains in strength from 20 lb lifted before the programme to 60 lb lifted after 36 days were seen.

The DeLorme and Watkins programme enables the movement to be rehearsed before a maximal contraction is required, perhaps recognizing the importance of neurogenic factors in strength performance.

Practically there are number of issues in determining 1 RM. Fatigue after each lift means than a rest period of 1–5 minutes has to be given after a single repetition before the test can be repeated to failure. Also, the relationship between the 1RM and 10RM changes with training: 7–10 RM has been shown to represent 68% of the 1RM for untrained subjects but 79% of the 1 RM for trained subjects (McArdle, Katch and Katch, 2001).

> **Keypoint**
>
> 1 RM is the maximum weight an athlete can lift once. 10 RM is the maximum weight lifted for 10 repetitions, and will be a percentage of the 1 RM value. *The percentage value is less for an untrained subject.*

Pyramid system

In this routine, the number of repetitions performed with each set is reduced as the weight increases, the subject working on a 'light to heavy' system. This results in the athlete performing a few repetitions to fatigue when the muscle is thoroughly warm. An example is given below:

1. 1st set, 12 repetitions at 50% maximum
2. 2nd set, 8 repetitions at 65% maximum
3. 3rd set, 6 repetitions at 75% maximum, or to fatigue.

Oxford technique (reverse pyramid)

This is the reverse of the pyramid system. Now the user adopts a 'heavy to light' system, starting by performing 10 repetitions at their 10 RM and reducing to 75% and 50% of this value.

1. 1st set, 10 repetitions at 100% 10 RM
2. 2nd set, 10 repetitions at 75% 10 RM
3. 3rd set, 10 repetitions at 50% 10 RM.

The Oxford technique (Zinovieff, 1951) works on the principle that as the muscle fatigues, the weight should be reduced to take account of the reduction in force output.

DAPRE technique

Knight (1979) recommended that the resistance to be lifted should be based on previous performance. The technique of daily adjusted progressive resistance exercise (DAPRE) determines when, and by how much, to increase the weight, and allows for individual differences in the rate of strength development, as shown below.

1. 1st set, 10 repetitions 50% working weight
2. 2nd set, 6 repetitions 75% working weight
3. 3rd set, maximum number of repetitions with working weight
4. 4th set, maximum number of repetitions with adjusted working weight.

Table 5.12 Guidelines for adjusting weight in the DAPRE technique

Number of repetitions performed in third set	Adjusted working weight (fourth set)	Next session
–2	Deduct 2.5–5 kg	Deduct 2.5–5 kg
3–4	Deduct 0–2.5 kg	Same weight
5–6	Same weight	Add 2.5–5 kg
7–10	Add 2.5–5 kg	Add 2.5–7.5 kg
10–11	Add 5–7.5 kg	Add 5–10 kg

Table 5.13 Timing in circuit training

Method of controlling timing	Description
Stopwatch	Time dictated by instructor and may vary depending on feedback from participants
Exercise station specific	Time set specific to exercise station type
Music	Change station as music changes
Lighting system	Use traffic light system built into gym
Repetitions (user)	User decides number of reps and records this
Repetition (instructor)	Instructor determines number of reps

Source Lawrence, D. and Hope, B. (2002) *Complete Guide to Circuit Training.* A C Black, London. With permission.

Four sets are performed as indicated in Table 5.12, the first two sets being 10 and then six repetitions with one half and then three-quarters of the 'working weight'. This is roughly a 6 RM, and is determined from previous performance. In the third set, the weight is adjusted depending on the number of repetitions which could be performed. For example, if in the third set the athlete is able to lift the weight only five times, the weight used in the fourth set will be the same. If he or she were able to perform 10 repetitions in the third set, the weight is increased by 2.5 to 5 kg. The number of repetitions performed during the fourth set with this adjusted weight determine the new working weight to be used in the next training session.

High intensity strength training

For a muscle to work maximally, during the final set an athlete should not stop training simply because a certain number of repetitions have been performed, but only when no more can be performed. In this way volitional fatigue rather than number of repetitions determines the extent of the set.

If maximal work can be performed in a single set, multiple sets may not be necessary. Hurley et al. (1984) showed strength increases of 33% for lower body and 50% for upper body, when using a single set of 8–12 repetitions performed to volitional fatigue. Silvester et al. (1982) found that one set of arm curls performed to volitional fatigue was as effective at increasing biceps strength as three sets at maximal weights.

Messier and Dill (1985) also showed a single set performed to volitional fatigue produced greater mean values of amount of weight lifted than three sets at sub-maximal weight. The duration of training in this study was 20 minutes, compared to 50 minutes required for a multiple set programme. Single set programmes have been compared to two set and four set programmes and found to be equally effective when compared for improvement of muscle size, strength and upper body power over a 10-week period (Ostrowski et al., 1997).

Hass et al. (2000) found a single set programme to be as effective as a three set programme (8–12 reps to volitional fatigue) over a 13-week programme. Importantly, they also reported that the single set programme took less time to perform (25 min) than the three set programme (60 min),

improving compliance. They encountered a 25% dropout rate for the three set programme. High intensity strength training, although effective, may not be appropriate for early rehabilitation when pain will limit the intensity of training which an athlete is capable of. In addition, single set programmes are probably better suited to beginners, or as a brief intense period of strength training within a more broadly based programme. Single set programmes do not offer the same training volume as multiple set programmes and have been shown to be less effective for long term training, especially when multiple set programmes are used with periodization (Kraemer, Stone and O'Bryant, 1997).

> **Definition**
>
> *Training volume* is the total amount of training performed in a single workout session. In weight training it is the amount of weight lifted in total, calculated by adding the total number of sets, repetitions and weights lifted.

Circuit training

Circuit training consists of a series of exercises performed in a continuous sequence, and a number of formats are available. Three variables are important in the construction of a circuit (Lawrence and Hope, 2002), *timing* (controlling movement from one station to another), *layout* (shape of circuit) and *exercise choice* (free exercise, resistance, functional).

Timing is used to control movement of subjects from one exercise station to another. A specific time may be performed at each station and this may vary between exercises, for example longer periods on a static cycle and shorter on resistance machines. Alternatively, the instructor may dictate the pace using a stopwatch, and vary this, depending on feedback from participants. Lighting systems (traffic light) and music may also be used to dictate time. The number of repetitions may also be used to set the time, dictated either by the instructor or by the user (Table 5.13).

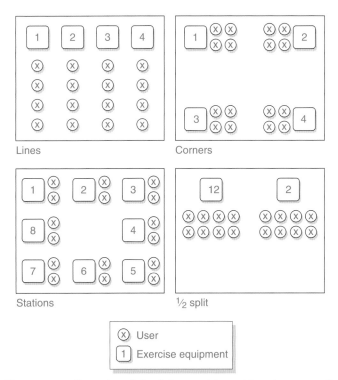

Figure 5.13   Examples of circuit layout. Adapted from Lawrence, D. and Hope, B. (2002) *Complete Guide to Circuit Training*. A C Black, London. With permission.

Circuit layout will be dictated by both safety and effectiveness. Typical examples include the line, corners, stations, and half split (Fig. 5.13). A variety of free exercises or apparatus may be chosen, incorporating different fitness components. Exercises for strength (push-ups, chins) may be interspersed with flexibility (straight leg raise), stamina (jogging), speed (throwing a medicine ball) and skill (flamingo balance). Specificity of training may be enhanced by mimicking the actions involved in a particular sport. For example, a circuit may be set up on a football pitch involving short sprints, zig-zag running, dribbling skills and shooting skills, in addition to upper body and trunk work. An example of a typical circuit is given in Fig. 5.14.

Circuit weight training (CWT)

Circuits may be designed using only one specific type of exercise. An example of this more specialized circuit is circuit weight training or circuit resistance training (CWT/CRT) using only resistance training apparatus. Less emphasis is placed on heavy overload or a single muscle group, and instead a more general fitness programme is obtained. CWT involves alternating the body part worked (arms/legs/trunk) to prevent fatigue of one muscle group. Various types of work–rest ratio may be used. Typical combinations would be eight or more exercises, with a weight of 40–55% 1 RM. A maximum number of repetitions may be performed for 30 seconds, with a rest of 15 seconds, to gain a more general body conditioning programme.

Increase in cardiopulmonary (CP) fitness has been shown with CWT, but it is dependent on rest period, exercise intensity, exercise type and total work. Allen, Byrd and Smith (1976) failed to show significant changes in VO_2 max using 30-second work and 60-second rest periods, the long rest period allowing too much recovery. A programme using a shorter rest period (15 seconds) showed an increase of 11% VO_2 max in women but no significant change in men (Wilmore, Parr and Girandola, 1978). Here, the rest period was short enough, but the exercise intensity for the men was not adequate. The women worked at 87.6% of their VO_2 max, but the men at only 78.2% of theirs. Longer training programmes have been shown to produce better results in terms of VO_2 max improvement (Pollock, Cureton and Greniger, 1969), and Gettman, Ayres and Pollock, (1978) showed a 3.5% increase in VO_2 max after a 20-week CWT programme. Subjects performed at 50% of their maximum strength in a 30-minute programme, which progressed from 10 to 20 repetitions with a rest period which was reduced from 30 to 20 seconds.

Slow speed (60°/s) isokinetic CWT has been shown to be better than high speed (120°/s) training at increasing cardiopulmonary fitness (Gettman and Ayres, 1978). This reflects the importance of the total work performed during the circuit. Athletes using slow speed training worked for a longer period than those using the high speed programme.

Improvements in VO_2 max are not as great with CWT as with running. Average values after a 20-week programme being 3.5% for CWT compared with 35% for running (Gettman and Pollock, 1981). However, the real value of CWT is to maintain cardiopulmonary fitness when an athlete is unable to run or perform other cardiopulmonary fitness activities due to lower limb injury. In a study comparing CWT with running, Gettman, Ayres and Pollock (1979) examined subjects who worked for 8-week periods, first at CWT, then on a running programme, and finally on either running or CWT. Improvements in VO_2 max obtained by running were preserved with CWT, and both groups maintained cardiopulmonary fitness to the same levels. Increases in lean body mass, reductions in bodyfat and strength improvements have all been shown with CWT (Gettman and Pollock, 1981).

One criticism of many of the studies into the cardiopulmonary effects of CWT is that the testing usually uses only treadmill assessment, whereas CWT uses upper body work as well (McArdle, Katch and Katch, 2001). One study which assessed CWT on both a treadmill and an arm crank dynamometer gave improvement in aerobic capacity after CWT of 7.8% with treadmill testing and 21.1% with arm crank dynamometry (Harris and Holly, 1987), illustrating the greater all-body conditioning (cross training) benefits of CWT.

Kinetic chain exercise

Movement of the limbs occurs as a kinetic chain. Several joints arranged in sequence move together to produce a complex motor action. If the terminal joint in the kinetic

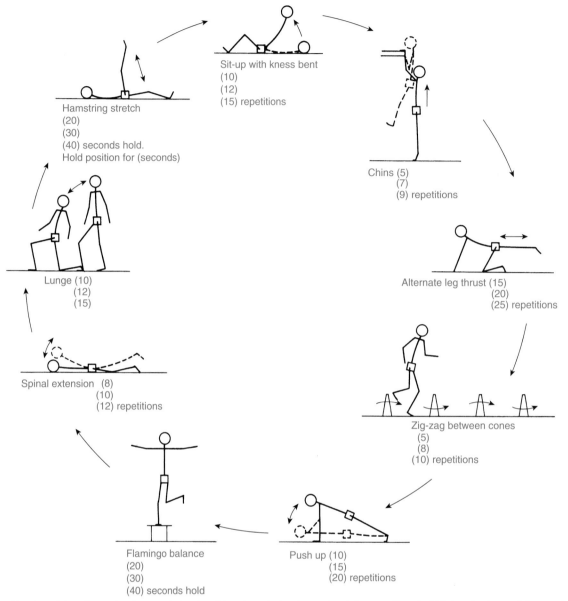

Figure 5.14   Circuit training. Example of general circuit, with values for beginners (top), intermediate (middle) and advanced (bottom) athletes.

chain can move freely, the chain is open. If this same joint is unable to move independently because it faces a significant resistance, the action constitutes a closed kinetic chain.

Definition

In a *closed chain* action, both the proximal and distal ends of the chain of movement are fixed, and motion occurs between the two. In an *open chain* action the proximal segment is fixed but the distal segment moves freely.

Most functional activities involving the lower limb in sport are performed using a closed kinetic chain. Walking, running, jumping, and rising from a sitting position are all examples of closed kinetic chain activities. One of the only

open kinetic chain activity of the lower limb normally used in sport is kicking.

We have seen the importance of exercise specificity in terms of muscle work and energy system, but the exercise must also be specific to the type of kinetic chain action used. To exercise the quadriceps on a leg extension bench (open chain) does not accurately reflect the demands placed on the lower limb with running and jumping (closed chain). As many of the adaptations produced during resistance training, particularly in the first 4 weeks of training, are neurogenic in nature, the mismatch in movement patterns could detrimentally affect the athlete's performance (Palmitier et al., 1991).

A common open chain movement used in knee training is the seated leg extension exercise. The muscles primarily responsible for this action are the quadriceps. Contrast this to the closed chain movement of the squat. When the leg extends to raise the body from the squatting position, the hamstrings extend the hip and assist in knee extension as the foot is stabilized. This co-contraction (co-activation) greatly reduces the anterior shear forces acting on the knee, and is of particular importance in the rehabilitation of anterior cruciate ligament (ACL) repairs (see p. 230).

Several additional differences exist between open (single joint or 'isolation') and closed chain (multi-joint or 'general') exercises in resistance training. In an open chain action, movement occurs mainly distal to the joint axis, whereas, with a closed chain action, motion is both proximal and distal to the joint. An open chain action primarily emphasizes concentric work, but a closed chain movement brings a more balanced action of concentric, eccentric and isometric contractions into play.

Implications for rehabilitation

The evidence on mixtures of sets, repetitions and types of muscle work indicates that no single combination yields optimal gains for everyone. In early rehabilitation, where range of motion is severely limited, isometric exercise is useful. Performing this type of exercise in inner range will contribute to joint stability, and it is important that this be obtained before resisted movement is begun.

Because isometric gains are joint angle specific, resistance training should progress rapidly to involve all types of muscle work. At the beginning of a weight-training programme we have seen that neurogenic changes predominate. Practising the skilled movement involved in the exercise is therefore important at this stage, so multiset regimes are likely to be more successful. As rehabilitation progresses, all the fitness components must be worked. Power and speed are important and should be combined with rapid eccentric contractions in plyometric routines. Cardiopulmonary fitness may be maintained using circuit weight training, where lower limb injury prevents activities such as running, cycling or swimming.

For pure strength gains, high intensity programmes are more suitable for well-motivated individuals. Those who are poorly motivated may not be able to perform maximally in one set and so would be better to stay on more traditional multiset programmes.

For a weight training exercise to be maximal throughout the range of motion, the resistance offered to the muscle must change. Some form of accommodating resistance provided by an asymmetric cam or electronic braking system may be useful. Alternatively, free weights using bodybuilding techniques such as 'forced repetitions' and 'cheating repetitions' can be used. Here, a training partner or body swing, respectively, is used to take the weight through the point of maximal leverage traditionally called the 'sticking point'.

Specificity of training makes it of paramount importance that exercise mimics as closely as possible the function which will be required of the athlete. At this stage, sports specific skills should be practised in preference to pure strength work.

MUSCLE PAIN

Muscle pain occurs under normal circumstances with exercise, and does not necessarily indicate injury. Two types of pain are generally recognized. First, pain which occurs during exercise but disappears when the activity stops (ischaemic pain). Secondly, with unaccustomed exercise, discomfort may not occur immediately afterwards, but pain comes on a number of days later (delayed onset muscle soreness).

> **Keypoint**
>
> *Ischaemic* muscle pain occurs during exercise but disappears when activity stops. *Delayed onset muscle soreness* (DOMS) does not occur immediately, but comes on a number of days later.

Ischaemic muscle pain

Pain of this type begins in the working muscle and increases in intensity as exercise continues. It disappears when exercise stops and generally leaves no after-effects. The rise in intramuscular pressure during exercise can compress the blood vessels running through a muscle, producing ischaemic pain.

The accumulation of metabolites is generally accepted to be the cause of the pain. Lactic acid is often cited as the culprit, but patients who are unable to produce lactic acid (McArdle's syndrome) still suffer ischaemic pain. Histamine, acetylcholine, serotonin (5-HT), potassium and bradykinin are the most likely agents to cause the pain of ischaemia (Newham, 1991).

Delayed onset muscle soreness

Delayed onset muscle soreness (DOMS) is residual muscle pain which occurs 24–48 hours following unaccustomed bouts of intense exercise. Eccentric muscle work and exercise with a long muscle length have been shown to increase the intensity of the delayed onset soreness (Clarkson and Byrnes, 1986; Jones, Newham and Torgan, 1989). A number of possibilities exist for the cause of this pain, and it is probable that it is the result of a combination of factors, the contribution of each being related to activity type and individual differences.

Mechanical trauma can develop as a result of the high tensions developed during eccentric contractions (Newman et al., 1983). More trauma is likely with eccentric work than with other muscle actions because the tensions created during eccentric contraction are usually greater. In a study of downhill running, increases in creatine kinase and myoglobin were seen, suggesting that structural damage was occurring within the muscle (Byrnes and Clarkson, 1985).

Disruption seems to be to the connective tissue elements, rather than the contractile tissue within the active muscles. Hydroxyproline, a product of connective tissue breakdown has been detected in the urine of subjects suffering from

DOMS (McArdle, Katch and Katch, 1986), suggesting connective tissue damage. The cytoskeleton of the muscle, when damaged, becomes more permeable, allowing excess leakage of muscle enzymes and an increased uptake of injected radio-isotopes (Newham, 1991). Further, changes in the sarcoplasmic reticulum of the muscle cell have been shown to depress calcium muscle metabolism, altering muscle contraction and causing pain (McBride, 1998).

Unaccustomed exercise can also produce a build-up of *metabolites* within the working muscle. This in turn will give rise to osmotic changes in the cellular environment of the muscle, resulting in fluid retention and subsequent pressure on sensory nerves. Similarly, ischaemia of the working muscle can occur, leading to an accumulation of pain (p) substance, bringing on reflex muscle spasm (DeVries, 1961; Abraham, 1977).

A number of methods have been suggested to relieve DOMS. Stretching has been shown to reduce pain in the anterior tibial muscles (DeVries, 1961), and would certainly seem to be able to reduce muscle spasm. Increasing the blood flow to the muscle during the warm-down period is also helpful. This can be achieved by gentle exercise, hot showers or massage. In each case, a possible mechanism of relief is that of flushing fresh blood through the muscle to remove metabolic wastes, and pumping the lymphatic vessels to remove local oedema and reduce interstitial pressure.

MUSCLE FATIGUE

Muscle fatigue can present as a loss of force or power output, slowing of relaxation, changes in contractile characteristics and alterations in electrical properties. Two basic mechanisms of fatigue have been described, central and peripheral. Central fatigue refers to changes occurring proximal to the motor neurone, and involves neural and psychological changes such as motivation and recruitment. Peripheral fatigue involves the motor unit itself, and occurs chiefly through exhaustion of the muscle energy supplies. The type and intensity of activity being performed will decide whether central and peripheral fatigue occur separately or in combination.

If a subject is told to push as hard as possible for as long as possible, without feedback, force output will fall due to fatigue. If central fatigue occurs, more force can only be generated when the muscle is stimulated electrically.

Traditionally, fatigue types have been studied by comparing forces generated by maximum stimulated contraction (MStC), with those of maximal voluntary contractions (MVC). In unfatigued muscle, the MVC is the same as the MStC. With central fatigue, the force produced during MVC is less than that from an MStC, while in peripheral fatigue there is no difference between force of MVC and MStC (Bigland-Ritchie, 1981).

Peripheral fatigue can be further categorized into high and low frequency types. The natural firing frequencies of normal voluntary contractions are approximately 5–30 Hz. High frequency fatigue occurs when a muscle is stimulated at high frequencies between 50 and 100 Hz, while low frequency fatigue is the loss of force at low stimulation frequencies between 10 and 40 Hz.

References

Abraham, W.M. (1977) Factors in delayed onset muscle soreness. *Medicine and Science in Sports*, **9**, (1) 11–20

Adams, J.A. (1961) The second facet of forgetting: a review of warm-up decrement. *Psychological Bulletin*, **58**, 257–273

Allen, T.E., Byrd, R.J. and Smith, D.P. (1976) Hemodynamic consequences of circuit weight training. *Research Quarterly*, **47**, 299–306

Alter, M.J. (1996) *Science of Flexibility*, 2nd edn. Human Kinetics, Champaign, Illinois, USA

American College of Sports Medicine (1978) The recommended quantity and quality of exercise for developing and maintaining fitness in healthy adults. *Medicine and Science in Sports and Exercise*, **10**, VII–X

American College of Sports Medicine (1990) The recommended quantity and quality of exercise for developing and maintaining cardiorespiratory and muscular fitness in healthy adults. *Medicine and Science in Sports and Exercise*, **22**, 265–274

American College of Sports Medicine (2002) Progression models in resistance training for healthy adults. *Medicine and Science in Sports and Exercise*, **34**, 364–380

Andzel W.D. (1982) One mile run performance as a function of prior exercise. *Journal of Sports Medicine*, **22**, 80–84

Andzel, W.D. and Gutin, B. (1976) Prior exercise and endurance performance: a test of the mobilisation hypothesis. *Research Quarterly*, **47**, (3) 269–276

Anshel, M.H. (1991) A psycho-behavioral analysis of addicted versus non-addicted male and female exercisers. *Journal of Sport Behaviour*, **14**, (2) 145–154

Ashton, D. and Davies, B. (1986) *Why Exercise?* Basil Blackwell, London

Astrand, P-O. and Rodahl, K. (1986) *Textbook of Work Physiology*, McGraw-Hill, Maidenhead

Bandy, W.D., and Irion, J.M. (1994) The effect of time on static stretch of the flexibility of the hamstring muscles. *Physical Therapy* 74, (9) 845–852

Bandy, W.D., Lovelace-Chandler, V. and McKitrick-Bandy, B. (1990) Adaptation of skeletal muscle to resistance training. *Journal of Orthopaedic and Sports Physical Therapy*, **12**, (6) 248–255

Barnard, R.J., Gardner, G.W., Diaco, N.V., MacAlpin, R.N. and Kattus, A.A. (1973) Cardiovascular responses to sudden strenuous exercise: heart rate, blood pressure, and ECG. *Journal of Applied Physiology*, **34**, 883

Bartlett, M.J. and Warren, P.J. (2002) Effect of warming up on knee proprioception before sporting activity. *British Journal of Sports Medicine*, **36**, 132–134

Behm, D.G., Button, D.C. and Butt, J.C. (2001) Factors affecting force loss with prolonged stretching. *Canadian Journal of Applied Physiology*, **26**, 261–272

Bergh, U. (1980) Human power at subnormal body temperatures. *Acta Physiologica Scandinavica*, **478**(Suppl.), 1–39

Bergh, U. and Ekblom, B. (1979a) Physical performance and peak aerobic power at different body temperatures. *Journal of Applied Physiology*, **46**, 885–889

Bergh, U. and Ekblom, B. (1979b) Influence of muscle temperature on maximal muscle strength and power output in human skeletal muscles. *Acta Physiologica Scandinavica*, **107**, 33–37

Bigland-Ritchie, B. (1981) EMG and fatigue of human voluntary and stimulated contractions. In *Human Muscle Fatigue: Physiological Mechanisms* (eds R. Porter and J. Whelan), Ciba Foundation Symposium 82, Pitman Medical, London

Bonner, H.W. (1974) Preliminary exercise: a two-factor theory. *Research Quarterly*, **45**, 138–147

Borms, J. (1984) Importance of flexibility in overall physical fitness. *International Journal of Physical Education*, **11**, 2

Bosco, C. and Komi, P.V. (1979) Potentiation of the mechanical behaviour of the human skeletal muscle through pre-stretching. *Acta Physiologica Scandinavica*, **106**, 467

Bray, J.J., Cragg, P.A., Macknight, A.D.C., Mills, R.G. and Taylor, D.W. (1986) *Lecture Notes on Human Physiology*, Blackwell Scientific, Oxford

Brown, B.S., Payne, T., Kim, C., Moore, G., Krebs, P. and Martin, W. (1979) Chronic response of rat brain norepinephrine and serotonin levels to endurance training. *Journal of Applied Physiology*, **46**, 19–23

Brown, R.D. and Harrison, J.M. (1986) The effects of a strength training program on the strength and self-concept of two female age groups. *Research Quarterly for Exercise and Sport*, **57**, (4) 315–320

Byrnes, W.C. and Clarkson, M.C. (1985) Delayed onset muscle soreness following repeated bouts of downhill running. *Journal of Applied Physiology*, **59**, 283

Carlile, F. (1956) Effect of preliminary passive warming on swimming performance. *Research Quarterly*, **27**, (2) 143–151

Clarkson, P.M. and Byrnes, K.M. (1986) Muscle soreness and serum creatine kinase activity following isometric, eccentric, and concentric exercise. *International Journal of Sports Medicine*, **7**, 152–155

Cornelius, W.L. and Hinson, M.M. (1980) The relationship between isometric contraction of hip extensors and subsequent flexibility in males. *Journal of Sports Medicine and Physical Fitness*, **20**, 75–80

Costill, D.L., Fink, W.J., Getchell, L.H., Ivy, J.L. and Witzmann, F.A. (1979) Lipid metabolism in muscle of endurance trained males and females. *Journal of Applied Physiology: Respiratory, Environmental and Exercise Physiology*, **47**, 787

Crossman, J., Jamieson, J. and Henderson, L. (1987) Responses of competitive athletes to lay-offs in training: exercise addiction or psychological relief? *Journal of Sport Behaviour*, **10**, (1) 28–38

Cureton, T.K. (1941) Flexibility as an aspect of physical fitness. *Research Quarterly*, **12**(Suppl.), 381–390

Darden, E. (1975) Positive and negative work. *Scholastic Coach*, **45**, 6–12 and 85–86

Davies, C.T.M. and Young, K. (1983) Effect of temperature on contractile properties and muscle power of triceps surae in humans. *Journal of Applied Physiology*, **55**, 191–195

DeLorme, T. and Watkins, A. (1948) Techniques of progressive resistance exercise. *Archives of Physical Medicine and Rehabilitation*, **29**, 263–273

DeVries, H.A. (1959) Effects of various warm-up procedures on 100 yard times of competitive swimmers. *Research Quarterly*, **30**, 11–20

DeVries, H.A. (1961) Prevention of muscular distress after exercise. *Research Quarterly*, **32**, 177

DeVries, H.A. (1962) Evaluation of static stretching procedures for improvement of flexibility. *Research Quarterly*, **33**, 222–229

DeVries, H.A. (1980) *Physiology of Exercise for Physical Education and Athletics*, William C. Brown, Dubuque

Dishman, R.K. and Gettman, L.R. (1981) Psychological vigour and self-perceptions of increased strength. *Medicine and Science in Sports and Exercise*, **13**, 73–74

Ekstrand, J., Gillquist, J., Moller, M. et al. (1983) Incidence of soccer injuries and their relation to training and team success. *American Journal of Sports Medicine*, **11**, (March–April) 63–67

Enoka, R.M. (1994) *Neuromechanical Basis of Kinesiology*, 2nd edn, Human Kinetics, Champaign, Illinois

Etnyre, B.R. and Abraham, L.D. (1986) H-reflex changes during static stretching and two variations of proprioceptive neuromuscular facilitation techniques. *Electroencephalography and Clinical Neurophysiology*, **63**, 174–179

Etnyre, B.R. and Lee E.J. (1987) Comments on proprioceptive neuromuscular facilitation stretching. *Research Quarterly for Exercise and Sport*, **58**, (2) 184–188

Farrell, P.A., Gates, W.K., Morgan, W.P. and Pert, C.B. (1983) Plasma leucine enkephalin-like radioreceptor activity and tension-anxiety before and after competitive running. In *Biochemistry of Exercise* (eds H.G. Knuttgen, J.A. Vogel and J. Poortmans), Human Kinetics, Champaign, Illinois

Fiatarone, M.A. (1994) Exercise training and nutritional supplementation for physical frailty in very elderly people. *New England Journal of Medicine*, **330**, 1769

Fowles, J.R., Sale, D.G., and Macdougall, J.D. (2000) Reduced strength after passive stretch of the human plantarflexors. *Journal of Applied Physiology*, **89**, 1179–1188

Gettman, L.R. and Ayres, J.J. (1978) Aerobic changes through 10 weeks of slow and fast speed isokinetic training (abstract). *Medicine and Science in Sports and Exercise*, **10**, 47

Gettman, L.R. and Pollock, M.L. (1981) Circuit weight training: a critical review of its physiological benefits. *Physician and Sports Medicine*, **9**, (1) 44–60

Gettman, L.R., Ayres, J.J. and Pollock, M.L. (1978) The effect of circuit weight training on strength, cardio-respiratory function, and body composition of adult men. *Medicine and Science in Sports and Exercise*, **10**, 171–176

Gettman, L.R., Ayres, J.J. and Pollock, M.L. (1979) Physiological effects on adult men of circuit strength training and jogging. *Archives of Physical Medicine and Rehabilitation*, **60**, 115–120

Glasser, W. (1976) *Positive Addiction*, Harper and Row, New York

Goldberg, B., Saranitia, A. and Witman, P. (1980) Preparticipation sports assessment: an objective evaluation. *Pediatrics*, **66**, 736–745

Gonyea, W.J., Sale, D.G., Gonyea, F.B. and Mikesky, A. (1986) Exercise induced increases in muscle fiber number. *European Journal of Applied Physiology and Occupational Physiology*, **55**, 137–141

Greist, J.H., Klein, M.H., Eischens, R.R., Faris, J., Gurman, A.S. and Morgan, W.P. (1979) Running as treatment for depression. *Comprehensive Psychiatry*, **20**, 41–53

Gutin, B. and Stewart, K. (1971) Prior exercise and endurance. Physiology meeting. Springfield, Mass. Cited in Gutin et al. (1976)

Gutin, B., Stewart, K., Lewis, S. and Kruper, J. (1976) Oxygen consumption in the first stages of strenuous work as a function of prior exercise. *Journal of Sports Medicine*, **9**, 60–65

Hardy, L. and Jones, D. (1986) Dynamic flexibility and proprioceptive neuromuscular facilitation. *Research Quarterly for Exercise and Sport*, **57**, 150–153

Harris, M.L. (1969) Flexibility: a review of the literature. *Physical Therapy*, **49**, (6) 591–601

Harris, K.A. and Holly, R.G. (1987) Physiological response to circuit weight training in borderline hypertensive subjects. *Medicine and Science in Sports and Exercise*, **19**, 246

Hartig, D.E. and Henderson, J.M. (1999) Increasing hamstring flexibility decreases lower extremity overuse injuries in military basic trainees. *American Journal of Sports Medicine*, **27**, 173–176

Hass, C.J., Garzarella, L., Hoyos, D. and Pollock, M.L. (2000) Single versus multiple sets in long-term recreational weightlifters. *Medicine and Science in Sports and Exercise*, **32**, (1) 235–242

Herbert, R.D. and Gabriel, M. (2002) Effects of stretching before and after exercising on muscle soreness and risk of injury: systematic review. *British Medical Journal*, **325**, 468–470

Holland, G.L. (1968) The physiology of flexibility: a review of the literature. In *Kinesiology Review*, pp. 49–62

Hollis, M. (1977) *Practical Exercise Therapy*, Blackwell Scientific, Oxford

Holt, L.E. and Smith, R. (1983) *The Effect of Selected Stretching Programs on Active and Passive Flexibility*, Research Center for Sport, Del Mar, CA, USA

Holt, L.E., Travis, T.T. and Okita, T. (1970) Comparative study of three stretching techniques. *Perceptual and Motor Skills*, **31**, 611–616

Hopper, D. (1986) A survey of netball injuries and conditions related to these injuries. *Australian Journal of Physiotherapy*, **32**, (4) 231–239

Hurley, B.F., Hagberg, J.M., Allen, W.K., Seals, D.R., Young, J.C., Cuddihee, R.T. and Holloszy, J.O. (1984) Effect of training on blood lactate levels during submaximal exercise. *Journal of Applied Physiology: Respiratory Environment, and Exercise Physiology*, **56**, 1260

Janda, V. (1992) *Muscle and Back Pain: Assessment and Treatment of Impaired Movement Patterns and Motor Recruitment*, associated course to the 5th International Symposium of the Physical Medicine Research Foundation, Oxford

Jaric, S., Gavrilovic, P. and Ivancevic, V. (1985) Effects of previous muscle contractions on cyclic movement dynamics. *European Journal of Applied Physiology*, **54**, 216–221

Johnson, B.L., Adamezyk, J.W., Tenmore, K.O. and Stromme, S.B. (1976) A comparison of concentric and eccentric muscle training. *Medicine and Science in Sports and Exercise*, **8**, 35–38

Jones, D.A., Newham, D.J. and Torgan, C. (1989) Mechanical influences on long standing human muscle fatigue and delayed onset muscle pain. *Journal of Physiology*, **224**, 173–186

Jones, R.J. and Wright, V. (1982) Relative importance of various tissues in joint stiffness. *Journal of Applied Physiology*, **17**, (5) 824–828

Kent, M. (1994) *Oxford Dictionary of Sports Science and Medicine*, Oxford University Press, Oxford

Knight, K.L. (1979) Knee rehabilitation by the daily adjustable progressive resistance exercise technique. *American Journal of Sports Medicine*, **7**, 336

Kokkonen, J., Nelson, A.G. and Cornwall, A. (1998) Acute muscle stretching inhibits maximal strength performance. *Research Quarterly for Exercise and Sport*, **69**, 411–415

Kraemer, W.J., Stone, M. and O'Bryant, H. (1997) Effects of single vs. multiple sets of weight training; impact of volume, intensity and variation. *Journal of Strength and Conditioning Research*, **11**, 143–147

LaBan, M.M. (1962) Collagen tissue: implications of its response to stress in vitro. *Archives of Physical Medicine and Rehabilitation*, **43**, 461–466

Lashville, A.V. (1983) Active and passive flexibility in athletes specialising in different sports. *Soviet Sports Review*, **18**, (1) 30–32

Lawrence, D. and Hope, B. (2002) *Complete Guide to Circuit Training*, A&C Black, London

Lees, A. and Graham-Smith, P. (1996) Plyometric training: a review of principles and practice. *Sport Exercise and Injury*, **2**, 24–30

Levine, M.G. and Kabat, H. (1952) Co-contraction and reciprocal innervation in voluntary movement in man. *Science*, **116**, 115–118

Lewit, K. (1991) *Manipulative Therapy in Rehabilitation of the Locomotor System*, 2nd edn, Butterworth-Heinemann, Oxford

McArdle, W.D., Katch, F.I. and Katch, V.L. (1986) *Exercise Physiology: Energy, Nutrition, and Human Performance*, 3rd edn, Lea and Febiger, Philadelphia

McArdle, W.D., Katch, F.I. and Katch, V.L. (1991) *Exercise Physiology*, 4th edn, Lippincott, Williams and Wilkins, Philadelphia

McArdle, W.D., Katch, F.I. and Katch, V.L. (2001) *Exercise Physiology, Energy, Nutrition, and Human Performance*, 5th edn, Lea and Febiger, Philadelphia

McArdle, W.D., Katch, F.I. and Katch, V.L. (2002) *Exercise Physiology*, 5th edn, Lippincott, Williams and Wilkins, Philadelphia

McBride, J.M. (1998) Effects of resistance exercise on free radical production. *Medicine and Science in Sports and Exercise*, **30**, 67

McCafferty, W.B. and Horvath, S.M. (1977) Specificity of exercise and specificity of training: a subcellular review. *Research Quarterly*, **48**, 358–371

MacDougall, J.D., Ward, G.R., Sale, D.G. and Sutton, J.R. (1977) Biochemical adaptation of human skeletal muscle in heavy resistance training and immobilization. *Journal of Applied Physiology*, **43**, 700–703

McNair, P.J. and Stanley, S.N. (1996) Effect of passive stretching and jogging on the series elastic muscle stiffness and range of motion of the ankle joint. *British Journal of Sports Medicine*, **30**, 313–318

Magnusson, S.P., Simonsen, E.B. and Kjaer, M. (1996) Biomechanical responses to repeated stretches in human hamstring muscle in vitro. *American Journal of Sports Medicine*, **24**, (5) 622–628

Mandell, A.J. (1979) The second wind. *Psychiatric Annals*, **9**, 57–69

Messier, S.P. and Dill, M.E. (1985) Alteration in strength and maximal oxygen uptake consequent to Nautilus circuit weight training. *Research Quarterly*, **56**, (4) 345–351

Moore, M.A. and Kukulka, C.G. (1991) Depression of Hoffman reflexes following voluntary contraction and implications for proprioceptive neuromuscular facilitation therapy. *Physical Therapy*, **71**, 321–333

Morgan, W.P. (1985) Affective beneficence of vigorous physical activity. *Medicine and Science in Sports and Exercise*, **17**, (1) 94–100

Nacson, J. and Schmidt, R.A. (1971) The activity-set hypothesis for warmup decrement. *Journal of Motor Behavior*, **3**, 1–15

Newham, D.J. (1991) Skeletal muscle pain and exercise. *Physiotherapy*, **77**, (1) 66–70

Newman, D.J., Mills, K.R., Quigley, B.M. and Edwards, R.H.T. (1983) Pain and fatigue after concentric and eccentric muscle contractions. *Clinical Science*, **64**, 55–62

Norris, C.M. (1996) *Stretching*, Physiotools compatable CD ROM programme, Physiotools, Helsinki, Finland

Norris, C.M. (1999) *The Complete Guide to Stretching*, A&C Black, London

Norris, C.M. (2002) *Bodytoning*, A&C Black, London

Ostrowski, K.J., Wilson, G., Weatherby, P. and Lyttle, A. (1997) The effect of weight training volume on hormonal output and muscular size and function. *Journal of Strength and Conditioning Research*, **11**, 148–154

Palmitier, R.A., An, K., Scott, S.G. and Chao, E.Y.S. (1991) Kinetic chain exercise in knee rehabilitation. *Sports Medicine*, **11**, (6) 402–413

Pert, C.B. and Bowie, D.L. (1979) Behavioral manipulation of rats causes alterations in opiate receptor occupancy. In *Endorphins in Mental Health* (eds E. Usdin, W.E. Bunney and N.S. Kline), Oxford University Press, Oxford

Pollock, M.L., Cureton, T.K. and Greniger, L. (1969) Effects of frequency of training on working capacity, cardiovascular function and body composition of adult men. *Medicine and Science in Sports*, **1**, 70–74

Potteiger, J.A. (1999) Muscle power and fiber characteristics following 8 weeks of plyometric training. *Journal of Strength and Conditioning Research*, **13**, (3) 275–279

Ranatunga, K.W., Sharpe, B. and Turnbull, B. (1987) Contractions of a human skeletal muscle at different temperatures. *Journal of Physiology*, **390**, 383–395

Reilly, T. (1981) The concept, measurement and development of flexibility. In *Sports Fitness and Sports Injuries* (ed. T. Reilly), Faber and Faber, London

Renstrom, P. and Kannus, P. (1992) Prevention of injuries in endurance athletes. In *Endurance in Sport* (eds R.J. Shephard and P.O. Astrand), IOC Medical Commission Publication, Blackwell Scientific, Oxford, pp. 325–350

Richards, D.K. (1968) A two factor theory of the warm-up in jumping performance. *Research Quarterly*, **39**, 668–673

Rigby, B. (1964) The effect of mechanical extension under the thermal stability of collagen. *Biochimica et Biophysica Acta*, **79**, 634–636

Roman, W.J. (1993) Adaptations in the elbow flexors of elderly males after heavy resistance training. *Journal of Applied Physiology*, **74**, 750

Rosenbaum, D. and Henning, E.M. (1995) The influence of stretching and warm up exercises on Achilles tendon reflex activity. *Journal of Sports Science*, **15**, 481–484

Rutherford, O.M. (1988) Muscular coordination and strength training: implications for injury rehabilitation. *Sports Medicine*, **5**, 196–202

Safran, M.R., Garrett, W.E., Seaber, A.V., Glisson, R.R. and Ribbecsk, B.M. (1988) The role of warmup in muscular injury prevention. *American Journal of Sports Medicine*, **16**, (2) 123–129

Sale, D.G. (1988) Neural adaptation to resistance training. *Medicine and Science in Sports and Exercise*, **20**, (5) 135–145

Sale, D.G. (1992) Neural adaptation to strength training. In *Strength and Power in Sport* (ed. P.V. Komi), IOC Medical Publication, Blackwell Scientific, Oxford

Sapega, A.A., Quedenfel, T.C., Moyer, R.A. and Butler R.A. (1981) Biophysical factors in range of motion exercise. *Physician and Sports Medicine*, **9**, (12) 57–65

Sargeant, A.J. (1987) Effect of muscle temperature on leg extension force and short term power output in humans. *European Journal of Applied Physiology*, **56**, 693–698

Sargeant, A.J. and Dolan, P. (1987) Effect of prior exercise on maximal short term power output in humans. *Journal of Applied Physiology*, **63**, 1475–1480

Schmidt, R.A. (1982) *Motor Control and Learning*, Human Kinetics, Champaign, Illinois

Seward, H.G. and Patrick, J. (1992) A three year survey of Victorian football league injuries. *Australian Journal of Medicine and Science in Sport*, **24**, (2) 51–54

Seyle, H. (1956) *The Stress of Life*, McGraw-Hill, New York

Shellcok, F.G. and Prentice, W.E. (1985) Warming up and stretching for improved physical performance and prevention of sports related injuries. *Sports Medicine*, **2**, 267–278

Silvester, L.J., Stiggins, C., McGown, C. and Bryce, G. (1982) The effect of variable resistance and free-weight training programs on strength. *National Strength and Conditioning Association Journal*, **3**, 30–33

Sipala, S. and Suominen, H. (1995) Effects of strength and endurance training on thigh and leg muscle mass and composition in elderly women. *Journal of Applied Physiology*, **78**, 334

Smith, L.L., Brunetz, M.H. and Chenier, T.C. (1993) The effects of static and ballistic stretching on delayed muscle soreness and creatine kinase. *Research Quarterly for Exercise and Sport*, **64**, 1438–1446

Taylor, D.C., Dalton, J., Seaber, A.V. and Garrett, W.E. (1990) The viscoelastic properties of muscle-tendon units. *American Journal of Sports Medicine*, **18**, 300–309

Thorstensson, A. (1977) Observations on strength training and detraining. *Acta Physiologica Scandinavica*, **100**, 491–493

Tucker, L.A. (1982) Effect of a weight training program on the self concept of college males. *Perceptual and Motor Skills*, **54**, 1055–1061

Verhoshanski, Y. and Chornonson, G. (1967) Jump exercises in sprint training. *Track and Field Quarterly*, **9**, 1909

Voight, M.L. and Draovitch, P. (1991) Plyometrics. In *Eccentric Muscle Training in Sports and Orthopaedics* (ed. M. Albert), Churchill Livingstone, London

Vujnovich, A.L., and Dawson, N.J (1994) The effect of therapeutic muscle stretch on neural processing. *Journal of Orthopedic and Sports Physical Therapy*, **20**, (3) 145–153

Warren, C.G., Lehmann, J.F. and Koblanski, J.N. (1971) Elongation of rat tail tendon: effect of load and temperature. *Archives of Physical Medicine and Rehabilitation*, **51**, 465–474

Weldon, S.M. and Hill, R.H. (2003) The efficacy of stretching for prevention of exercise-related injury: a systematic review of the literature. *Manual Therapy*, **8**, (3) 141–150

Westing, S.H., Seger, J.Y. and Thorstensson, A. (1991) Isoacceleration: a new concept of resistive exercise. *Medicine and Science in Sports and Exercise*, **23**, (5) 631–635

Wilmore, J.H., Parr, R.B. and Girandola, R.N. (1978) Physiological alterations consequent to circuit weight training. *Medicine and Science in Sports and Exercise*, **10**, 79–84

Wolpaw, J.R., Lee, C.L. and Carp, J.S. (1991) Operantly conditioned plasticity in spinal cord. *Annals of the New York Academy of Sciences*, **627**, 338–348

Yarasheski, K.E. (1993) Acute effects of resistance exercise on muscle synthesis in young and elderly adults. *American Journal of Physiology*, **265**, 210

Zinovieff, A.N. (1951) Heavy resistance exercise, the Oxford technique. *British Journal of Physical Medicine*, **14**, 129

Chapter 6

Exercise therapy

CHAPTER CONTENTS

STRUCTURE VS FUNCTION

Often, student physiotherapists new to soft tissue injury management will focus attention purely on structure. Equipped with a wide knowledge of anatomy, they try to find which single structure has been injured. If it is a muscle tear, for example, they may note the muscle's origin and insertion and treat the muscle in isolation. When it comes to exercise, they consider the muscle's action and give this action as an exercise of some type. For example, if the hamstring muscles are torn, exercises are often given which simply involve flexing the knee against resistance and performing a toe-touching movement to stretch the muscle.

As experience is gained, the clinical physiotherapist realizes the error of this *reductionist* approach. If the body is reduced to a number of simple components, rehabilitation of a sporting injury is largely ineffective. The muscle may strengthen or increase in flexibility, for example, but the ability of the patient to perform the adaptations of daily living (ADL), and the athlete to participate in sport, often remains poor. The athlete with a hamstring tear treated in this way will very often find pain relieved mainly through the passage of time, but on return to sport the injury simply recurs.

Definition
A *reductionist* approach seeks to understand complex items (in this case the body) in terms of their more simple component parts.

Rather than reducing the body to simple structural components, if movement quality is the starting point for rehabilitation, the athlete's ability is rapidly enhanced. Instead of considering the textbook anatomy of an area, if the therapist asks the simple question 'how does this injury affect the athlete?' the answer will often guide the rehabilitation programme perfectly.

The functional decrement which the patient is suffering becomes the central focus, rather than the structural damage, and as a consequence, rehabilitation is considerably more successful. The athlete with the hamstring injury described above may well lack strength and flexibility, and in the early stages of rehabilitation, simple single plane motions may suffice. But if the therapist considers the function of the hamstrings in the closed kinetic chain position, the action of the muscle in ballistic movements, and the stresses imposed on a two-joint muscle, a whole series of exercises become available.

Through this approach the therapist can break away from standard lists of exercises which fail to take account of the needs of the individual. Instead of the athlete grinding away in boredom at endless repetitions of a movement, exercise therapy can become vibrant and challenging. The end result is a more rewarding period of rehabilitation for both athlete and therapist.

The aim of this chapter is therefore to develop the theme of 'functional exercise therapy', and we will begin by looking at muscle imbalance. Further details of these concepts maybe found in Norris (2000) and Norris (2002).

MUSCLE IMBALANCE

Basic concepts

Changes in muscle length or strength occur throughout the body in set patterns rather than purely at random. The relationship between the tone and length of muscles around a joint is known as muscle imbalance and has been described by a number of authors (Janda and Schmid, 1980; Sahrmann, 1987; Richardson, 1992; Kendall, McCreary and Provance, 1993; Comerford, 1995; Norris, 1995a). Muscles may be broadly classified into two types, those whose actions are mainly to stabilize a joint and approximate the joint surfaces, and those responsible more for movement, which more effectively develop angular rotation. The main differences between the two types of muscles are shown in Table 6.1.

The stability muscles tend to be more deeply placed, while the mobilizers are superficial. In addition, mobilizers are often biarticular muscles. For example, in the leg the rectus femoris is classified as a mobilizer, while the quadriceps are stabilizers. Stabilizer function is more slow twitch (type I) or tonic in nature, while that of the mobilizers tends towards fast twitch (type II) phasic action. This physiology suits the functional requirements of the muscles, enabling mobilizers to contract and build maximal tension rapidly, but fatigue quickly. The stabilizers build tension slowly and

perform well at lower tensions over longer periods, being more fatigue resistant.

Stabilizer muscles are better activated in closed kinetic chain actions, where movement occurs proximally on a distally stabilized segment. Mobilizer function is more effective in an open chain situation, where free movement occurs without distal fixation. The structure and functional characteristics of the two muscle categories make the stabilizers better equipped for postural holding and anti-gravity function. The mobilizers are better set up for rapid ballistic movements.

Two of the fundamental changes seen in the muscle imbalance process include tightening of the mobilizer (two-joint) muscles and laxity/loss of endurance within the inner range for the stabilizer (single-joint) muscles. These two changes are used as tests for the degree of muscle imbalance. The combination of length and tension changes alter muscle pull around a joint and so pull the joint out of alignment. Changes in body segment alignment and the ability to perform movements which dissociate one body segment from another form the bases of the third type of test used when assessing muscle imbalance (Fig. 6.1).

> **Keypoint**
>
> Through misuse or injury, stabilizing muscles tend to become lax (sagging) while movement muscles tend to tighten.

The mixture of tightness and weakness seen in the muscle imbalance process alters body segment alignment and changes the equilibrium point of a joint. In addition, imbalance leads to lack of accurate segmental control. The combination of stiffness (hypoflexibility) in one body segment and laxity (hyperflexibility) in an adjacent body segment leads to the establishment of relative flexibility (White and Sahrmann, 1994). In a chain of movement the body seems to take the path of least resistance, with the more flexible segment moving first and furthest. If we take as an illustration two pieces of rubber tubing (Fig. 6.2) of unequal strengths. When the movement begins at C and A is fixed, the more flexible area B–C moves more. This will still be the case if C is held still and A moves.

Table 6.1 Muscle types (basic classification)

Stability	Movement
Deep	Superficial
Slow twitch	Fast twitch
One joint	Two joint
Weaken and lengthen	Tighten and shorten
Inhibited	Preferential recruitment

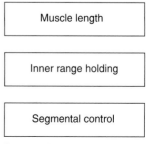

Figure 6.1   Assessing muscle imbalance.

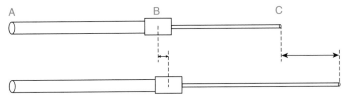

Figure 6.2 Relative stiffness. When the cord is stretched, the tighter segment (A–B) moves less than the looser segment (B–C).

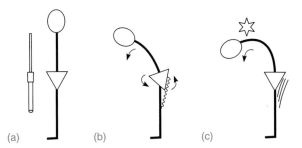

(a)   (b)   (c)

Figure 6.3 Relative stiffness in the body. (a) Tighter hamstrings, more lax spinal tissues. (b) Forward flexion should combine pelvis tilt and spinal flexion equally. (c) Tight hamstrings limit pelvic tilt, throwing stress on the more lax spinal tissues.

Taking this example into the body, Figure 6.3 shows a toe-touching exercise. The two areas of interest with relation to relative stiffness are the hamstrings and lumbar spine tissues. As we flex forwards, movement should occur through a combination of anterior pelvic tilt and lumbar spine flexion (see p. 143). Subjects often have tight hamstrings and looser lumbar spine tissues due to excessive bending during everyday activities. During this flexion action, greater movement, and therefore greater tissue strain, will always occur at the lumbar spine. Relative stiffness, in this case, makes the toe-touching exercise ineffective as a hamstring stretch unless the trunk muscles are tightened to stabilize the lumbar spine.

Definition

Relative flexibility (relative stiffness) occurs when the body takes the path of least resistance in a movement. Tighter tissues will allow less movement while looser (lax) tissues allow more.

Muscle adaptation

Muscle adaptation to reduced usage has been extensively studied using immobilized limbs (Appell, 1990). The greatest tissue changes occur within the first days of disuse. Strength loss has been shown to be as much as 6% per day for the first 8 days with little further loss after this period (Muller, 1970). Greater reduction in size and loss of numbers is seen in type I fibres, with a parallel increase in type II fibres, demonstrating selective atrophy of type I fibres (Templeton et al., 1984). However, not all muscles show an equal amount of type I fibre atrophy. Atrophy is largely related to change in use

relative to normal function, with the initial percentage of type I fibres that a muscle contains being a good indicator of likely atrophy pattern. Those muscles with a predominantly anti-gravity function, which cross one joint and have a large proportion of type I fibres, show greatest selective atrophy (e.g. soleus and vastus medialis). Those predominantly slow anti-gravity muscles which cross multiple joints are next in order of atrophy (e.g. erector spinae); last are phasic, predominantly fast type II muscles which can be immobilized with less loss of strength (e.g. biceps) (Lieber, 1992).

Keypoint

Following immobilization, muscles with a large number of type I (slow) fibres will show more marked atrophy.
Muscles with predominantly type II (fast) fibres show less loss of cross-sectional area (CSA) and strength.

These three categories of muscles have led to stabilizers being subdivided into *primary* and *secondary* types (Jull, 1994) as shown in Figure 6.4. Examples of the three types include multifidus, transversus abdominis and vastus medialis oblique as primary stabilizers. The gluteals and oblique abdominals are classified as secondary stabilizers, while rectus femoris and the hamstrings are mobilizers, only acting as stabilizers in conditions of extreme need.

The primary stabilizers have very deep attachments, lying close to the axis of rotation of the joint. In this position they are unable to contribute any significant torque, but will approximate the joint. In addition, many of these smaller muscles have important proprioceptive functions (Bastide, Zadeh and Lefebvre, 1989). The secondary stabilizers are the main torque producers, being large monoarticular muscles attaching via extensive aponeuroses. Their multipennate fibre arrangement makes them powerful and able to absorb large amounts of force through eccentric action. The mobilizers are fusiform in shape, with a less powerful fibre arrangement, but one which is designed for producing large ranges of motion. In addition, the mobilizers are biarticular muscles, which have their own unique biomechanical characteristics (see p. 17).

Selective changes in muscle may also occur as a result of training (Richardson and Bullock, 1986). In the knee, rapid flexion – extension actions have been shown to selectively increase activity in the rectus femoris and hamstrings (biarticular) but not in the vasti (monoarticular). In this study, comparing speeds of 75°/s and 195°/s, mean muscle activity for the rectus femoris increased from 23.0 uV to 69.9 uV. In contrast, muscle activity for the vastus medialis increased from 35.5 uV to only 42.3 uV (Fig. 6.5). The pattern of muscle activity was also noticeably different in this study after training. At the fastest speeds the rectus femoris and hamstrings displayed phasic (on and off) activity while the vastus medialis showed a tonic (continuous) pattern (Fig. 6.6).

Even in the more functional closed kinetic chain position, similar changes have been found (Ng and Richardson, 1990).

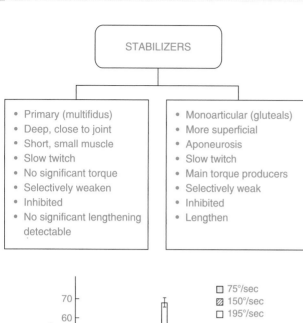

Figure 6.4 Muscle types (extended classification). After Jull (1994).

STABILIZERS

- Primary (multifidus)
- Deep, close to joint
- Short, small muscle
- Slow twitch
- No significant torque
- Selectively weaken
- Inhibited
- No significant lengthening detectable

- Monoarticular (gluteals)
- More superficial
- Aponeurosis
- Slow twitch
- Main torque producers
- Selectively weak
- Inhibited
- Lengthen

MOBILIZERS

- Biarticular (Hamstrings)
- Superficial
- Fusiform
- Fast twitch
- Multi-joint activity
- Strong
- Preferential recruitment
- Shorten

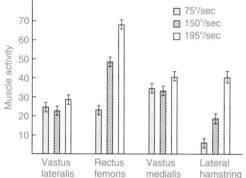

Figure 6.5 Changes in muscle activity with increases in speed. From Richardson, C.A. and Bullock, M.I. (1986) Changes in muscle activity during fast, alternating flexion–extension movements of the knee. *Scandinavian Journal of Rehabilitation Medicine*, **18**, 51–58. With permission.

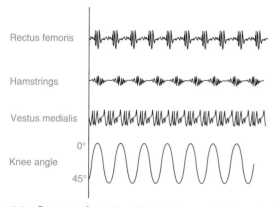

Figure 6.6 Patterns of muscle activity during rapid alternating knee flexion–extension. Biarticular muscles are phasic, monoarticular muscles are tonic. Redrawn from Richardson, C.A. and Bullock, M.I. (1986) Changes in muscle activity during fast, alternating flexion-extension movements of the knee. *Scandinavian Journal of Rehabilitation Medicine*, **18**, 51–58. With permission.

A 4-week training period of rapid plantarflexion in standing gave significant increases in jump height (gastrocnemius, biarticular) but also significant loses of static function of the soleus (monoarticular).

CHANGES IN MUSCLE LENGTH

Chronic muscle lengthening

Stabilizer muscles tend to 'weaken' (sag) whereas mobilizers tend to 'shorten' (tighten). Taking these responses further, primary stabilizers will react quickly to pain and swelling, by inhibition. Swelling has been shown to cause a reflex inhibition of muscles in the knee (de Andrade, Grant and Dixon, 1965; Stokes and Young, 1984). In addition, marked asymmetry of the multifidus has been shown using real-time ultrasound imaging.

Adaptation of primary stabilizers of the spine

Multifidus   The cross-sectional area (CSA) of the multifidus has been shown to be substantially reduced at the level of lumbar lesion (Hides et al., 1994). The authors suggested that the mechanism for the CSA reduction was inhibition through perceived pain via a long loop reflex.

In addition to changes in muscle bulk, alteration in fibre type has been shown in the multifidus in patients with low back pain (LBP) (Biedermann et al., 1991). A reduced ratio of slow twitch to fast twitch muscle fibres was shown, possibly as an adaptive response by the muscle to changes in functional demand placed upon it. Furthermore, injury may have caused a shift in the recruitment patterns of the motor units of the paraspinal muscles, with the fast twitch motor units being recruited before the slow twitch units.

Posture has also been shown to affect the multifidus. In a study of 20 healthy subjects, O'Sullivan et al. (2002) showed a reduction in activity of the multifidus (together with internal oblique and the thoracic erector spinae) in a sway-standing posture (see p. 139), indicating the importance for postural retraining when facilitating the muscle for rehabilitation. Prolonged flexion activities initially result in a reflex spasm of the multifidus, which reduces substantially if the posture is maintained. Williams et al. (2000) used a cat model to investigate sustained moderate flexion stress on seven preparations. They showed a reduction to 5% of this initial value within 3 minutes of taking up the posture, leading to tissue laxity and a loss of reflex protective muscle activity. Prolonged flexion (20 minutes, using cat preparation) has also been shown to result in multifidus spasm (Jackson et al. 2001), with full recovery not seen for 7 hours after initiation of rest.

Transversus abdominis   The transversus abdominis shows a similar response in the chronic LBP patient. Normally, this muscle acts as a primary stabilizer of the lumbar spine (Jull, 1994). It is active in both flexion and extension of the lumbar spine (Cresswell, Grundstrom and Thorstensson, 1992) and during action of the upper limb and lower limb in multiple directions (Hodges, Richardson and Jull, 1996). In addition, contraction of transversus abdominis precedes that of the other abdominal and lumbar extensor muscles (Cresswell, Oddsson and Thorstensson, 1994; Hodges and Richardson, 1996). Its primary function would seem to be to contract in response to forces applied to the trunk. In this way it is anticipating the requirement of stability and providing it.

Following LBP, transversus abdominis function changes considerably (Hodges and Richardson, 1995; Hodges, Richardson and Jull, 1996). Timing of onset of transversus contraction is delayed by a mean of 129 ms, while the action of the other abdominals is largely unchanged. When assessed in a hollowing action (see p. 130) the transversus muscle shows a smaller increase in thickness measured by real-time ultrasound (between rest and contraction) in patients with low back pain than in normal subjects. Normal subjects showed a mean thickness increase of 49.7% while low back patients showed mean values of 19.15% (Critchley and Coutts, 2002).

Quadratus lumborum   The quadratus lumborum (QL) is a muscle which has been described both as a movement muscle tending towards tightness (Janda, 1993) and as an important stabilizer in functional lifting tasks (McGill, Juker and Kropf, 1996). The medial fibres of the muscle connect directly to the lumbar transverse processes, therefore having the potential to stabilize the spine. The lateral fibres run between the ilium and iliolumbar ligament and the 12th rib, spanning the spine and acting as a movement muscle. The muscle is therefore separated into two functional components (Bergmark, 1989). The medial fibres can contribute directly to segmental support of the spine (Richardson et al., 1999), while the lateral portion may tend towards tightness and developing trigger points (Janda, 1993; Gunn, 2000).

The QL has been shown to be an important stabilizer of the spine in side carrying tasks especially (McGill, Juker and Kropf, 1996; McGill, 2000). It is important to note that when the spine fails (buckles) due to compressive loads, it does so laterally in the first instance, so a muscle which resists lateral forces is likely to be an important stabilizer when carrying loads. In addition, the QL functions differently to the erector spinae in forward bending, as it does not demonstrate a flexion relaxation response (Andersson et al., 1996). Whether the muscle reacts to injury and underusage in the same way as the transversus or multifidus is as yet uncertain. Categorization of the medial portion of the

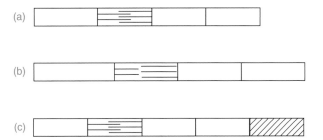

Figure 6.7   Muscle length adaptation. (a) Normal muscle length. (b) Stretched muscle – filaments move apart and muscle loses tension. (c) Adaptation by increase in serial sarcomere number (SSN), normal filament alignment restored, muscle length permanently increased.

muscle as a stabilizer is certain, but sub-categorization into a primary or secondary stabilizer will require more evidence (Bullock-Saxton et al., 2000).

Keypoint

Primary stabilizers adapt to reduced usage by (i) a shift in the recruitment patterns and timing of the synergistic muscle actions they are linked to, (ii) a reduction in cross-sectional area (CSA) and (iii) pathological changes to their muscle structure.

Adaptation of secondary stabilizers

The secondary stabilizer muscles show a tendency to *lengthen* and *weaken*. As postural muscles they almost seem to give way to the pull of gravity and 'sag'. This reaction has been termed stretch weakness (Kendall, McCreary and Provance, 1993). The muscle has remained in an elongated position, beyond its normal resting position, but within its normal range. This is differentiated from overstretch where the muscle is simply elongated or stretched beyond its normal range.

The length–tension relationship of a muscle (see p. 18) dictates that a stretched muscle, where the actin and myosin filaments are pulled apart, can exert less force than a muscle at normal resting length. Where the stretch is maintained, however, this short-term response (reduced force output) changes to a long-term adaptation. The muscle tries to move its actin and myosin filaments closer together, and to do this, it must add more sarcomeres to the ends of the muscle (Fig. 6.7). This adaptation, known as an increase in serial sarcomere number (SSN), changes the nature of the length–tension curve.

Definition

Serial sarcomere number (SSN) is the number of sarcomere units along an individual muscle fibre. Muscles held in a lengthened position for a prolonged period will adapt by increasing their SSN.

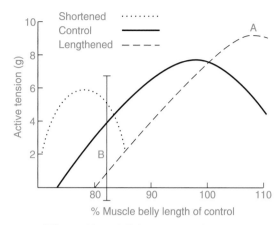

Figure 6.8 Effects of immobilizing a muscle in shortened and lengthened positions. The normal length–tension curve (control) moves to the right for a lengthened muscle, giving it a peak tension some 35% greater than the control (point A). When tested in an inner-range position (point B), however, the muscle tests weaker than normal. Reprinted from Gossman, M.R., Sahrmann, S.A. and Rose, S.J. (1982) Review of length associated changes in muscle. *Physical Therapy*, **62**(12), 1799–1808. With permission.

Long-term elongation of this type causes a muscle to lengthen by the addition of up to 20% more sarcomeres (Gossman, Sahrmann and Rose, 1982). The length–tension curve of an adaptively lengthened muscle moves to the right (Fig. 6.8). The peak tension that such a muscle can produce in the laboratory situation is up to 35% greater than that of a normal length muscle (Williams and Goldspink, 1978). However, this peak tension occurs at approximately the position where the muscle has been immobilized (point A, Fig. 6.8). If the strength of the lengthened muscle is tested with the joint in mid-range or inner-range (point B, Fig. 6.8), as is common clinical practice, the muscle cannot produce its peak tension, and so the muscle appears 'weak'. For this reason, manual muscle tests have been described as being more accurate indicators of positional (rather than total) strength (Sahrmann, 1987).

In the laboratory situation the lengthened muscle will return to its optimal length within approximately 1 week if once more placed in a shortened position (Goldspink, 1992). Clinically, restoration of optimal length may be achieved by either immobilizing the muscle in its physiological rest position (Kendall, McCreary and Provance, 1993) and/or exercising it in its shortened (inner-range) position (Sahrmann, 1990). Enhancement of strength is not the priority in this situation; indeed, the load on the muscle may need to be reduced to ensure correct alignment of the various body segments and correct performance of the relevant movement pattern.

Immobilization of cat hind limb in a lengthened position (4 weeks) showed a 19% increase in SSN of the soleus muscle but no change in individual sarcomere length. Immobilizing in a shortened position gave a 40% decrease in SSN, again with no change in sarcomere length (Tabary, 1972). It has been argued that this type of adaptation enables the muscle to develop maximum tension when movement of the muscle is limited (Jaspers, Fagan and Tischler, 1985).

SSN may be partly responsible for changes in muscle strength without parallel changes in hypertrophy (Koh, 1995). SSN exhibits marked plasticity and may be influenced by a number of factors. For example, immobilization of rabbit plantarflexors in a lengthened position showed an 8% increase in SSN in only 4 days, while applying electrical stimulation to increase muscle force showed an even greater increase (Williams et al., 1986). Stretching a muscle appears to have a greater effect on SSN than does immobilization in a shortened position. Following immobilization in a shortened position for 2 weeks, the mouse soleus has been shown to decrease SSN by almost 20% (Williams, 1990). However, stretching for just 1 hour per day in this study not only eliminated the SSN reduction but actually produced nearly a 10% increase in SSN.

An *eccentric stimulus* may cause a greater adaptation of SSN than a concentric stimulus. Morgan and Lynn (1994) subjected rats to uphill or downhill running, and showed SSN in the vastus intermedius to be 12% greater in the eccentric trained rats after 1 week. In contrast to this, however, Koh and Herzog (1998) used the dorsiflexor muscles of the rabbit to assess the effect of eccentric training on SSN. Using a 2 week training session over a total of 12 weeks, they found little effect on SSN or fibre length, but the variation between the studies may well be related to species or training protocol differences.

It has been suggested that if SSN adaptation occurs in humans, strength training might produce such a change if it were performed at a joint angle different from that at which the maximal force is produced during normal activity (Koh, 1995).

Rather than being weak, the lengthened muscle lacks the ability to maintain a full contraction within inner range. This shows up clinically as a difference between the active and passive inner ranges. If the joint is passively placed in full anatomical inner range, the subject is unable to hold the position. Sometimes the position cannot be held at all, but more usually the contraction cannot be sustained, indicating a lack in slow twitch endurance capacity.

Shortening posturally lengthened muscle

Clinically, reduction of muscle length is seen as the enhanced ability to hold an inner-range contraction. As the muscle is already strong, the focus is not on resistance but on position (alignment) and holding time. The muscle is passively positioned within its inner range and the patient is instructed to hold this position. Initially this will not be possible and the limb will fall away from the inner-range joint position. The patient should be encouraged to slow the rate of limb fall to initiate an eccentric contraction. Once this is achieved, the eccentric action is emphasized, with the therapist placing the joint within its inner range and the patient using an eccentric action to guide the limb descent. Over time (sometimes within one treatment session, more normally 2–3 sessions), the patient will be able to hold the inner-range position for a short period of time (seconds only). The next phase in the

Keypoint

Keypoint

Shortening a posturally lengthened muscle is achieved by working within inner range only. The initial muscle work is eccentric followed by isometric contractions with minimal loading.

restoration of muscle balance is to emphasize the inner-range holding ability, building to 10–30 seconds holding. Finally, the patient uses a concentric action to pull the limb into its inner range position, holds using an isometric action, and lowers under control (eccentric). At this point, muscle control through full range has been achieved.

Inner-range holding may or may not represent a reduction in SSN, but is a required functional improvement in postural control. Muscle shortening may certainly be achieved through splinting. Muscles immobilized in a shortened position in this way show loss of sarcomeres in series within 14–28 days (Tabary, 1972; Williams and Goldspink, 1978). With training, there is less evidence for reduction in SSN. Muscle shortening has been shown in the dorsiflexors of horseriders. Clearly, this position is not held permanently as with splinting, but rather shows a training response. Following pregnancy, SSN increases in the rectus abdominis in combination with diastasis. Again, the length of the muscle gradually reduces in the months following birth. It is generally thought that inner-range training is likely to shorten a lengthened muscle, although the precise method through which this adaptation is achieved is not certain (Goldspink, 1996). The treatment aim for a posturally lengthened muscle must ultimately be to change its resting length and therefore correct segmental alignment. In so doing the joints within a body region will be able once more to move through an optimal movement range (Sahrmann, 2002).

Keypoint

To restore the serial sarcomere number (SSN) and shorten a chronically lengthened muscle, it can be (i) splinted in a shortened position, (ii) worked within inner range, (iii) subjected to eccentric loading. A combination of these procedures will give the best result.

Inner-range holding ability

The ability of a stabilizer muscle to maintain an isometric contraction at low load over a period of time is vital to its anti-gravity function (Richardson, 1992). This may be assessed by using the classic muscle test position (see Appendix) and asking the subject to maintain a contraction in full inner range (Richardson and Sims, 1991). The important factor in the assessment is the length of time a static hold can be maintained without jerky (phasic) movements

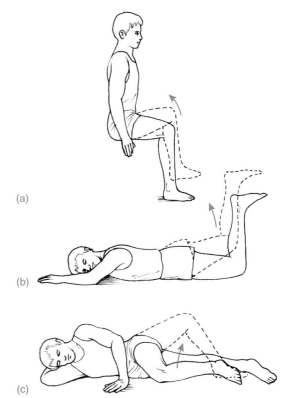

(a)

(b)

(c)

Figure 6.9   Inner-range holding of the lower limb. (a) Iliopsoas. (b) Gluteus maximus. (c) Gluteus medius.

occurring. In each case the limb is placed passively into full inner range. When released, if the limb drops, the passive range of motion differs from the active range, which is an important indicator of poor stabilizer function. Full stabilizing function is achieved when a subject can maintain the inner-range position for 10 repetitions, each of 10 seconds duration (Jull, 1994). Often the first two or three repetitions are performed normally, and it is only with further repetition that the deficit becomes apparent.

Keypoint

Inner-range holding ability is assessed by holding the test position for 10 seconds and repeating this action 10 times.

Tests for the major stabilizing muscles

Tests for the major stabilizing muscles of the trunk, pelvic and shoulder girdle areas, including transversus abdominis, gluteus medius, gluteus maximus, the deep neck flexors and the lower trapezius are described below

Lower limb

Iliopsoas   The iliopsoas (IP) is assessed in the sitting position. The patient flexes the hip while maintaining a 90° knee flexion so that the foot is lifted clear of the ground (Fig. 6.9a).

Where the IP is lengthened the thigh may drop down from the inner range position, or more commonly the pelvis is tilted backwards while the knee position is maintained. Backward tilting of the pelvis accompanied by flattening of the lumbar lordosis moves the origin of the muscle away from its insertion and lengthens the IP.

Gluteus maximus   The gluteus maximus is assessed in prone lying with the knee flexed to 90°. Flexing the knee shortens the hamstring muscles, placing them at a physiological disadvantage and making hamstring substitution less likely. The hip is lifted to inner-range extension and held (Fig. 6.9b). In this position, the gluteus maximus may be palpated; often, with a chronic low back pain patient, little activity is noted. Where the muscle is working, it may still not be able to maintain the inner range position over time. Here, the inner range position is held for 1–2 seconds and the limb slowly sinks to a lower position and is held at this mid-range angle. As endurance of the muscle fails, muscle shaking is evident as the large diameter fast twitch fibres of the muscle are used.

Gluteus medius   The gluteus medius is tested in side lying with the knee flexed. The action is combined with hip abduction, with slight lateral rotation to emphasize the posterior fibres of the muscle (Fig. 6.9c). Two starting positions may be used, both with the foot supported to work the limb in closed chain format. In the *first* the feet are placed together; in the *second* the foot of the upper leg is placed on the couch at mid-shin level. The action is to keep the foot still and lift the knee while keeping the trunk still. Rotation of the trunk at the pelvis must be avoided. The therapist should monitor the position of the greater trochanter of the upper leg and ensure that it points to the ceiling and does not move forwards or backwards.

Cervical spine

For the cervical spine the essential stabilizers are the deep neck flexors. These are retrained in the supine position using pressure biofeedback, with the cuff placed behind the head or upper cervical spine (Jull, 1994). The aim is to achieve suboccipital rather than lower cervical flexion. The action is a minimal flexion or 'nodding' action of the head alone, avoiding forceful actions or lifting the head from the couch (see p. 358).

Overactivity of the superficial muscles with trigger point development is common. The sternomastoid and anterior scalene especially may be shortened in a head held forward (HHF) posture. In addition, tightness and thickening are seen in the splenius capitis and splenius cervicis, as well as the semispinalis capitis and levator scapuli (Gunn, 1996).

> **Keypoint**
>
> The stabilizers of the cervical spine are the deep neck flexors (see also p. 358). These are retrained using suboccipital flexion (nodding) rather than lower cervical flexion.

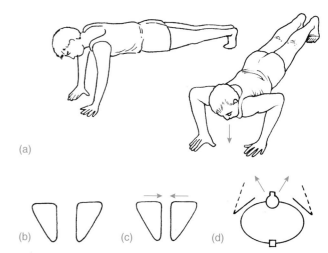

Figure 6.10   Eccentric push-up as a global assessment of scapulothoracic stability. (a) Athlete slowly lowers from a push-up position – note position of scapula. (b) Scapulae should remain apart and fixed to the ribcage as the body is lowered. (c) Scapulae fall together if rhomboids and levator scapulae are dominant. (d) True winging. The medial edges of the scapulae lift.

Upper trunk

A blanket assessment of scapular stability may be usefully made in prone falling (Fig. 6.10). Slowly lowering (eccentric push-up) will often reveal inappropriate movement of the scapulae in the first phase of the action. The scapulae should remain apart, and firmly fixed to the thoracic wall throughout the movement. Scapular movement outward and upward indicates lack of stability (Janda, 1994). If the scapulae fall together, the rhomboids and levator scapulae are dominant (Kendall, McCreary and Provance, 1993). True winging, apparent through lifting of the medial edge of the scapula, represents serratus anterior inactivity.

Retraining scapular stability   Scapular stability is enhanced by restoring the functional capacity of the lower trapezius and serratus anterior, which, as stability muscles, often show reduced activity and lengthening. Surface electromyography (sEMG) may be used with the active electrode placed over the lower trapezius or serratus anterior. The patient is placed in prone lying and the scapula is passively positioned into its neutral position by the therapist. This often requires retraction and depression to neutralize the protraction/elevation often found (Fig. 6.11). The patient is encouraged to hold this position through his or her own muscle activity, gaining feedback from the sEMG readout. Enough muscle activity

> **Keypoint**
>
> The main scapular stabilizers are serratus anterior and the lower trapezius. These muscles are worked using low load scapular depression and retraction. The inner range scapular position is held to build postural endurance.

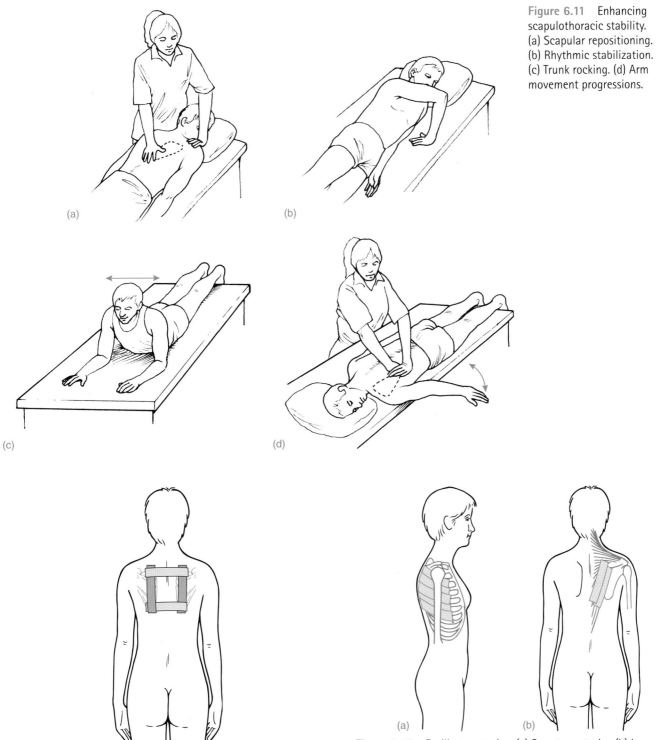

Figure 6.11   Enhancing scapulothoracic stability. (a) Scapular repositioning. (b) Rhythmic stabilization. (c) Trunk rocking. (d) Arm movement progressions.

Figure 6.12   Box taping to facilitate correct scapular alignment.

Figure 6.13   Facilitatory taping. (a) Serratus anterior. (b) Lower trapezius.

should be used to keep the anterior aspect of the shoulder off the treatment couch, but not to retract the scapulae. Once this position can be maintained actively, the holding time is built up until the patient can perform 10 repetitions, holding each for 10 seconds.

Taping may be used to give feedback about the position of the scapula and lengthened muscle. A positional box tape may be used to facilitate position of the scapula (Fig. 6.12). The tape has two horizontal strips to draw the medial borders of the scapulae together and two vertical strips to facilitate thoracic extension. Non-elastic taping is used to take up skin tension and act as a feedback system for the patient. Facilitatory taping may be used over the serratus anterior (Fig. 6.13a), lower trapezius (Fig. 6.13b), or to increase patient awareness of body segment position and facilitate underlying muscle action.

The scapular force couples may be maximally challenged using a side lying, braced position (Wilk and Arrigo, 1993). The patient begins in side lying with the arm flexed/abducted to 90° and internally rotated. The hand is now flat on the couch with the fingers pointing towards the patient. Scapular fixation is maintained against the rhythmic stabilization provided by the therapist in all planes.

The next stage is to introduce a limited range of movements of the humerus onto the now stable base of the scapular thoracic joint. Initially, the patient assumes elbow support prone lying to work the shoulder in closed kinetic chain format. He or she moves the body over the arm forward and backwards and side to side to create closed chain flexion/extension and abduction/adduction. At all times the scapula must remain in contact with the thorax. The patient is now moved to the edge of the couch so the affected arm hangs over the couch side. Maintaining scapula thoracic stability, inner-range movements in all three planes are used in an attempt to automatize stability (see p. 320).

The starting position is now changed to sitting or standing and inner-range movements are used with sEMG monitoring of the lower trapezius. Home exercises may be used by asking the patient to place the thumb of the opposite hand beneath the inferior scapular angle. The patient then gently keeps the inferior ankle pressed against the thumb (retraction and depression) while performing inner-range movements.

These initial actions, where stabilization ability is being re-educated, must keep the arm below 30° abduction to prevent scapular movement. Later, greater glenohumeral range may be used as the patient can control scapulothoracic movement.

The scapulothoracic muscles may be selectively strengthened using the individual exercises shown in Figure 6.14.

Lower trunk

Inner-range holding of the trunk begins with the abdominal hollowing action. This is the fundamental action for the initiation of core stability. Core stability itself is re-educated in three phases, *muscle isolation*, *stability control* and *reduced attention demand* (Norris, 1995c). Abdominal hollowing for muscle isolation is described here. Progressions from this movement for stability control and reduced attention demand are covered in Chapter 14.

Abdominal hollowing   For the abdominal hollowing action, the patient begins in the prone kneeling position. As the transversus has horizontally aligned fibres, this action allows the abdominal muscles to sag, giving stretch facilitation. The patient focuses attention on the umbilicus and is instructed to pull the umbilicus 'in and up' while breathing normally (Fig. 6.15a). This action has been shown to dissociate activity in the internal obliques and transversus from that of rectus abdominis (Richardson et al., 1992). This makes the exercise useful for re-educating the stabilizing function of the

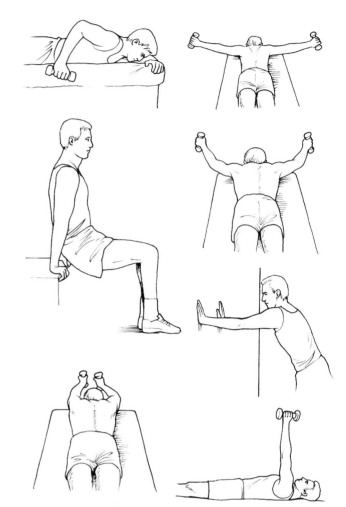

Figure 6.14   Exercises to selectively strengthen the scapulothoracic muscles. After Kamkar, Irrang and Whitney (1993).

Muscle	Suggested exercises
Serratus anterior	Scapular plane abduction, pushup, end-range shoulder flexion in prones, serratus anterior punch
Upper trapezius	Shoulder shrugs, scapular plane abductions
Middle trapezius	Rowing, shoulder elevation and hyper extension in standing, shoulder abduction and flexion in prones, scapular retraction with horizontal abduction of the externally rotated shoulder in prone
Lower trapezius	Scapular plane abduction and rowing, shoulder depression and retraction in sitting, elevation of the externally rotated arm which is positioned diagonally between flexion and abduction
Levator scapulae	Shoulder elevation, abduction, flexion, rowing
Rhomboids	Rowings, shoulder retraction, elevation and abduction, scapular retraction with horizontal abduction of the internally rotated shoulder in prone
Latissimus dorsi	Press-ups, lateral pull
Pectoralis major	Press-ups
Pectoralis minor	Press-ups

abdominals where rectus abdominis has become the dominant muscle of the group.

To facilitate learning, multisensory cueing is used (Miller and Medeiros, 1987) to increase the sensory input to the patient. Auditory cues can be provided by the therapist speaking to the subject and giving feedback about performance. Visual cues are given by encouraging the subject to look at the muscles as they function, and by using a mirror. Kinaesthetic cueing is accomplished by encouraging the subject to 'feel' the particular action, for example, to 'feel the stomach being pulled in'. Tactile cues are provided by the therapist touching the subject's abdomen as muscle contraction begins.

Errors in the abdominal hollowing action   Several errors can occur when a patient practises abdominal hollowing. Essentially, the rib cage, shoulders and pelvis should remain still throughout the action. The contour of the abdomen will flatten if a deep breath is taken and held, but the therapist should see the chest expansion involved (Fig. 6.15b). Where this occurs, the patient is instructed to exhale and hold this chest position as the exercise is performed. Placing a belt around the lower chest is useful to give feedback about chest movement (Richardson and Hodges, 1996).

Another substitution action is to use the external oblique to brace the abdomen. However, these muscles will pull on the lower ribs and depress them at the same time, slightly flexing the thoracic spine. A horizontal skin crease is often visible across the upper abdomen (Fig. 6.15c). Where this occurs, the patient is encouraged to perform pelvic floor contraction at the same time as abdominal hollowing. Simultaneous contraction of the gluteus maximus must be avoided with this action, as this will teach an inappropriate motor pattern for trunk stability during dynamic sports activity.

Keypoint

When performing the abdominal hollowing action, monitor the patient's lower ribs. As the action is performed the ribs should stay still and neither raise nor lower.

Use of pressure biofeedback   Restoration of the abdominal hollowing mechanism can also be enhanced by the use of pressure biofeedback (Chattanooga Group Limited, Bicester, England). The biofeedback unit consists of a rubber bladder and pressure gauge similar to a sphygmomanometer.

Prone lying   In prone lying, the pressure biofeedback unit is placed beneath the abdomen with the lower edge of the bladder level with the anterior superior iliac spines, and the centre of the bladder over the umbilicus (Fig. 6.16a). The unit is inflated to 70 mmHg, and abdominal hollowing is performed. The aim is to reduce the pressure reading on the biofeedback unit by 6–10 mmHg, and to be able to maintain this contraction to repetition (10 repetitions of 10-second hold) to ensure that endurance of the target muscles is adequate (Richardson and Hodges, 1996).

Crook lying   As a further test, a crook lying position is used. The bladder of the unit is placed beneath the subject's lumbar spine and inflated to show a constant figure of 40 mmHg. The subject is instructed to contract the abdominal muscles without performing a posterior pelvic tilt (Fig. 6.16b). If the lordosis is unchanged, a constant pressure is shown on the pressure unit. Increasing pressure shows flattening of the

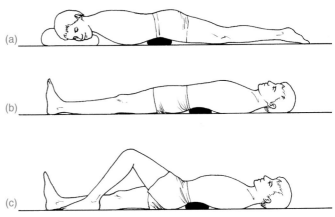

Figure 6.16   Use of pressure biofeedback. (a) Prone lying abdominal hollowing assessment. (b) Assessing change in the depth of the lordosis during abdominal hollowing. (c) The heel slide to test lumbar stability.

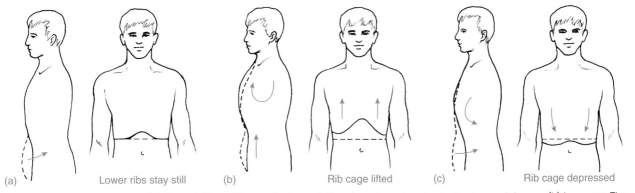

Figure 6.15   Abdominal hollowing. (a) Normal. The subject pulls the umbilicus in and up, drawing in the lower abdomen. (b) Incorrect. The subject takes a deep breath in, raising the ribs to stretch the abdominal muscles to produce flattening. (c) Incorrect. The subject uses the external oblique to brace the abdomen. The lower ribs are depressed and the slight flexion causes a horizontal skin crease across the upper abdomen.

lordosis (lumbar flexion), while reducing pressure shows increased lordosis (lumbar extension). Excessive motion in either direction represents loss of lumbar stability. Alteration of starting position and the addition of simultaneous limb movement encourages body awareness and movement control.

Heel slide The ability of the deep abdominals to maintain spinal stability may be accurately assessed using the heel slide manoeuvre (Fig. 6.16c). The subject starts in crook lying with the spine in a neutral position and the pressure biofeedback unit positioned beneath the lower spine. One leg is then gradually straightened, sliding the heel along the ground to take the weight of the leg. During this action, the hip flexors are working eccentrically and pulling on the pelvis and lumbar spine. If the strong pull of these muscles is sufficient to displace the pelvis, the pelvic tilt is noticeable by palpation of the anterior superior iliac spine (ASIS) and by an alteration of the pressure biofeedback unit. The action must be completed without using the substitution actions described above.

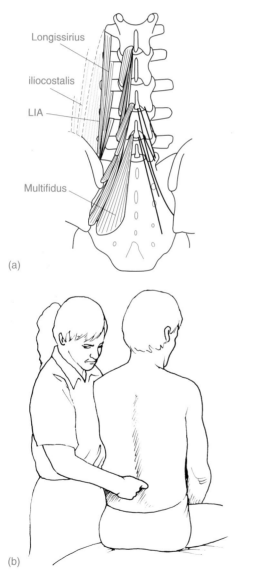

(a)

(b)

Figure 6.17 Multifidus retraining. (a) The fascicles of multifidus in the lumbar spine. (b) Multifidus facilitation in sitting.

Multifidus muscle retraining Measurement and enhancement of multifidus function is begun in prone lying. The fibres of multifidus (Fig. 6.17a) are palpated medial to the longissimus at L4 and L5 levels. The spinous processes are identified and the fingers then slide laterally into the hollow between the spinous process and the longissimus bulk. The difference in muscle consistency is assessed, and then the patient's ability to isometrically contract the multifidus in a 'setting' action is determined. The patient is encouraged to use multifidus setting in a sitting position with a neutral lumbar spine. Palpation is with the therapist's thumb and knuckle of the first finger placed on either side of the lumbar spinous process at any one level. The instruction to the patient is to 'feel the muscle swelling' without actively flexing the lumbar spine (Fig. 6.17b). The patient's own thumbs may be used to give feedback for home practice. sEMG can also be used as the multifidus is superficial at this level. Multifidus function may also be enhanced using manual therapy techniques such as rhythmic stabilization (for details see Norris 2000, pp. 90–91).

Spasm of the multifidus has been proposed as a factor in many instances of chronic low back pain (Gunn, 1996). In addition to manual therapy techniques and dry needling (see Norris 2001), muscle re-education may be used to restore normal function of the muscle. Contraction and relaxation of muscle is a familiar treatment protocol for pain reduction in muscles such as the upper trapezius for example. The same method would seem to apply to the multifidus.

Muscle shortening

Mobilizer muscles have long fusiform shapes and, as such, show a tendency to tighten. Tightness in the hamstrings, for example (mobilizers, biarticular), is often seen, while tightness in the gluteals (stabilizers, monoarticular) is rare. As well as reducing range of motion, the tightened muscle is more likely to develop painful trigger points (Travell and Simons, 1983) These are small hypersensitive regions within a muscle which stimulate afferent nerve fibres, causing pain. The sensation created is a deep tenderness with an overlying increase in tone creating a palpably tender band of muscle. When palpated deeply, the trigger point creates a local muscle spasm, giving the 'jump sign' (Janda, 1993). The irritability threshold of a tight muscle is lowered, causing it to be activated earlier than normal in a movement sequence. One of the reasons for this is that, being tight, there is less 'slack' to take up in the muscle before contraction begins. In addition, the muscle shows an increased afferent input via the stretch receptors (Sahrmann, 1990).

Tightness of mobilizer muscles is an important factor in muscle balance assessment. Rather than simply range of motion, however, we are interested in a subject's ability to maintain body segment alignment while the stretch is put on. Using the straight leg raise (SLR) as an example of range measurement for the hamstrings, the point which indicates full range from a muscle imbalance perspective is not necessarily the end of available motion for the leg, but the point at which hamstring tension is sufficiently high to cause the pelvis to tilt (see below).

The lower limb

The tests used to assess muscle length may also be used to stretch a muscle if it is found to be tight. The three key movements to assess restriction of pelvic motion are the modified Thomas test, the SLR, and the Ober test. If any movement reproduces the patient's pain it is relevant, and if the range is significantly less than the optimal value given, the muscle will require specific stretching.

Thomas test   The Thomas test used here is modified from the original test first described by Jones and Lovett (1929). With the modified Thomas test (Fig. 6.18), the patient begins in crook lying at the end of the couch. The knees are brought to the chest and the back flattened to a point where the sacrum just begins to lift away from the couch surface but no

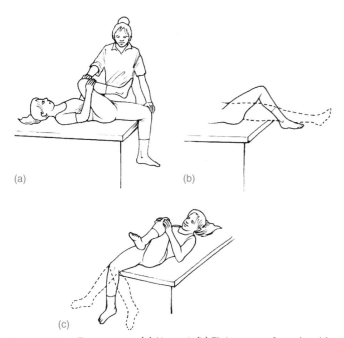

Figure 6.18   Thomas test. (a) Normal. (b) Tight rectus femoris – hip flexed, but femur drops down as leg is straightened. (c) Tibia should be vertical – deviation from this position indicates femoral rotation.

further. One leg is held close to the chest to maintain the pelvic position and the other leg is straightened over the couch end. An optimal alignment exists when the femur lies horizontally, and aligned to the sagittal plane (no abduction). The tibia should lie vertically (90° knee flexion) and be aligned with the sagittal plane (no hip rotation), as shown in Fig. 6.18. If the femur rests above the horizontal and the knee is flexed less than 90°, tightness may be present in either the iliopsoas or rectus femoris. If the rectus is tight, straightening the knee will take the stretch off the muscle and the leg will drop down. If the knee is straightened and the leg stays in place, it indicates tightness in the iliopsoas. Deviation of the knee laterally (the 'J' sign) indicates a possible tightness in the iliotibial band (ITB), indicating that the Ober test should be performed to confirm the tightness. The Thomas test has been shown to be a repeatable measure using 11 subjects over a sequence of 10 trials (Bullock-Saxton and Bullock, 1994).

Ober test   The modified Ober test (Ober, 1936) begins in side lying (Fig. 6.19). The test assesses the length of the tensor fascia lata (TFL), providing the pelvis remains in a neutral position. In side lying, the lower leg is bent to improve stability and the therapist stabilizes the pelvis to avoid lateral pelvic dipping. The couch should be low enough to allow pressure to be placed through the iliac crest in the direction of the lower shoulder. Maintaining the neutral pelvic position, the hip is abducted and extended to 15°. It is then adducted while maintaining extension. An optimal length for an athlete would be seen when the upper leg is able to lower to couch level. This differs from the original test which was described with the knee flexed. Testing with the knee straight, however, places a greater stretch on the femoral nerve and the rectus femoris, which makes the test less precise. In addition the ITB has a greater stretch placed on it with the knee extended providing the hip remains in extension, as in this position the ITB is stretched over the greater trochanter (Magee, 2002).

Where the TFL may be tight, causing friction syndromes (p. 222), knee flexion may be added to localize the stretch towards or away from the knee. To differentiate pain in this case from that of neural origin from femoral nerve impingement, the prone knee bend test (PKB) may be used.

Figure 6.19   Ober test. (a) With pelvis neutral, upper leg should stay in extension and adduct past the horizontal. (b) A false reading is obtained if the pelvis is allowed to tip and the lumbar spine to laterally flex.

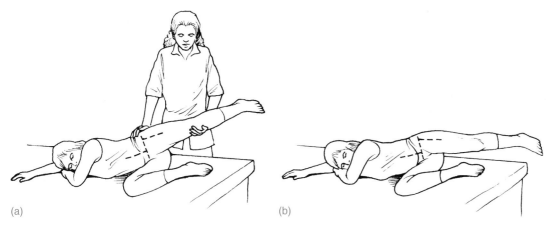

(a)   (b)

> **Definition**
>
> For the *prone knee bend (PKB) test*, the patient lies on their front, and the examiner flexes the knee maximally on the painful side to provoke pain in the low back, buttock or leg. This indicates an L2 or L3 nerve lesion, or involvement of the femoral nerve itself. Pain must be distinguished from quadriceps tightness.

Where hip extension is limited, the test can still be carried out, but the hip tightness must be assessed further to determine if it is muscular, capsular, or osteological in nature.

Hamstring length tests   The hamstrings are assessed by three actions: the straight leg raise (SLR), active knee extension (AKE), and the tripod test. The *SLR test* (Fig. 6.20a) is used to assess flexibility of the hamstrings but also as a clinical test for sciatic nerve entrapment. Although useful clinically to determine associated symptoms from neural involvement, the accuracy of the test as a muscle length measure may be questioned (Bohannon, 1982; Urban, 1981). To use the SLR as a muscle imbalance test, the anterior rim of the pelvis is palpated to note the point at which the pelvis begins to posteriorly tilt due to hamstring tightness. This is the point at which a stable base is no longer being provided for the hamstrings to stretch against, and is perhaps more relevant than full passive range pressing against a fully posteriorly tilted pelvis.

The *AKE test* (Fig. 6.21) is performed with the subject lying supine on a couch. The knee and hip are flexed to 90° and held in this position by the subject or therapist. The subject then straightens the leg using quadriceps action and holds the maximum knee extension for 3–5 seconds while the knee angle is measured. This test has been shown to be reliable in both the laboratory (Gajdosik and Lusin, 1983) and clinical settings (Norris and Mathews, in press).

The *tripod test* (Fig. 6.20b) again assesses the interplay between hamstring flexibility and lumbar stability. In the sitting position (feet off the floor), one leg is straightened. Two measures are noted: first, the point at which posterior pelvic tilting occurs, and second, the total range of combined motion at both hip and knee. For optimal performance, the lumbar spine should remain neutral and allow the knee to straighten to within 10° of full extension while the femur remains horizontal.

Stretching tight muscles   Where muscle tightness is found, the test exercises may be used as starting positions for stretching. Before stretching tight muscles, we must ensure that excessive strain will not be placed on adjacent body parts through relative stiffness. This often requires some stability work before beginning the stretch. Passive static stretching is used initially, followed by contract – relax (see p. 102). Finally, the opposing muscles are shortened to full inner range to stretch the antagonist actively. From the Thomas test position, the hip is flexed slightly and the knee extended against the resistance of limb weight alone. The position is held for 20–30

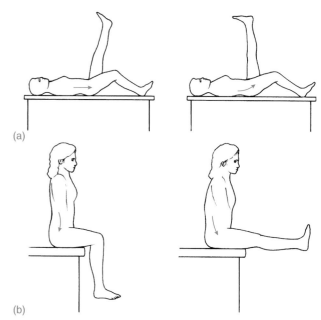

(a)

(b)

Figure 6.20   Assessing the effect of hamstring tightness on pelvic tilt. (a) Straight leg raise – the beginning of posterior pelvic tilt marks the loss of alignment. (b) Tripod test – as the leg is straightened the pelvis posteriorly tilts.

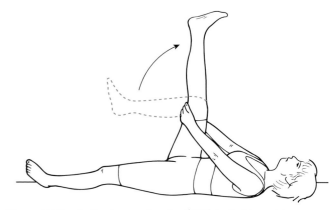

Figure 6.21   Active knee extension (AKE) test of hamstring muscles. From Norris, C.M. (1999) *The Complete Guide to Stretching*. A C Black, London. With permission.

seconds and the leg is then lowered to a new stretched position. The opposing knee must remain tightly gripped to the chest to ensure the posterior pelvic tilt is maintained throughout the exercise. An alternative exercise to stretch the hip flexors while re-educating spinal stability is the half lunge (Fig. 6.22a). The half-kneeling position is taken up, with one hand placed on a chair to aid balance, the other pressing into the lumbar spine on the side of the dependent leg. The abdominal hollowing procedure is performed and is held throughout the exercise to maintain a neutral position of the lumbar spine. To impart the stretch, the body lunges forwards, forcing the dependent hip into extension while avoiding increasing the lordosis.

In the Ober test position, the iliotibial band (ITB) is stretched. However, this exercise is only effective if the subject is able to stabilize the pelvis against frontal movement by maintaining a contraction of the quadratus lumborum and ipsilateral obliques. To re-educate this action, the subject is first taught a hip-hitching action in standing (Fig. 6.22b) to be repeated in lying. Finally, hip-hitching is performed and the subject maintains the contraction of the trunk side flexors on the side of the upper leg, as this leg is lowered into adduction and slight extension (Fig. 6.22c).

The hamstrings are initially stretched in the SLR test position. Exercise one (Fig. 6.22d) is the active knee extension (AKE) manoeuvre, where the upper leg is held in 90° hip flexion and the leg is straightened. An alternative is to straighten the leg in 160° hip flexion and then actively pull the straight leg up to 90° hip flexion without allowing the knee to bend (Fig. 6.22e). This combines inner-range shortening of the hip flexors with lengthening of the hip extensors.

Finally, the tripod test position combines lumbar stability with mobilizer lengthening in a functional starting position (Fig. 6.22f). The subject begins sitting on the edge of a couch with the feet off the floor. An upright sitting posture is taken with the lumbar spine in its neutral position. This position is maintained throughout the exercise by performing abdominal hollowing. The leg is now straightened to stretch the hamstrings against the stable base of the unmoving pelvis.

Longer periods of stretching are generally recommended (see p. 101), with holding times of 30 seconds being optimal. Some authors, however, recommend even longer holding times for combining stretch of the shortened muscle with shortening of the lengthened muscle. Using the tripod stretch position above, the patient would be instructed to sit with the back slightly lordosed (hollow) using minimal contraction of the erector spinae to anteriorly tilt the pelvis. They would then extend the knee to the point where tightness is felt and

support the heel on a low stool. This low level stretch would be maintained for 20–30 minutes and repeated six times throughout the day (Sahrmann, 2002). Obviously, patient compliance is a large factor with this type of intervention, so the method of functional stretching must be built into a patient's daily living. The stretch above, for example, may be given as an adaptation of the normal sitting position for an office worker.

The upper limb

Neck side flexion combined with other movements is a key movement for the trapezius, sternomastoid and anterior scalenes (Fig. 6.23).

Upper trapezius and levator scapulae   The upper trapezius may be tight if the scapula is held in a downwardly rotated position. However, more normally the upper trapezius is hypertonic, its overactivity trying to compensate for underactivity of the lower trapezius and serratus anterior. Stretching consists of side flexion away from the tight muscle, combined with neck flexion. For this to be effective the scapula must be fixed. Clinically, many patients with an overactive upper trapezius also present with neck pain. For this reason scapular fixation is normally used as overpressure, rather than neck movements which would throw stress onto the painful cervical spine. To stretch the right muscle, the patient sits on a chair and elevates the right scapula. The patient then flexes the cervical spine and laterally flexes it to the left. This neck position is held by reaching over the head with the left arm and hand. Maintaining the cervical position, the right scapula is depressed and retracted to place the stretch on the muscle. Painful trigger points are often found within the upper trapezius muscle at the highest point of the muscle belly.

The levator scapulae is stretched using a similar movement, but this time adding rotation away from the muscle being stretched (in this case rotate to the left). A trigger point is often present in the levator scapulae, and this can be found by palpating the superior angle of the scapula and tracing the muscle distally from this point towards the upper cervical spine.

Sternomastoid   The sternomastoid is stretched by combining side flexion away, and rotation towards, the muscle being tested. Where the right sternomastoid is stretched, the head is turned to the left and side flexed to the right. Painful trigger points may be found in the centre of the muscle, level with the Adam's apple (laryngeal prominence).

Anterior scalene and rhomboids   The anterior scalene is stretched initially by manual pressure on the first rib

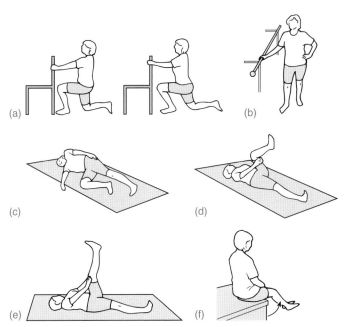

Figure 6.22   Hip flexibility exercises. (a) Half lunge. (b) Hip hitching in standing. (c) Hip hitching is maintained (pull pelvis up against hand) as upper leg is lowered into adduction. (d) Active knee extension (holding thigh). (e) Active knee extension (press thigh against hand). (f) Active knee extension in sitting – the tripod test.

combined with side flexion away from the muscle. Further stretch is placed on the muscle by rotating towards the muscle and extending the lower cervical spine by performing a full chin-tuck action. The rhomboids are stretched by actively stabilizing the scapula and flexing the arms to 90° and protracting. The arms are then crossed to the elbows. Trigger points for the anterior scalene muscles lie over the anterior aspect of the neck, close to the clavicle, and for the rhomboid muscles along the medial edge of the scapula.

Pectoralis major and minor In supine lying, the pectoralis major and minor and latissimus dorsi may be tested (Fig. 6.24). When lying supine, the posterior border of the acromion should rest no more than 2–3 finger breadths above

Figure 6.23 Neck side flexion tests. (a) Trapezius and levator scapulae (see text). (b) Sternomastoid. (c) Anterior scalene.

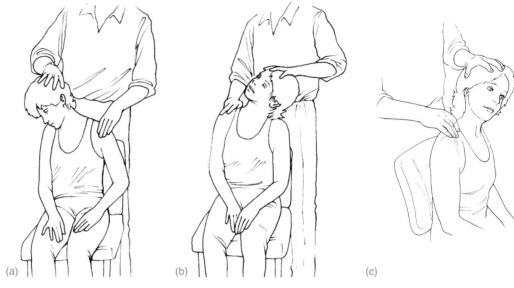

(a) (b) (c)

Fig. 6.24 Supine lying tests. (a) Pectoralis minor. (b) Pectoralis major (sternal portion). (c) Pectoralis major (clavicular portion). (d) Latissimus dorsi.

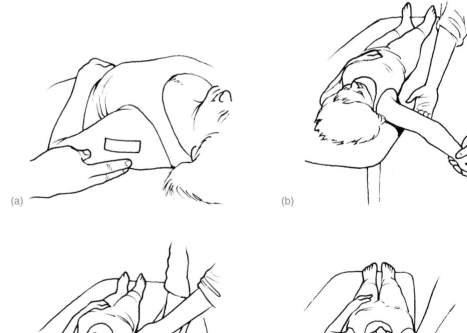

(a) (b)

(c) (d)

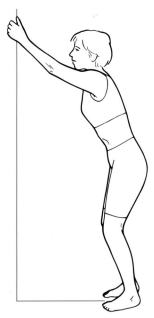

Figure 6.25   Latissimus dorsi stretch. From Norris, C.M. (1999) *The Complete Guide to Stretching.* A C Black, London. With permission.

the surface of the couch. A greater gap, combined with resistance to posterior shoulder girdle glide and painful direct palpation, represents tightness in the pectoralis minor. Trigger points may be located by palpating the corocoid process and tracing the muscle distally towards the upper ribs.

The pectoralis major is assessed by arm abduction. The sternal portion of the muscle is assessed with the arm at 120° abduction. When released, it should rest level with the couch. The clavicular portion is evaluated by lowering the arm over the couch side into extension/abduction: 80–90° extension is the norm. Painful trigger points are often found along the lateral edge of the muscle with the arm placed in an abducted position.

Latissimus dorsi   Latissimus dorsi is stretched by taking the arm overhead into flexion/abduction to couch level. In addition, latissimus dorsi may be stretched in standing. The back is flattened against the wall and the shoulder flexed, adducted and externally rotated (Koala stretch). In sport, a more useful stretch is to hold onto a piece of apparatus above shoulder level and flex the knees and hips to stretch the latissimus and traction it simultaneously (Fig. 6.25). Trigger points may be found within the muscle but more commonly they are located at the insertion of the muscle into the iliac crest.

POSTURE

The combination of altered muscle length and function will be noticeable as a change in body alignment to both static (posture) and dynamic (segmental control) assessment.

Standing posture is assessed in comparison to a standard reference line (Kendall, McCreary and Provance, 1993). The subject is positioned with a plumb-line passing just in front of

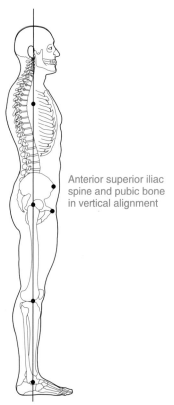

Anterior superior iliac spine and pubic bone in vertical alignment

Figure 6.26   The standard reference line for posture. After Kendall, F.P., McCreary, E.K. and Provance, P.G. (1993) *Muscles. Testing and Function*, 4th edn. Williams and Wilkins, Baltimore. With permission.

the lateral malleolus. In an ideal posture, this line should pass just anterior to the mid-line of the knee, and then through the greater trochanter, bodies of the lumbar vertebrae, shoulder joint, bodies of the cervical vertebrae, and the lobe of the ear (Fig. 6.26).

When viewed from the front, with the feet 3 inches apart, the line should bisect the body into two equal halves. The anterior superior iliac spines (ASIS) should be approximately in the same horizontal plane, and the pubis and ASIS should be in the same vertical plane (Kendall, McCreary and Provance, 1993). This alignment defines the neutral lumbopelvic alignment as one of 5° to the horizontal.

Anatomical landmarks are compared for horizontal level on the right and left sides of the body, and include the knee creases, buttock creases, pelvic rim, inferior angle of the scapulae, acromion processes, ears, and the external occipital protuberances. In addition, the alignment of the spinous processes and rib angles are observed, with minor scoliosis becoming more evident when assessed in Adam's position. The distance between the arms and the trunk (keyhole), skin creases, and unequal muscle bulk are indicators of asymmetry requiring closer examination. Foot and ankle alignment are also assessed.

When compared to this standard line, four major posture types are commonly seen (Fig. 6.27): lordotic, sway back, kyphotic and flat back.

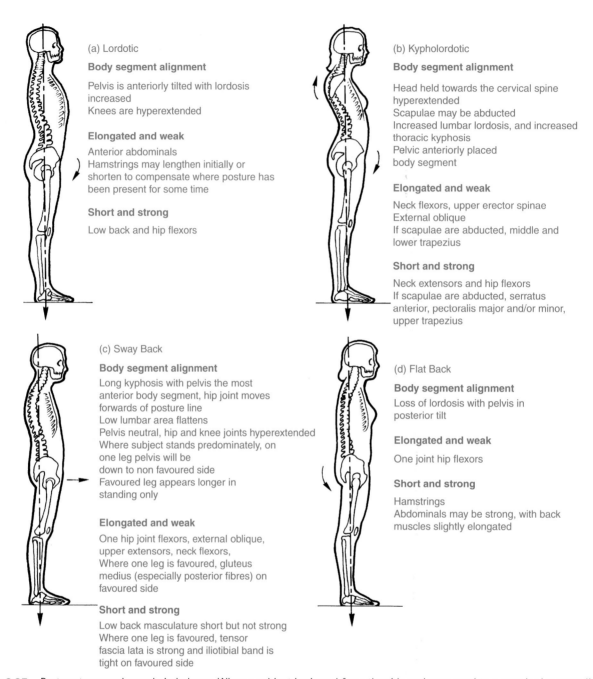

(a) Lordotic

Body segment alignment

Pelvis is anteriorly tilted with lordosis increased
Knees are hyperextended

Elongated and weak

Anterior abdominals
Hamstrings may lengthen initially or shorten to compensate where posture has been present for some time

Short and strong

Low back and hip flexors

(b) Kypholordotic

Body segment alignment

Head held towards the cervical spine hyperextended
Scapulae may be abducted
Increased lumbar lordosis, and increased thoracic kyphosis
Pelvic anteriorly placed body segment

Elongated and weak

Neck flexors, upper erector spinae
External oblique
If scapulae are abducted, middle and lower trapezius

Short and strong

Neck extensors and hip flexors
If scapulae are abducted, serratus anterior, pectoralis major and/or minor, upper trapezius

(c) Sway Back

Body segment alignment

Long kyphosis with pelvis the most anterior body segment, hip joint moves forwards of posture line
Low lumbar area flattens
Pelvis neutral, hip and knee joints hyperextended
Where subject stands predominately, on one leg pelvis will be down to non favoured side
Favoured leg appears longer in standing only

Elongated and weak

One hip joint flexors, external oblique, upper extensors, neck flexors,
Where one leg is favoured, gluteus medius (especially posterior fibres) on favoured side

Short and strong

Low back masculature short but not strong
Where one leg is favoured, tensor fascia lata is strong and iliotibial band is tight on favoured side

(d) Flat Back

Body segment alignment

Loss of lordosis with pelvis in posterior tilt

Elongated and weak

One joint hip flexors

Short and strong

Hamstrings
Abdominals may be strong, with back muscles slightly elongated

Figure 6.27 Posture types and muscle imbalance. When a subject is viewed from the side and compared to a standard posture line, four main posture types may be found. These are associated with shortened and lengthened muscles as shown. After Kendall, McCreary and Provance (1993). Muscles. Testing and Function, 4th edn., Williams and Wilkins, Baltimore. With permission.

Lordotic posture

In the lordotic posture, anterior pelvic tilt is excessive. The abdominal muscles and gluteals are typically lengthened and of poor tone. The hip flexors may shorten, and pelvic tilt is limited by tightness in the overactive and tight hamstrings. In an extreme lordotic posture, seen in chronic obesity, the lumbar spine rests in extension with the lumbar facet joints impacted and the elastic recoil of the hamstrings allowing the pelvis to hang. This posture equates with the pelvic crossed syndrome described by Janda and Schmid (1980). With obesity, the deep abdominal muscles become stretched and the viscera move forwards and downwards (visceral ptosis). In so doing they move anterior of the posture line (the gravity line), increasing the leverage acting upon them and effectively making them 'heavier'. The combination of weight and leverage forces acting on the viscera makes the act of visceral compression by the deep abdominal muscles harder.

The lordotic posture is commonly seen in sport in young gymnasts and dancers. In addition, it is the posture most noticeable after childbirth and during obesity.

Sway back posture

In the sway back posture the pelvis remains level, but the hip joint is pushed forward of the posture line. The hip is effectively extended, lengthening the hip flexors, and the body 'hangs' on the hip ligaments. The lordosis is now longer and more shallow than in the lordotic posture, and may extend up to the mid-thoracic spine. In addition, there is typically a noticeable crease where the direction of movement changes at a single spinal level, rather than through several, as is the case with the lordotic posture. A patient with this posture will often be able to point to the exact point of pain which normally occurs after prolonged standing.

The sway back posture may be combined with dominance of one leg in standing ('hanging on the hip'), especially in the adolescent. Now, weakness in the gluteus medius allows the pelvis to tip laterally, a situation partially compensated by increased tone in the tensor fascia lata. Shortening is seen in the iliotibial band (ITB), with a prominent groove apparent on the lateral aspect of the thigh.

> **Keypoint**
>
> With the *lordotic* posture the lumbar curve is increased but the greater trochanter remains on the posture line. With the *sway back*, the lumbar curve is again increased but the greater trochanter moves forwards of the posture line.

Flat back posture

With the flat back posture, the main problem is lack of mobility in the lumbar spine and a flattening of the lordosis. This posture reflects the extension dysfunction described by McKenzie (1981). The pelvis may be posteriorly tilted in comparison to the reference line, and the lumbar tissues are often thickened and immobile.

Flattening associated with repeated flexion movements of the trunk (manual handling) will show more mobility to flexion in the *upper* lumbar spine. Flattening associated with prolonged sitting will show greater flexion mobility in the *lower* lumbar spine.

Kyphotic posture

In the kyphotic posture, the shoulder joint moves anteriorly to the posture line and the thoracic kyphosis is increased. A number of pathological conditions may give rise to this condition (Table 6.2), and these should be differentiated from simple soft tissue imbalance.

In an optimal upper body alignment (Table 6.3), the scapulae should be approximately three finger breadths from the spine and the medial borders of the scapulae should be vertical. Optimal positioning of the shoulder is

Table 6.2 Pathological conditions giving rise to kyphotic posture

Scheuermann's disease
Vertebral compression fracture
Ankylosing spondylitis
Senile osteoporosis
Tuberculosis
Congenital abnormalities
partial segmental defect
centrum hypoplasia
aplasia

Source Magee (2002) with permission.

Table 6.3 Alignment of the shoulder girdle

From behind	From the side
Medial border of scapula vertical	Line from ear canal to centre of shoulder joint
Medial border of scapula no more than three finger breadths from the spinous processes	No more than one third of head of humerus anterior to acromion
Spine of scapula T3/T4 level, inferior angle at T7	Humerus held with cubital fossa 45° to sagittal plane
Scapula flat against chest wall	

assessed by comparing the head of the humerus in relation to the acromion process. In optimal positioning, no more than one-third of the humeral head should be anterior to the point of the acromion. The humerus should be held with the cubital fossa at 45° to the sagittal plane in relaxed standing. A greater angle than this indicates excessive medial rotation, indicative of tightness in the medial rotators (especially the pectoralis major) and lengthening of the lateral rotators.

Deviation from this ideal is often described as a 'round shouldered' posture, a blanket term which covers a number of scenarios. Tightness in the anterior structures will pull the shoulder forwards, away from the posture line. The weight of the arm moves further from the centre of gravity of the upper body, dramatically increasing the leverage forces transmitted to the thorax. Eventually, the thoracic kyphosis will increase as a result. Tightness in the pectoralis minor pulls on the coracoid process tilting the scapula forwards superiorly (Fig. 6.28a). Tightness in the pectoralis major causes a combination of excessive medial rotation at the glenohumeral joint with anterior displacement of the humeral head (Fig. 6.28b). Excessive abduction of the scapula (Fig. 6.28c) and downward rotation (Fig. 6.28d) may result from lengthening of the lower trapezius and serratus anterior. Excessive elevation (Fig. 6.28e) and upward rotation (Fig. 6.28f) may result from tightness in the upper fibres of trapezius.

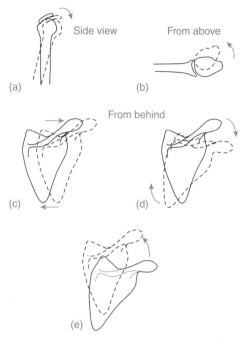

Figure 6.28 Postural changes around the shoulder. (a) Superior tilt of the scapula. (b) Medial rotation and anterior displacement of the glenohumeral joint. (c) Abduction. (d) Downward rotation. (e) Elevation and upward rotation.

SEGMENTAL CONTROL

Segmental control is the ability to dissociate the movement of one body segment from that of a neighbouring segment. It is dependent on stabilization ability and adequate mobilizer length. Where imbalance exists, lengthened muscle will fail to act sufficiently and will be dominated by shortened overactive movement muscles. This imbalance leads to an alteration in the movement pattern controlled by the muscles, giving subtle changes seen on examination.

Definition

Segmental control is the ability to dissociate the movement of one body segment from another. It is dependent on stabilization ability and adequate mobilizer length.

The central features of segmental control require the pelvis to tilt independently of the lumbar spine in both frontal and sagittal planes, the shoulder girdle and thoracic spine to move in relation to each other (see Ch. 18 p. 373), and the upper and lower portions of the cervical spine to move in a controlled fashion.

Treatment note 6.1   Therapist posture during treatment

Posture is normally seen from the perspective of the patient, either being part of their condition or their treatment. However, posture has another important aspect, that of the therapist's health. Treatments carried out in a suboptimal posture over a period of time can result in musculoskeletal pain in the therapist.

In a study of physical therapists (PTs), over 62% had complained of back pain in the last year and of those, nearly 8% had been prevented from working by this (Cromie, Robertson and Best, 2000). In addition, 36% of PTs with musculoskeletal pain reported that maintaining a position for a prolonged time (for example massage) made their pain worse (Holder et al., 1999). Optimizing therapist posture is therefore a primary consideration before treatment begins.

Low back
Maintaining lumbopelvic alignment is the key to safer treatment from the point of view of the therapist's low back. The lumbar lordosis should be preserved and prolonged flexion avoided. The first factor in achieving this is to adjust the couch height to the correct level for the height of the therapist and to adjust it as the treatment techniques vary. For example, cervical techniques may require a high couch level (Fig. 6.29a) and lumbar techniques (Fig. 6.29b) a low level. Forgetting to adjust the couch between treatments may place considerable stress on the spine.

When the therapist has to lean over the couch, placing the knee on the couch surface will serve to support the spine and

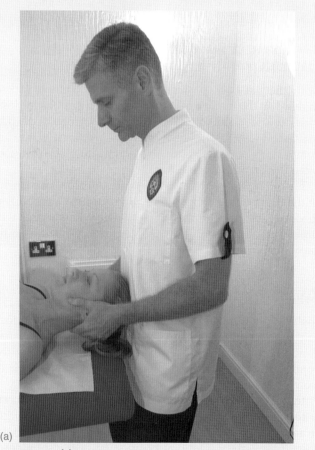

(a)

Figure 6.29   (a) High couch height to avoid excessive bending.

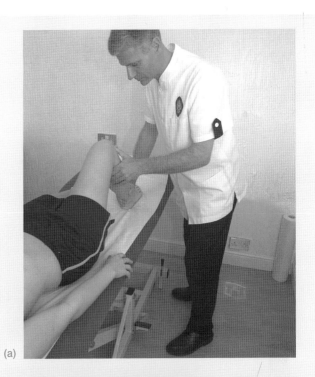

(a)

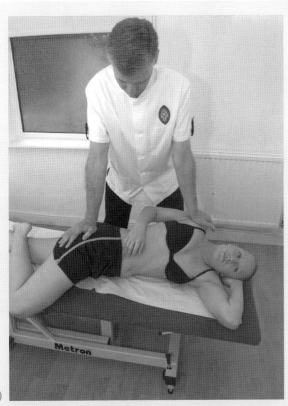

(b)

Figure 6.29   (Continued) (b) Low for lumbar treatments.

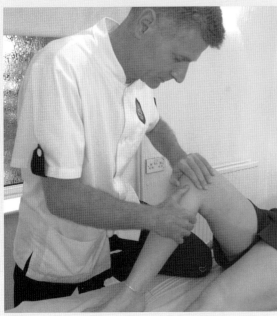

Figure 6.30   Supporting the spine by leaning onto the treatment couch.

reduce leverage effects (Fig. 6.30). In addition, standing close to the couch rather than at a distance will reduce leverage and allow some of the weight to be supported by the couch itself (Fig. 6.31).

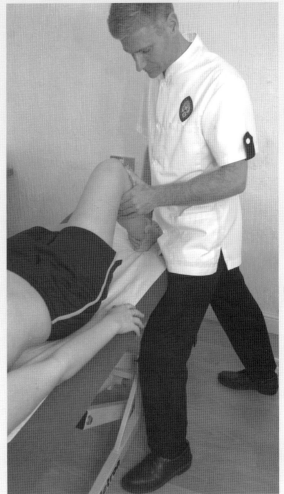

(b)

Figure 6.31   Standing close to the couch reduces stress on the therapist's spine. (a) Incorrect. (b) Correct.

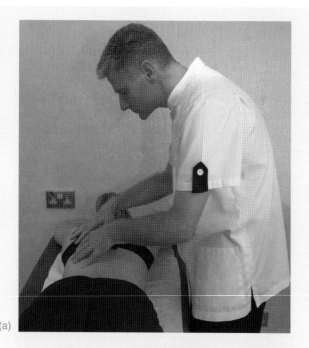

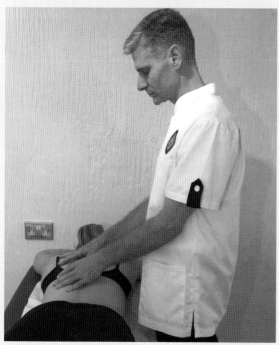

Figure 6.32 Avoiding thoracic flexion by optimizing scapular position. (a) Incorrect. (b) Correct.

Thoracic spine

The major factor in the thoracic spine is scapular abduction and thoracic flexion. This occurs particularly with mobilization techniques on a low couch (Fig. 6.32) where upper body alignment is lost. The aim should always be to 'think tall' and extend the thoracic spine while drawing the scapulae down and in (depression and retraction).

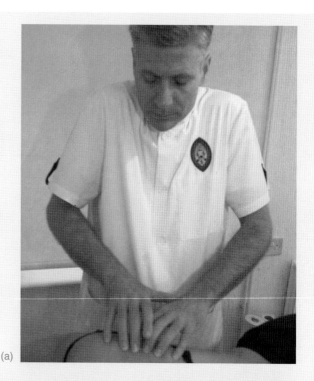

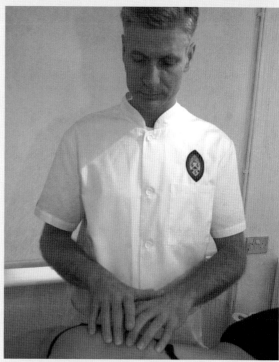

Figure 6.33 Reducing muscle stress by avoiding shoulder shrugging. (a) Incorrect. (b) Correct.

Another factor in the upper body is overactivity in the upper portion of the trapezius muscle. This can occur when holding the arms away from the sides of the body and allowing the point of the shoulder (acromion process) to creep upwards towards the ear (Fig. 6.33). The aim should be to maintain the

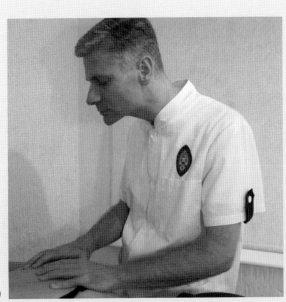

(a)

(b)

Figure 6.34   Cervical posture. (a) Incorrect. (b) Correct.

distance between the shoulder and ear and to keep the upper trapezius more relaxed.

Cervical spine

In the cervical spine, the chin should be drawn in slightly to avoid a forward head posture (Fig. 6.34). This posture commonly occurs when the therapist is focusing closely on a small object. Intense concentration leads to loss of cervical alignment which may ultimately cause tension headaches.

Lumbopelvic rhythm

The combination of movements of the hip on the pelvis and the lumbar spine on the pelvis increases the range of motion of this body area. In forward flexion in standing, for example, when the legs are straight, movement of the pelvis on the hip is limited to about 90° hip flexion. Any further movement, allowing the subject to touch the ground, must occur at the lumbar spine. In this example the body is acting as an open kinetic chain and the pelvis and lumbar spine are rotating in the same direction. Anterior tilt of the pelvis is accompanied by lumbar flexion (Fig. 6.35a). In the upright posture, the foot and shoulders are static and so spinal movement acts in a closed kinetic chain. In this situation, movements of the pelvis and lumbar spine (lumbopelvic rhythm) occur in opposite directions (Fig. 6.35b). Now, an anteriorly tilted pelvis is compensated by lumbar extension to maintain the head and shoulders in an upright orientation. The relationship between various pelvic movements and the corresponding hip joint action is shown in Table 6.4.

For lumbopelvic rhythm to function correctly, hip flexion should be greater than lumbar flexion, and occur first during functional activities. In subjects where there is a history of back pain, however, the reverse situation often occurs, leading to stress through repeated flexion of the lumbar spine.

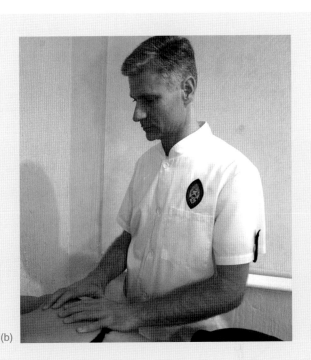

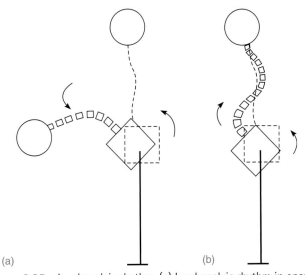

(a)   (b)

Figure 6.35   Lumbopelvic rhythm. (a) Lumbopelvic rhythm in open chain formation occurs in the same direction. Anterior pelvic tilt accompanies lumbar flexion. (b) Lumbopelvic rhythm in closed kinetic chain formation occurs in opposite directions. Anterior pelvic tilt is compensated by lumbar extension. From Norris, C.M. (1995b) Spinal stabilisation, 2. Limiting factors to end range motion in the lumbar spine. *Physiotherapy*, **81**, 4–12. Chartered Society of Physiotherapy. With permission.

Table 6.4 Relationship of pelvis, hip joint, and lumbar spine during right lower-extremity weight-bearing and upright posture

Pelvic motion	Accompanying hip joint motion	Compensatory lumbar motion
Anterior pelvic tilt	Hip flexion	Lumbar extension
Posterior pelvic tilt	Hip extension	Lumbar flexion
Lateral pelvic tilt (pelvic drop)	Right hip adduction	Right lateral flexion
Lateral pelvic tilt (hip hitch)	Right hip abduction	Left lateral flexion
Forward rotation	Right hip MR	Rotation to the left
Backward rotation	Right hip LR	Rotation to the right

MR – medical rotation, LR – lateral rotation. From Norkin, C.C. and Levangie, P.K. (1992) *Joint Structure and Function*, 2nd edn. FA Davis, Philadelphia. With permission.

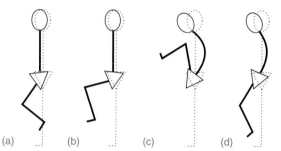

Figure 6.36 Lumbopelvic rhythm: standing. (a) Hip flexes, no pelvic or lumbar movement. (b) Posterior rotation of pelvis begins as hip approaches 90°. Lordosis flattens. (c) Maximum hip and pelvic motion. Lumbar flexion completes movement. (d) Incorrect: pelvic rotation and lumbar flexion occur immediately.

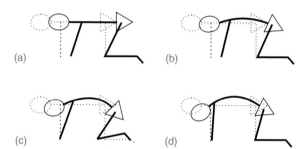

Figure 6.37 Lumbopelvic rhythm: kneeling. (a) Phase I. Hip flexion alone. (b) Phase II. Posterior pelvic tilt and hip flexion combined. (c) Phase III. Lumbar flexion completes movement. (d) Incorrect: lumbar flexion and posterior pelvic tilt occur immediately.

In the lower trunk, the ability to dissociate lumbar movement from pelvic movement is important, and is often lost in the chronic low back pain patient. Three exercises are used to assess lumbopelvic rhythm: standing hip flexion, kneeling sit-back, and the hip hinge.

Standing hip flexion

In the first (Fig. 6.36), the subject stands side on to a wall-bar for support. Hip flexion is then performed to beyond 90°. The movement should ideally occur in three phases. Initially, there should be no pelvic movement, with phase I consisting of hip flexion alone. During phase II the pelvis should begin to posteriorly tilt but the lumbar spine movement should not be excessive. In phase III no further hip or pelvic movement is available and the final position is obtained by lumbar flexion alone. Where control of lumbopelvic rhythm is poor, lumbar flexion often occurs early in phase I, with thoracic movement noticeable as the subject dips the chest downwards towards the knee. Once detected, this same movement is used to re-educate pelvic control, with the subject actively stabilizing the pelvis and initially performing hip flexion to only 10–20°.

Kneeling sit back

Lumbopelvic rhythm is further assessed in prone kneeling (Fig. 6.37). From this position the subject sits back onto the ankles. Again, the action should occur in three phases. In phase I no lumbar or pelvic movement should occur. In phase II hip, pelvis and lumbar spine should all move, and in phase III lumbar flexion and some thoracic flexion finishes the action. Faulty lumbopelvic rhythm often shows up as lumbar flexion occurring immediately.

Hip hinge

The hip hinge movement is the final action (Fig. 6.38), and the most important in terms of function as it mimics the bending action used in daily living activities. Lumbar spine to hip flexion (L/H) ratios for early (0–30°) middle (30–60°) and late (60–90°) forward bending are 2:1, 1:1, and 1:2 respectively (Esola et al., 1996). There is therefore an *increase* in the contribution of pelvic tilt to forward bending as the action proceeds. Subjects with a history of low back pain (LBP) tend to have a changed pattern of forward bending compared to normal subjects, although the total range of

> **Keypoint**
>
> During forward bending two motions occur, anterior pelvic tilt and spinal flexion. In patients with LBP, tightness in the hamstrings may delay the onset of pelvic tilt, altering the *timing* of this action rather than the total motion range.

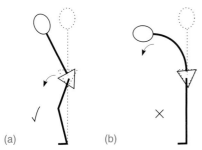

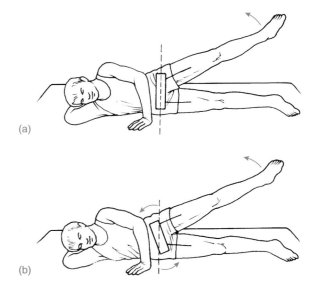

Figure 6.38   Hip hinge movement. (a) Correct: knees unlock, pelvis rotates anteriorly. Neutral lumbar position maintained. (b) Incorrect: pelvis fixed, flexion occurs to spine only.

motion for both groups is generally the same. In LBP subjects, hamstring flexibility is reduced (Esola et al., 1996; Rose, Sahrmann and Norton, 1988) and greater electrical activity in the hamstring muscles is seen (Mooney and Robertson 1976). A reduction in the contribution of pelvic tilt to the total range of forward bending leads to earlier lumbar motion in the activities of daily living (ADL). This in turn may increase the repetitive stress imposed on the low back tissues and could be an important factor in the re-occurrence of low back pain.

The hip hinge test measures the subject's ability to isolate pelvic motion from that of the lumbar spine. Initially, forward flexion is assessed, and the relative contribution of anterior pelvic tilt to this movement is important. With normal lumbopelvic rhythm, anterior pelvic tilt reduces the amount of lumbar flexion required to reach downwards to waist height. Where pelvic tilt is limited, greater lumbar flexion is required, and throughout the day the number of lumbar flexion movements is greatly increased, leading to accumulated stress on the body tissues in this area. The subject is retrained to maintain the neutral lumbar position and flex the hip on the fixed foot. To release tension from the hamstrings, the knees should be slightly unlocked as the movement begins.

Pelvic motion in the frontal plane

Pelvic motion control in the frontal plane represents the Trendelenburg sign (see Fig. 8.10, p. 187). When the bodyweight is supported on one leg, the hip abductors (mainly gluteus medius) of the supporting leg work to prevent the pelvis dipping. Their action, combined with that of quadratus lumborum of the contralateral leg, can dip the pelvis upwards on the free leg side, effectively adducting the hip on the supporting side. Where these muscles are unable to hold an inner-range contraction, the pelvis is seen to dip downwards towards the lifted leg, effectively adducting the weight-bearing limb.

In the non-weight-bearing situation, inactivity of the gluteus medius shows as a false hip abduction movement. Normally, when the upper leg is lifted from side lying, the pelvis remains level and the hip moves on this stable base (Fig. 6.39). When the hip abductors are weak, the subject is unable to abduct the leg correctly. Instead, the pelvis is

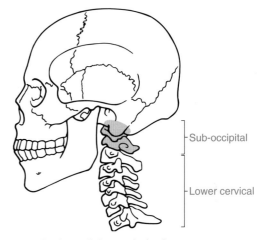

Figure 6.39   Pelvic alignment during hip abduction. (a) Correct: pelvis remains stable as hip abducts. (b) Incorrect: pelvis tilts laterally on spine giving false appearance of hip abduction.

Figure 6.40   Regions of the cervical spine.

laterally tilted through the action of the trunk side flexors. Although the leg lifts, the relationship between the femur and pelvis remains unchanged, with close inspection showing the movement isolated to the lower spine.

The cervical and thoracic spines

Observation of segmental control of the cervical spine is used to determine the division into suboccipital and lower cervical movement (Fig. 6.40).

Definition
The *suboccipital* region consists of the occiput of the skull with the first and second cervical vertebrae (C1 and C2). The *lower cervical* region is made up of the remaining cervical and first thoracic vertebrae (C2 to T1).

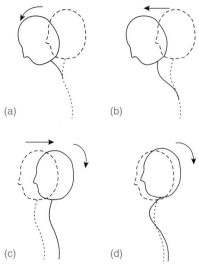

Figure 6.41 Movement of the cervical spine. (a) Upper cervical flexion – axial rotation. (b) Lower cervical flexion, upper extension with translation of joints. (c) Extension occurs in upper and lower cervical region. (d) Extension in upper cervical region only.

Cervical spine

As flexion is initiated, movement should occur in the upper cervical spine first. Where a protracted head posture is present, the lower cervical spine will often move first, with the upper region remaining extended in a lordosis (Fig. 6.41). As extension is performed, the head should move back over the shoulders before the upper cervical spine extends, indicating that both the upper and lower regions of the cervical spine are moving. If the head pivots to initiate the movement, extension may be limited to the upper region alone. If this occurs, a further test is to assess the degree of head retraction, which should show the ability of the lower cervical spine to extend.

During rotation, the movement should be pure and accompanied by only slight lateral flexion. Excessive lateral flexion indicates a possible tightness in the levator scapulae and/or the scalenes. If these muscles are tight and are limiting rotation, shrugging the shoulders (and so relaxing the muscles) will increase the available range of rotation.

Thoracic spine

The thoracic spine is assessed with the subject sitting over the couch end. The subject should be able to reverse (flatten) the thoracic kyphosis as extension is attempted. Rotation movements should be symmetrical. Emphasis is placed on the upper thoracic region when thoracic rotation is combined with cervical rotation. The mid-thoracic region is tested with the arms folded, while the lower thoracic region is emphasized by placing the patient's arms overhead and pulling through the thoracolumbar fascia.

Restoration of muscle balance

Three elements combine to restore muscle balance: correction of *muscle length,* increasing *core stability* and correction of

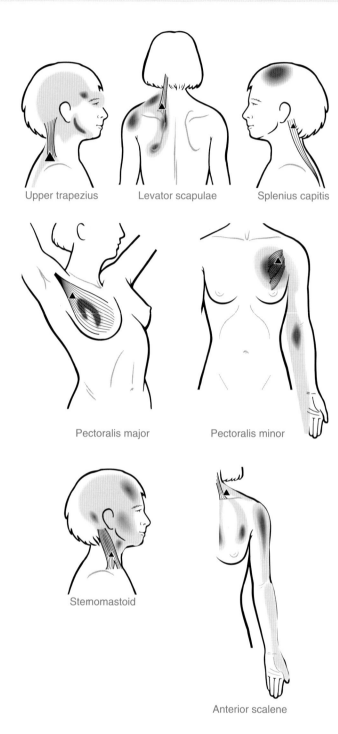

Figure 6.42 Trigger points within hyperactive upper limb muscles. From Petty and Moore (2001) with permission.

segmental control. The order in which these are used will depend on the patient's symptoms.

Muscle length

Tight muscles may inhibit their antagonists (Jull and Janda, 1987) and often develop painful trigger points. This is especially the case in the upper limb (Fig. 6.42). A trigger point (myofascial trigger point) is often located within a tight band of muscle. The point is painful to palpation and the muscle will often go into spasm if the trigger point is palpated briskly or flicked (the jump sign). For more information on trigger point pathology and treatment see Norris (2001).

Definition

A *trigger point* (TrP) is a highly sensitive local area within a taut band of muscle fibres. TrPs are thought to result from: (i) muscle ischaemia, (ii) a hyperactvie muscle spindle, (iii) excessive release of acetylcholine at the muscle motor end plate.

Furthermore, through relative flexibility (see p. 123), a tight muscle will throw stress onto a hyperflexible body segment causing tissue stress and pain. Elimination of tightness and redevelopment of stability, coupled with correction of segmental movement, is therefore a key aim of treatment.

Where pain is a prominent factor, the elimination of this pain may be the primary aim of treatment. Pain which occurs through muscle spasm, or through trigger points in tight muscle, may be relieved by treatment aimed at reducing muscle tone. This can be achieved by modalities or manual therapy, and will often involve the use of stretching (Table 6.5).

Stability

Where pain is the result of persistence over stress on a hypermobile segment, the initial treatment should be aimed at segmental control and stability. Stability may have to be applied passively at first (through taping or splinting) until sufficient control of the muscular stabilizing system has been gained.

Table 6.5 Methods of treating trigger points

Deep massage
Sustained local finger point pressure
Deep local circular massage (finger/probe)
Local and regional finger point pressure (acupressure)
Ice massage
Static stretching
PNF stretching
Muscle energy technique (MET)
Spray stretch (Vapocoolant spray)
Dry needling: shallow
Dry needling: deep (intramuscular stimulation, IMS)
Electrical point stimulation (non-invasive electroacupuncture)
Electrotherapy
transcutaneous electrical nerve stimulation (TENS)
interferential therapy (IF)
low level laser therapy (LLLT)
ultrasound (U/S)
vibration massage

Core stability itself is divided into three overlapping phases: *muscle isolation* (above, p. 131), *stability control* and *reduced attention demand* (see p. 320).

Segmental control

Finally, where the tissues themselves are normal, but poor alignment has become habitual (particularly in adolescent athletes), coordination and alignment training may be all that is required. This will necessitate close inspection and regular feedback, and the use of a video in these cases is of great value.

Segmental control of the spine has been described on page 143, and that of scapular motion is covered in Chapter 18. Further segmental control of hip during a prone lying hip extension action is shown on pages 143 and 196.

PROPRIOCEPTIVE TRAINING

Background to proprioceptive training

Proprioception has been defined as a specialized variation of touch encompassing the sensations of both joint movement and joint position (Lephart and Fu, 1995). Practically, it is the ability of the body to use position sense and respond (consciously or unconsciously) to stresses imposed on the body by altering posture and movement (Houglum, 2001).

Definition

Proprioception is the awareness of the body in space. It is the use of joint position sense and joint motion sense to respond to stresses placed upon the body by alteration of posture and movement

---

Proprioception encompasses three aspects, known as the 'ABC of proprioception'. These are: agility, balance and coordination. *Agility* is the capacity to control the direction of the body or body part during rapid movements, while *balance* is the ability to maintain equilibrium by keeping the line of gravity of the body within the body's base of support. *Coordination* is the smoothness of an activity. This is produced by a combination of muscles acting together with appropriate intensity and timing (Houglum, 2001).

Proprioceptive exercise is progressed in terms of skill and complexity rather than pure overload. The aim is to perform gradually more challenging actions while maintaining movement accuracy. The emphasis therefore is on *quality* of motion rather than quantity (volume) of muscle work.

Proprioception and injury

During acute injury, proprioception may play a protective role by reflex muscular splinting. The reflex, initiated by displacement of mechanoreceptors and muscle spindles, occurs far more rapidly than that brought about by pain (nociception) (Barrack and Skinner, 1984). Joint effusion contributes to a reduction in mechanoreceptor discharge, resulting in inhibition of muscular contraction. This is especially seen in the vastus medialis (VMO) of the knee, for example, where just 60 ml of intra-articular effusion may result in 30–50% inhibition of quadriceps contraction (Kennedy, Alexander and Hayes, 1982). Proprioceptive deficits have also been shown to parallel joint degeneration (Barrett, Cobb and Bentley, 1991), but it is unclear whether this occurs as a result of degeneration, or is in fact part of its aetiology (Lephart and Fu, 1995).

> **Keypoint**
>
> Following injury, an athlete's proprioceptive ability will be impaired. Training to restore this is an essential part of sport rehabilitation.

From a clinical standpoint, proprioception may be seen to consist of three interrelating components (Beard et al., 1994) (Fig. 6.43), representing activity at spinal, brainstem, and higher centre levels (Tyldesley and Grieve, 1989). Each component is assessed by a variety of different tests (Lephart and Fu, 1995).

Static joint position sense

First, static joint position sense is used to maintain posture and balance at brainstem level. Input for these actions is from joint proprioception, the vestibular centres in the ears, and from the eyes. Balance and postural exercise with the eyes open and/or closed may be used to enhance static joint position sense. This component is commonly measured by tests which address reproduction of passive positioning (RPP) and reproduction of active positioning (RAP). The subject is required to return the joint to its start position after either an active or passive movement.

Movement sense

Secondly, kinaesthetic awareness or 'movement awareness' is a result of higher centre activity. This component encompasses the detection of both joint displacement and velocity change. It is commonly assessed by measuring the threshold to detection of passive motion (TTDPM), the subject simply stating when he or she feels movement has begun. Once movement has been detected through kinaesthetic

awareness, motor programmes may be performed automatically in many cases (see p. 150). Consciously performed joint positioning activities, especially at end-range, will enhance the development of automatic control and cognitive awareness (Lephart and Fu, 1995).

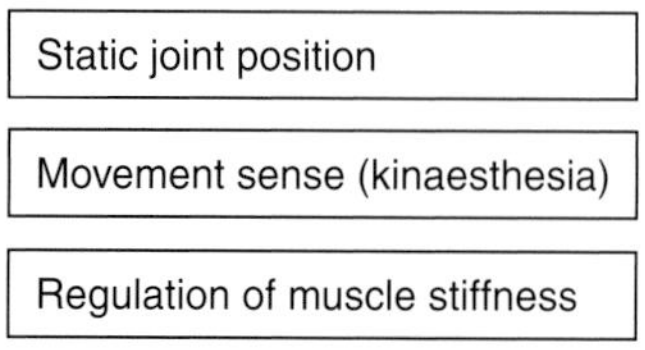

Regulation of muscle stiffness

Finally, closed loop efferent activity is required for reflex (spinal) activity and regulation of muscle stiffness, leading to dynamic joint stability. This type of activity underlies all movements by supplying reflex splinting when a joint is stressed. Damage to joint receptors has been shown to affect co-contraction of muscles and reduce joint stability. This, in turn, can lead to an increase in the likelihood of injury (Tyldesley and Grieve, 1989).

Proprioception is enhanced at this level through the initiation of reflex joint stabilization, using activities which involve sudden alterations in joint position. Reflex stabilization is therefore assessed through measurement of the onset of muscle contraction in relation to joint displacement. The aim is to see if the muscles are able to limit joint displacement and effectively stabilize the joint.

> **Keypoint**
>
> Train static *joint position sense* using balance exercises with the eyes open/closed, *movement sense* with joint positioning activities at end-range, and *muscle stiffness* with sudden alteration of joint angle.

Proprioceptive research

Using TTDPM and RPP, Barrack and Skinner (1984) found decreased kinaesthesia with increasing age. In general, our highly mechanized Western society may fail to impose the variety of movements which an individual requires for optimal musculoskeletal health. This reduced movement 'vocabulary' decreases the proprioceptive stimulation needed for skilled motor action (Jull and Janda, 1987). After injury, proprioceptive input is further reduced due to prolonged inactivity and damage to proprioceptive nerve endings within the injured tissues. A number of authors have stressed the importance of proprioceptive training in rehabilitation following injury to the knee (Barrack and Skinner, 1984; Beard et al., 1994), ankle (Freeman, Dean and Hanham, 1965; Lentell, Katzman and Walters, 1990; Konradsen and Ravn, 1990) and shoulder (Smith and Brunolli, 1990; Lephart et al., 1994). The functional importance of proprioceptive training has also been emphasized during rehabilitation of the spine (Lewit, 1991; Irion, 1992; Norris, 1995a), although its use in spinal rehabilitation is less common than for other areas of the body.

Proprioception may be enhanced with training. Barrack and Skinner (1984) found enhanced kinaesthesia in trained

| Static joint position |
| Movement sense (kinaesthesia) |
| Regulation of muscle stiffness |

Figure 6.43 Components of proprioception.

dancers, and Lephart and Fu (1995) demonstrated the same in intercollegiate gymnasts. Both of these types of athletes practice free exercise using bodyweight as resistance, and use complex multijoint activities. This type of training would seem appropriate for proprioceptive rehabilitation.

Training techniques

Proprioceptive training involves highly skilled actions, often performed at speed, with the aim of making the movement less attention-demanding (automatic). Proprioceptive exercises are progressed in terms of speed and complexity aiming at quality of movement execution rather than simple overload. Multiple sensory inputs are used to improve the sense of both static position and movement. Once this has been achieved, dynamic stability exercises may be used.

Proprioceptive training may be performed by following the general stages by which and athlete actually learns any skilled action (Table 6.6).

How athletes learn skilled movements

Proprioceptive exercises are highly skilled, and in order to effectively prescribe this type of training we need to understand the way that an athlete actually learns a skilled movement. There are three overlapping stages to motor skill (movement) learning (Fitts and Posner, 1967; Schmidt, 1991).

Stage I (cognitive)

The first stage is the stage of *understanding*, where the athlete attempts to form an idea of the whole skill. The process is cognitive (thinking) rather than motor (doing) in nature, and hence the title of this learning stage. The athlete is learning what to do (and importantly, what not to do), and how to do it.

Environmental cues which later will go unnoticed are important to this early stage of learning. They provide an important frame of reference for building the new skill. For example, when learning a new dance step, a person will often focus attention on the foot position, which they later take for granted.

In this stage movements will be poorly coordinated. The athlete must concentrate intensely and will therefore tire easily. The therapist can assist by providing clear instructions and feedback. Complex actions should be split up into more simple components. For example, a single leg hop and twist would be learned as a single leg balance first in stage I. This would be followed by straight line hopping, and, eventually, hopping and twisting on the spot and finally hopping and twisting over a distance, in stages II and III.

Demonstration of the movement is important, and the athlete will need constant coaching and correction of the skill to prevent them practising mistakes.

One of the ways we can help learning in this stage is to use *cueing*, to paint a mental picture of an action in terms which an athlete can easily understand. For example, an abdominal hollowing action may be cued by asking the athlete to pull the tummy button in (visual), or use the fingers to feel the abdomen tightening (tactile). The instructor may use the

---

Definition

A *cue* is a signal which facilitates a particular action, and may be verbal, visual or tactile in nature. When a number of cues facilitate an action, *multisensory* cueing is being used.

Table 6.6 Learning motor skills

Stage of learning		
Stage (I) – understanding	**Stage (II) – effective movement**	**Stage (III) – automatic action**
Understand what is required from action	Refine action	Less attention required
Environmental cues important	Able to recognize own mistakes	Movement seems to 'run by itself'
Movements poorly coordinated	Movements more consistent and efficient	Speed of movement increased
Demonstration and movement cueing important	Energy expenditure lower	
Practical implication		
Split complex movement sequences into simple components	Correct movement pattern when/if it erodes	Distract athlete to ensure less attention is used
Increase movement awareness by cueing	Stop if athlete becomes fatigued	Progress speed of movement while maintaining accuracy
Use palpation and passive movement to facilitate learning	Link simple actions together into sequences	Increase repetitions
Slow precise actions	Reduce environmental cues	Alter environmental cues
Progress only when athlete can perform action independently of therapist	Increase repetitions as endurance improves	Perform multiple actions
	Require athlete to recognize their own mistakes (self-monitoring)	

voice intonation (auditory) to indicate the intensity of the movement.

Stage II (motor)

This is the stage of *effective movement*, when the athlete will try to make the motor programme more precise and refine the action. It is as though the original clumsy action is 'whittled down' to a smoother defined movement. Through practice, the athlete is now able to recognize mistakes, and so self-practice (unsupervised) can now be allowed.

The dependence on visual and verbal cues (stage I) now gradually gives way to the reliance on proprioceptive information. Movements become more consistent and the athlete is able to work on the finer details of an action. As the action becomes more efficient, energy expenditure is reduced because the athlete does not have to work as hard to produce the action. Environmental cues are used for timing and as anticipation develops, movements become smoother and less rushed.

> **Keypoint**
>
> As a motor skill becomes more efficient, energy expenditure is reduced and movements become smoother.

The individual movement sequences used in stage I are now linked together to give a longer skill sequence. The actions must still be slow and precise, with progression made only when the movement sequence is correct.

Stage III (automatic)

In this stage the action 'runs by itself' or becomes *automatic* (grooved). Movements in this stage demand less attention to perform and so the athlete can now perform other actions at the same time. The speed of the movement may be increased, and functions such as muscle reaction time become important. Here, the body is challenged (for example, knocking it off balance) and the athlete must react quickly with appropriate changes in posture and movements. This type of final training is used with balance balls and gymballs, for example.

Practical aspects of proprioceptive training

Training begins by splitting complex movements into a number of simple component sequences (Table 6.7), with the choice of exercise being determined by the functional requirements of the patient. Splitting the movement in this way enables the athlete to focus their attention selectively on a single action, making learning far easier. Initially actions must be slow and precise with the emphasis on control of the correct body position. The rate of movement is progressed, while maintaining accuracy, and the simple movement components are linked together to form the total activity sequence (Tropp, Alaranta and Renstrom, 1993). The athlete

must stop when they become fatigued, failure to do so will often lead to practice of incorrect exercise technique and negative transfer effects.

> **Definition**
>
> A *negative transfer* effect occurs when an activity in training is learned to such a degree that it actually interferes with a skilled movement in sport performance.

Movement of other body parts draws the athlete's attention away from the conscious control of the core action, and assists in the development of automatic actions. To gain true automaticity of a movement sequence, thousands of repetitions are needed. Rather than practising isolated exercises to repetition, functional activities should be built into an athlete's activities of daily living (ADL).

Using proprioceptive training of the ankle as an example, single leg standing may begin, followed by single leg standing with 1/4 squat activities, and finally, the same base activity with throwing and catching. This could be built into an athlete's daily activities (ADL) by performing simple home exercises such as cleaning the teeth while standing on one leg!

Once an action can be performed correctly on a stable surface, the subject may be positioned on a moving base of support. The subject must now use not just joint position and movement sense, but anticipation of body displacement, requiring reflex stabilization. Initially, the labile surface should involve uniaxial movements, for example a rocker

Table 6.7 Proprioceptive training

Increase awareness of correct pattern
Split complex movement sequence into simple components
Increase awareness by passive movement using
  multisensory input

Gain voluntary control of movement pattern
Use multisensory stimulation during demonstration and
  performance of exercise
Start with slow precise movements
Stop exercising when patient becomes fatigued
Continually correct movement pattern passively
Progress exercise only when movement pattern is correct
Patient must perform independently before proceeding to more
  advanced actions
Link simple tasks to form more complex actions

Gain automatic control of movement
Progress speed while maintaining accuracy of movement
Perform multiple repetitions of movement sequence
Perform actions with other body parts while maintaining accurate
  stability in the affected body part

From Norris, C.M. (1995b) Spinal stabilisation, 2. Limiting factors to end range motion in the lumbar spine. *Physiotherapy*, **81**, 4–12. Chartered Society of Physiotherapy. With permission.

board. Placing the pivot of this type of board in the frontal plane will work the flexion and extension reaction, while placing the pivot in the sagittal plane will work abduction and adduction. If the pivot is then placed diagonally, movements will be biaxial in nature. Progression is made to the wobble board where the pivot point is dome-shaped to allow triaxial motion. Other apparatus useful for balance work and muscle reaction includes the large diameter (65 cm) gymnastic ball, the mini-trampette, the 'Fitter' ski-training device (Fitter International Inc., Calgary, Alberta, Canada) and the 'slide trainer' (Forsa Fitness Equipment, London, England). In each case, as the athlete is pushed off balance, the aim is to maintain stabilization and enhance both movement detection and closed-loop reflex muscular stabilization. These actions must be built into an athlete's normal training programme rather than isolated from it.

Examples of proprioceptive training for the ankle, knee, shoulder and spine are given in the relevant clinic chapters for these body parts.

References

Andersson, E.A., Oddsson, L., Grundstrom, O., Nilsson, J. and Thorstensson, A. (1996) EMG activities of the quadratus lumborum and erector spinae muscles during flexion-relaxation and other motor tasks. *Clinical Biomechanics*, **11**, 392–400

Appell, H.J. (1990) Muscular atrophy following immobilisation: a review. *Sports Medicine*, **10**, 42

Barrack, R.L., Skinner, B.L., Brunet, M.E. and Cook, S.D. (1984) Joint kinesthesia in the highly trained knee. *Journal of Sports Medicine and Physical Fitness*, **24**, 18–20

Barrett, D.S., Cobb, A.G. and Bentley, G. (1991) Joint proprioception in normal, osteoarthritic, and replaced knees. *Journal of Bone and Joint Surgery*, **73B**, 53–56

Bastide, G., Zadeh, J. and Lefebvre, D. (1989) Are the 'little muscles' what we think they are? *Surgical and Radiological Anatomy*, **11**, 255–256

Beard, D.J., Kyberd, P.J., O'Connor, J.J., Fergusson, C.M. and Dodd, C.A.F. (1994) Reflex hamstring contraction latency in anterior cruciate ligament deficiency. *Journal of Orthopaedic Research*, **12**, (2) 219–228

Bergmark, A. (1989) Stability of the lumbar spine: a study in mechanical engineering. *Acta Orthopaedica Scandinavica*, **230**, 20–24

Biedermann, H.J., Shanks, G.L., Forrest, W.J. and Inglis, J. (1991) Power spectrum analyses of electromyographic activity. *Spine*, **16**, (10) 1179–1184

Bohannon, R.W. (1982) Cinematographic analysis of the passive straight leg raising test for hamstring muscle length. *Physical Therapy*, **62**, (5) 1269–1274

Bullock-Saxton, J., Murphy, D., Norris, C., Richardson, C. and Tunnell, P. (2000) The muscle designation debate: the experts respond. *Journal of Bodywork and Movement Therapies*, **4**, (4) 225–227

Bullock-Saxton, J.E. and Bullock, M.I. (1994) Repeatability of muscle length measures around the hip. *Physiotherapy Canada*, **46**, (2) 105–109

Comerford, M. (1995) *Muscle Imbalance*, course notes, Nottingham School of Physiotherapy, Nottingham

Cresswell, A.G., Grundstrom, H. and Thorstensson, A. (1992) Observations on intra-abdominal pressure and patterns of abdominal intra-muscular activity in man. *Acta Physiologica Scandinavica*, **144**, (4) 409–418

Cresswell, A.G., Oddsson, L. and Thorstensson, A. (1994) The influence of sudden perturbations on trunk muscle activity and intra abdominal pressure while standing. *Experimental Brain Research*, **98**, 336–341

Critchley, D.J. and Coutts, F.J. (2002) Abdominal muscle function in chronic low back pain patients. *Physiotherapy*, **88**, (6) 322–332

Cromie, J., Robertson, V. and Best, M. (2000) Work related musculoskeletal disorders in physical therapists. *Physical Therapy*, **80**, (4) 336–351

de Andrade, J.R., Grant, C. and Dixon, A. (1965) Joint distension and reflex muscle inhibition in the knee. *Journal of Bone and Joint Surgery*, **47(A)**, 313–322

Esola, M.A., McClure, P.W., Fitzgerald, G.K. and Siegler, S. (1996) Analysis of lumbar spine and hip motion during forward bending in subjects with and without a history of low back pain. *Spine*, **21**, (1) 71–78

Fitts, P.M. and Posner, M.I. (1967) *Human Performance*, Greenwood Press, Westport, Connecticut

Freeman, M.A.R., Dean, M.R.E. and Hanham, I.W.F. (1965) The etiology and prevention of functional instability of the foot. *Journal of Bone and Joint Surgery*, **47B**, 678–685

Gajdosik, R. and Lusin, G. (1983) Hamstring muscle tightness: reliability of the active knee extension test. *Physical Therapy*, **63**, (7) 1085–1090

Goldspink, G. (1992) Cellular and molecular aspects of adaptation in skeletal muscle. In *Strength and Power in Sport* (ed. P.V. Komi), Blackwell, Oxford

Goldspink, G. (1996) Personal communication

Gossman, M.R., Sahrmann, S.A. and Rose, S.J. (1982) Review of length associated changes in muscle. *Physical Therapy*, **62**, (12) 1799–1808

Gunn, C.C. (1996) *Treatment of Chronic Pain*, 2nd edn, Churchill Livingstone, Edinburgh

Gunn, C.C. (2000) *The Gunn Approach to the Treatment of Chronic Pain*, course notes, Westminster Hospital, London

Hides, J.A., Stokes, M.J., Saide, M., Jull, G.A. and Cooper, D.H. (1994) Evidence of lumbar multifidus muscle wasting ipsilateral to symptoms in patients with acute/subacute low back pain. *Spine*, **19**, (2) 165–172

Hodges, P., Richardson, C. and Jull, G. (1996) Evaluation of the relationship between laboratory and clinical tests of transversus abdominis function. *Physio-therapy Research International*, **1**, (1) 30–40

Hodges, P.W. and Richardson, C.A. (1995) Neuromotor dysfunction of the trunk musculature in low back pain patients. In *Proceedings of the World Confederation of Physical Therapists Congress*, Washington

Hodges, P.W. and Richardson, C.A. (1996) Contraction of transversus abdominis invariably precedes movement of the upper and lower limb. In *Proceedings of the 6th International Conference of the International Federation of Orthopaedic Manipulative Therapists (IFOMT)*, Lillehammer, Norway

Holder, N., Clark, H., DiBlasio, J., Hughes, C. and Scherpf, J. (1999) Causes prevalence and response to occupational musculoskeletal injuries reported by physical therapists. *Physical Therapy*, **79**, (7) 642–652

Houglum, P.A. (2001) *Therapeutic Exercise for Athletic Injuries*, Human Kinetics, Champaign, Illinois

Irion, J.M. (1992) Use of the gym ball in rehabilitation of spinal dysfunction. *Orthopaedic Physical Therapy Clinics of North America*, Oxford, pp. 375–398

Jackson, M., Solomonow, M., Zhou, B., Baratta, R.V. and Harris, M. (2001) Multifidus EMG and tension-relaxation recovery after prolonged static lumbar flexion. *Spine*, **26**, (7) 715–723.

Janda, V. (1993) Muscle strength in relation to muscle length, pain and muscle imbalance. In *Muscle Strength: International Perspectives in Physical Therapy* (ed. K. Harms-Ringdahl), 8, Churchill Livingstone, Edinburgh

Janda, V. (1994) Muscles and motor control in cervicogenic disorders: assessment and management. In *Physical Therapy of the Cervical and Thoracic Spine* (ed. R. Grant), 2nd edn, Churchill Livingstone, Edinburgh

Janda, V. and Schmid, H.J.A. (1980) Muscles as a pathogenic factor in backpain. *Proceedings of the International Federation of Orthopaedic Manipulative Therapists*, 4th conference, New Zealand, pp. 17–18

Jaspers, S.R., Fagan, J.M. and Tischler, M.E. (1985) Biomechanical response to chronic shortening in unloaded soleus muscles. *Journal of Applied Physiology*, **59**, 1159–1163

Jones, R. and Lovett, R.W. (1929) *Orthopedic Surgery*, William Wood and Co., New York

Jull, G.A. (1994) Headaches of cervical origin. In *Physical Therapy of the Cervical and Thoracic Spine* (ed. R. Grant), Churchill Livingstone, New York

Jull, G.A. and Janda, V. (1987) Muscles and motor control in low back pain: assessment and management. In *Physical Therapy of the Low Back* (ed. L.T. Twomey), Churchill Livingstone, New York

Kamkar, A., Irrgang, J.L. and Whitney, S.L. (1993) Nonoperative management of secondary shoulder impingement syndrome. *Journal of Orthopedic and Sports Physical Therapy*, **17**, (5) 212–224

Kendall, F.P., McCreary, E.K. and Provance, P.G. (1993) *Muscles. Testing and Function*, 4th edn, Williams and Wilkins, Baltimore

Kennedy, J.C., Alexander, I.J. and Hayes, K.C. (1982) Nerve supply of the human knee and its functional importance. *American Journal of Sports Medicine*, **10**, 329

Koh, T.J. and Herzog, W. (1998) Eccentric training does not increase sarcomere number in rabbit dorsiflexor muscles. *Journal of Biomechanics*, **31**, 499–501

Koh, T.J. (1995) Do adaptations in serial sarcomere number occur with strength training? *Human Movement Science*, **14**, 61–77

Konradsen, L. and Ravn, J.B. (1990) Ankle instability caused by prolonged peroneal reaction time. *Acta Orthopedica Scandinavica*, **61**, (5) 388–390

Lentell, G.L., Katzman, L.L. and Walters, M.R. (1990) The relationship between muscle function and ankle stability. *Journal of Orthopaedic and Sports Physical Therapy*, **11**, 605–611

Lephart, S.M. and Fu, F.H. (1995) The role of proprioception in the treatment of sports injuries. *Sports Exercise and Injury*, **1**, (2) 96–102

Lephart, S.M., Warner, J.P., Borsa, P.A. and Fu, F.H. (1994) Proprioception of the shoulder in normal, unstable, and surgical individuals. *Journal of Shoulder and Elbow Surgery*, **3**, (4) 371–381

Lewit, K. (1991) *Manipulative Therapy in Rehabilitation of the Locomotor System*, 2nd edn, Butterworth-Heinemann, Oxford

Lieber, R.L. (1992) *Skeletal Muscle Structure and Function*, Williams and Wilkins, Baltimore

Magee, D.J. (2002) *Orthopedic Physical Assessment*, 4th edn, W.B. Saunders, Philadelphia

McGill, S.M., Juker, D. and Kropf, P. (1996) Quantitative intramuscular myoelectric activity of quadratus lumborum during a wide variety of tasks. *Clinical Biomechanics*, **11**, 170–172

McGill, S. (2000) Biomechanics of the thoracolumbar spine. In *Clinical Biomechanics* (ed. Z. Dvir), Churchill Livingstone, Edinburgh

McKenzie, R.A. (1981) *The Lumbar Spine: Mechanical Diagnosis and Therapy*, Spinal Publications, Lower Hutt, New Zealand

Miller, M.I. and Medeiros, J.M. (1987) Recruitment of internal oblique and transversus abdominis muscles during the eccentric phase of the curl-up exercise. *Physical Therapy*, **67**, 1213–1217

Mooney, V. and Robertson, J. (1976) The facet syndrome. *Clinical Orthopaedics and Related Research*, **115**, 149–156

Morgan, D.L. and Lynn, R. (1994) Decline running produces more sarcomeres in rat vastus intermedius muscle fibers than does incline running. *Journal of Applied Physiology*, **77**, 1439–1444

Muller, E.A. (1970) Influence of training and of inactivity on muscle strength. *Archives of Physical Medicine and Rehabilitation*, **51**, 449–462

Ng, G. and Richardson, C.A. (1990) The effects of training triceps surae using progressive speed loading. *Physiotherapy Practice*, **6**, 77–84

Norkin, C.C. and Levangie, P.K. (1992) *Joint Structure and Function*, 2nd edn, F.A. Davis, Philadelphia

Norris, C.M. (1995a) Spinal stabilisation. *Physiotherapy*, **81**, (2) 1–4

Norris, C.M. (1995b) Spinal stabilisation, 2. Limiting factors to end range motion in the lumbar spine. *Physiotherapy*, **81**, 4–12

Norris, C.M. (1995c) Spinal stabilisation, 5. An exercise programme to enhance lumbar stabilisation. *Physiotherapy*, **81**, (3) 31–39

Norris, C.M. (1999) *The Complete Guide to Stretching*, A&C Black, London

Norris, C.M. (2000) *Back Stability*, Human Kinetics, Champaign, Illinois

Norris, C.M. (2001) *Acupuncture: Treatment of Musculoskeletal Conditions*, Butterworth-Heinemann, Oxford

Norris, C.M. (2002) *Back Stability*, video, Human Kinetics, Champaign, Illinois

Norris, C.M. and Mathews M. (in press) The influence of a hamstring stretching programme on pelvic tilt during forward bending: an initial evaluation.

Ober, F.B. (1936) The role of the iliotibial and fascia lata as a factor in the causation of low back disabilities and sciatica. *Journal of Bone and Joint Surgery*, **18**, 105–110

O'Sullivan, P.B., Grahamslaw, K.M., Kendell, M., Lapenskie, S.C., Moller, N.E. and Richards, K.V. (2002) The effect of different standing and sitting postures on trunk muscle activity in a pain free population. *Spine*, **27**, (11) 1238–1244

Petty, N.J. and Moore, A.P. (2001) *Neuromusculoskeletal Examination and Assessment*, Churchill Livingstone, Edinburgh

Richardson, C.A. (1992) Muscle imbalance: principles of treatment and assessment. *Proceedings of the New Zealand Society of Physiotherapists Challenges Conference*, Christchurch, New Zealand

Richardson, C.A. and Bullock, M.I. (1986) Changes in muscle activity during fast, alternating flexion – extension movements of the knee. *Scandinavian Journal of Rehabilitation Medicine*, **18**, 51–58

Richardson, C.A. and Hodges, P. (1996) *New advances in exercise to rehabilitate spinal stabilisation*, course notes, Edinburgh

Richardson, C.A. and Sims, K. (1991) An inner range holding contraction: an objective measure of stabilizing function of an antigravity muscle. *Proceedings of the World Confederation for Physical Therapy*, 11th International Congress, London

Richardson, C., Jull, G., Toppenburg, R. and Comerford, M. (1992) Techniques for active lumbar stabilisation for spinal protection: a pilot study. *Australian Journal of Physiotherapy*, **38**, (2) 105–112

Richardson, C., Jull, G., Hodges, P. and Hides, J. (1999) *Therapeutic Exercise for Spinal Segmental Stabilisation in Low Back Pain*, Churchill Livingstone, Edinburgh.

Rose, S.J., Sahrmann, S.A. and Norton, B.T. (1988) Quantitative assessment of lumbar-pelvic rhythm. *Physical Therapy*, **68**, 824

Sahrmann, S.A. (1987) Posture and muscle imbalance: faulty lumbar-pelvic alignment and associated musculoskeletal pain syndromes. *Postgraduate Advances in Physical Therapy*, Forum Medicum, Berryville, Virginia

Sahrmann, S.A. (1990) *Diagnosis and treatment of movement-related pain syndromes associated with muscle and movement imbalances*, course notes, Washington University

Sahrmann, S.A. (2002) *Diagnosis and Treatment of Movement Impairment Syndromes*, Mosby, St Louis

Schmidt, R.A. (1991) *Motor Learning and Performance*, Human Kinetics, Champaign, Illionis

Smith, R.L. and Brunolli, J. (1990) Shoulder kinaesthesia after anterior glenohumeral joint dislocation. *Physical Therapy*, **69**, 106–112

Stokes, M. and Young, A. (1984) The contribution of reflex inhibition to arthrogenous muscle weakness. *Clinical Science*, **67**, 7–14

Tabary, J.C. (1972) Physiological and structural changes in the cat's soleus muscle due to immobilisation at different lengths by plaster casts. *Journal of Physiology*, **224**, 231–244

Templeton, G.H., Padalino, M., Manton, J., Glasberg, M. and Silver, C.J. (1984) Influence of suspension hypokinesia on rat soleus muscle. *Journal of Applied Physiology*, **56**, 278–286

Travell, J.G. and Simons, D.G. (1983) *Myofascial Pain and Dysfunction*, Williams and Wilkins, Baltimore

Tropp H., Alaranta, H. and Renstrom, P.A.F.H. (1993) Proprioception and coordination training in injury prevention. In *Sports Injuries. Basic Principles of Prevention and Care* (ed. P.A.F.H. Renstrom), IOC Medical Commission, Blackwell Scientific, London

Tyldesley, B. and Grieve, J.I. (1989) *Muscles, Nerves and Movement: Kinesiology in Daily Living*, Blackwell Scientific, Oxford

Urban, L.M. (1981) The straight leg raising test: a review. *Journal of Orthopaedics and Sports Physical Therapy*, **2**, (3) 117–133

White, S.G. and Sahrmann, S.A. (1994) A movement system balance approach to management of musculoskeletal pain. In *Physical Therapy of the Cervical and Thoracic Spine* (ed. R. Grant), Churchill Livingstone, New York

Wilk, K.E. and Arrigo, C. (1993) Current concepts in the rehabilitation of the athletic shoulder. *Journal of Orthopedic and Sports Physical Therapy*, **18**, (1) 365–378

Williams, M., Solomonow, M., Zhou, B.H., Baratta, R.V. and Harris, M. (2000) Multifidus spasms elicited by prolonged lumbar flexion. *Spine*, **25**, (22) 2916–2924

Williams, P., Watt, P., Bicik, V. and Goldspink, G. (1986) Effect of stretch combined with electrical stimulation on the type of sarcomeres produced at the ends of muscle fibers. *Experimental Neurology*, **93**, 500–509

Williams, P.E. (1990) Use of intermittent stretch in the prevention of serial sarcomere loss in immobilised muscle. *Annals of the Rheumatic Diseases*, **49**, 316–317

Williams, P.E. and Goldspink, G. (1978) Changes in sarcomere length and physiological properties in immobilized muscle. *Journal of Anatomy*, **127**, 459–468

Chapter **7**

First contact management

CHAPTER CONTENTS

INJURY PREVENTION

Injury prevention should perhaps be the most important topic within the field of sports medicine. The term 'prevention' is normally used in the context of sports injuries to refer to any measure which can stop an injury occurring. But the processes of prevention also play an important role in arresting the exacerbation of a current injury, and ensuring that the same injury does not recur.

The causes of sports injuries are many and varied. Items such as technique failure, faulty sports equipment, poor physical fitness, inadequate warm-up and psychological factors can all act as co-factors. Taimela, Kujala and Osterman (1990) divided injury risk factors into intrinsic and extrinsic groups as shown in Table 7.1.

Some factors will clearly affect athletes differently, and certain elements are more important in one sport than another. However, in general, the more risk factors an athlete shows, the more likely he or she is to be injured.

Table 7.1 Injury risk factors

Extrinsic
Organization and management
Type of sport
Training errors
Environment
Equipment
Intrinsic
Age
Gender
Somatotype
Local anatomy and biomechanics
Fitness
Physical symmetry
Joint integrity
Motor control (skill)
Psychological/psychosocial factors

Adapted from Taimela, S., Kujala, U.M. and Osterman, K. (1990) Intrinsic risk factors and athletic injuries. *Sports Medicine*, **9**(4), 205–215. With permission.

Consequently, the aim of the coach or practitioner should be to reduce these risk factors to a minimum.

Warm-up

The subject of warm-up is dealt with in depth in Chapter 5. A general warm-up, intense enough to induce mild sweating without causing fatigue, is important for injury prevention. The general activity should be followed by a specific warm-up designed to produce a suitable arousal level in the athlete, and to rehearse any complex skills which will be used later in competition.

Joints, muscles, and other soft tissues should be extended through their full physiological range before competition, using maintenance stretching. However, it is important that developmental stretching be separate to, and follow, a warm-up.

Keypoint

Maintenance stretching may form part of a warm-up. Developmental stretching must be preceded by a warm-up.

It is also important that vigorous exercise does not end abruptly, but slows gradually during a cool-down period. This period allows the cardiopulmonary system to return to resting levels without placing undue stress on the body. In addition, delayed onset muscle soreness (DOMS) may be reduced by flushing fresh blood into the muscles previously worked during exercise, and removing waste products. To achieve an increase in muscle perfusion, the activity must involve rhythmic muscle pumping actions of low intensity. The use of post-event massage in this context is described in Chapter 3.

Fitness

All the components of fitness are required for injury prevention (see p. 93), and importantly, a balance should exist between each. For example, increased flexibility without a similar increase in strength may leave a joint hypermobile or unstable and increase the risk of injury. Similarly, strength and muscle bulk increases without adequate flexibility and skill can leave an athlete 'muscle bound' and lacking agility.

Symmetry of muscle development and range of motion is also important. Athletes who exercise unilaterally, for example throwers, must take care that they redress the imbalance caused by their sport with a suitable strength-training programme. Unequal muscle development across a single joint or series of joints may alter specific body segment alignment and general posture. Similarly, unequal training within an antagonistic pair of muscles will cause imbalance.

It is also important that training accurately reflects the physical demands of a sport, and exercise is specific to the physiological adaptations that the sport requires (SAID principle, see p. 93). Sports requiring speed and power, for example, will suffer if only strength is included in training.

Table 7.2   Psychological characteristics of injury-prone athletes

Counter-phobia
Athletes attempt to counter anxiety by being overtly aggressive and fearless. They repeatedly test their indestructibility

Sign of masculinity
Athlete uses injury as a mark of courage. Needs 'visible scars of battle' to show manhood. Continues to play despite injury, but exaggerates pain to seek admiration

Masochism
Punish themselves for feelings of guilt, often about failure to reach their own unrealistic targets

Injury as a weapon
Tries to punish others, for example the young athlete who is forced to play by overzealous parents

Escape
The 'training room athlete' who fears competition because of feelings of inferiority, but cannot opt out for fear of isolation

Psychosomatic injury
No physical injury, or slight injury made worse by emotional factors

Adapted from Sanderson, F.H. (1981) The psychology of the injury-prone athlete. In *Sports Fitness and Sports Injuries* (ed. T. Reilly). Faber and Faber, London. With permission.

The 'strong' athlete who has trained exclusively with heavy weight training is open to injury when rapid explosive actions are used in sport. This is because the skills involved in the two actions are very different.

Keypoint

Physical training must aim to give a balanced overall development.

Psychological factors

A variety of psychological factors may predispose an athlete to injury. Personality tests (Cattell 16PF) performed on footballers have shown that tender-minded players were more likely to be injured, and those who were reserved/detached or apprehensive to suffer more severe injuries (Jackson et al., 1978). Anxiety, and the unconscious attempt to cope with it, can cause abnormal behaviour in the athlete (Sanderson, 1981) and may also increase the likelihood of injury. Coping mechanisms for tension or anxiety can in some instances create a distortion of reality. An example is the overly tense athlete who simply denies that he/she is anxious, yet loses composure easily and in some cases actually becomes violent. Individuals of this type may harbour a sense of guilt which they try to reduce by self-punishment. A number of visible characteristics are displayed by the injury-prone athlete (Table 7.2).

Table 7.3 Examples of life change units (LCUs)

Positive	Negative
Marriage	Bereavement
Getting a better job	Redundancy
Passing an examination	Divorce

Table 7.4 Age, size and performance variables of youth ice-hockey players

Variable	Small (Mean)	Large (Mean)
Age (years)	13.4	14.0
Weight (kg)	37.1	74.3
Stature (cm)	147.4	178.9
Grip strength (kg)	27.7	56.5
Maximal speed (m/s)	7.6	8.3
Impact force (N)	1010.0	1722.0
Speed at impact (m/s)	3.2	3.7

Adapted from Roy, M.A. et al. (1989) Body checking in Pee Wee hockey. *Physician and Sportsmedicine*, **17**(3), 119–126. ©The McGraw-Hill Companies. With permission.

Stressful events in a player's life can also be a factor in injury. These can be measured as life change units (Table 7.3), and injured players tend to have significantly more of these in the period preceding injury (Kerr and Minden, 1988). One of the reasons for this increased risk is that the athlete's attention may be affected, with life events hindering concentration. To perform well, an athlete must 'let go' and allow automatic or grooved motor actions to 'flow' freely (see p. 149). Stressful life events could lead to worry about performance which may prevent an athlete from letting go. In a study of gymnasts, those who had experienced recent stressful life events were 4 times more likely to be injured and the severity of injury was 4.5 times greater. The subjects in this study reported 'lack of concentration' and 'thinking of other things' as the major causes of their injuries (Kerr and Minden, 1988).

Stressful life events may ultimately lead to mental fatigue, which may present as apathy where an athlete is 'not interested' and 'lacks concentration'. Remedial action could involve a period of attention training from a sport psychologist, to enable the athlete to focus on a task or shift attention between different tasks rapidly. Coaches and therapists must recognize that an athlete is vulnerable to injury after a stressful life event. Training should be modified by reducing its intensity and concentrating on basic skills rather than introducing new ones.

> **Keypoint**
>
> Athletes are more vulnerable to injury after a stressful life event. Training must be adapted to take this into account.

Equipment and environment

All athletes are under pressure to buy particular sportswear. Professional athletes may receive sponsorship, and amateur athletes (particularly children) will respond to changing fashions. It is important to emphasize to the athlete that sports equipment should be comfortable and functional. If a particular shoe or item of clothing does not fit correctly, another should be tried, the fit being more important than the type.

The field of play should also be the focus of attention, particularly in amateur sport. Before training, both the environment and equipment should be inspected by the coach. If, for example, a child falls on a broken bottle that no one realized was there, part of the responsibility lies with the coach for not checking the area beforehand.

Another aspect of 'environment' that warrants attention is the other players. Variability of young athletes grouped by chronological age rather than biological (physiological) age may be tremendous. This is especially true at the onset of puberty, where a relatively narrow age range of 2 years in a grouping of 9–11-year-olds will give a large size variation. It was these variations (at the time within the child labour market) which gave rise to the use of physiological age groupings based on pubic hair development (Crampton, 1908).

Table 7.4 shows the difference between age, size and a selection of performance variables in small and large youth ice hockey players in the same league. It is clearly a risk to have a 37 kg athlete able to produce an impact force of just over 1000 N competing against a 74 kg athlete capable of producing an (almost double) impact force of 1700 N.

Self-assessment of maturity can be made using secondary sex characteristics, including external genitalia and pubic hair in males, and breasts, pubic hair and menarche in females (Malina and Beunen, 1996). There is obviously a potential problem of under- and overestimation (by the athlete or others) to remain with peers or to gain a competitive advantage, but the possibility of random testing by medical staff should control this.

> **Keypoint**
>
> Children in sport should be matched for biological age, body build and skill level, rather than chronological age alone.

Rules

In professional sport, rule changes have had a dramatic effect, particularly with head injuries. However, the local youth club under-12 team must also have a firm policy of sports regulation. Where children are involved, it is important to lay down firm rules concerning safety and equipment. The coach who tries to be popular by allowing a 'free for all' is really being irresponsible and is likely to be the cause of injury.

Alteration of rules in sport has been shown to have a positive effect on injury rate and intensity (Table 7.5). Changes in the rules in *ice hockey*, making the wearing of helmets compulsory, significantly reduced the number of head and eye injuries (Vinger, 1981). In *American football*, the banning of 'spear tackles' (hitting an opponent with the vertex of the head) has reduced the number of head and neck injuries (Torg, Truex and Quedenfield, 1979). In *hockey*, banning high sticking (lifting the stick above shoulder level) has reduced eye injuries (Tator and Edmonds, 1984); and in *karate*, banning round-house kicks in competition (a rapid kick aimed at the side of the head) has prevented injury (McLatchie, Davis and Caulley, 1980). Allowing free substitution (permitting injured players to be substituted immediately) in *soccer* has been shown to reduce injury (Jorgensen, 1989).

Screening

The subject of physical screening of youngsters in sport is one which attracts much discussion. A variety of anatomical abnormalities may develop largely unnoticed to the layperson. However, these can often be readily identified by the sports medicine practitioner with a series of annual screening tests. Posture, flexibility and strength can all be measured

Table 7.5 Influence of rules in injury

Failure to apply rules strictly (rugby, soccer)
Not allowing free substitution (soccer)
Foul play (hockey, rugby)
Type of tackle allowed (rugby and American football)
Status of equipment (skiing)
Compulsory protective equipment (cricket, martial arts)
Limits to performance (ultra-endurance events)

Adapted from Jorgensen, U. (1989) Free substitution in soccer. *Nitz*, 3, 155–158. With permission.

Table 7.6 Examples of measures for pre-season screening

Medical history
Psychological questionnaire
Cardiopulmonary health
Body composition
Strength
Range of motion
Posture and segmental alignment
Balance and coordination

using fairly simple field tests. These can be incorporated into a training session and educational period for youngsters, at the beginning of a season.

Pre-season screening may involve tests of a number of measures (Table 7.6). Tests should be performed 6–8 weeks prior to competition to allow for the effects of training to take place. In addition, pre-event screening should be performed to assess a player's suitability to compete.

FIRST AID

First aid treatment marks the beginning of the rehabilitation process. Correct management at this stage can reduce the severity of an injury and so shorten the time an athlete is away from sport. More importantly, effective first aid can save lives. In this section, a number of first aid methods relevant to the injured sportsperson are described. All therapists involved with sports injuries management are recommended to obtain certification in cardiopulmonary resuscitation (CPR) and basic first aid.

The unconscious athlete

Unconsciousness is the result of an interruption of normal brain activity. The most common cause in sport is *concussion*.

Definition
Concussion is the sudden loss of consciousness due to a blow to the head.

Concussion occurs when the brain is rapidly 'shaken', and the condition can be present even though the patient is still conscious. Often, the period of unconsciousness is so brief that it may go unnoticed, and there is only transient memory loss. This is frequently the case with contact injuries where an athlete collides with another and hits his or her head.

The danger from any head injury is an expanding intracranial lesion resulting from a torn blood vessel, causing epidural (extradural) haemorrhage, subarachnoid haemorrhage or subdural haematoma (Fig. 7.1).

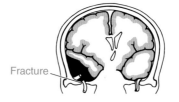
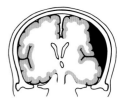

Fracture

Extradural haemorrhage   Subdural haemorrhage

Figure 7.1   Intracranial haematoma.

The conditions are indicated by an alteration in consciousness (lucid state) and the signs and symptoms shown in Table 7.7. Normally, the intracranial pressure is 4–15 mmHg and an intracranial pressure of 40 mmHg will cause neurological impairment.

After such an incident, an athlete should only be allowed to continue providing he or she did not lose consciousness. Tests such as the ability to stand up without assistance, stand alone with eyes closed and run to a mark and change direction rapidly are all useful for initial assessment.

The first decision to be made with an unconscious athlete is whether he or she is still breathing. If not, resuscitation must be started *immediately*. If the athlete regains consciousness, the level of potential damage should be assessed. Response of the eyes, body movements and speech all give clues to the level of consciousness, and the Glasgow Coma Scale is the standard examination method.

The Glasgow Coma Scale

The Glasgow Coma Scale (Teasdale and Jennett, 1974) is a series of tests which are given a numerical value which can then be used to objectify an athlete's state of consciousness (Table 7.8). The first test relates to the eyes, and determines whether the athlete opens the eyes spontaneously or in response to sound (verbal command) or pain. Opening the eyes to verbal command merely means that the person has registered sound; it does not imply that they necessarily understand the command. The second test is of verbal response, and assesses the athlete's reaction to simple questions such as 'where are you' or 'what is your name'. The test assesses whether the athlete is aware of him/herself and the environment. The third test is of motor response. The maximum score is 6 if the athlete is able to perform actions correctly to verbal commands such as 'move your arm'. If the athlete fails to respond, a painful stimulus is applied by the practitioner pressing their knuckles into the athlete's sternum, or pressing the athlete's fingers together around a pen. Painful stimuli to the face or palm of the hands should be avoided as these can give reflex eye closing and hand closing respectively (Magee, 2002). Where reflex responses alone result, flexion of the arms and hands together with adduction of the upper limb and extension of the lower limb with plantarflexion of the feet (decorticate posturing) indicates a lesion above the red nucleus. Extension of the arms with pronation of the forearm (decerebrate posturing) indicates a lesion of the brainstem. The time of the test should be noted and the test repeated every 15–30 minutes to note any degeneration of results.

Where the score is between 3 and 8 on the coma scale, emergency care is required immediately as a severe head injury is present. Scores of 9–11 are considered to have a moderate head injury, and those with a score of 12 or higher are considered to have a mild head injury.

Caution must always be exercised with concussion injuries. Unfortunately, the practitioner or coach who has to decide whether to allow an athlete to continue playing has no way of knowing if secondary brain damage is going to develop. At the time of injury, bleeding may have occurred which could accumulate and give rise to a subdural haematoma.

Table 7.7 Signs of an expanding intracranial lesion

Altered state of consciousness (dizzy/drowsy)
Changes in normal eye movements
nystagmus
pupil inequality
irregular eye movements
Slow heart rate
Irregular respiration
Altered coordination
Weakness
Severe, and often increasing, headache
Vomiting (may be projectile)
Convulsion (fits)

After Magee (2002), with permission.

Table 7.8 The Glasgow Coma Scale

Function	Response	Score
Eye opening	Spontaneous eye opening	4
	Eyes open to command	3
	Eyes open to pain	2
	No eye opening	1
Verbal response	Coherent appropriate response	5
	Coherent but inappropriate response	4
	Incoherent speech	3
	Non-speech noises (moans and groans)	2
	No vocalization	1
Motor response	Obeys commands	6
	Localizing purposeful response to pain	5
	Non-localising purposeful withdrawal from pain	4
	Reflex flexion to pain (arm, decorticate posturing)	3
	Reflex extension to pain (arm, decerebrate posturing)	2
	No motor response	1
Total score		**46**

An athlete who remains unconscious should be placed in the recovery position until an ambulance is available to take him or her to hospital. If there is bleeding or discharge from an ear, the athlete should be turned so that the affected ear is dependent. Nothing should be given by mouth, and the athlete should not be left unattended. Testing for responses should continue regularly (every 10 minutes or more frequently) and any changes in the athlete's condition should be recorded.

Multiple concussion incidents

The cumulative effects of concussion are important in sports such as boxing, steeplechase and football (Corsellis, 1974; Sortland, Tysvaer and Storli, 1989; McLatchie, 1993). EEG disturbances due to neuronal damage through repeated trauma are seen, especially where a series of EEGs are performed. In addition, neuropsychological performance is impaired, often in the presence of a normal CT scan (McLatchie, Brooks and Galbraith, 1987).

Failure to allow adequate recovery from a concussion incident may result in *second impact syndrome* (SIS), where a second blow to the head causes further swelling and bleeding. The second blow may be minor and may not appear sufficient to affect the brain. However, the two combined insults cause rapid and profuse swelling. Athletes usually develop respiratory failure and collapse. The mortality rate for this condition is as high as 50% (Cantu, 1998).

Definition

Second impact syndrome occurs when a second blow is received before the effects of the first concussion have worn off. Massive swelling develops in the brain, the athlete collapses and may go into respiratory failure. The syndrome is often fatal.

Because of the risk of persistent swelling or late bleeding, the return to sport should be delayed. All athletes sustaining a head injury, however minor, should be given an advice card (Table 7.9), and the return to sport will depend on the degree of concussion (Table 7.10). Medical examination is recommended where there is a failure to remember the event which gave the concussion (memory loss). All cases of severe concussion, that is where consciousness has been lost for longer than 3 minutes, warrant X-rays of the skull and cervical spine (Buxton and Firth, 1999).

Epilepsy

Epilepsy is due to a disturbance in the electrical activity in the brain. There are two major types, convulsions or *generalized seizures* (grand mal) and *absence seizures* (petit mal). In a grand mal attack the person loses consciousness, begins to convulse, and the back may arch into extension. Rigidity may last for a few seconds and cyanosis of the mouth and lips can occur. Fitting athletes should be protected by clearing a space around them. Any tight clothing around the neck should be loosened, and something soft placed under the head.

No attempt should be made to move or restrain the fitting athlete, and nothing should be given by mouth until there is full recovery. No object should be placed in the mouth, as the athlete may choke. In addition, it has been known for an epileptic to break a tooth in this way and inhale it.

Absence seizures (petit mal) may also occur, particularly in young athletes. In these cases the person appears to suddenly go distant or 'switch off'. There may be slight twitching of the eyelids or lips. Again, clear a space and remove any potentially dangerous items such as hot drinks or sharp

---

Table 7.9 Care of athletes who have sustained a head injury

Name _____

Sustained a head injury at (*time*) _____ On (*date*) _____

For the rest of today he/she should
Rest quietly at home
Not consume alcohol
Not drive
Not be left alone

He/she should be taken to hospital if he/she
Vomits repeatedly
Develops a severe headache
Becomes restless or irritable
Shows dizziness
Becomes drowsy or difficult to rouse
   (*Children should be woken every 2 hours during the first 12 hours after the injury to make sure that they are still rousable*)
Has a fit (convulsion)
Experiences anything unusual

Table 7.10 Return to sport after concussion

Mild	
• No loss of consciousness (LOC) or memory loss	Continue playing after being checked
• No LOC but with memory loss	Leave field. Resume playing or training only after medical examination
Moderate	
• LOC less than 2 minutes	Leave field. No playing or training for 15 days
Severe	
• LOC less than 3 minutes	Leave field. No playing or training for 22 days. Resume only after medical examination
• LOC longer than 3 minutes	Admit to hospital. No playing or training for 29 days. Resume only after medical examination

Source Buxton, N. and Firth, J. (1999) Head and neck injury. In *Sports Medicine Handbook* (eds R. Hackney and A. Wallace). BMJ Publishing, London. With permission.

objects. Give reassurance and, if the person is unaware of their condition, ensure that they seek medical advice.

Diabetic coma

In diabetes mellitus, both hyperglycaemia and hypoglycaemia may give rise to unconsciousness. Hyperglycaemia usually develops gradually and so is rarely a first aid problem.

With intense unaccustomed exercise, the blood sugar level may fall, and hypoglycaemia can then result. An athlete may initially feel faint, dizzy or light-headed, and may be confused or disorientated. The skin becomes pale, the pulse rapid, and sweating occurs. Breathing often becomes shallow, and muscle tremor may be apparent. The level of consciousness drops rapidly.

If the athlete is conscious, a rapidly metabolized sugar (glucose tablet, sugary drink, or glucose gel) will help, together with some slowly absorbed carbohydrate (bread) to prevent recurrent blood glucose fall. If the athlete is unconscious, nothing should be given and hospital treatment should be sought as a glucagon injection may be required.

If the coma is due to hypoglycaemia, the response to sugar is usually rapid and the danger of secondary symptoms is averted. If hyperglycaemic coma is present, slightly more sugar will not harm the patient (Sperryn, 1985).

Where someone collapses and it is not known whether they have simply fainted or are hypoglycaemic, a *glucometer* may be used. This measures the blood sugar level from a finger pinprick. Normal blood sugar values are in the region of 4–7 mmol/litre. A reading of 1–2 mmol/litre indicates a possible hypoglycaemic state.

Definition
Glucagon is a hormone secreted by the pancreas which increases blood glucose levels. A *glucometer* is a battery-operated blood sugar meter which uses a finger pinprick drop of blood.

Asthma

Asthma is a condition in which the small airways in the lung (bronchioles) narrow. This results from spasm in the muscles of the wall of the bronchioles. Patients have a difficultly breathing out and this may be accompanied by an audible wheeze. Someone who suffers an attack during which the bronchioles go into spasm will show the features of *hypoxia*, where insufficient oxygen reaches the body tissues. The skin of the lips, ear lobes and nailbeds goes grey-blue.

Definition
Hypoxia occurs when insufficient oxygen reaches the body tissues. The skin of the lips, ear lobes and nailbeds goes grey-blue, a discoloration called *cyanosis*. As the condition worsens, cyanosis will affect the whole body.

In sport, the two factors to consider in connection with asthma are cold air and dry (dusty) environments, as these may both trigger an asthma attack. Studies on asthmatic athletes (Harries, 1994) show that bronchoconstriction (narrowing of the airways) occurs after exercise (Fig. 7.2). At room temperature (14°C), normal subjects show an increase in peak flow (rate of air entering the lungs) after a 3-minute treadmill run which returns to normal after exercise. Asthmatic athletes, however, show a 20% fall in peak flow. With cold air (−10°C) normal subjects show a 15% fall in peak flow, whereas asthmatic athletes show a 35% fall. At −20°C normal athletes again show a peak flow fall, this time by 20%, but with asthmatic athletes the intensity of cold at this temperature is sufficient to induce brochospasm, even at rest.

Asthmatic athletes will often have an inhaler and carry it with them. These will give a dose of drug, either to prevent an attack coming on (*preventive inhaler – brown or white cap*) or to relieve the symptoms of wheeze and chest tightness when they happen (*reliever inhaler – blue cap*).

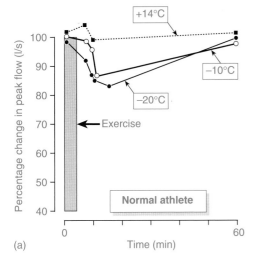

(a)

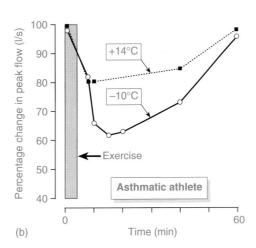

(b)

Figure 7.2 Bronchoconstriction after exercise at different temperatures. From Harries, M. (1994) Asthma. In *Oxford Textbook of Sports Medicine* (eds M. Harries et al.). Oxford Medical Publications. With permission.

Athletes who have an asthma attack may wheeze and have difficulty in breathing and speaking. They will appear exhausted and may have cyanosis to the lips and ear lobes. The aim is to calm them and make them comfortable, and encourage them to breathe slowly. They should sit and lean forwards slightly with the arms supported (sitting the wrong way round on a chair for example). If they have a reliever inhaler they should use it but not a preventive inhaler. If the athlete shows no sign of improvement in 5–10 minutes, an ambulance should be called.

Resuscitation

With an unconscious subject who is not breathing, or in whom no heart beat can be detected, it is vital that these processes be restored or sustained until hospital treatment is available. In all cases, help must be summoned as soon as possible. A basic mnemonic usefully describes the course of action: ABC – airway, breathing, circulation.

Airway

If breathing is noisy, or not present, the airway may be blocked. This can occur if the tongue has fallen back and is covering the airway, or if the airway is narrowed due to the position of the head. Absence of the gagging reflex may allow saliva or vomit to accumulate at the back of the throat and block the airway.

Definition
The gagging reflex occurs when the throat or pharynx is stimulated by an object or substance. Vomiting may result.

The subject's chin should be pulled forwards and the head tilted back (Fig. 7.3a). This will open the airway. If breathing is still noisy, the head should be turned to one side, keeping the head well back, providing cervical injury is not suspected. If foreign matter is in the mouth, clear any obvious obstructions such as broken teeth or dislodged dentures but do not place your fingers in the subject's mouth (First Aid Manual, 2002), as you risk your finger being bitten and the skin broken. The practitioner should look, listen and feel for signs of respiratory movements (Fig. 7.3b). If these are not present, artificial ventilation is required.

Breathing

When the airway is cleared, the subject should be laid supine, and mouth-to-mouth, or mouth-to-nose ventilation given. In small children, the nose and mouth may be used together. The subject's mouth is opened wide and the nose pinched close, at the same time keeping the head well back (Fig. 7.4a). The practitioner breathes out directly into the subject's mouth, making sure a good seal is maintained between his or her own lips and the subject's mouth. The chest should be observed, to assess lung inflation, which will normally take about 2 seconds (Fig. 7.4b). If this does not occur, the airway may still be blocked, in which case the head should be readjusted and the artificial ventilation resumed. If no chest movement occurs this time, the subject should be treated with an abdominal thrust as though choking (see below).

After two lung inflations, check for visible signs of circulation such as breathing, coughing or movement. If circulation is present, but breathing has not commenced, artificial ventilation should be continued at a rate of 10 inflations per minute, re-checking for circulation after each 10 breaths. If circulation is not detected, external chest compression is required.

Circulation

For external chest compression, the subject should be supine on a firm surface. The practitioner kneels to one side, and places the heel of one hand, reinforced by the other, over the subject's lower sternum (Fig. 7.5a). Keeping the

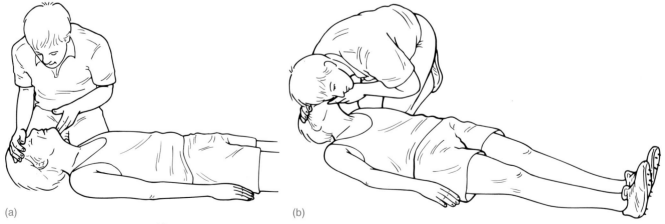

(a)   (b)

Figure 7.3   Opening the airway. (a) Pull the athlete's chin forwards, tilt the head back and look into the mouth to check for obstructions. (b) Look, listen and feel for signs of respiratory movements.

elbows locked, a downwards pressure is exerted onto the patient's sternum by the practitioner leaning downwards and pushing through straight arms (Fig. 7.5b). The force used should be sufficient to depress the sternum by 4–5 cm. The pressure is released and the procedure repeated 15 times. Following this, attention is again focused on the mouth and two breaths of artificial ventilation are given. This sequence of 15 repetitions of external chest compression and two breaths of artificial ventilation continues until hospitalization is available, or the subject recovers. Check for circulation after 1 minute and then after each third minute. When circulation returns, chest compression is stopped. If breathing returns and is sustained, the subject is placed into the recovery position.

If an assistant is available, resuscitation may be carried out with one person performing chest compression and the other artificial respiration. The rate is then five compressions to one inflation (Fig. 7.5c).

A number of resuscitation aids are available. Some consist of a plastic sheet, mouthpiece and valve which covers

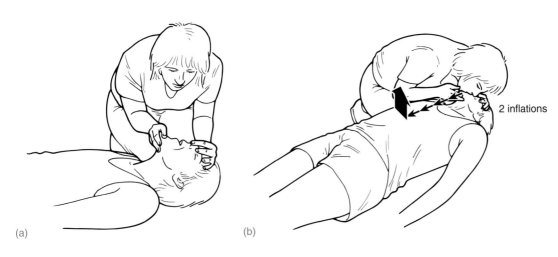

(a)   (b)   2 inflations

Figure 7.4   Breathing. (a) Open the athlete's mouth, pinch the nose closed and tilt the head back. (b) Breathe directly into the athlete's mouth and observe chest movements.

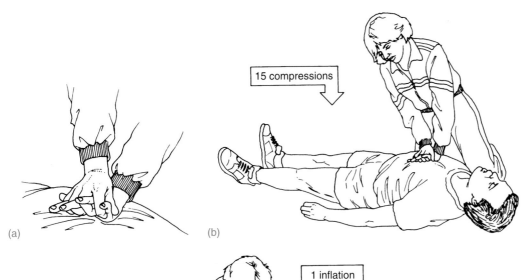

15 compressions

(a)   (b)

5 compressions   1 inflation

(c)

Figure 7.5   Circulation. (a) One hand, reinforced by the other, is placed over the athlete's sternum. (b) Keeping the elbows locked, a downward pressure is exerted to depress the sternum by 4–5 cm. (c) With an assistant, one person performs chest compression, and the other artificial respiration.

Table 7.11   Using an automated external defibrillator (AED)

- Switch machine on and check that the electrodes are plugged in
- Remove or cut away clothing covering the chest
- Wipe away any sweat
- Shave any excessive chest hair as this will prevent the adhesive pads from sticking
- Remove backing paper from electrode pads and attach them to the athlete's chest in the position indicated on the pads themselves
- The AED will start to analyse the heart rhythm
- *Make sure that no one is touching the athlete as this will interfere with the machine*
- Follow the spoken/visual machine prompts
- If the athlete begins to breathe, place them into the recovery position
- Leave the AED attached

Source *First Aid Manual* (2002), 8th edn. Dorling Kindersley, London. With permission.

the face of the subject and holds the mouth open. Plastic airways themselves are helpful to hold the tongue away from the back of the throat, and airways with a valve to stop the passage of saliva to the practitioner are also available. All airways have the potential to damage the soft palate and should only be used after appropriate training.

Many major sporting venues have portable defibrillators (automated external defibrillator or AED) and the practitioner working with a sports team must know how to use these. The AED analyses the athlete's heart rhythm and tells you what action to take at each stage of resuscitation (Table 7.11).

Recovery position

When an unconscious athlete is breathing and shows a regular pulse, he or she should be placed into the recovery position (First Aid Manual, 1995, 2002). In this position, the chin is lifted forwards to keep the airway clear and open, the head is lower than the body so fluids will drain from the mouth, avoiding the possibility of them being inhaled. The athlete's hand supports the head and protects it from the ground, and the arm and leg are bent, increasing stability and preventing the body rolling forwards. The side-lying position avoids the chest compression of the prone position, making breathing easier.

The athlete is rolled into the recovery position in five stages (Fig. 7.6), making sure that the open airway remains a priority throughout the movement. In stage I, the practitioner kneels to the side of the athlete at waist level. The athlete's airway is opened (gum shield removed) by pulling the chin forwards and tilting the head back. If there is time, objects such as the athlete's spectacles, keys in the pocket, and any cord in or around the neck (stopwatch, whistle, etc.) should be removed. The nearest arm is bent to 90° at the elbow and shoulder, and supinated to bring the palm

forward facing at the side of the head ('oath' position). For stage II, the athlete's other arm is brought across the chest and the hand held, palm outwards, against the near cheek throughout the remaining stages to support and protect the head. In stage III the far leg is grasped over the lower hamstrings to flex it and pull the bent knee towards the practitioner. The foot remains on the floor to take the weight of the limb and avoid lifting stress on the practitioner. In stage IV the knee is pulled towards the practitioner to roll the athlete onto the side. The practitioner's knees prevent the athlete from rolling too far. Finally, in stage V, the athlete's chin is pulled forwards to clear the tongue from the throat and assist drainage. Final adjustments are made to the hand beneath the cheek to maintain correct head alignment, and to the upper leg (flexed at 90° to both hip and knee) for maximum stability.

Skin wounds

Skin wounds are common injuries in sport, especially when athletes train on hard surfaces. When treating skin wounds, practitioners must protect themselves against contact with blood or tissue fluids. If the practitioner has grazes, sores or open wounds on the hands or forearms, these must be covered with a waterproof adhesive dressing. Disposable gloves should always be used when treating skin wounds of any type. Where gloves are not available, ask the athlete to dress the wound under your supervision. If the athlete is unconscious and gloves are not available, you should improvise and place your hands in plastic bags.

As described in Chapter 2, wounds may be either open or closed, depending on whether the epidermis has been completely penetrated. With closed wounds, such as abrasions and gravel burns, the aim is to prevent infection and remove any foreign material. Grit may cause *ingrained tattooing* where embedded particles remain beneath the surface. The material is covered by epithelium, giving a hypertrophic scar. The injured area is cleaned with 0.5% chlorhexidine or a mixture of chlorhexidine and cetrimide, and grit or other material removed with sterile forceps. Where the material is too fine and profuse, the area may be scrubbed with a sterile nailbrush. If an athlete is known to be allergic to chlorhexidine, sterile water should be used instead.

Exposed areas may be left without a dressing, as air will assist healing. If an abrasion cannot be left exposed, it should be dressed with a single layer of paraffin gauze and a dry dressing (or a dry dressing alone for small wounds). The area should be checked every 48 hours to ensure there is no infection and that healing is progressing. When a practitioner decides that a player must continue until the end of the match, a wound may be sprayed with antiseptic dry spray, and the area bandaged with a cohesive (non-adhesive) tape which is impermeable to blood.

Blisters are caused by pressure or friction where the epidermal surface of the skin is detached from the underlying tissue. The gap between the two layers is filled with lymph,

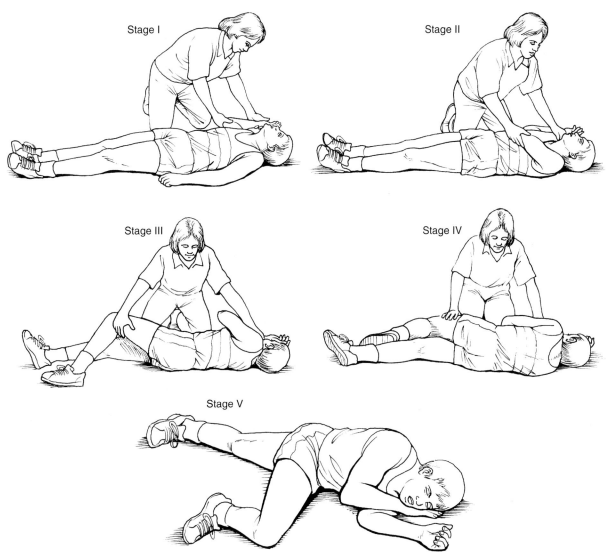

Figure 7.6   Moving the athlete into the recovery position. Stage I: open airway, remove any obstructing objects, straighten legs and kneel at the athlete's waist, bend near arm into oath position. Stage II: bring far arm across chest to side of face, and maintain this position throughout. Stage III: grasp far leg, bend knee and pull it towards you. Stage IV: roll the athlete towards you, blocking him or her with your knees. Stage V: adjust the head position to ensure a clear airway, adjust upper leg position to ensure whole body stability.

exposing nerve endings to fluid pressure and therefore pain. Blisters may be treated by cleaning the wound site with antiseptic solution and padding. If the blister is blood-filled, do not aspirate it, as this runs the risk of infection. Cover the area with a protective sterile dressing. Where the blister is large, clear, and fluid-filled it may be aspirated. Use a sterile needle introduced into the side of the blister sac. Clean the area again with antiseptic solution and cover with an antiseptic dressing.

Keypoint

If a blister is blood-filled, it should not be aspirated (drained) as this risks infection.

Open wounds, such as lacerations and puncture wounds, are more serious. The amount of bleeding which occurs is dependent on the site of the injury and the depth of the wound – arterial damage will obviously result in profuse bleeding. The first priority is to stop bleeding with direct pressure over the wound and elevation of the injured limb. Pressure should be given with a sterile (or at least clean) dressing, or the patient's hand, and maintained for at least 10 minutes to allow blood clotting.

Some minor lacerations may be cleaned and closed with sterile adhesive strips or dumb-bell sutures. These have the advantage that no local anaesthetic is needed for their application, and they avoid the risk of stitch marks and suture tearing of the skin.

More extensive wounds may require suturing. When deeper tissues have been damaged, suturing in layers may be required, the deep layers being sutured with catgut and the skin closed with silk. Because of the risk of infection, all but the most minor open skin wounds should be managed in a hospital casualty department. In cases where bleeding is profuse, the patient may need to be treated for shock by lying them flat and elevating the lower limbs, until they can be removed to hospital.

All skin wounds run the risk of tetanus infection, so an injured athlete who sustains a major injury may require a full course of tetanus prophylaxis. This consists of three injections of 0.5 ml tetanus toxoid. The first is given at the time of injury, the second 6 weeks later and the third 6 months after the first. If an athlete is not sure of the time interval since his last tetanus injection (or if a course has been given within the last 12 months), a booster dose of 0.5 ml toxoid may be given after injury as a precaution. A synopsis of simple skin wound management is given in Table 7.12.

Soft tissue injury

The initial aim with a soft tissue injury is to protect the area from further harm and slow the inflammatory process. A simple mnemonic for first contact treatment is RICE: rest, ice, compression, elevation. This mnemonic is sometimes given as 'PRICE', the 'P' standing for protection. However, in this book the shorter mnemonic is preferred, as protection is included within the remit of rest.

Rest

The immediate first aid concern (assuming a life-threatening situation does not exist) is to protect the injured body part from further injury. This may simply mean rest, or splinting/strapping in the case of an injured joint to limit movement.

Inflatable splints are invaluable here for fast immobilization to permit safe removal to hospital. Details on strapping are given in Chapter 4.

During the acute phase of inflammation, the athlete should rest. However, rather than complete rest, 'functional rest' is to be preferred. Here, any activity which stresses the injured tissue is avoided, but other activities are allowed. In the subacute phase, the injured tissues themselves should be allowed to move gently, to produce a strong mobile scar, and to allow collagen fibres to align in the direction of stress. As collagen synthesis does not begin until the 4th or 5th post-injury day (see p. 39), range of motion (ROM) exercise does not need to start until that time. After this period, total rest of an injured body part may lead to increased adhesions. In addition, a haphazard arrangement of collagen fibres within the newly formed scar will result in a reduction of tensile strength.

More vigorous general exercise is to be encouraged, with the injured body part still protected. This will help maintain general cardiopulmonary fitness and the condition of the non-injured tissues.

Ice

Ice, or cold application, is used to slow the metabolic rate of the injured tissue and reduce hypoxic tissue damage (Knight, 1989). Furthermore, the production of cold-induced analgesia is desirable. An ice pack should be kept on for 15–20 minutes and reapplied every 2 hours for the first 2 days following injury.

If no ice is available, cold water is of use, but the tissue temperature changes are not as great as with ice, and so hypoxic damage is not prevented as efficiently. The use of ice is covered later in this chapter.

Compression

Compression is used in combination with cold to reduce swelling. Compression should be sufficient to limit the formation of oedema but not to compromise the blood flow to the area. The circulation distal to the compression should be checked by observing skin coloration. In addition, a fingernail or toenail should be squeezed on the injured limb which has been compressed. The subungual skin will go white with compression and the normal pink coloration should return a few seconds after pressure is released, illustrating that adequate circulation is reaching the nailbed.

Table 7.12	Treatment of common skin injuries in sport*
Injury	**Action**
Abrasion	Clean and remove all visible contaminants using an antiseptic wash and brush. Cover with a sterile dressing. Refer for a tetanus booster if needed
Blister	Clean wound site with antiseptic solution If blood-filled, do not aspirate. Cover with a protective sterile dressing If the blister is large, clear, and fluid-filled, aspirate using a sterile needle introduced into the side of the blister sac. Clean the area again with antiseptic solution and cover with an antiseptic dressing
Cut	Clean wound and surrounding site. Use spray adhesive on small wounds or adhesive strips on larger wounds. Dress the wound with a non-stick sterile dressing. Refer for a tetanus booster if needed

*With all skin injuries there is a risk of infection from body fluids, and for this reason the practitioner should always wear gloves.

> **Keypoint**
>
> Check the athlete's circulation distal to any compression by squeezing the finger- or toenail until the nailbed goes white. The normal pink colour should return within a few seconds when the pressure is released. If it does not, remove the compression and reapply it less tightly.

Elevation

Gravity will pull swelling into a dependent limb, so elevation should be used to aid lymphatic drainage. The limb need only be elevated above the level of the heart. Athletes with lower limb injuries, particularly to the ankle, should be encouraged to keep the leg elevated on a stool when sitting throughout the day. In addition, gentle isometric or short range isotonic exercise is useful to stimulate the muscle pump and aid venous return and lymphatic drainage.

A combination of the above treatment techniques will produce the best results. Cold compresses can easily be applied with lint soaked in iced water and wrapped around the limb. A polythene bag covers the wet lint and an elastic tubular bandage covers both. The compress is reapplied every 2 or 3 minutes as its temperature rises. The limb is elevated and isometric exercise performed at a rate of one contraction every 3–5 seconds. Various cryogel impregnated bandages are commercially available which perform a similar job. Flaked ice in a towelling bag may be applied flat with an elastic bandage over the top. Once more, elevation and muscle pump exercise is required. Various machines are available which circulate cold/iced water through an inflated cuff. Again, these combine cold, elevation and compression.

Fractures

Fractures should only receive treatment after breathing has been restored and bleeding stopped. If a fracture is present, squeezing the area, or gentle limb movements, will usually cause pain. If the accident was not seen, and the athlete has not moved, a screening examination is required. The 'squeeze technique' is used. This procedure, where a body area is compressed to assess pain and bony contour, starts at the head, and then moves to the neck, shoulders and arms, and so on until the whole body has been assessed. The experienced practitioner can carry out such an examination in 30–60 seconds (Table 7.13).

If a fracture is found, the injured bone should be immobilized by splinting. A number of options exist. Several emergency splints are on the market, and sports clubs should be encouraged to have these available. The various types include inflatable splints, cardboard splints, backslabs and slings. If none of these is available, improvisation is the order of the day. Broom handles, hockey sticks and ski poles are all useful splints, and with lower limb fractures, using the uninjured leg is also effective. In each case the limb should be gently straightened (if pain is not intense) and immobilized.

Injuries to the shoulder/clavicle and forearm fractures are best immobilized across the chest in a sling. Where the elbow cannot be bent, the straight arm is fixed at the side of the chest, by straps around the pelvis, waist and chest.

The question of whether an injury is a fracture or not often arises in sport. Observation will show any obvious deformity, and palpation by squeezing will usually elicit intense pain, considerably more than with a soft tissue injury. In addition, bleeding is normally more profuse. However, the only way to be totally sure is to view a radiograph of the affected limb.

Dislocations and subluxations

The most common joints dislocated in sport are the fingers and shoulder. No attempt should be made to reduce a shoulder dislocation because of the danger of damage to the axillary nerve (but see p. 395). Finger dislocations may be reduced easily, and this can lead to an underestimation of their potential severity. If light traction applied along the length of the bone causes the joint to relocate, this action is justified. Reduction later will need to be carried out under anaesthetic, as muscle spasm will have set in. There are two potential dangers of injury management on the field using the age-old 'pull it, tape it, and play on' attitude. First, a fracture may have occurred near the joint line which will only reveal itself on X-ray. For this reason, even if the joint is successfully reduced, an X-ray is desirable (Walkden, 1981). Secondly, the final injury result may be jeopardized by early aggressive management (Reid, 1992). Misplaced taping may subject the injury to rotatory or angulatory stress, leading to malalignment, and increased/accumulating swelling may lead to additional joint stiffness.

> **Keypoint**
>
> The danger of simply pulling a joint back into place and playing on is that: (i) a hairline fracture may have occurred close to the joint which may go unnoticed, and (ii) the final cosmetic appearance of the limb may be compromised.

Genital injury

Injury to the genitalia is common in the male, and a suitable box should be worn to offer some degree of protection. Bruising to the scrotum may occur by direct contact with another player or with apparatus. The pain from such an

Table 7.13 The squeeze technique of emergency examination

Test	Identifies
Abnormal joint angulation	Joint subluxation or dislocation
Bony palpation	Fracture
Soft tissue palpation	Swelling, tissue indentation, muscle spasm
Skin temperature	Shock (cold and clammy), fever (hot and sweaty)

Table 7.14 Some medical causes of haematuria (blood in the urine)

Lesion of urinary tract
Blood diseases
Contamination during menstruation
Prostate conditions
Trauma
Tumour
Poisoning
Malaria
Toxaemia (poisons produced by bacteria)
Calculus (stones) in urinary tract

injury is often incapacitating. Application of a cold sponge or ice may give some relief. If blood occurs in the urine after this injury, the player should seek medical attention.

Torsion of the testicles may occur in cycling, particularly in teenagers, and priapism (persistent erection) has been reported due to vascular obstruction (Sperryn, 1985). In both cases, medical attention is required.

Injury to the female genitalia may similarly occur through direct trauma causing contusion and possible pubic fracture, especially after a fall onto gymnastic apparatus. In addition, water-skiing may cause vaginal injury through forced douching. Female water-skiers are well-advised to protect the pudendal region by wearing a wet suit and not a bathing costume. Immediate gynaecological assistance is required.

Blood in the urine (haematuria) varies from a slightly smoky tea colour to profuse redness. *Initial haematuria* is blood appearing in the urine at the start of normal flow and normally indicates a urethral source, while *terminal haematuria* is blood appearing at the end of normal flow and can indicate a source from the bladder or higher (Reid, 1992). A number of medical conditions may cause this (Table 7.14) and athletes may need to seek medical opinion in the conditions persists. In sport, agitation of the bladder and kidneys may give rise to *runner's haematuria*. This condition is seen in endurance athletes and has been shown to be present in 20% of marathon runners and as many as 70% of ultra distance athletes (Reid, 1992). Repeated trauma of the bladder through the shock of running causes microscopic lesions in the bladder wall. The condition usually resolves in up to 3 days and is less common when athletes do not run with an empty bladder.

Choking

Choking occurs when the act of swallowing forces something over the entrance to the trachea rather than into the oesophagus. Two first aid procedures may be used. Initially, the athlete should be bent forwards and firmly slapped with the flat of the hand between the shoulder blades five times. If this fails to dislodge the item, an abdominal thrust (Heimlich manoeuvre) may be used. Here, sharp pressure is placed over the upper abdomen in an attempt to rapidly increase abdominal pressure and simulate a cough.

The victim may be lying supine, in which case the thrust can be through the straight arms of the practitioner. In standing, the practitioner wraps his or her arms around the victim and forces the heels of the hands up and into the victim's abdomen. The manoeuvre must be sharp and hard, and may be repeated five times (Fig. 7.7).

Five back slaps may be used, alternating with five abdominal thrusts until the obstruction is removed. If the athlete loses consciousness, relaxation of muscle spasm may release the obstruction, so check to see if spontaneous breathing has resumed.

Cramp, stitch and winding

A sudden blow to the solar plexus may affect the sympathetic nerve centre in this region, causing a transient contusion (Reid, 1992). A momentary paralysis of the diaphragm may occur, with spasm of the abdominal muscles, causing the player to be 'winded' (Fowler, 1981). Respiration is impaired and nausea may ensue. The player will almost always fall to the ground if the blow was severe, and should be left in the side lying position until recovered. Reassurance is all that is required, and a cold sponge to the nape of the neck may sometimes help. The injury occurs when the athlete is off-guard and the abdominal muscles are relaxed, so there is a danger of intra-abdominal injury (rib or visceral). For this reason, a winded player should be carefully observed for the remaining practice period or game.

Cramps can be a particular problem to athletes because they are so unpredictable. The terms 'cramp' or 'spasm' are used to imply a painful, sustained and involuntary muscle contraction. It is important to realize that cramps are symptoms of some underlying fault. They may be the result of nerve entrapment, or metabolic disorder, and so, if persistent, the athlete should seek medical attention.

A number of possible causes have been suggested (Benda, 1989). Fluid loss, low glucose, electrolyte imbalance, training faults and fatigue have all been implicated. Cramps affect many different categories of people. Well-conditioned athletes are at risk, as are sedentary individuals who often complain of cramps in bed at night. The unfit individual who suddenly embarks on a vigorous keep-fit routine is particularly at risk.

Fluid loss will occur with profuse sweating, and athletes are best advised to take small amounts of water throughout a training period. Large amounts taken when cramp has occurred are not generally as effective, and lead to a bloated feeling.

Electrolyte imbalance altering the excitability of motor units is another possible cause (Fowler, 1981), and both potassium and salt may be involved. Some athletes use electrolyte drinks, but those containing a lot of sugar should be avoided, as should salt tablets. Salt will draw fluid out of the circulatory system, and sugar will slow fluid absorption.

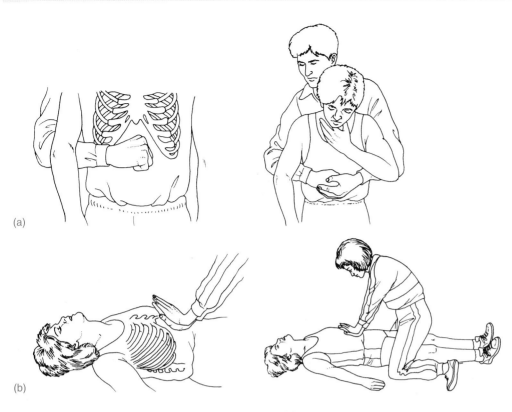

Figure 7.7 Abdominal thrust technique for choking (Heimlich manoeuvre). (a) Standing position, (b) lying position.

If salt or potassium is to be taken, it should be incorporated into the diet as a preventive measure. Potassium-rich foods such as bananas and oranges, and salty foods are suitable.

Pain relief and reduction of muscle spasm may be achieved by the use of ice and stretching. Ice is used to produce cold analgesia, and then slow stretching is carried out. Contraction of the antagonist muscle will help relax the cramped muscle through reciprocal inhibition. Direct pressure over the pain trigger point of the muscle, and deep massage using kneading techniques can both be effective with some athletes.

Stitch is pain which occurs in the upper abdomen. It occurs more often after a heavy meal and is common in runners. It is generally made worse by expiration and relieved slightly by inspiration. A number of possibilities exist as to its cause. After a heavy meal, the mesentery must bear excessive weight, and the liver is full of blood. This may give rise to minor internal bleeding. A reduction in oxygen supply to the diaphragm, or alterations in blood flow to the spleen and liver have also been suggested (Peterson and Renstrom, 1986).

A similar condition is the precordial catch sydrome (Sparrow and Bird, 1978). Pain is usually in the anterior chest to the left side and lasts from 30 seconds to up to 3 minutes. The condition is usually aggravated by deep breathing and alleviated by shallow breaths and standing upright. History and examination reveal that the pain is not from cardiac origin, and the likely cause is intercostal muscle spasm or entrapment of the pleura.

With all forms of stitch, diaphragmatic breathing should be encouraged, allowing the abdominal wall to protrude during inspiration. The athlete should either lean away from the affected side or reach overhead with the arm on the affected side, to stretch the area out. Some athletes report relief by squeezing a hard object in the hand, but the relief mechanism for this technique is puzzling.

Spinal injury

Sport accounts for 10–15% of severe spinal injuries, and unfortunately a significant number of these are made worse by incorrect management. Descriptions exist of patients who became quadriplegic after being able to move their limbs at the time of accident, and of individuals presenting with unstable neck fractures 2 weeks after injury (Garrick and Webb, 1990). A lack of neurological signs does not rule out spinal injury, and the safest approach is to assume that any player who has sustained substantial head or neck trauma has an unstable fracture until this has been disproven radiologically. Even with more minor trauma, unless the athlete is alert and able to demonstrate full range pain-free neck motion without neurological signs, he or she may still have sustained bony injury. The advice is clear: when in doubt immobilize the neck and refer the athlete for further investigation.

Where severe trauma to the spine has occurred, the athlete should not be moved unless he or she is in a life-threatening situation. If movement is necessary, the aim is to prevent further injury to the spine. The position in which the athlete is found should be maintained unless priorities of airway or circulation demand otherwise. Initial treatment follows the ABC protocol, and if movement is required, the head and body should be fully supported and moved as one. The therapist maintains the head position by placing his or her hands over the patient's ears. Three assistants kneel at one side of the athlete and two at the other side. The patient may be rolled in one piece (log roll) onto the side, into the recovery position.

When an athlete is wearing a helmet (motorcycle or football) it should only be removed where airway obstruction or fire occurs (Meyer and Daniel, 1985). An assistant stabilizes the head by placing his or her hands around the athlete's neck. The practitioner unfastens the chin strap and grips the helmet at either side of the rim, spreading this outwards. The helmet is slowly removed by applying traction from below as the assistant continues to stabilize the athlete's neck. When the helmet has been removed, traction is reapplied to the head and maintained until a backboard is in place.

ENVIRONMENT AND INJURY

Thermal stress

The human functions best at temperatures between 36.5 and 40.0°C (Astrand and Rodahl, 1986), and the body will try to keep itself within this region, to maintain equilibrium in the body core. When the external temperature rises, sweating occurs to try to lower body temperature, and when the external temperature is lower than the ideal, shivering starts in an attempt to increase body temperature through metabolic activity.

Heat is exchanged between the body and external environment through convection, conduction and radiation, and through the evaporation of water from the skin surface and respiratory passages. Heat loss through radiation occurs without contact between the body and the object

---

Treatment note 7.1   Subjective examination

In terms of general treatment, the first contact a therapist has with the patient as regards examination should be a subjective examination or 'history'. This forms part of a general clinical diagnosis (Table 2.11, p. 57), and consists of a number of elements (Table 7.15). The aim is to establish a chronological description of the development of the condition and also to learn how the condition behaves. However, although specific headings may be used as a framework for assessment they must not interrupt the fluency of the patients description. Studies on data collection by physicians have shown that continued interruption and the consistent use of closed questions will prevent the patient presenting the true nature of their problem (Blau 1989, Kesson and Atkins 1998).

Age and occupation
The age of the patient is relevant because certain conditions are more common at certain ages (osteochondrosis in children for example), and activities pursued by the patient (occupation, leisure activities) can suggest postures and joint loading. In sport, the exact physical requirements of an activity help to plan a suitable (and specific) rehabilitation programme.

Site and spread
The site(s) of symptoms and their spread may be recorded on a body chart or simply listed, and give information about referred pain especially. The current position of pain and the area into which it travels should be noted, and compared to dermatomal charts to give an indication of the level of a spinal lesion or the body part affected. For example, back pain from a lower lumbar (L4/L5) lesion will give pain into the foot and big toe but not the heel, while that of a sacral lesion (S1/S2) does not give toe pain but does give heel pain. Where a body part is within a dermatome, it may refer pain distally. The hip, for example, is within the L3 dermatome and is capable of referring pain down the front of the thigh and into the knee, misleading the practitioner into thinking that the patient has a knee problem (Fig. 7.8).

The previous position of pain is also important, as it may indicate *centralization* or *peripheralization* (Fig. 7.9). A more irritable lesion will create a greater stimulus and refer further into a dermatome. For example, an acute L5 disc lesion may refer down the leg and into the big toe. As it resolves, pain may be referred only into the shin or front of the knee. The same dermatome is involved, but the reduced stimulus refers for a shorter distance.

As conditions resolve, the length of pain referral will reduce, and the symptoms are said to be centralizing. As a condition worsens, the length of pain referral will increase and the symptoms are peripheralizing. This phenomenon may be used as a guide to the effectiveness of treatments, especially with mechanical therapy (p. 307).

Onset and duration
The onset and duration of a lesion will give an indication of fast onset (trauma) and slow onset (overuse). A knee injury which occurred suddenly on the football field where the

---

Table 7.15   Subjective examination

Age, occupation, activities
Site and spread
Onset and duration
Symptoms and behaviour
Past medical history (PMH)
Other joint involvement
Drug history (medication) (DH)

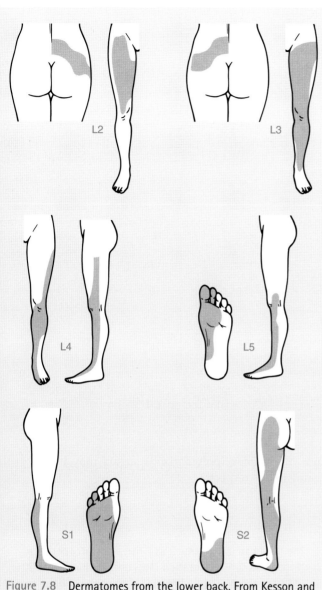

Figure 7.8   Dermatomes from the lower back. From Kesson and Atkins (1998).

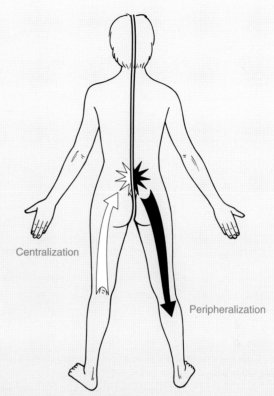

Figure 7.9   Symptom behaviour.

manner. For example, a mechanical joint lesion (torn ligament) is generally worse with activity as movement stresses the injured tissues. However, an injury which is resolving and has left chronic inflammation is generally better for movement as it mobilizes the joint. Most musculoskeletal injuries in sport do not give continual pain. Constant unremitting pain suggests a more serious pathology which warrants medical investigation.

Other considerations
A patient's past medical history is important, and a serious pathology may have recurred. In addition, previous medical history will give information about fractures which may be giving rise to arthritic changes or alterations in gait, for example. Other joints which are affected could also indicate alterations in general body alignment, and medications may be important as they may contraindicate certain treatment protocols (anticoagulants and manipulation or dry needling, for example).

player was unable to continue suggests trauma (e.g. meniscal tear), whereas a knee injury which gradually built up over a period of weeks in a runner indicates overuse (e.g. tendinitis).

Symptoms and behaviour
The type of symptoms (pain, tingling, locking) assists diagnosis, and certain symptoms behave in a predictable

receiving the heat, providing the environment is cooler than the body. In situations where the temperature of the environment exceeds that of the body, radiant heat energy is absorbed from the surroundings, and heat loss must occur by evaporation. Conduction involves direct contact between objects, and is particularly important in water. The rate of heat loss by convection is largely dependent on the rate of movement of air (or water) over the body surface. Accidental

immersion in cold water will result in rapid heat loss. This will be made worse by attempting to swim rather than waiting for help, as the moving water passing the body results in greater heat loss through convection. The cooling effect of temperature and wind speed combined is represented by the wind chill factor. When it is cold and windy, air touching the body surface becomes warmed by body heat, but is immediately taken away to be replaced by cold air once

Table 7.16 The wind chill index

	Ambient temperature (°F**)														
	40	35	30	25	20	15	10	5	0	−5	−10	−15	−20	−25	−30
	Equivalent temperature (°F)														
Calm	40	35	30	25	20	15	10	5	0	−5	−10	−15	−20	−25	−30
5	37	33	27	21	16	12	6	1	−5	−11	−15	−20	−26	−31	−35
10	28	21	16	9	4	−2	−9	−15	−21	−27	−33	−38	−46	−52	−58
15	22	16	11	1	−5	−11	−18	−25	−36	−40	−45	−51	−58	−65	−70
20	18	12	3	−4	−10	−17	−25	−32	−39	−46	−53	−60	−67	−76	−81
25	16	7	0	−7	−15	−22	−29	−37	−44	−52	−59	−67	−74	−83	−89
30	13	5	−2	−11	−18	−26	−33	−41	−48	−56	−63	−70	−79	−87	−94
35	11	3	−4	−13	−20	−27	−35	−43	−49	−60	−67	−72	−82	−90	−98
*40	10	1	−6	−15	−21	−29	−37	−45	−53	−62	−69	−76	−85	−94	−101

Wind speed (mph) [row label, left axis]

Little danger / Danger / Great danger [zones marked within table]

*Convective heat loss at wind speeds above 40 mph have little additional effect on body cooling.
**°C = 0.556 (°F − 32).
From McArdle, Katch and Katch (1986), with permission. Exercise Physiology: Energy, Nutrition and Human Performance, Lea and Febiger, Philadelphia.

more. Table 7.16 shows the wind chill index at various temperatures and wind speeds. It can be seen that a temperature of 10°F is equivalent to −25°F when the wind is blowing at 20 m.p.h. This speed can easily be achieved on a blustery winter's day by running at 8 m.p.h. into a 12 m.p.h. headwind. In addition, when more body surface is exposed heat total loss is greater. Thirty to forty percent of the loss of body heat occurs through the head, so wearing a hat in a cold windy environment is essential.

Evaporation provides the most effective means of heat loss from the body. For each litre of water lost by evaporation of sweat and moisture from the respiratory passages, 580 kcal is lost from the body (McArdle, Katch and Katch, 1986). The total amount of sweat lost will be determined largely by the amount of skin exposed, the air temperature and humidity, and the speed of air currents surrounding the body. Water loss through sweating can be as much as 2 litres per hour. This must be compensated for by fluid intake, but during vigorous exercise only about 800 ml of fluid can be emptied by the stomach (McArdle, Katch and Katch, 1986), so the payback is never complete. In addition, various factors can affect the ability of the body to take fluids up. A 10% glucose solution, for example, will reduce the rate of fluid uptake by 40%, so the use of glucose drinks to replace fluid alone is not logical. When glucose loss rather than fluid loss is the concern, these drinks may be of use, but it should be noted that it can take as much as 30 minutes for the ingested glucose to reach the working muscle. The use of complex (polymerized) sugars may be of greater value in this respect.

> **Keypoint**
>
> The body can lose as much as 2 litres of water per hour through sweating. Ingestion rates dictate than only 800 ml of water can be emptied from the stomach per hour, so fluid loss can easily outweigh fluid gain.

Heat illness

Heat illness occurs in the form of rash, collapse, cramp, exhaustion and finally, heat stroke (Table 7.17). *Heat rash* (prickly heat or miliaria) presents as a red raised skin rash accompanied by a tingling or itching sensation. It usually occurs in areas of the skin where sweat builds up rather than it 'wicking' away through evaporation. The sweat glands may become blocked, preventing normal free vapour movement. A variety of popular remedies are reputed to be of benefit including daily ingestion of vitamin C, rubbing lemon juice on the skin after showering and calamine lotion to reduce the itch.

Heat collapse (syncope) is sudden fatigue or fainting when overheating. This is normally caused by prolonged standing or exercising in the heat when not accustomed to doing so.

Table 7.17 Heat illness

Illness	Signs and symptoms	Treatment
Rash (prickly heat)	Red raised skin rash accompanied by tingling when sweating	Prevent sweat build up by regular towelling down
Collapse (syncope)	Sudden fatigue or fainting when overheating	Lie athlete down in cool room and give fluids
Cramps	Most common in calf and abdomen	Electrolyte replacement drinks
Exhaustion	Sweating, pale, dizzy, hyperventilate, rapid pulse	Water, initially by mouth but if collapsed, intravenously
Heat stroke	Collapse, flushed hot skin, reduced sweating, core temperature of 40°C or higher. *Life-threatening*	Lower body temperature by removing clothing and sponging athlete down with tepid water. *Do not immerse in iced water as this will constrict blood vessels in the skin and reduce heat loss.* Hospitalize

The athlete should lie down in a cool room and fluids should be given.

Heat cramps occur after exercise in the particular muscles worked, probably due to electrolyte imbalance. The most common areas are the calf and abdomen. Adding salt to meals in the periods before heat exposure is a useful precaution, but taking salt once cramp has occurred is not effective. Furthermore, ingestion of large amounts of salt is not well tolerated unless accompanied by large amounts of water which in turn results in a bloated feeling. The cramp itself will usually respond to stretching and heat massage to release it.

In those not acclimatized to hot weather, *heat exhaustion* can occur. This is thought to occur by ineffective adjustment of the circulation, combined with excessive fluid loss, which in turn results in lowered blood volume (McArdle, Katch and Katch, 1986). Blood pooling results, usually in the periphery, leading to a reduction in cardiac output. Symptoms include a weak rapid pulse, low blood pressure, headache, dizziness and general malaise. Athletes show sudden strength loss and may feel dizzy. They will recover on stopping exercise and removal to a cool environment. Fluids should be given.

Heat-stroke is a much more serious condition, requiring medical attention. It is a failure of the thermoregulatory system of the body, causing sweating to cease, and the skin to become dry and hot. The body temperature rises to dangerous levels, and death can result if the condition progresses. Body core temperature must be lowered, and treatment includes sponging down with tepid water and hospitalization. Whole body immersion in iced water should be avoided

as this may constrict blood vessels in the skin and reduce heat loss. The athlete should be hospitalized immediately.

Cold illness

In water, athletes with greater body fat percentages perform well as they have additional insulation, as witnessed by the endomorphic tendencies of most cross-Channel swimmers. However, most humans do not acclimatize well to cold, and the response is usually one of avoidance, by producing a warmer microclimate with clothing and local environmental changes. Heat loss can be reduced by shunting blood from the periphery (shell) to the central area (core) of the body. However, prolonged peripheral vasoconstriction during cold causes circulatory deprivation to the exposed parts and can cause severe tissue damage through ischaemic cold injury. Early sensations include numbness, tingling and burning sensations in the fingers, toes, nose and ear lobes. Neuromuscular function deteriorates, so that motor performance is impaired, as witnessed by a loss of finger strength and dexterity.

Frost-bite

Frost-bite may occur when ice crystals form in the peripheral tissues, giving ulceration. First degree frost-bite affects the superficial layer of the skin, while second degree frost-bite involves the formation of skin blisters filled with exudate. Third degree frost-bite results when the deeper areas are frozen, including the subcutaneous tissues and muscle. Rapid freezing causes ice crystals to form within the cells, resulting in cellular damage and, ultimately, necrosis. Slow freezing occurs to the tissue fluids, but solutes are not involved in the freezing process. This increases the osmotic pressure of the extracellular fluid, and pulls liquid out from the cells causing exudate formation (Astrand and Rodahl, 1986).

> **Keypoint**
>
> Frost-bite occurs when ice crystals form in the tissues, giving skin ulceration. If severe, the subcutaneous tissue and muscle may also be affected.

If first and second degree damage has occurred, gentle re-warming is required, with any blisters being left untouched. The athlete should be sheltered, any restricting clothing should be loosened, and warm drinks given. Activity to increase metabolic heating is useful. Third degree frost-bite requires urgent hospitalization.

In addition to general cold injury, damage to the eyes may occur in events such as cross-country skiing and downhill skiing, with the combination of severe cold and wind. The blinking reflex may be impaired, reducing the nourishment to the cornea, and causing transitory damage (Kolstad and Opsahl, 1979).

Hypothermia

Hypothermia occurs when the body core temperature drops below 35°C (Astrand and Rodahl, 1986), the temperature being measured rectally. Initial exposure to cold causes shivering, an autonomic response to generate heat through muscular activity. As the temperature drops further, the athlete may become disorientated and may hallucinate. Further temperature reduction can cause loss of consciousness, with weak pulse and respiration. Reflexes are lost, pupil dilation occurs, and cardiac arrhythmias can occur.

Management in the field is by gradual body re-warming. Rapid re-heating can cause the core temperature to fall lower, due to the return of cold venous blood from the extremities to the core.

Clothing and temperature regulation

As the body temperature rises with exercise, sweating should be aided by wearing loose clothing which encourages air circulation around the body, and by clothing which allows the passage of moisture through it and away from the body (wicking). In addition, dark clothing radiates and absorbs heat well, whereas light clothing reflects heat.

In a cold climate, the athlete should wear fibrous materials and a number of layers of clothing to try to trap air as an insulation within the material of the garment. A hat should be worn to reduce heat loss from the head. As clothing becomes wet, it can lose as much as 90% of its insulating properties, because water conducts heat much more effectively than air. Cold weather clothing should ideally permit the passage of water vapour, but not air.

Sports clothing can be effectively combined in three layers. The inner layer consists usually of shorts and a vest made of a fibre which is water permeable but non-absorbent. The seams of the inner layer must be positioned so that no abrasion is caused between the clothing and the athlete's skin.

The intermediate layer offers greater heat insulation properties, and is usually fibrous (wool or cotton) or fleecy. Modern materials have removed the need for bulk to provide insulating properties, and the intermediate layer should not restrict movement. The outer or 'shell' layer is waterproof, but should preferably still allow the passage of moisture from the body. This layer should also be strong enough to resist ripping, and be conveniently removed. Zips or other fasteners around the ankles facilitate the removal of the shell garment without the need to remove sports shoes.

Altitude

At high altitudes, the air density reduces with height. At a height of 5500 metres the air pressure is about half that at sea level, and this gives a corresponding reduction in partial pressure of oxygen (PO_2). The amount of oxygen carried by the blood reduces, and exercise performance is impaired.

The body's immediate response to the thinner air at altitude is an increase in respiratory drive, giving hyperventilation and an increase in blood flow, witnessed by an increased cardiac output (especially heart rate) by as much as 50% above resting sea-level values.

During the first few days of training at altitude, *acute mountain sickness* (AMS) may occur at altitudes above 3000 metres. The most common symptom is headache, sometimes accompanied by dizziness, nausea and (rarely) vomiting. The condition is exacerbated by intense exercise on the first day at altitude. Headache is thought to be the result of an alteration in cerebral haemodynamics brought on by hyperventilation (Jansen, 1999). Appetite can become suppressed, and a diet low in salt but high in carbohydrate is best tolerated. The cool dry air of mountainous regions can give mild dehydration resulting in soreness and drying of the mouth, lips and throat.

In rare (1–2%) instances, AMS may progress to *high altitude pulmonary oedema* (HAPE) or *high altitude cerebral oedema* (HACE) at altitudes above 3000 metres (McArdle, Katch and Katch, 2001). Fluid accumulates in the brain and lungs giving a wheeze and rasp, a symptom known as 'rales'. An enlarged cerebral fluid volume distorts the brain, resulting in coma and eventually death. Practitioners should become suspicious of these conditions when the symptoms of AMS have not subsided after 1 day of rest. Treatment includes administering supplemental oxygen and using the drug nifedipine, a calcium channel blocker, normally used in the treatment of angina.

Acclimatization periods to high altitudes are largely dependent on the altitude itself. Improvements may be seen within a few days, but total acclimatization may take between 4 and 6 weeks. Two weeks is normally sufficient for altitudes up to 2300 metres, with an additional week added for every 610 metres increase (McArdle, Katch and Katch, 1986).

Keypoint

Acclimatization to high altitude normally takes 2 weeks for heights up to 2300 metres and an extra week for every 610 metres after that.

Cryotherapy

Cold or ice is probably the most convenient modality available for the treatment of sports injuries. Ice is a low-cost and effective treatment, but its ready availability can lead to misuse, with the potential for injury.

Effects

Cryotherapy may be used both in the immediate treatment of sports injuries, and in later rehabilitation. During immediate treatment, the aim is to limit the body's response to injury, in particular hypoxic tissue damage, swelling, pain and muscle spasm. Later, during the rehabilitation phase, the aims change. Then the goal is to restore function, and at that stage, the effects of other techniques such as exercise and manual therapy can be augmented by ice application.

Ice is often used in combination with rest, compression and elevation (RICE) as an effective initial treatment of sports injuries. Ice alone has been shown to be effective in the treatment of ankle injuries (Hocutt et al., 1983), but is usually more effective when used to treat soft tissue injuries in conjunction with compression (Santiesteban, 1990). As shown in Fig. 7.10, a combination of mild pressure and cooling (10 mmHg and 15–25°C) has been shown to produce significant reductions in artificially induced inflammation (Sloan, Giddings and Hain, 1988). The main effects of cryotherapy are outlined in Table 7.18.

During immediate treatment, the most important effect is often claimed to be a reduction in blood flow through the local capillary network. However, blood clotting will usually seal these damaged vessels within 3–5 minutes of injury (Knight, 1989), about the same time as it takes to get an athlete off the sports field and into the treatment room. Consequently, when an athlete is first seen, local bleeding may have stopped. For this reason, decreased tissue metabolism is now thought to be a more important effect of cryotherapy during the immediate treatment of sports

injuries (Knight, 1989; McLean, 1989). After injury, further tissue damage occurs through local hypoxia secondary to a disruption in blood flow. A reduction in metabolic rate and oxygen requirement is seen with ice treatment (Abramson et al., 1957), and this gives the body cells a better chance to survive for the period they are without oxygen, almost in a state of 'temporary hibernation' (Knight, 1989).

> **Keypoint**
>
> One of the main effects of cold/ice application is a 'temporary hibernation' of the tissues brought on through a reduction in metabolic rate and oxygen requirement.

Circulatory changes occur during ice application, and are the subject of some debate. Blood flow has been shown to decrease during cold application and remain reduced for up to 45 minutes after treatment (Knight, Bryant and Halvorsen, 1981). Cold applications produce an easily observed reactive hyperaemia of the skin, but deeper vasodilatation may not occur during therapeutic cooling (Knight, 1989). Certainly the cyclical skin changes (the hunting response), originally described by Lewis (1930), have been shown to occur only in fingers which have been cooled to 20°C prior to ice water immersion (Knight et al., 1980).

The immediate response to ice application is a short-lived (5–60 seconds) dull pain, which is more intense with some individuals than others. Following this, pain reduction occurs through a reduction in nerve conductivity (Tepperman and Devlin, 1983), and stimulation of pain receptors (Halvorson, 1990). With immersion in iced water a second pain sensation is sometimes felt, followed by after-pain when the body part is removed from the ice bath. The intensity of pain that an athlete feels is related to both the temperature imposed on the tissues and the rate of temperature change or 'thermal gradient' (Wolf and Hardy, 1941; Croze and Duclaux, 1978). A slow application of ice immersion will normally abolish cold-induced pain (Knight, 1995).

Local cooling depresses muscle spindle activity (Mense, 1978; Halvorson, 1990), and so muscle spasm initiated through gamma nerve stimulation can be reduced. Inflammation is thought to be reduced by ice application (Schmidt et al., 1979), and joint viscosity has been shown to increase, and with it joint stiffness (Knight, 1989).

Cryotherapy techniques

Common cold applications include the use of flaked ice in towelling or plastic bags, cold compression, ice massage, cold sprays, ice baths, cryogel or chemical packs, and cold gas modalities.

The choice between the various methods is often dependent on cost and convenience. Ice soaks are better for uneven and small body parts, such as the hand and foot.

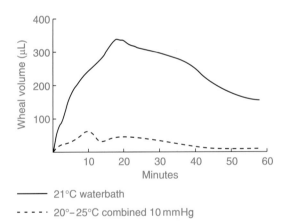

— 21°C waterbath

- - - - 20°–25°C combined 10 mmHg

Figure 7.10   Combined pressure and cooling to reduce swelling. From Sloan, J.P., Giddings, P. and Hain, R. (1988) Effects of cold and compression on edema. *Physician and Sportsmedicine*, **16**, 116–120, The McGraw-Hill Companies, with permission, and Reid (1992).

Table 7.18   Physiological changes within cooled tissue

Decreased metabolism
Decreased circulation
Transient increase followed by decreased pain
Decreased muscle spasm
Decreased inflammation
Increased stiffness

From Knight (1989) with permission.

With this technique some ice should be left floating on the surface of the water throughout the treatment to ensure that a low enough temperature is maintained.

Ice packs are better for larger tissue areas such as the knee, hip and shoulder. Flaked ice in a plastic bag will give a lower tissue temperature than ice in a towelling bag, with the towelling providing insulation. Although mild frost-bite is unusual (Knight, 1989), the body part should be regularly inspected. Wet towelling provides less insulation, but will still not give tissue temperatures as low as ice within a plastic bag. Knight (1989) claimed that two layers of dry wrap placed below an ice pack resulted in ankle temperatures which were 16°C higher after a 30-minute application than when ice was applied directly to the skin. Wetting the wraps gave temperatures which were 5.7°C higher than direct application. These temperature differences may, however, be of use where a patient demonstrates ice sensitivity.

Cryogel bags usually give a lower temperature than flaked ice, depending on the freezer setting used. Placing this type of pack directly on the skin should be avoided, as mild frost-bite has been repeatedly observed (Knight, 1989).

> **Keypoint**
>
> Cryogel bags can give a lower skin temperature than melting flaked ice. Do not place the bag directly on the athlete's skin as blistering and skin damage may occur. Wrap the bag in a wet cloth or sheath.

Chemical packs have the advantage of convenience, and are easily carried by athletes themselves. However, they rarely produce temperatures which are low enough, and the temperature reduction which does occur is usually too short-lived. Some packs also have the potential for chemical burns if punctured.

Similarly, temperature changes produced by cold sprays are slight and short-term. The place of cold sprays is really as a stimulant for use with spray stretch techniques. Here, the vapocoolant spray (usually fluromethane) is applied as a jet, either to overcome guarding muscle spasm or to treat irritable trigger points (Travell and Simons, 1983).

Ice or cold can be combined with compression to good effect. Several methods exist, including the use of elasticated bandage around a layer of ice, or a similar ice layer below a compression (IPC) boot. Machines which produce continuous cold air, or iced water and compression are also available.

Ice massage is particularly useful for pain relief of smaller tissue areas. Massage is carried out until cold anaesthesia ensues. Usual sensations are of cold, then burning, deep aching and finally numbness (Halvorson, 1990). Once numbness has occurred, no additional skin sensation follows with more prolonged treatment, but underlying tissue temperature will continue to fall.

During the immediate treatment of sports injuries ice should preferably be applied within 5–10 minutes of injury, but certainly as soon as possible, and kept on for 20–30 minutes. Re-application is made every 2 hours, it taking 2–4 hours for the ankle, knee, forearm and thigh to return to pre-application temperature (Knight, 1989). Ice may have no effect on joint swelling once intra-articular effusion has formed (McLean, 1989).

> **Keypoint**
>
> After a sports injury, apply ice for 20 minutes every 2 hours throughout the waking day.

Cryostretch and cryokinetics are additional rehabilitation procedures involving the use of ice (Knight, 1995). Cryostretch is the combination of cold application to relieve pain (Kowal, 1983) and reduce muscle spasm, and stretching to increase mobility. Ice is applied until cold anaesthesia is present, and stretching is carried out for as long as numbness lasts. Cryokinetics is the combination of cold therapy with active exercise. Cold is used to reduce pain and allow active exercise to be performed earlier than would otherwise be possible. The benefits of the therapy are from the exercise itself rather than the ice application.

Dangers of ice application

The two main dangers with ice application are frost-bite and nerve palsy. Frost-bite occurs when local tissues freeze. Direct cellular damage occurs due to ice crystal formation and indirect damage occurs due to dehydration as water moves out of the cells to form extracellular crystals. In addition, vascular damage may also occur during the thawing process due to platelet aggregation and vessel occlusion. The intensity of the tissue response can also vary from minor erythema and swelling (frost-nip), blister formation (second degree or superficial frost-bite), damage to subcutaneous tissues (third degree or full thickness frost-bite) and tissue damage so severe that the body part is lost (fourth degree or deep frost-bite). Ebholm et al. (1957) reported mild frost-bite in subjects following ice water immersion of the forearm, and Proulx (1976) reported frost-bite in the first metatarsal following continuous ice pack application. Frost-bite is far more common when cold gel packs are used (Stevens and D'Angelo, 1978). These will often be cooled far below 0°C, and so should not be applied for longer than 30 minutes, and should not be used in conjunction with compression. Gel packs should be wrapped in a damp cloth to reduce the likelihood of injury (Knight, 1995).

Nerve palsy has been reported by several authors, at the fibular head, elbow and shoulder (Drez, Faust and Evans, 1981; Collins, Storey and Peterson, 1986; Green, Zachazewski and Jordan, 1989; Malone et al., 1992). Total motor and sensory loss can occur when tissue temperatures reduce to between 0 and 5°C. Nerve palsy is more common when compression is used with ice, and when chemical ice packs are used rather than crushed ice packs. Most incidences recover quickly providing no necrosis has occurred, with sensory function returning before motor function (Knight, 1995).

References

Abramson, D.L., Kahn, A., Tuck, S., Turman, G.A., Rejal, H. and Fleisher, C.J. (1957) Relationship between a range of tissue temperature and local oxygen consumption in the resting forearm. *Laboratory Clinical Medicine*, **59**, 789–793

Astrand, P-O. and Rodahl, K. (1986) *Textbook of Work Physiology*, 3rd edn, McGraw-Hill, Maidenhead

Benda, C. (1989) Outwitting muscle cramps – is it possible? *Physician and Sports Medicine*, **17**, (9) 173–178

Blau, J.N. (1989) Time to let the patient speak. *British Medical Journal*, **298**, 39

Buxton, N. and Firth, J. (1999) Head and neck injury. In *Sports Medicine Handbook* (eds R. Hackney and A. Wallace), BMJ Publishing, London

Cantu, R.C. (1998) Second impact syndrome. *Clinics in Sports Medicine*, **17**, 37–44

Collins, K., Storey, M. and Peterson, K. (1986) Peroneal nerve palsy after cryotherapy. *Physician and Sports Medicine*, **14**, 105–108

Corsellis, J.A.N. (1974) Brain damage in sport. *Lancet*, **i**, 401–402

Crampton, C.W. (1908) Physiological age: a fundamental principle. *American Physical Education Review*, **13**, 141–154

Croze, S. and Duclaux, R. (1978) Thermal pain in humans: influence of the rate of stimulation. *Brain Research*, **157**, 418–421

Drez, D., Faust, D.C. and Evans, I.P. (1981) Cryotherapy and nerve palsy. *American Journal of Sports Medicine*, **9**, 256–257

Ebholm, O.G., Fox, R.H., Lewis, H.E. and MacPherson, H.E. (1957) Cold injury. *Journal of Physiology*, **139**, 14–15

First Aid Manual (1995) 6th edn, Dorling Kindersley, London

First Aid Manual (2002) 8th edn, Dorling Kindersley, London

Fowler, J.A. (1981) First aid in sport. In *Sports Fitness and Sports Injuries* (ed. T. Reilly), Faber and Faber, London, pp. 253–258

Garrick, J.G. and Webb, D.R. (1990) *Sports Injuries: Diagnosis and Management*, W.B. Saunders, Philadelphia

Green, G.A., Zachazewski, J.E. and Jordan, S.E. (1989) Peroneal nerve palsy induced by cryotherapy. *Physician and Sports Medicine*, **17**, 63–70

Halvorson, G.A. (1990) Therapeutic heat and cold for athletic injuries. *Physician and Sports Medicine*, **18**, (5) 65–67

Harries, M. (1994) Asthma. In *Oxford Textbook of Sports Medicine* (eds M. Harries, C. Williams, W.D. Stanish and L. Micheli), Oxford Medical Publications, Oxford

Hocutt, J.E., Jaffe, R., Rylander, C.R. and Bebbe, J.K. (1983) Cryotherapy in ankle sprains. *American Journal of Sports Medicine*, **10**, 316–319

Jackson, D.W., Jarrett, H., Bailey, D., Kausek, J., Swanson, J. and Powell, J.W. (1978) Injury prediction in the young athlete: a preliminary report. *American Journal of Sports Medicine*, **6**, 6–14

Jansen, G.F. (1999) Cerebral vasomotor reactivity at high altitude in humans. *Journal of Applied Physiology*, **86**, 681

Jorgensen, U. (1989) Free substitution in soccer. *Nitz*, **3**, 155–158

Kerr, G. and Minden, H. (1988) Psychological factors related to the occurrence of athletic injuries. *Journal of Sports Psychology*, **10**, 167–173

Kesson, M. and Atkins, E. (1998) *Orthopaedic Medicine: A Practical Approach*, Butterworth-Heinemann, Oxford

Knight, K.L. (1989) Cryotherapy in sports injury management. In *International Perspectives in Physical Therapy*, 4 (ed. V. Grisogono), pp. 163–185

Knight, K.L. (1995) *Cryotherapy in Sport Injury Management*, Human Kinetics, Champaign, Illinois

Knight, K.L., Bryant, K.S. and Halvorsen, J. (1981) Circulatory changes in the forearm in 1, 5, 10 and 15°C water (Abs). *International Journal of Sports Medicine*, **4**, 281

Knight, K.L., Aquino, J., Johannes, S.M. and Urban, C.D. (1980) A reexamination of Lewis' cold induced vasodilation in the finger and the ankle. *Athletic Training*, **15**, 24–27

Kolstad, A. and Opsahl, R. (1979) Cold injury to the corneal epithelium: a case of blurred vision in cross-country skiers. *Acta Ophthalmology*, **48**, 789

Kowal, M.A. (1983) Review of the physiological effects of cryotherapy. *Journal of Orthopaedic and Sports Physical Therapy*, **5**, 66–73

Lewis, T.S. (1930) Observations upon the reactions of the vessels of the human skin to cold. *Heart*, **15**, 177–208

McArdle, W.D., Katch, F.I. and Katch, V.L. (1986) *Exercise Physiology: Energy, Nutrition, and Human Performance*, Lea and Febiger, Philadelphia

McArdle, W.D., Katch, F.I. and Katch, V.L. (2001) *Exercise Physiology*, 5th edn, Lippincott, Williams and Wilkins, New York

McKenzie, R.A. (1981) *The Lumbar Spine*, Spinal Publications, New Zealand

McLatchie, G.R. (1993) Risks and injuries in combat sports. In *The Soft Tissues: Trauma and Sports Injuries* (eds G.R. McLatchie and C.M.E. Lennnox), Butterworth-Heinemann, Oxford

McLatchie, G.R., Brooks, N. and Galbraith, S. (1987) Clinical neurological examination, neuropsychology, electroencephalography and computed tomographic head scanning in active amateur boxers. *Journal of Neurology, Neurosurgery and Psychiatry*, **50**, 96–99

McLatchie, G.R., Davis, J.E. and Caulley, H. (1980). Injuries in karate. *Journal of Trauma*, **20**, 56–58

McLean, D.A. (1989) The use of cold and superficial heat in the treatment of soft tissue injuries. *British Journal of Sports Medicine*, **23**, (1) 53–54

Magee, D.J. (2002) *Orthopedic Physical Assessment*, 4th edn, W.B. Saunders, Philadelphia

Malina, R.M. and Beunen, G. (1996) Matching of opponents in youth sports. In *The Child and Adolescent Athlete, Encyclopaedia of Sports Medicine* (IV) (ed. O. Bar-Or), Blackwell Scientific, Oxford

Malone, T., Englehardt, D.L., Kirkpatrick, J.S. and Bassett, F.H. (1992) Nerve injury in athletes caused by cryotherapy. *Journal of Athletic Training*, **27**, 235–237

Mense, S. (1978) Effects of temperature on the discharges of muscle spindles and tendon organs. *Pflugers Archives*, **374**, 159–166

Meyer, R.D. and Daniel, W.W. (1985) The biomechanics of helmets and helmet removal. *Journal of Trauma*, **25**, 329–332

Peterson, L. and Renstrom, P. (1986) *Sports Injuries*, Martin Dunitz, London

Proulx, R.P. (1976) Southern California frostbite. *Journal of American College of Emergency Physicians*, **5**, 618

Puffer, J.C. and Zachazewski, J.E. (1988) Management of overuse injuries. *American Family Physician*, **38**, (3) 225–232

Reid, D.C. (1992) *Sports Injury Assessment and Rehabilitation*, Churchill Livingstone, London

Roy, M.A., Bernard, D., Roy, B. and Marcotte, G. (1989) Body checking in Pee Wee hockey. *Physician and Sports Medicine*, **17**, (3) 119–126

Sanderson, F.H. (1981) The psychology of the injury-prone athlete. In *Sports Fitness and Sports Injuries* (ed. T. Reilly), Faber and Faber, London

Santiesteban, A.J. (1990) Physical agents and musculoskeletal pain. In *Orthopaedic and Sports Physical Therapy*, 2nd edn (ed. J.A. Gould), C.V. Mosby, St Louis

Schmidt, K.L., Ott, V.R., Rocher, G. and Schaller, H. (1979) Heat cold and inflammation (a review). *Zeitschrift fur Rheumatologie*, **38**, 391–404

Sloan, J.P., Giddings, P. and Hain, R. (1988) Effects of cold and compression on edema. *Physician and Sports Medicine*, **16**, 116

Sortland, U., Tysvaer, A.T. and Storli, O.V. (1989) Association football injuries to the brain: a neurological and encephalographic study of former football players. *Neuroradiology*, **31**, 44

Sparrow, M.J. and Bird, E.L. (1978) Precordial catch: a benign syndrome of chest pain in young persons. *New Zealand Medical Journal*, **88**, 325

Sperryn, P.N. (1985) *Sport and Medicine*, Butterworth-Heinemann, Oxford

Stevens, D.M. and D'Angelo, J.V. (1978) Frostbite due to improper use of frozen gel packs. *New England Journal of Medicine*, **299**, 1415

Taimela, S., Kujala, U.M. and Osterman, K. (1990) Intrinsic risk factors and athletic injuries. *Sports Medicine*, **9**, (4) 205–215

Tator, C.H. and Edmonds, V. (1984) National survey of spinal injuries in hockey players. *Canadian Medical Association Journal*, **130**, 875–880

Teasdale, G. and Jennett, B. (1974) Assessment of coma and impaired consciousness. *Lancet*, **ii**, 81–84

Tepperman, P.S. and Devlin, M. (1983) Therapeutic heat and cold. *Postgraduate Medicine*, **73**, 69

Torg, J.S., Truex, R. and Quedenfield, T.G. (1979) The national football head and neck injury registry. *Journal of the American Medical Association*, **241**, 1477–1479

Travell, J.G. and Simons, D.G. (1983) *Myofascial Pain and Dysfunction: The Trigger Point Manual*, Williams and Wilkins, Baltimore

Vinger, P.F. (1981) Sports eye injuries: a preventable disease. *American Academy of Ophthalmology*, **88**, (2) 108–113

Walkden, L. (1981) Immediate post-injury considerations in games. In *Sports Fitness and Sports Injuries* (ed. T. Reilly), Faber and Faber, London, pp. 247–252

Wolf, S. and Hardy, J.D. (1941) Studies on pain: observations on pain due to local cooling and factors involved in the 'Cold pressor' effect. *Journal of Clinical Investigation*, **20**, 521–533

Chapter **8**

Lower limb motion during walking, running and jumping

Most sporting activities involve the movement of the human body over distance. An understanding of the biomechanical factors which affect gait is therefore fundamental to the prevention and management of sports injuries. Abnormal forces placed on the body through alterations in normal running or walking can cause injury. In addition, rehabilitation of lower limb injuries, if it is to be successful, must involve the restoration of correct gait. Failure to do so may impair performance and leave the athlete open to further problems.

Injuries to the lower limb, especially those to the ankle and knee, tend to occur when weight bearing. Typically this is a twist on the fixed foot, or when landing from a jump. Brief analysis of this action will again help to understand injury causality, and to better structure rehabilitation programmes.

CLOSED AND OPEN MOTION

Motion at a joint is often described anatomically as though it occurred in isolation, yet functionally, isolated joint movements rarely occur. The limbs or trunk may be considered as moveable chains, the links of which are the joints themselves. Movement of one of the joints causes an effect on the other links in the chain, and so other joints respond.

Open chain motion occurs when the proximal bone segment in a limb is fixed but the distal segment remains free. Closed chain motion is the reverse. Both the proximal and distal bone segments are fixed, and movement occurs between the two. When we evaluate a joint within a limb in open chain motion, the movement of the bony segment occurs distal to the joint being studied. Movement within a closed chain will occur both proximally and distally to the joint being studied.

Muscle function is also different in open and closed chain motion. Take, as an example, dorsiflexion of the foot. Open chain dorsiflexion, for example sitting in a chair and pulling the foot upwards, results from concentric action of the anterior tibial muscles. Closed chain dorsiflexion, such as occurs in walking as the bodyweight moves forward over the foot, involves eccentric action of the calf muscles.

> **Keypoint**
>
> *Open chain motion* occurs when the proximal bone segment in a limb is fixed but the distal segment remains free. *Closed chain motion* occurs when both the proximal and distal bone segments are fixed, and movement occurs between the two.

JOINT MOVEMENTS

Hip joint

The hip joint is the articulation between the head of the femur and the acetabulum. In standing, the femoral head is not completely covered by the acetabulum. This occurs in a position which mimics a quadruped stance, hip flexion to 90°, abduction to 5°, and lateral rotation to 10°. Hip flexion is free, being limited by soft tissue contact, but extension is usually limited to about 20–30°, depending on the amount of anterior pelvic tilt which occurs. Common values for abduction and adduction are 45° each, given a total range of rotation of 90°.

In single leg standing, vertical compression forces of 1.8–3.0 times bodyweight have been recorded at the hip, while in the stance phase of walking, forces between 3.3 and 5.5 times bodyweight have been measured. In running, the forces are higher still. Although the major force on the hip is vertical, anteroposterior forces (AP or 'shearing') are still present. At heel-strike and toe off, the AP forces acting on the hip actually exceed bodyweight (Palastanga, Field and Soames, 1998).

> **Keypoint**
>
> In running, *compression* forces on the hip joint are as much as three times total bodyweight (210 kg in a 70 kg athlete). *Shearing* forces may exceed total bodyweight.

The hip passes through one flexion/extension movement during the running cycle. The limit of flexion occurs within the middle of the swing phase, and the limit of extension just before the end of the stance phase.

Knee joint

The knee joint articulation is between the condyles of the femur and tibia. The posterior surface of the patella and the patellar surface of the femur is usually considered in the knee complex. The neutral position of the knee is full extension. From this position, approximately 140° of flexion is possible in the average subject. In full extension, no transverse plane motion is possible, but as the knee flexes rotation can occur.

During the last 15° of extension, the femur medially rotates on a fixed tibia, or if the tibia is free it will laterally rotate to bring the bones into close pack formation and lock the knee (the *screw home mechanism*). Flexion progresses as a combination of rolling and gliding movements of the femoral condyles. At the beginning of flexion, rolling occurs alone, and as flexion increases the amount of gliding increases, until at the end of range, gliding is the only movement present.

> **Definition**
>
> The *screw home mechanism* is the method by which the knee locks passively into extension. When the foot is on the floor (tibia fixed) the femur medially rotates tightening the knee ligaments and securing the joint.

The medial condyle only rolls for the first 10–15° of flexion, while the lateral condyle continues until 20° flexion, and at the same time the two menisci deform. This range of motion is the amount required during normal gait, and means that the knee is more stable (no gliding movement) during this functional range. Beyond 20° flexion, the knee becomes looser as the part of the femoral condyles now involved in the articulation is smaller. As a result the knee ligaments relax, and a wider range of rotation is available.

During walking, forces between two and four times bodyweight are taken by the knee. Peak forces correspond to hamstring, quadriceps and gastrocnemius contraction, and occur at heel strike and during propulsion. In jumping, forces may approach 24 times bodyweight on the knee (tibiofemoral) joint and 20 times bodyweight on the patellofemoral joint (Palastanga, Field and Soames, 1998). When walking down stairs, the intense eccentric activity in the quadriceps results in joint forces on the patellofemoral joint which are up to six times greater than those seen when walking on a flat surface.

The knee flexes and extends twice during running. At initial contact the knee is extended, and it flexes during midstance to absorb shock. As toe-off is reached, the knee extends again to provide propulsion and flexes as part of the swing phase.

> **Keypoint**
>
> Forces on the knee joint in *walking* are 2–4 times bodyweight. In *jumping*, forces may approach 24 times bodyweight on the knee joint, and 20 times bodyweight on the patellofemoral (PF) joint.

Ankle joint

The ankle or talocrural joint consists of the trochlear surface of the talus and the distal ends of the tibia and fibula. The talar trochlea is wider anteriorly, and so plantarflexion is more free than dorsiflexion, average values being 30–50° and 20–30°, respectively. Marked variations occur both between individuals and following injury, and normal foot function can be achieved with as little as 20° of plantarflexion and 10° of dorsiflexion (McPoil and Brocato, 1990).

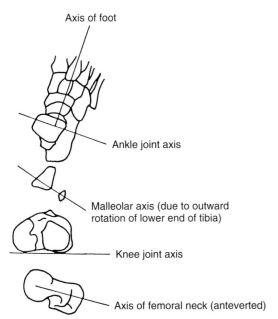

Figure 8.1   Relationship between the ankle, knee and hip joint axes. From Palastanga, Field and Soames (1998) with permission.

The ankle is essentially a hinge, externally rotated to between 20 and 25° with the malleoli (Fig. 8.1). In the neutral position, with the foot perpendicular to the lower leg, there is very little frontal or transverse plane motion. With dorsiflexion, abduction of the foot is possible, and during plantarflexion, adduction can occur. In dorsiflexion the broad anterior part of the talus is forced into the narrower mortice between the tibia and fibula. The interosseous and transverse tibiofibular ligaments are stressed, as the bones part slightly, and the joint moves into close pack position.

Plantarflexion sees the narrow posterior part of the trochlear surface of the talus moving into the broader tibiofibular mortice. Recoil of the above ligaments causes the malleoli to approximate and maintain contact with the talus.

During running, the ankle is dorsiflexed at heel strike, and plantarflexes to bring the forefoot to the ground. Plantarflexion occurs again at push-off, and the foot dorsiflexes throughout the swing phase. As the speed of gait increases, the total range of motion at the ankle decreases, the range reducing by 10% when changing from a cadence of 40 strides/min to one of 60 strides/min. Joint forces at the ankle (Palastanga, Field and Soames, 1998) at heel strike are three times bodyweight for compression and 80% bodyweight for AP shear. At heel lift, muscle force creating the plantarflexion force to lift the body increase compression at the ankle to five times bodyweight (Fig. 8.2). Patients with ankle pain modify their gait pattern to reduce these forces, but in so doing stress other areas of the kinetic chain.

Subtalar joint

The subtalar joint (STJ) lies between the concave undersurface of the talus and the convex posterior portion of the upper

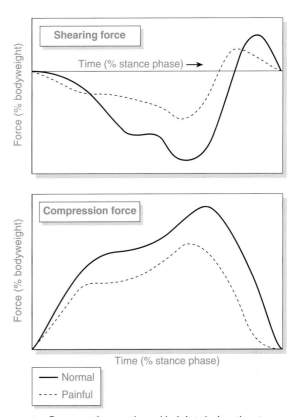

Figure 8.2   Forces acting on the ankle joint during the stance phase of walking. Adapted from Stauffer, R.N., Chao, E.Y.S. and Brewster, R.C. (1977) Force and motion analysis of the normal diseased, and prosthetic ankle joint. *Clinical Orthopaedics and Related Research*, **127**, 189–196.

surface of the calcaneum. The STJ is said to be in neutral position when the posterior aspect of the heel lies vertical to the supporting surface of the foot, and parallel to the lower one-third of the leg (Subotnick, 1989).

Determining neutral position of the STJ

Neutral position of the STJ is its optimal alignment and this is used as a starting point or *baseline* to determine foot and leg alignment faults. Neutral STJ position may be obtained in standing, supine lying and prone lying. In standing, the practitioner palpates the head of the talus on the doral aspect of the foot. The athlete then twists the trunk, forcing the tibia to internally and externally rotate. In the neutral position, the head of the navicular bone may be palpated on the medial edge of the foot. The distance between the navicular and the floor should not exceed 1 cm (Mueller, Host and Norton, 1993).

The neutral position is the point at which the head of the talus appears to bulge equally under each palpating finger. In lying (prone or supine), the practitioner grasps the athlete's foot over the 4/5th metatarsal head and presses the foot into dorsiflexion. Again, the practitioner palpates the head of the talus and swings the foot into inwards and outwards to stop at the point where the talar head seems not to bulge more on one side.

> **Keypoint**
>
> *Neutral position* of the subtalar joint (STJ) is determined by palpating the head of the talus and moving the foot. When the talus appears to bulge equally at each side, the STJ is in neutral.

Biomechanics of the STJ

An essential feature of the STJ is its ability to perform triplane motion. This occurs when movement of one joint is in all three body planes, because the joint axis is oblique.

Pronation of the foot is a triplane movement of the calcaneum and foot consisting of calcaneal eversion (frontal plane), abduction (transverse plane) and dorsiflexion (sagittal plane). Supination is an opposing movement of calcaneal inversion, adduction and plantarflexion in the same planes. These are both open chain movements in their pure forms. Functionally, the movements occur in closed chain formation with the foot on the ground. Abduction and adduction cannot occur owing to friction with the floor, and dorsiflexion and plantarflexion will not occur in their pure form as they are no longer free to move. Instead, the talus takes over these movements with supination consisting of calcaneal inversion with abduction and dorsiflexion of the talus, while pronation combines calcaneal eversion with adduction and plantarflexion of the talus (Fig. 8.3).

> **Definition**
>
> In the weight-bearing foot, *supination* (high arched foot) consists of calcaneal inversion with abduction and dorsiflexion of the talus, while *pronation* (flattened foot) combines calcaneal eversion with adduction and plantarflexion of the talus.

The foot has two important functions during the gait cycle. The first is to act as a *mobile adaptor*, adjusting to alterations in the ground surface and reducing the shock travelling up to the other lower limb joints. Secondly, the foot must efficiently transmit force from the muscles of the lower leg to provide propulsion to push off. For this, the foot must change into a *rigid lever*. These two diametrically opposed functions of mobile adaptor and rigid lever are achieved by changing the bony alignment of the foot joints, and 'locking' or 'unlocking' the foot.

Mid-tarsal joint

The movement of the STJ alters the alignment of the two components of the mid (transverse) tarsal joint (MTJ). These are laterally the calcaneal cuboid joint, and medially the talo-calcaneonavicular joint. The mid-tarsal joint has two axes of motion, one oblique and one longitudinal. The longitudinal axis primarily allows inversion and eversion of the forefoot, while the oblique axis permits adduction/abduction and plantarflexion/dorsiflexion. The direction of the motions at the mid-tarsal joint causes the dorsiflexion force created by weight bearing to lock the forefoot against the rearfoot.

The position of the STJ alters the neutral alignment of the mid-tarsal joint axes (Fig. 8.4b). Supination of the STJ causes the axes to become more oblique (Fig. 8.4c), and less motion can take place. The foot is said to be locked, and acts as a rigid lever ideal for propulsion. Pronation of the STJ causes the mid-tarsal joint axes to become more parallel (Fig. 8.4a), and therefore more mobile. Now the foot is unlocked, and acts as a mobile adaptor capable of accommodating to changes in the ground surface.

First ray complex

The first ray is a functional unit consisting of the first metatarsal and the first cuneiform. Its axis is at 45° to the sagittal and frontal planes. The joint does have triplane motion, but little abduction and adduction occur functionally. Dorsiflexion of the first ray is accompanied by inversion, and plantarflexion is combined with eversion.

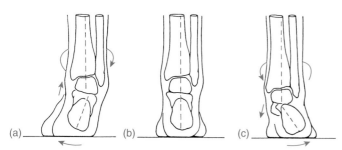

Figure 8.3 Weight-bearing motion of the sub-taloid joint. (a) Supination. (b) Neutral position. (c) Pronation. From Gould (1990) with permission.

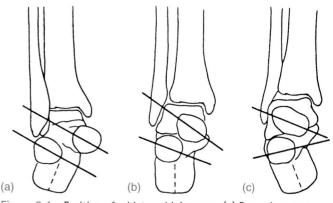

Figure 8.4 Position of mid-tarsal joint axes. (a) Pronation, axes parallel increasing mobility. (b) Neutral. (c) Supination, axes oblique reducing mobility. From Gould (1990) with permission.

Jumping

A jumping activity usually involves a wind-up period where the body is lowered before the jump is initiated. This period enables the push phase of the jump to last longer and the power for lift off comes from hip and knee extension accompanied by ankle plantarflexion. This leg sequence is reversed to absorb shock as the body lands. The whole jump may be divided into seven phases (Durward, Baer and Rowe, 1999; Fig. 8.5).

In phase 1 the body moves downwards to pre-stretch the extensor muscles of the hip and knee, and the plantarflexors of the ankle. In phase 2 the downward motion of the body decelerates and stops in the lowest position. The negative vertical force of the body dropping is equalled by the positive vertical force of the body coming to a halt in the low position. The two areas are shaded on Figure 8.5. In phase 3 we see the main propulsive action of the body as it accelerates upwards until at phase 4 the body leaves the ground to enter the flight phase. During the flight phase there is no vertical force registered on the force plate because the body is off the ground; there will be some vertical force acting on the body but this will be minimal. Phase 5 sees the body landing with initial contact being made by the foot, and the body and rest of the leg decelerate rapidly. Once the body and leg have flexed to absorb shock, the subject straightens the leg and body to stand upright again (phase 6) and finally comes to a halt (phase 7). In a non-athletic individual, body control is not as skilled, and so additional movements or 'overshoots' may appear where the individual tries to regain balance.

The action of flexing or 'softening' the legs when landing from a jump greatly affects the forces acting on the body (Fig. 8.6). This occurs especially in '*drop jumps*' where the body is lowered from a height rather than simply moved upwards in a jumping action. This occurs in plyometrics (pp. 109–110) in sport, and also in daily activities such as stepping down from a kerb or single step. As there is no acceleration phase as with the traditional jump, the body must anticipate the landing surface and prepare accordingly. In a soft landing, flexion of the lower limb attenuates some of the compression forces acting on the body by using the muscles eccentrically as 'springs'. Where the landing is hard, the time taken to stop is approximately 50% of that of a soft landing (Durward, Baer and Rowe, 1999), so the landing is more abrupt, giving a jolting effect. The combination of shorter time and higher forces in a hard landing makes injury more likely. Athletes performing jumping actions should always be encouraged to use a soft landing 'going through' the leg and foot.

Keypoint

A *hard landing* from a jump is *more abrupt* and gives higher reaction forces acting on the joints. Injury is therefore more likely.

THE GAIT CYCLE

The gait cycle can be conveniently divided into two phases. The *stance phase* occurs when the foot is on the floor,

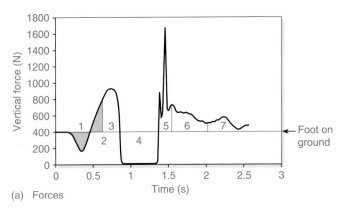

(a) Forces

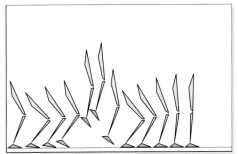

(b) Movement

Figure 8.5   Vertical jump. Adapted from Durward, Baer and Rowe (1999), with permission.

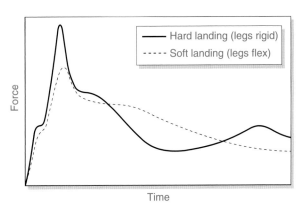

Figure 8.6   Vertical forces on landing from a jump. Adapted from Durward, Baer and Rowe (1999), with permission.

Figure 8.7 (a) The walk cycle and (b) the run cycle. From Subotnick (1989).

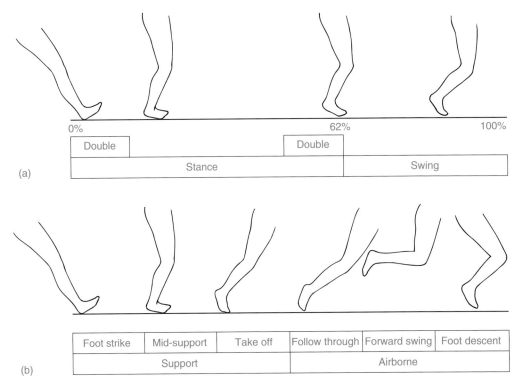

(a)

Foot strike	Mid-support	Take off	Follow through	Forward swing	Foot descent
	Support			Airborne	

(b)

supporting the bodyweight. Closed chain motion occurs in the lower limb, as it decelerates. The *swing phase* takes place as the foot comes off the ground and open chain motion follows. This time the limb is accelerating.

The foot moves through four positions in three phases during stance. Initially, the heel strikes the ground (contact phase) and as the bodyweight moves forwards, the foot flattens (mid-stance). Forward movement continues and the heel lifts off the ground; finally the toes push off (propulsion) and the leg moves into the swing phase.

At the start of the swing phase the limb is accelerating. In the mid-swing position the speed is constant, and finally the leg decelerates, and is lowered to the ground where heel strike again occurs and the cycle is repeated (Fig. 8.7).

The stance phase in walking is approximately 60% of the total gait cycle, while the swing phase is 40%. Walking at a normal rate of 120 steps/min, the total cycle takes 1 second, so stance occurs for 0.6 s while swing takes only 0.4 s. With running, the movements occur more rapidly, and the stance phase occupies less of the total cycle time. A runner with a pace of 6 min/mile has a total cycle time of only 0.6 s. The stance phase would last for 0.2 s, and so events occurring within this phase are performed three times faster.

During the walking gait cycle, overlap of the stance phases of both legs occurs so that, for a short period, both feet are on the ground at the same time (double leg support). As walking speed increases, the double leg support period reduces. When the stance leg 'toes-off' before the swinging leg contacts the ground, double leg support is eliminated and an airborne period is created. Walking has now progressed to running.

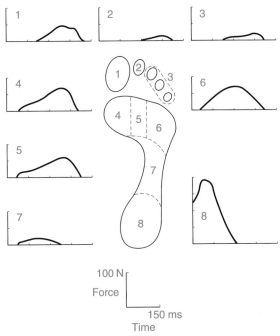

Figure 8.8 Force acting through the foot during walking. From Reid (1992), with permission.

Stance phase

During the stance phase, the forces taken by the various areas of the foot will vary from a peak at the heel during the contact phase, to a more gradual and later occurring force curve at the first metatarsophalangeal region at toe-off (Fig. 8.8).

Contact

With the contact phase, the lateral aspect of the calcaneum strikes the ground. The ankle joint is close to its neutral (90°) position, and the subtalar joint is slightly supinated. The hip is flexed to about 30°. The pelvis and the body's centre of gravity are moving laterally over the weight-bearing leg, producing closed chain adduction of the hip. Total lateral motion of the trunk is 4–5 cm (Whittle, 1996).

The STJ starts to pronate, and the mobility of the mid-tarsal joint is increased. The ankle begins to plantarflex to bring the foot flat onto the ground for mid-stance. Pronation causes the tibia to internally rotate, and this in turn unlocks the knee, allowing it to flex to about 20°, in a movement opposite to the screw home effect. The hip begins to extend and internally rotate and this continues until heel raise.

The anterior tibials contract eccentrically to stop the foot slapping at heel strike, and the posterior tibials decelerate pronation. The quadriceps work eccentrically to allow the knee to bend, and the hamstrings prevent trunk flexion at the hip. Later, the hamstrings work concentrically to extend the hip (closed chain extension). The hamstrings are used in preference to the gluteals here, possibly because they have been prestretched. When the knee bends, the hamstrings can no longer produce hip extension, and the gluteals take over.

The hip abductors work eccentrically to control lateral movement over the supporting leg and then concentrically to pull the bodyweight back again in preparation for the next cycle.

Mid-stance

In mid-stance, the transition of the foot from mobile adaptor to rigid lever occurs. The STJ starts to supinate, reducing mid-tarsal mobility and locking the foot. When hip adduction is completed, closed chain abduction occurs for the rest of the stance phase.

The action of the calf is eccentric to control dorsiflexion and with it forward motion of the body, and the posterior tibials contract concentrically to supinate the foot.

Propulsion

The heel rises with plantarflexion at the ankle and the propulsion phase begins, the knee reaching its point of maximal extension. At toe-off, dorsiflexion again occurs at the ankle to prevent toe drag, and the hip begins to flex. The calf now works concentrically to actively plantarflex the ankle, and the peroneus longus and brevis are eccentric to control supination. The peroneus longus also stabilizes the first ray. The quadriceps work eccentrically to control the knee.

Swing phase

During the swing phase, the maximally supinated STJ moves back to its position of slight supination just before heel strike. The knee continues to flex during the acceleration position

of the swing phase, and starts to extend again before heel strike. The hip continues to flex, until it has reached its 30° position to begin the cycle again. The quadriceps continue to contract eccentrically to stop the knee 'snapping' back, and the hip flexors are concentric to accelerate the leg forwards. Phasic muscle action during running is summarized in Figure 8.9.

ABNORMAL GAIT PATTERNS

Several abnormalities of gait are commonly seen in clinical practice, and the reader is referred to Whittle (1996), and Magee (2002) for a more detailed description.

Painful and stiff leg gait

Painful (*antalgic*) gait and stiff leg (*arthrogenic*) gait patterns are among the most common walking patterns seen following injury. In the antalgic gait the patient tries to reduce pain by altering his/her walking pattern. The stance (weight-bearing) phase of the affected leg is shortened as the patient tries to take the weight off the leg as quickly as possible. The swing phase of the unaffected leg shortens, the patient attempting to get this leg back on the ground as quickly as possible so that it can again take the weight off the painful side. The overall effect is that the step length on the affected side is reduced. Where the hip is the source of pain, the bodyweight is often shifted over this side to reduce the leverage effect of the hip abductors and so reduce the consequent compression forces on the femoral head (Fig. 1.5, p. 7).

With an arthrogenic gait, the affected leg is unable to flex during the gait cycle. This may be a result of either knee or hip pathology or simply following immobilization. Four gait changes may occur as a consequence (Table 8.1) Circumduction, hip hiking, and high stepping are all modifications of the swing phase. Vaulting is a modification of the stance phase (Whittle, 1996). *Circumduction* involves swinging the leg out to the side to clear the ground, and is best noticed by viewing the subject from behind. Where weakness of the hip flexors is present, circumduction will move the leg forwards via action of the hip abductors. *Hip hitching* (hiking) achieves ground clearance by lifting the pelvis on the side of the moving leg (the opposite of the Trendelenburg gait). Often, this pelvic lift is accompanied by excessive pelvic rotation to thrust the leg forwards. *High stepping* gait sees an increase in both knee and hip flexion to exaggerate the ground clearance. This is especially common in patients with foot drop. Finally, *vaulting* increases ground clearance by lifting onto the toes of the support leg, and therefore increasing the vertical displacement of the body.

Trendelenburg gait

One of the most universally recognized faults is the Trendelenburg gait. An excessive lateral flexion of the trunk

Figure 8.9 Phasic muscular activity during normal ambulation. From McGlamry, J.G. (1987) *Fundamentals of Foot Surgery*. Williams and Wilkins. Baltimore. With permission.

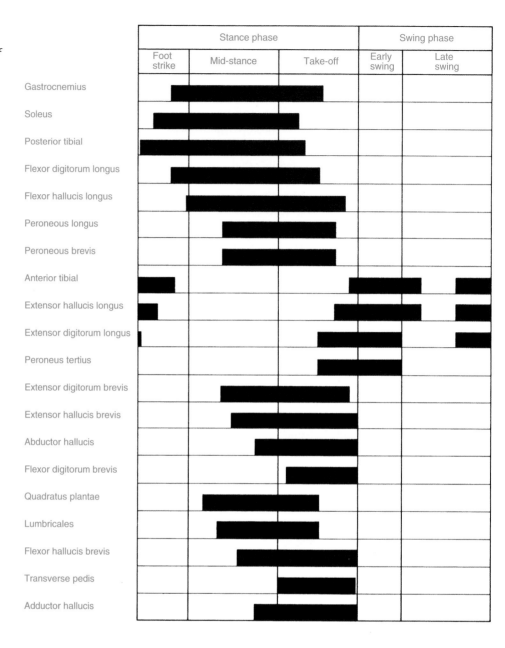

Table 8.1 Changes seen in stiff leg gait patterns

Fault	Characteristic
Circumduction	Swinging the leg out to the side to clear the ground
Hip hitching	Lifting the pelvis on the side of the moving leg
High stepping	Increase in both knee and hip flexion to exaggerate ground clearance
Vaulting	Lifting onto the toes of the support leg

occurs to reduce forces on the hip joint and hip abductor muscles. During normal standing, the weight of the body is taken evenly on both legs (Fig. 8.10a) and the weight of the legs passes through the ground. As one leg is

lifted, the bodyweight and the weight of the opposite leg must be taken by the weight-bearing leg (Fig. 8.10b). If the trunk is laterally flexed towards the weight-bearing leg, the reduction in leverage forces enables the hip to be stabilized by less abductor force, and the resultant compression over the hip joint itself is reduced (Fig. 8.10c). The Trendelenburg gait is typically seen as a result of a painful or abnormal hip joint, weakness of the hip abductor muscles (especially gluteus medius) or unequal leg length.

Where weak abductors are present, the Trendelenburg sign may be seen (Fig. 8.10d). As one leg is lifted, the hip abductors of the supporting leg are unable to maintain the neutral position of the pelvis. As a result, the pelvis dips towards the lifted leg.

the subject *flexes the trunk* at the hip to move the bodyweight anterior to the knee joint axis, and so eliminate the flexion moment (Fig. 8.11b). Similarly, the line of force during early stance passes *in front* of the hip joint axis, tending to flex it. This moment is normally resisted by the hip extensors. At heel strike, the hip extensors work to pull the hip back and in so doing propel the body forwards by pushing the pelvis through. Where the hip extensors (especially the gluteus maximus) are weak, the trunk will be *thrust back* to bring the line of force posterior to the hip joint axis (Fig. 8.11c). The other cause of posterior trunk bending is an increased lordosis due to hip flexor tightness (see pp. 133 and 138).

> ### Keypoint
>
> Where the *gluteus medius* (hip abductor) is weak, the body will lurch to one side to compensate. Where the *gluteus maximus* (hip extensor) is weak, the trunk is thrust backwards to push the hips through at heel strike.

ABNORMAL BIOMECHANICS OF THE FOOT

Excessive pronation/supination

These conditions occur if the normal pronation and supination periods of the gait cycle are extended, or when there is a change in the angulation of the foot segments. Causes may be *extrinsic*, such as tight muscles or abnormal lower leg rotation, or *intrinsic*, as occurs with fixed deformities of the STJ and MTJ.

Severe pronation causes foot flattening. The range of motion at the STJ is increased, making the mid-tarsal joint axes more parallel and unlocking the foot. The foot can then remain pronated and mobile after the stance phase, hence the terms 'hypermobile' or 'weak' foot.

With excessive supination, the MTJ is locked, the foot is more rigid and the arch higher (cavus). In time the plantar fascia and intrinsic foot muscles become tight, reducing the capacity of the foot to dissipate shock.

Rearfoot varus

The rearfoot and forefoot can both move outward (valgus) or inward (varus) giving the four alignment faults shown in Table 8.2. The first is rearfoot varus. With this condition, the calcaneus appears inverted when the foot is examined in the neutral position. Left uncompensated the forefoot would invert and leave the medial side of the foot off the ground. To compensate, the STJ pronates excessively on ground contact. This deformity has been associated with an increased number of lateral ankle sprains (Weil, 1979).

Rearfoot varus is usually a result of developmental abnormality. From the eight to twelfth fetal week the calcaneum lies at the side of the talus. As the fetus develops, the

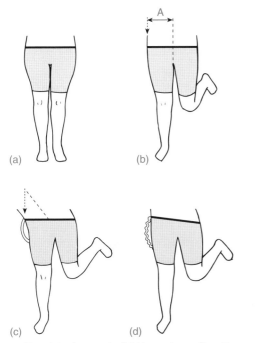

Figure 8.10 Trendelenburg gait. (a) Normal standing. Even weight distribution between both legs. (b) Normal single-leg standing. (c) Trunk lateral flexion eliminating lever arm. (d) Weak hip abductors allow pelvis to dip.

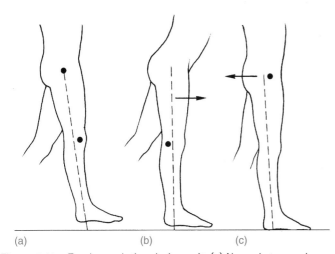

Figure 8.11 Trunk angulation during gait. (a) Normal stance phase. Knee joint axis in front of force line, hip joint axis behind. (b) Flexing the trunk brings the force line anterior to the knee axis. (c) Extending the trunk moves the force line posterior to the hip axis. Adapted from Whittle (1996), with permission.

Trunk angulation

Excessive trunk bending in the sagittal plane is normally a result of inadequate muscle control in the knee and hip. During the normal stance phase, the line of force (gravity line) passes *behind* the knee joint axis, producing a flexion moment (Fig. 8.11a). This must be resisted by the quadriceps to maintain stability of the knee. If the quadriceps contraction is inadequate (either in terms of force generation or timing), calcaneum rotates to a more plantar position, so that it lies below the talus. However, the calcaneus may not be completely perpendicular to the ground until the child is 6 years old, and in some cases the rotation is never complete. In

Table 8.2 Common alignment faults in the foot

Deformity	Foot position
	With the STJ neutral, compare the ***calcaneal line*** with the ***tibial line***
Rearfoot varus (a)	Tibial line — Calcaneal line — Heel appears inverted
Rearfoot valgus (b)	Heel appears everted
	With the STJ neutral and the midtarsal joint maximally pronated, compare ***heel*** with the plane of the ***metatarsal heads***
Forefoot varus (c)	Plane of metatarsal heads — Medial side of foot raised
Forefoot valgus (d)	Lateral side of foot raised

addition to the subtalar deformity, the condition is also associated with tibial varum.

Rearfoot valgus

This condition can occur if the calcaneum rotates excessively in its development, or following a Pott's fracture. The posterior surface of the calcaneum will appear everted, and the foot will hyperpronate, giving a severe flatfoot. The condition is associated with genu valgum (knock knees) and the medial longitudinal arch appears flattened.

Forefoot varus

In this deformity (Table 8.2) the forefoot is inverted in respect to the rearfoot, when the STJ is in a neutral position. To compensate, and bring the forefoot to the ground, the STJ everts and the entire plantar surface of the foot becomes weight-bearing, flattening the medial longitudinal arch. The head of the talus bulges proximally to the tuberosity of navicular. Plantar calluses are apparent over the second and third metatarsal heads, and an associated hallux valgus deformity may be present.

If the STJ is unable to pronate sufficiently, the entire plantar surface of the foot will be unable to touch the ground. Weight bearing will therefore be lateral, with callus formation this time over the fourth and fifth metatarsal heads.

Abnormal pronation continues into the propulsive phases of the gait cycle, and the foot tries to push off without becoming a rigid lever. This instability causes shearing forces between the metatarsal heads, giving rise to associated pathologies. Interdigital neuroma, postural fatigue, fasciitis, chondromalacia and shin pain have all been described as resultant to this deformity (McPoil and Brocato, 1990).

Forefoot valgus

Here, there is an eversion of the forefoot in relation to the rearfoot, a situation exactly opposite to that above. The medial foot structures are in contact with the ground while the lateral side is suspended. Deformities greater than 6° (McPoil and Brocato, 1990) will require STJ and MTJ compensations. To place the foot flat on the ground, the calcaneus will invert pulling the talus into an abducted-dorsiflexed position. During the contact phase of gait, the foot will pronate more than normal, and remain pronated and therefore mobile into the propulsive phase. Symptoms associated with hypermobility of the metatarsophalangeal and interphalangeal joints occur.

Plantarflexed first ray

This condition is present when the first metatarsal lies below the level of the other metatarsals in neutral position, causing the forefoot to appear slightly everted relative to the rearfoot. When forefoot eversion continues, a forefoot valgus is present.

Various conditions may give rise to this problem. If the first metatarsal phalangeal (MP) joint is rigid (hallux rigidus, see pp. 283–284) the foot is forced rapidly into supination (a supinatory rock) to allow the lateral side of the foot to bear weight. In so doing, the fifth metatarsal head strikes the ground rapidly (Wernick and Langer, 1985). In addition, weakness of the tibialis anterior will allow the peroneus longus to pull the first ray into plantarflexion unopposed. Deformity occurs over time, and is particularly exaggerated in certain neuromuscular diseases.

BIOMECHANICAL EXAMINATION AND TREATMENT

Examination of the lower limb may reveal problems with the spine, pelvis, hip or knee. The aim of this section, however, is to deal with the examination of the limb in relation to foot problems, assessment procedures for the other body parts being covered in the sections describing injuries to these areas. Equally, foot examination in isolation is not enough. Forces acting through the kinetic chain, and referral of pain from other structures, make holistic evaluation of lower limb function essential.

Subjective examination and inspection of the lower limb will act as pointers to further assessment, and give clues about any additional tests which may be required.

Objective examination is made both with the athlete weight bearing and then non-weight bearing. Positions include standing, sitting, walking and then running. With walking and running, video analysis is often used to slow the motion down and aid in the identification of faults. In each case the examination may be carried out with the athlete in shorts and bare feet, and then while wearing their normal training shoes. The wear pattern of the shoes (Fig. 8.12) is often a useful general guide to the existence of underlying biomechanical faults.

In standing, the alignment of the various body segments is assessed. Starting from the top of the body and working down, viewed from behind, the head and shoulder positions are noted, as is the symmetry of the spine. Shoulder and pelvic levels are assessed. Buttock and knee creases are examined for equal level. Knee position gives a clue to the presence of coxa valga/vara and genu vara/valga (Fig. 8.13).

Tibial vara can be measured in standing by comparing the line of the distal third of the leg to a line perpendicular to the supporting surface which passes through the posterior contact point of the calcaneus (Fig. 8.14).

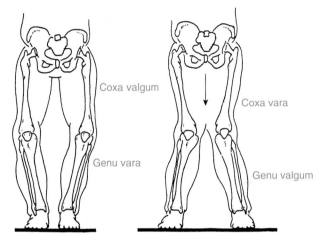

Figure 8.13   Femoral and tibial alignment. From Subotnick (1989).

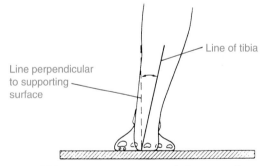

Figure 8.14   Tibia vara measurement made from standing position.

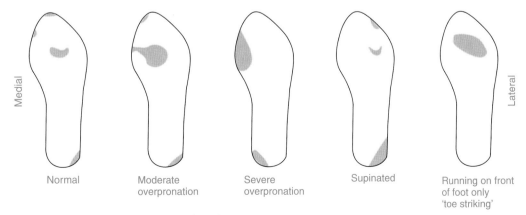

Figure 8.12   Wear pattern on sports shoes. From Reid (1992), with permission.

From the front, similar comparisons of shoulder, pelvic, spinal and leg alignments are made. The position of the patella relative to the foot will suggest any tibial torsion. Tibial torsion can be further assessed with the patient in sitting with the knee flexed to 90° over the end of the couch. The examiner places his or her thumbs over the patient's malleoli and compares an imaginary line connecting these two points with the knee axis.

In supine lying, active and passive range of movement at the knee and hip are measured and any asymmetry or alteration in normal end-feel is noted. Resisted strength is measured and limb girths measured. The distribution of any pain or alteration in sensation is mapped. The appearance of the foot is observed and any skin abnormalities noted. In prone lying, range of movement of the foot is measured and compared to normal values.

Calcaneal inversion and eversion are measured by marking a line bisecting the back of the calcaneus (*calcaneal line*) and comparing this to a line bisecting the calf and Achilles (*tibial line*).

Definition

The *tibial line* joints two points on the midline of the lower third of the tibia. The *calcaneal line* joints the midpoint of the calcaneus at the insertion of the Achilles with a midpoint 1 cm distal to this point.

Forefoot position is assessed by placing the STJ in its neutral position. A goniometer is then placed over the metatarsal heads, and its line compared to one perpendicular to the line of calcaneal bisection. Alternatively, a forefoot measuring device (FMD) may be used. This has a slit which is placed over the line of calcaneal bisection, the plateau on the front of the FMD is placed over the plantar surface of the foot in line with the met heads, and a value for forefoot–rearfoot alignment read from the scale. Using both goniometry and the FMD, the most common forefoot–rearfoot relationship is one of varus, with average values being 7.5° (Garbalosa, Donatelli and Wooden, 1989).

Significant biomechanical faults of the foot can be managed by using a functional orthotic device.

Orthotics

An orthotic device is usually made after taking a plaster impression of the foot in the neutral position. This may be sent to an orthotic laboratory where a device is fabricated according to the practitioner's prescription and laboratory assessment of the cast. Alternatively, a number of temporary heat moulded orthotics are available which have the advantage that they are fitted in the functional standing (weight-bearing) position.

The orthotic aims to alter the mechanical functioning of the foot, and so is more than a simple arch support. When worn, the device changes the foot's alignment to make the lower limb function more normally. There are generally few long-term benefits, and much like with a pair of spectacles, once the orthotic is removed, the body returns to its previous state.

References

Durward, B., Baer, G. and Rowe, P. (1999) *Functional Human Movement*, Butterworth-Heinemann, Oxford

Garbalosa, J.C., Donatelli, R. and Wooden, M.J. (1989) Dysfunction, evaluation and treatment of the foot and ankle. In *Orthopaedic Physical Therapy* (eds R. Donatelli and M.J. Wooden), Churchill Livingstone, London, pp. 533–553

Gould, J.A. (1990) *Orthopaedic and Sports Physical Therapy*, 2nd edn, Mosby, St Louis

McGlamry, J.G. (1987) *Fundamentals of Foot Surgery*, Williams and Wilkins, Baltimore

McPoil, T.G. and Brocato, R.S. (1990) The foot and ankle: biomechanical evaluation and treatment. In *Orthopaedic and Sports Physical Therapy*, 2nd edn (ed. J.A. Gould), Mosby, St Louis, pp. 293–321

Magee, D.J. (2002) *Orthopedic Physical Assessment*, 4th edn, W.B. Saunders, Philadelphia

Mueller, M.J., Host, J. and Norton, B. (1993) Navicular drop as a composite measure of excessive pronation. *Journal of the American Podiatric Medical Association*, **83**, 198–202

Palastanga, N., Field, D. and Soames, R. (1998) *Anatomy and Human Movement*, 3rd edn, Butterworth-Heinemann, Oxford

Reid, D.C. (1992) *Sports Injury Assessment and Rehabilitation*, Churchill Livingstone, London

Subotnick, S.I. (1989) *Sports Medicine of the Lower Extremity*, Churchill Livingstone, London

Weil, L.S. (1979) A biomechanical study of lateral ankle sprains in basketball. *Journal of the American Podiatry Association*, **69**, 687

Wernick, J. and Langer, S. (1985) *A Practical Manual for a Basic Approach to Biomechanics*, Langer Biomechanics Group, Stoke-on-Trent

Whittle, M.W. (1996) *Gait Analysis*, 2nd edn, Butterworth-Heinemann, Oxford

SECTION 2

Management

Chapter 9

The hip and thigh

THE HIP JOINT

Whereas the glenohumeral joint functions mainly in a open kinetic chain position, the hip (coxofemoral) joint functions mainly in a closed chain position. For this reason, its structure is one of stability for weight bearing. In the standing position, however, the joint is not fully congruent, the antero-superior portion of the cartilage of the head being exposed. It is only when the joint is taken into a position equivalent to that of the quadruped (90° flexion, 5° abduction, and 10° lateral rotation) that maximum articular contact of the head with the acetabulum occurs (Palastanga, Field and Soames, 1994).

The femoral neck makes an angle (the angle of inclination) with the shaft of 120–130° in the adult, representing the adaptation of the femur to the parallel position of the legs in gait (Fig. 9.1a). This changes from 150° in the newborn to 142° by age 5, 133° by age 15, and 125° in the adult (Reid, 1992; Palastanga, Field and Soames, 1994). Greater angles than these are termed coxa valga, lesser angles as coxa vara.

Definition

In *coxa vara* the angle between the neck and shaft of the femur is *reduced*, and a knock-knee position results. In *coxa valga* the angle is *increased* and a bowleg position results.

Similarly, the axis of the femoral head and neck make an angle with the axis of the femoral condyles (Fig. 9.1b). This angle (angle of torsion, or angle of anteversion) is normally 10° in the adult, having reduced from 25° in the infant. Increased anteversion is linked to squinting or kissing patellae (p. 217) and this condition is twice as common in girls as in boys.

Craig's test may be used to assess the angle of anteversion; it compares the angle of the femoral neck to that of the femoral condyles at the knee. The patient lies prone on a couch with the knee flexed to 90°. The therapist palpates the

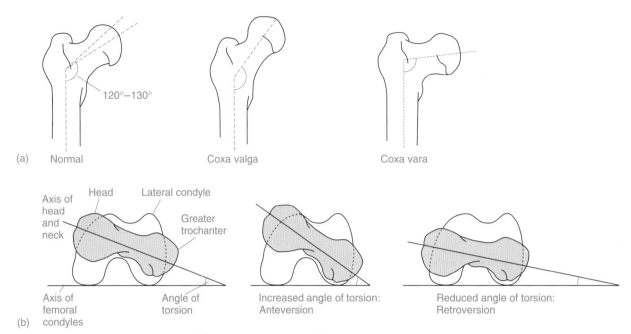

Figure 9.1   Angulation of the femoral neck. (a) Angle of inclination. (b) Angle of torsion.

greater trochanter (posterior aspect), and the femur is medially and laterally rotated until the trochanter is parallel with the horizontal plane. The angle of anteversion is estimated from the angle of the lower leg to the vertical, and angles greater than 15° are considered abnormal (Sahrmann, 2002). Interestingly, this test has been found to be more reliable than radiological assessment (Ruwe et al., 1992).

Weight bearing

In standing, each hip takes roughly 0.3 times bodyweight, increased to 2.4 times body weight when standing on one leg. Weight bearing forces of up to 4.5 times bodyweight may be taken on the hip in running (Magee, 2002). In order to take weight most effectively, bony trabeculae line up in the direction of imposed stress. Two major systems exist within the femur (Fig. 9.2). The medial trabecular system travels from the medial cortex of the upper femoral shaft to the superior aspect of the head. This system takes vertically aligned forces created by weight bearing, and is aligned with the superior aspect of the acetabulum, the main weight-bearing region. The lateral trabecular system begins from the lateral cortex of the upper femoral shaft, crosses the medial system, and terminates in the cortical bone on the inferior aspect of the head. The lateral system is aligned to take oblique forces created by contraction of the hip abductors during gait.

In addition to the medial and lateral trabecular systems, the upper femur is reinforced by medial and lateral accessory systems which take forces created about the trochanters. A zone of weakness is left within the femoral neck which is susceptible to bending forces and is the site of femoral neck fracture (Norkin and Levangie, 1992).

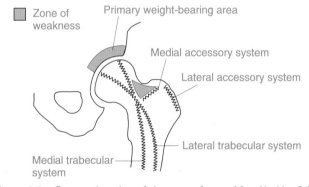

Figure 9.2   Bony trabeculae of the upper femur. After Norkin, C.C. and Levangie, P.K. (1992) *Joint Structure and Function*, 2nd edn. FA Davis, Philadelphia. With permission of the publisher FA Davis.

Hip ligaments

The hip joint is strengthened by three capsular ligaments: the iliofemoral ligament and the pubofemoral ligament are on the anterior aspect of the joint, while the ischiofemoral ligament is on the posterior aspect (Fig. 9.3). As the hip is flexed, all three ligaments relax. However, in extension all three ligaments are tight, with the inferior band of the iliofemoral ligament being placed under greatest tension as it runs almost vertically. It is this ligamentous band which limits posterior tilt of the pelvis (Palastanga, Field and Soames, 1994).

Keypoint
The inferior (lower) band of the iliofemoral ligament runs almost vertically. With hip extension it is under greatest tension and it limits posterior tilting of the pelvis.

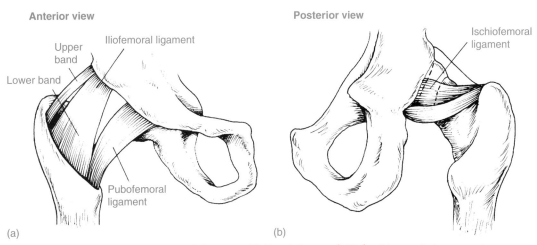

Figure 9.3 Capsular ligaments of the hip joint. After Palastanga, Field and Soames (1994), with permission.

During adduction, it is the turn of the superior band of the iliofemoral ligament to become tighter while the pubofemoral ligament and ischiofemoral ligament relax. In abduction the opposite occurs. In lateral rotation both the iliofemoral ligament and pubofemoral ligament are taut, while in medial rotation the ischiofemoral ligament tightens.

SCREENING EXAMINATION

Hip conditions may refer pain anywhere within the L3 dermatome, over the front of the thigh and down to the knee. Initial observation includes resting position, muscle wasting, leg length and gait. Functional activities may also be revealing. Lying in bed with the affected side uppermost (hip adduction and medial rotation) places a stretch over the iliotibial band (ITB) and lengthens the posterior portion of the gluteus medius. This may be a consideration in ITB friction syndrome (p. 222) and for muscle imbalance over the hip (p. 127). Pain on squatting (hip flexion), as when sitting on the toilet or sitting down into a low chair, warrants closer examination of flexion movements.

Examination for range of motion may be carried out in a supine position for flexion, abduction and adduction and both rotations. Medial and lateral rotation are best compared between the affected and unaffected hip in a prone position with the knees flexed to 90°. Resisted abduction is better tested in a side lying position with the affected joint uppermost.

Compression of the joint through the flexed knee and circumduction with compression to 'scour' the femoral head into the acetabulum is an important assessment for arthritic changes. Both the lumbar spine and the sacroiliac joints must be examined, to eliminate them as a potential cause of pain referral. The straight leg raise and slump test should be used to eliminate the possible involvement of neural tissue. Cyriax (1982) warned that serious pathology may be present if the sign of the buttock is positive. Here, hip flexion with the knee bent is more painful and more limited than straight leg raising. A non-capsular limitation is present, and pain may make the end-feel empty. As straight leg raising is full the sciatic nerve is unimpinged, and the non-capsular limitation precludes the hip joint. Possibilities include an inflammatory disease state, neoplasm and fracture.

> **Keypoint**
>
> With the sign of the buttock, hip flexion with the knee bent is more painful and more limited than straight leg raising. Serious hip pathology may be present and further investigation is required.

Muscle imbalance around the hip

The concept of muscle imbalance was covered in Chapter 6. In the hip region, the Thomas test and the Ober manoeuvre are used to assess for muscle tightness of the hip flexors (rectus femoris and iliopsoas) and hip abductors (tensor fascia lata and iliotibial band – TFL/ITB). Inner range holding ability of the gluteus medius is assessed with side-lying hip abduction (p. 127) and of the gluteus maximus with the prone-lying hip extension movement described below. Segmental control tests include standing hip flexion, standing hip abduction and the hip hinge (Table 9.1). All tests are described in Chapter 6.

MUSCLE INJURIES

Quadriceps

On the whole, strains occur mostly in two-joint muscles, due to the more complex coordination involved in controlling movement of two body segments simultaneously. Direct trauma, however, can be imposed on any muscle. In the hip region, this means that the rectus femoris, hamstrings and gracilis muscles tend to suffer strain. The more anterior position of the quadriceps, however, exposes these muscles to

Table 9.1 Muscle imbalance around the hip

	Muscle length	Inner range holding	Segmental control
Figure			
Test	Thomas	Gluteus medius	Standing hip flexion
Figure			
Test	Ober	Gluteus maximus	Standing hip abduction
Figure			
Test	Active knee extension (AKE)	Iliopsoas	Hip hinge

risk during contact sports, and to blunt trauma through collision with sports apparatus. A quadriceps contusion is often referred to colloquially as a 'dead leg' or 'charley horse'.

Initially, there is local swelling over the front of the thigh, with some superficial bruising appearing later, often tracking down to the knee. The main danger with this injury is the development of myositis ossificans traumatica (MOT, see p. 54). Thigh contusions may be rated as grade 1 (mild), in which knee flexion beyond 90° is possible, grade 2 (moderate), in which motion is restricted to 45–90°, or grade 3 (severe), in which swelling and pain limit movement to less than 45°. This grading system can be an accurate predictor of the likelihood of MOT development. Jackson and Feagin (1973) assessed quadriceps contusions in 65 subjects, and found that none of the subjects with grade 1 injuries had developed MOT. However, 13 out of 18 subjects who had been graded 2 or 3 later went on to develop the condition, so the amount of movement present in the initial stages is an important indicator of the severity of the lesion, and the prognosis.

> **Keypoint**
>
> Following a quadriceps haematoma or 'dead leg', myositis (muscle calcification) is more likely to occur if an injured athlete is unable to flex the knee to 90°.

It is important to limit movement in grade 1 and 2 injuries and to discourage the use of massage, vigorous stretching or exercise and ultrasound, as these are contraindicated in the early post-injury stage. The RICE protocol is used to limit the tissue damage. Ice is applied with compression with the knee and hip flexed as far as is comfortable. Internal compression is therefore applied by fascial tightening (Reid, 1992), while external compression comes from the elastic bandage.

The athlete resuming contact sports should wear padding over the damaged area, to reduce the risk of secondary injury. It is important that full broadening of the muscle belly be obtained during rehabilitation. This will involve resisted quadriceps exercises, beginning with low intensity and building eventually to maximum voluntary contractions (MVC). This is equally important to endurance athletes as to power athletes. Often, distance runners, for example, do not use weight training, focusing instead on stretching. For this injury, however, longitudinal movement of the muscle is less important than lateral movement (broadening). This is because the rectus femoris, being a two-joint muscle, may limit movement, but the vasti, being single-joint muscles, do not. As the vasti form the bulk of the injured tissue, stretching, although important with this injury, is secondary to strength training.

In cases of MOT, calcification is slow, with fibroblasts beginning to differentiate into osteoblasts about 1 week after

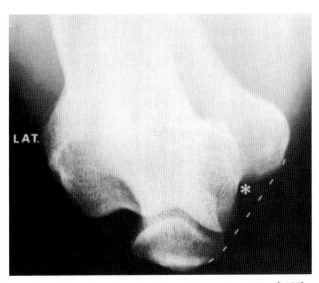

Figure 9.4   X ray showing myositis ossificans traumatica (MOT). From Magee (2002) with permission.

injury. Radiographic evidence of bone formation is usually visible after 3 weeks (Fig. 9.4). By 6–7 weeks after injury, the calcified mass generally stops growing. Total reabsorption may occur with minor lesions, but more major conditions may continue to show remnants of the mass. The mass rarely interferes with muscle contraction, so excision is not normally required (Estwanik and McAlister, 1990).

Rectus femoris

The rectus femoris is frequently injured by a mistimed kicking action. On examination, pain is usually apparent to resisted knee extension and hip flexion. Passive stretch into knee flexion coupled with hip extension and adduction is also painful. Injury is usually to either the upper insertion or the mid-belly. Upper insertion injuries are palpated with the patient half-lying to relax the muscle. The area of injury is usually the musculotendinous junction approximately four finger widths below the anterior superior iliac spine.

> **Keypoint**
>
> The most common point of injury to the rectus femoris is at the musculotendinous (MT) junction four fingerbreadths below the anterior superior iliac spine (ASIS).

Tenderness to the reflected head attaching to the anterior inferior iliac spine in a youth should raise the question of avulsion injury and may require X-ray confirmation.

Mid-belly tears are less common and are usually sited within the middle third of the thigh. Here, the muscle is subcutaneous and any swelling is immediately apparent. The athlete should flex the hip and knee to 45° against

Figure 9.5   (a) Rectus femoris strengthening combining hip flexion and knee extension against elastic band resistance. (b) Rectus stretch. (i) Correct with pelvis fixed. (ii) Incorrect, anterior pelvic tilt throws stress on lumbar spine. (c) Alternate leg lunge. Front leg stresses quadriceps and gluteals, rear leg stresses hip flexors and knee extensors.

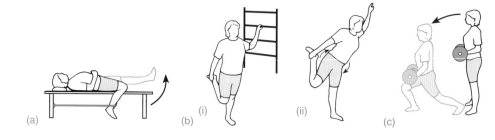

resistance, and as the muscle stands out any abnormality will become apparent.

The rectus femoris can be worked concentrically by flexing the hip against a resistance supplied by a weight bag attached to the knee. Two-joint action of the muscle can be worked with the athlete in supine with the injured leg over the couch side, flexed at both the knee and hip. Manual resistance is applied to the foot of the athlete as he or she extends the knee and flexes the hip simultaneously (Fig. 9.5a).

Stretching must involve both knee flexion and hip extension and can be carried out in a side-lying position by the athlete, or by the therapist. When performing a rectus femoris stretch in standing (Fig. 9.5b), the abdominal muscles must be tightened to stabilize the pelvis before the hip stretch is applied. Failure to do so will increase the apparent range of motion by anterior tilt of the pelvis with stress thrown on the lumbar spine. Lunging actions are also useful, for both general flexibility and eccentric control (Fig. 9.5c).

> **Keypoint**
>
> The rectus femoris muscle must be stretched and strengthened at both the knee and hip simultaneously.

Results are generally very good, even with complete tears (Fig. 9.6), where full function may be regained even though a marked muscle deformity is present.

Sartorius

Injury to the sartorius is usually an avulsion from the anterior superior iliac spine. There is usually immediate pain, often radiating into the anterior thigh. Swelling and bruising is seen over the iliac crest, often tracking down the thigh. Flexion/adduction of the hip with flexion of the knee causes pain. Displacement of the bone fragment may be from a few mm to 3 cm, but although surgical reattachment of the bone fragment has been described (Veselko and Smrkolj, 1994), conservative treatment normally suffices. The athlete should be non-weight bearing initially, followed by partial weight-bearing ambulation for 3–6 weeks, depending on the intensity of pain. Full strength and flexibility must be regained before competitive sport is resumed.

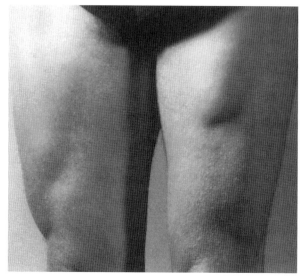

Figure 9.6   Rectus femoris tear. From Reid (1992) with permission.

The hamstrings

The hamstrings may be injured either at their attachment to the ischial tuberosity or within their mid-bellies and, less commonly, at the knee (see below). The hamstring pull is the classic sprinting injury, with the athlete spectacularly pulling up in mid-flight with obvious pain.

Pain is apparent on straight leg raising and resisted knee flexion. Resisted flexion and tibial rotation will determine whether the biceps femoris or semimembranosus and semitendinosus is affected.

To palpation, the structure of the muscles differentiates them. The semitendinosus and long head of biceps have a combined attachment on the lower medial facet of the ischial tuberosity, the two muscles travelling together for a short distance until they form fusiform muscle bellies. The semitendinosus almost instantly forms into a long slender tendon, and travels around the medial condyle of the tibia to attach to the medial surface of the tibia below gracilis. The biceps has two proximal attachments; the long head, as described, and the short head from the lower linea aspera. The muscle swings downwards and laterally across the posterior aspect of the thigh and around the lateral ligament to insert into the head of the fibula. The biceps has a dual innervation, and asynchronous stimulation of the two heads has been described as a factor in injury (Burkett, 1975). The semimembranosus comes from the lateral facet of the ischial tuberosity and travels down and medially, becoming flattened and broader as it does so. The semimembranosus is deep to both the semitendinosus and biceps, and divides into five components when it reaches the knee (p. 249). The principal insertion is to the posterior aspect of the medial tibial tubercle.

> ### Keypoint
>
> The semimembranosus attaches from the *lateral* aspect of the ischial tuberosity, the semitendinosus and biceps from the medial. At the knee the biceps is *lateral*, the semitendinosus (medial) is *cord-like* and the semitendonosus (medial) is *flat*.

Biomechanics and hamstring injury

During the running cycle (p. 123), the hamstrings contract eccentrically to decelerate the leg in late forward swing. This action also helps to stabilize the knee. During the support phase, the hamstrings act concentrically to extend the hip, and continue to stabilize the knee by preventing knee extension. During push-off, the hamstrings and gastrocnemius, both two-joint muscles, paradoxically extend the knee (see p. 17, action of two-joint muscles). This action is necessary because the mechanical efficiency of the quadriceps is reducing at this point (Sutton, 1984).

The ratio of the strength of the hamstrings to that of the quadriceps muscles (HQ ratio) is important. Normally, the quadriceps is the stronger of the two muscle groups (Table 9.2), as demonstrated by its greater volume. However, any disturbance to this natural balance may leave the weaker muscle group open to injury. The optimum value of the HQ ratio varies from 50% to 80% (Kannus, 1989), with average values in the region of 60%. After knee injury, quadriceps wasting may result in the two muscle groups producing the same power, giving an HQ ratio of 100% (Burnie and Brodie, 1986a).

Strength measures comparing quadriceps to hamstrings are traditionally carried out with an isometric dynamometer. However, the disadvantages of joint specificity and lack of movement make isokinetic testing more desirable. During isokinetic testing the speed of movement should match the speed of the sport as closely as possible. The speed must be quoted, as the absolute value of the HQ ratio increases as velocity of movement increases (Burnie and Brodie, 1986b). Slow speeds (45°/s) have been shown to give ratios of 60% and high speeds (300°/s) ratios of 80% (Sutton, 1984). Isokinetic testing in the standard sitting position does not allow hip motion, and movement of the limb does not occur in a closed kinetic chain, so testing is not ideal.

Aetiology of hamstring injury

Tears tend to occur when there is a breakdown in the reciprocal action of the quadriceps and hamstrings, and happen

Table 9.2 Percentage of strength relative to quadriceps at 100%

Hamstrings	50–60%
Adductors	90%
Abductors	60%
Hip flexors	55%

From Reid (1992) with permission.

at one of two instances in the running cycle. First, during late forward swing as the hamstrings are decelerating the limb and the athlete feels the muscle 'stretch', and secondly, during the take off phase as the athlete 'pushes'. Changes in muscle coordination as a result of an alteration in the sensitivity of muscle spindles have been cited as a contributory factor to injury. It has been suggested (Sutton, 1984) that an athlete who is fatigued unconsciously increases the sensitivity of the muscle spindles, which respond to stretch with an exaggerated contraction, and this in turn causes injury.

Lack of flexibility may predispose to hamstring injury, and may be assessed with the athlete lying supine with one hip flexed to 90°. Maintaining this position by gripping the leg with the hands, the athlete attempts to straighten the leg with quadriceps power only (AKE test). Adequate flexibility is indicated by an ability to lock the leg out while maintaining 90° hip flexion. Alterations in the normal 60% strength ratio between the quadriceps and hamstrings and a deficit greater than 10% between the two sets of hamstrings has also been cited as a predisposing factor (Burkett, 1970).

Many hamstring injuries tend to recur, and lack of full rehabilitation may be one cause. After injury, athletes are usually aware of lack of mobility in the hamstrings and are often conscientious about stretching exercises. However, muscle wasting is not so obvious in the hamstrings as it is in the quadriceps, and so many athletes forget to spend time regaining hamstring strength. In addition, using eccentric exercises as part of a general leg conditioning programme may strengthen the series elastic components within the hamstrings (the non-contractile portion of the muscle, including the muscle tendon and the connective tissue framework of the muscle itself; see Ch. 1), making them better equipped to withstand loading at heel strike (Stanton and Purdam, 1989). The inclusion of plyometric training in late stage rehabilitation of hamstring injury is therefore essential.

Exercise therapy following hamstring injury

Strength

Exercise therapy aims to progressively increase the function of all the fitness components relevant to hamstring function. Strength restoration begins with isometric contractions within the pain-free range to facilitate muscle broadening

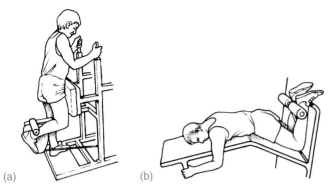

Figure 9.7 Hamstring isolation exercises. (a) Standing leg curl. (b) Lying leg curl. These are non–functional movements which must be used with caution.

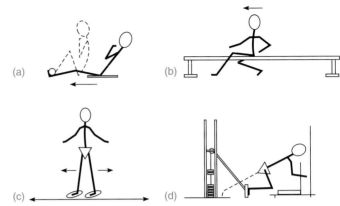

Figure 9.8 Hamstring exercises in closed kinetic chain. (a) Athlete sits on a towel on a wooden floor with feet fixed. Pull body forwards by flexing the knees and hips. (b) Sitting astride a gym bench, grip the feet against the floor and pull the body forwards. (c) Using a commercial slide trainer, straight leg hip flexion and extension is performed. (d) Kneeling on a seated leg press machine, hip and knee extension is performed.

and reduce adhesion formation. Concentric strength is later introduced against limb resistance initially, followed by therapist resistance and later light-weight resistance. Knee flexion may be used in both lying and standing. Hip extension (from outer to inner range) is used in prone lying and also standing. The two may be worked in PNF patterns using hip extension, abduction and external rotation combined with knee extension, and the reverse using hip flexion, adduction and internal rotation combined with knee flexion. Both patterns are used initially against controlled therapist resistance but may be later usefully modified against elastic band or pulley resistance.

Where isokinetics are available, a variation of speeds is important. Slow speeds of 60° and 120°/s may be used to begin with, progressing to 240° and 300°/s as pain allows. Hamstring isolation exercises, such as leg curls in lying and standing (Fig. 9.7), have their place in initial rehabilitation to ensure maximal muscle broadening, but have distinct limitations which must be recognized. First, these exercises work only the knee flexion function of the hamstrings, with little activity over the hip. Secondly, the action is open chain only, when the predominant function of the hamstrings occurs in closed chain format. Thirdly, the exercises are often performed with the emphasis placed on inner-range contraction, which may tend to shorten the muscle. The hamstrings are unlikely to be posturally lengthened so that they require shortening. It is more likely that the muscles will already lack flexibility, so full range resisted work is preferable.

Keypoint

Weight training machines often work the hamstrings only in open chain format. This type of action often shortens the hamstrings and works them at the knee only. Closed chain actions involving simultaneous knee and hip movement are more functional.

Closed chain actions

Closed chain exercises may be performed by modifying many common exercises. Leg rowing (Fig. 9.8a) is a useful exercise. The athlete sits on a towel (on a wooden floor) or plastic tray (on a carpeted floor) with the feet fixed. The action is to pull the body forwards by hamstring action, mimicking a rowing position. Sitting astride a gym bench or 'form' (Fig. 9.8b), the athlete digs the heels into the ground and again pulls the body forwards using leg strength alone. Both of these actions may be performed unilaterally or bilaterally. The slide trainer may also be used for sagittal leg pumping actions with the knees straight or bent (Fig. 9.8c). The sitting leg press weight training apparatus may be used for the sprint kick exercise (Fig. 9.8d). Instead of sitting on the bench, the athlete turns around and places the shoulder against the chair back, and the ball of the foot on the machine pedal. The action is to press the machine pedal with a combined hip and knee extension action.

Speed, power and flexibility

Speed and power are worked using plyometric activity. Stepping, jumping, lunging and hopping actions are all useful and are progressed for range and speed against body weight resistance and for power against weight resistance. For this later aspect, a weighted jacket is easier (and safer) than holding weights.

Flexibility exercises for the hamstrings must take account of pelvic action and the action of the two-joint muscle. In addition, relative flexibility (p. 123) may dictate that the majority of the stretching force is imposed on the lumbar spine in toe-touching type movements (Fig. 9.9a).

Flexibility may begin with active knee extension (Fig. 9.9b). The advantage of this movement is the reciprocal innervation gained from quadriceps action, and the control

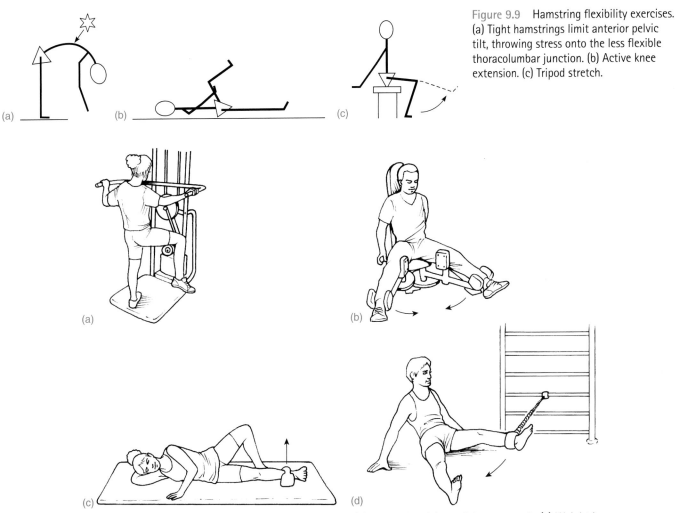

Figure 9.9   Hamstring flexibility exercises. (a) Tight hamstrings limit anterior pelvic tilt, throwing stress onto the less flexible thoracolumbar junction. (b) Active knee extension. (c) Tripod stretch.

Figure 9.10   Hip adductor strengthening. (a) Unilateral weight-training. (b) Bilateral weight-training approach. (c) Weight bag. (d) Resistance tubing.

that the athlete has over the movement. In addition, the back is supported throughout the action. The tripod stretch (Fig. 9.9c) is also a useful exercise which requires a combination of pelvic stability with hamstring flexibility.

Adductor strain

Variously called groin strain and rider's strain, a tear of the adductor muscles gives pain to resisted adduction, and abduction stretch. Damage is usually to the musculotendinous junction about 5 cm from the pubis, or more rarely the teno-osseous junction, giving pain directly over the pubic tubercle (adductor longus) or body of the pubis.

The condition is more common in sports requiring a rapid change of direction, and where the adductors are used for propulsion. Pain is often experienced with sprinting, lunging and twisting on the straight leg.

Ultrasound must be used with caution because of the proximity of this area to the genitalia. Isometric contractions may be carried out by gripping a foam pillow between the knees. During the subacute phase, transverse frictions may be applied with the athlete in a supine position, with the affected leg abducted and the knee flexed and supported on a pillow.

Strength and flexibility

The adductor muscles are often neglected with respect to strengthening and flexibility, particularly in the male athlete. Sagittal plane leg movements are common in weight training, and although frontal plane actions are possible, they are infrequently used.

Treatment for the condition must therefore involve stretching and strengthening the adductors. Initially, strength exercises such as side-lying (injured limb down), hip adduction with a weight bag over the knee (early) or ankle (more advanced) are useful. Later, adduction may be performed using a weight and pulley apparatus (Fig. 9.10). Power training may be carried out by flicking a medicine ball with the foot with an adduction action. Swimming exercises, such a breast stroke, and hip adduction with a paddle secured to the lower leg are also of benefit. Closed kinetic chain actions using running, side stepping, jumping and hopping are included during late stage rehabilitation.

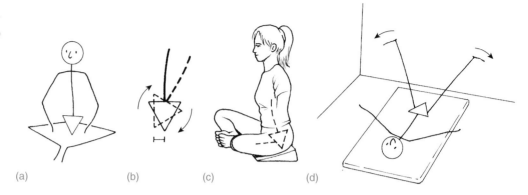

Figure 9.11 Adductor stretching. (a) Common adductor stretch. (b) Allowing the pelvis to posteriorly tilt pushes the pubis forwards. (c) Sitting on a wedge maintains the neutral lordosis. (d) Long adductor stretch.

Adductor stretching may be used for both the short adductors with the knee bent, and gracilis with the knee straight. One common exercise is the 'tailor position' stretch (Fig. 9.11a), where the soles of the feet are together and the knees are pressed down with the hands or elbows. Although a useful movement, athletes often allow the pelvis to posteriorly tilt, flexing the lumbar spine (Fig. 9.11b). The posterior tilt of the pelvis pushes the pubic bone forwards, allowing a greater apparent range of motion and the knee to drop down further. A neutral pelvic position may be maintained by sitting on a wedge (Fig. 9.11c), or alternatively placing a rolled towel beneath the ischial tuberosities. As the knees are pressed down, the spine should be lengthened ('reach the top of your head to the ceiling'). The gracilis may be stretched in the stride sitting position with the leg straight, the same cautions concerning pelvic tilt applying. A more advanced gracilis stretch can be performed against a wall (Fig. 9.11d). The hips are flexed to 90° and the legs straight. Contract–relax (CR) stretching is performed by closing the legs (adduction resisted by limb weight) and then relaxing them into abduction.

> **Keypoint**
>
> When stretching the adductor muscles, take account of the degree of pelvic tilt. Posterior pelvic tilt will draw the pubic bone forwards and release tension from the adductor muscles in many stretches. Ensure that the athlete maintains lumbopelvic alignment throughout the stretch.

One complication of the disorder is the formation of myositis ossificans traumatica within the adductor origin. This is usually a consequence of inadequate rest during the acute stage of the condition. This condition is often described, somewhat inaccurately, under the general term 'osteitis pubis' (see below).

Osteitis pubis

True osteitis pubis is a condition affecting the pubic symphysis rather than the pubis itself, although the two conditions often coalesce. It is an inflammatory reaction of the bone adjacent to the symphysis pubis. In sport the condition is sometimes called *traumatic aseptic osteitis pubis* (Reid, 1992) to differentiate it from osteitis pubis occurring as a result of urological surgery. Shearing stress is placed on the pubic symphysis during mid-stance as the non-weight-bearing hip drops, tilting the pelvis. With distance runners, and particularly after pregnancy when the pubic symphysis is still mobile, this repetitive stress may inflame the pubic symphysis, a condition known as *pubis stress symphysitis* (Rold and Rold, 1986).

With osteitis pubis no instability of the pubic symphysis occurs, but there is tenderness over the area with rarefaction of the pubic bones and widening of the symphysis pubis apparent on X-ray. Erosion of the superior and inferior aspects of the symphysis may also occur (Fig. 9.12). The athlete often has a waddling gait, and may describe occasional crepitus. Severe (long-term) cases may progress to sclerosis and eventual narrowing of the symphysial joint space requiring wedge resection (Grace, Shives and Coventry, 1989). Differential diagnosis between the various persistent groin conditions calls for radiographic investigation and, possibly, bone scan.

Palpation may be used to differentiate true osteitis pubis from tendinitis of the gracilis or avulsion injury to the gracilis attachment. The gracilis muscle attaches to the inferior aspect of the symphysis and local palpation may reveal spot tenderness (Fig. 9.13). Both of these conditions give pain to resisted adduction as well as to local palpation. Importantly, osteitis pubis often gives pain to pelvic springing tests to the iliac crest whilst gracilis conditions do not.

> **Keypoint**
>
> Palpation of the groin reveals the attachment of rectus abdominis at the top of the symphysis and adductor longus as a tight cord at the bottom. Gracilis attaches to the inferior portion of the symphysis away from the mid-line.

Treatment is through functional rest, avoiding resisted exercise and ballistic stretching to the adductors and rectus

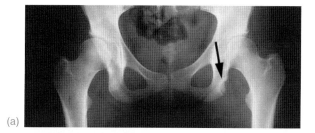

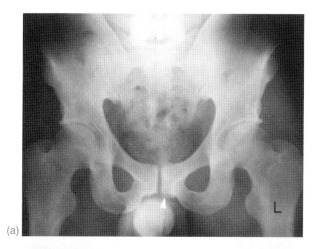

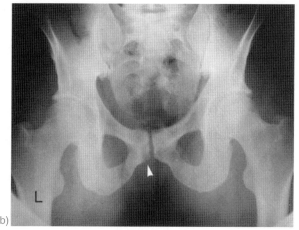

Figure 9.12   Osteitis pubis. (a) Anterior and (b) posterior view showing bone fragment. From Magee (2002) with permission.

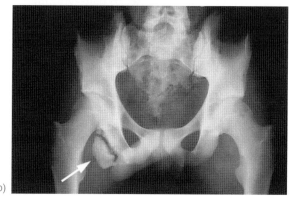

Figure 9.14   Avulsion injury around the hip. From Read (2000) with permission.

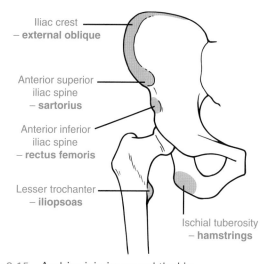

Figure 9.15   Avulsion injuries around the hip.

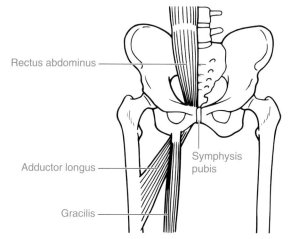

Figure 9.13   Palpation of the groin.

abdominis. Fitness may be maintained with static cycling and aquajogging. As pain subsides exercises progress, avoiding mid- to end-range abduction. After 3–4 weeks, training may begin to involve controlled side step actions and zig-zag runs. This should be used in parallel with adductor stretches. Stretching must target the gracilis, which, as it attaches below the knee, must involve abduction movements with the knee straight.

Avulsion injuries around the hip

Avulsion injuries occur when a rapid muscle contraction pulls on the bony origin of the muscle. This may occur if the contracting muscle suddenly meets an unexpected resistance, such as kicking and catching the ground. Alternatively, avulsion may occur through uncontrolled stretching, particularly unsupervised full-range ballistic stretching (Fig. 9.14). This may occur to the sartorius at the anterior superior iliac spine, the rectus femoris at the anterior inferior iliac spine, the hamstrings at the ischial tuberosity or, less commonly, to the iliopsoas at the lesser trochanter (Fig. 9.15).

Avulsion usually occurs at the apophysis in a young (14–17 years) athlete. However, as the ischial apophysis unites later (20–25 years), avulsion of the hamstrings at the ischial tuberosity may be seen up until this age and has been described in judo exponents (Kurosawa et al., 1996). At this time the tenoperiosteal junction is generally stronger than the unfused growth centre. There is usually little displacement due to the thickness of the periosteum. Athletes usually complain of a sudden onset of pain with limitation of movement over the affected joint. Treatment involves RICE, and, importantly, protection from tension forces over the muscle. X ray is used to confirm the injury and bone healing usually occurs within 3–6 weeks where displacement has not occurred. With displacement of the hamstring origin, suturing may be required (Oravo and Kujala, 1995).

Bursitis

The main sites of bursitis around the hip are the trochanteric bursa, and, to a lesser extent, the ischial bursa and psoas bursa (Fig. 9.16).

Trochanteric bursitis

The trochanteric bursa lies between gluteus maximus and the posterolateral surface of the greater trochanter. Bursitis may arise if flexibility of the iliotibial band (ITB) is reduced. Normally, the ITB moves forwards with flexion and backwards with extension of the hip. The bursa may be irritated if the movement of the ITB is limited, a cause of 'snapping hip syndrome' (see below). Biomechanical faults in running which tax the gluteus maximus or alter pelvic tilt in the frontal plane are also a causal factor. Running on a banked surface with one foot lower than the other, and excessive posterolateral heel wear, which increases supination at heel strike, will increase pressure on the bursa via the ITB. Muscle imbalance between the adductors and abductors, especially in an athlete with a wide pelvis, or in young athletes with a

tendency to run with the feet crossing, may also be a contributory factor.

Pain often comes on gradually over the lateral aspect of the hip, in some cases radiating down to the knee. It may be aggravated by crossing the legs, climbing stairs and getting into and out of a car. Pain may be elicited by passively flexing, adducting, and medially rotating the affected hip, and with resisted hip abduction allowing muscle tension to compress the bursa beneath the gluteus maximus. Palpation for tenderness is carried out in a side-lying position, with the injured limb uppermost and slightly flexed. The patient can often feel the injury while lying in this position because of the hip adduction involved. Pressure for palpation should be directed behind, rather than on top of, the trochanter. The Ober manoeuvre (p. 133) is often positive.

> **Keypoint**
>
> Trochanteric bursitis gives pain over the lateral aspect of the hip. Palpation is carried out in a side-lying position, with the injured limb uppermost and slightly flexed. Pressure for palpation should be directed behind, rather than on top of, the trochanter.

Treatment aimed at reducing pain and inflammation must be linked to a removal of the cause, be it training or biomechanically related. Phonophoresis with hydrocortisone gel may be useful as the bursa is fairly superficial. If the ITB is shortened (the Ober manoeuvre will confirm this), stretching is obviously called for.

In patients where pain is referred and point tenderness is not present, trochanteric bursitis may be differentiated from arthritis by the absence of a capsular pattern.

Ischial and psoas bursitis

Psoas bursitis usually occurs as a result of excessive activity. Pain is reproduced by passive hip flexion and adduction. In addition, slight pain can occur on contraction of the psoas in a position of maximal hip flexion. Palpation over the lesser trochanter is made easier by flexing the hip and knee to 45° and externally rotating the hip. The limb is supported on a pillow.

Ischial bursitis (weavers' bottom) gives pain after prolonged sitting, and may be set off by direct trauma, such as a fall onto the backside when ice-skating. There is pain on palpation of the bursa between the ischial tuberosity and the gluteus maximus. This condition may be mistaken for a hamstring pull but is differentiated by the absence of pain to resisted knee flexion. The condition is aggravated by tight hamstrings, speed work and excessive hill running.

Treatment is by rest from the aggravating movement, and anti-inflammatory modalities. Where ischial bursitis has developed through overuse, hamstring stretching may be required.

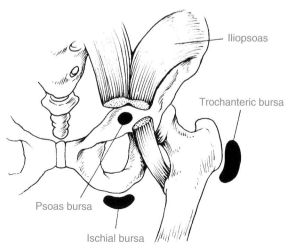

Figure 9.16   Common sites for bursitis around the hip.

Keypoint

Psoas bursitis presents as pain to passive hip flexion and adduction, with discomfort to contraction of the psoas in maximal hip flexion. *Ischial bursitis* gives pain after prolonged sitting.

NEURAL STRUCTURES AND POSTERIOR THIGH PAIN

Discal involvement

The hip is an L3 structure and so can refer pain down the front of the thigh. However, posterior thigh pain frequently accompanies low back pain and may be a result of nerve entrapment in the absence of accompanying symptoms in the back. Distinguishing between sciatic impingement and hamstring injury is not always straightforward. A history of trauma is important, and if straight leg raising (SLR) causes pain but resisted knee flexion does not, the spine should be examined further. Weakness on resisted knee flexion could be through intramuscular trauma, pain inhibition or impaired neural conduction. Lasegue's sign (straight leg raise) will cause pain from sciatic and hamstring stretch; however, adding neck flexion will not affect the hamstrings but will stretch the dural covering of the cord and nerve roots. Pain of discal origin will therefore be worse and that of hamstring origin unchanged.

The slump test is helpful both diagnostically and therapeutically (see p. 307), and is used to assess tension in the pain-sensitive structures around the vertebral canal and/or intervertebral foramen. During the slump test, a hamstring tear will give pain as the leg is straightened, but will not be made worse by slumping the spine, providing the pelvis does not tilt.

Kornberg and Lew (1989) assessed athletes with grade I hamstring tears using the slump test. Where positive, they used the slump therapeutically as a stretching exercise, and found that the addition of the slump procedure to standard physiotherapy management of the injuries (which had included stretching exercises) was significantly more effective in returning a player to full function. They argued that abnormal neural tension had produced symptoms which mimicked hamstring injury. In addition, they made the point that increased tension in the neural structures could elevate the resting tone of the hamstrings, predisposing them to intrinsic injury.

Keypoint

Use the slump test to distinguish between pain from a hamstring injury and that of sciatic nerve involvement.

Piriformis syndrome

The piriformis muscle (Fig. 9.17) attaches from the front of the second to fourth sacral segments, the gluteal surface of the ileum and the sacrotuberous ligament. It then travels through the greater sciatic notch to attach to the upper medial side of the greater trochanter. Its position is such that the sciatic nerve rests directly on the muscle, and in 15% of the population (Calliet, 1983) the muscle is divided into two with the sciatic nerve passing between the two bellies.

Piriformis syndrome occurs in women more frequently than men (ratio 6:1). If the muscle is inflamed, shortened, or in spasm it will impinge on the sciatic nerve, giving pain and tingling in the posterior thigh and buttock. Pain is deep and localized and examination of the lumbar spine and sacroiliac joints is unrevealing. Palpation of the muscle may be carried

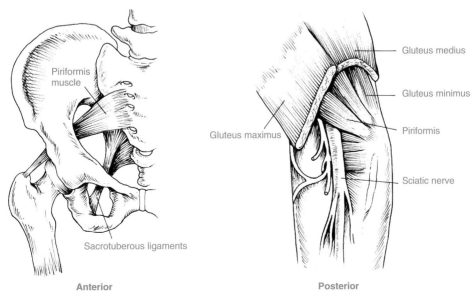

Figure 9.17 Position of the piriformis muscle.

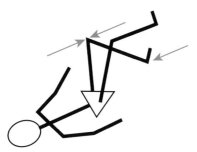

Figure 9.18   Gluteal stretch.

out with the patient prone in the frog position (hip flexed and abducted bringing knee to chest), or rectally. Resisted lateral rotation of the affected hip gives pain, and passive stretch into internal rotation is painful and may be limited.

Management involves pain-relieving modalities and stretching the external rotators of the hip. A simple self-stretch can be taught to the patient. If the right hip is affected, the left hip is flexed to 90° and the right foot is placed on the left knee. The right hip is pushed gently into abduction and external rotation (Fig. 9.18).

Gluteus medius tendinitis

Pain over the insertion of the gluteus medius into the greater trochanter has been reported as a common cause of hip pain (Lloyd-Smith, Clement and McKenzie, 1985). Pain from the gluteus medius itself can be differentiated from trochanter bursitis by palpation (tendinitis gives pain proximal to the trochanter, bursitis directly over it) and resisted movements. Pain to resisted abduction will define tendinitis, while bursitis will generally not give pain to resistance. However, the two conditions may coexist.

Although the exact cause of this condition is unclear, lengthening of the posterior fibres of the gluteus medius (PGM) has been proposed as part of a hip adduction syndrome (Sahrmann, 2002). Here, the PGM and hip lateral rotator muscles are long and weak due to single leg standing in a swayback posture with the hip held adducted and medially rotated. The trunk may be laterally flexed over the stance leg.

The condition is more common in women than in men due to the width of the pelvis, and muscle overstretch also occurs at night with the affected leg on top (adduction and

---

Treatment note 9.1   Trigger point treatment of buttock structures

Pain from muscle origin may be treated by direct pressure and dry needling. Dry needling or trigger point acupuncture involves inserting a sterile acupuncture needle into the muscle which is normally overactive and may be in spasm. As the needle enters the muscle, it meets tissue resistance. The needle may gradually be pressed into the firmer tissue as the tissue gives way. Precise surface marking is required for this technique and knowledge of underlying structures is essential.

In the hip, the major hip muscles treated in this way are the piriformis, gluteus medius and quadratus femoris. The lumbar multifidus may be treated as it thickens between the sacrum and medial aspect of the ilium, an area called the multifidus triangle. In addition, the quadratus lumborum and erector spinae may be needled at their insertion onto the iliac crest (Gunn 1996, 2000).

Surface marking
To visualize important structures in the buttocks, three lines may be drawn joining the sacral dimple (posterior superior iliac spine, PSIS) greater trochanter, and ischial tuberosity (Borley, 1997). The *sciatic nerve* emerges from the pelvis midway along a line drawn from the sacral dimple and the ischial tuberosity. It then runs in a semicircle to a point halfway along a line joining the ischial tuberosity and the greater trochanter of the femur. The *superior gluteal nerve and artery* pass a point 1/3 along a line joining the sacral dimple to the greater trochanter. The *inferior gluteal nerve and artery* pass a point 1/3 along a line joining the ischial tuberosity and the sacral dimple (Fig. 9.19).

Trigger points
To facilitate palpation, the patient should be placed in side lying with the painful side on top and the hip flexed. The *gluteus medius* may be treated about 5 cm along a line from the iliac crest to the greater trochanter. It is sometimes easier to palpate the greater trochanter and allow the palpating finger to move backwards and upwards until a painful point is located. The *quadratus femoris* can only be located with the gluteal muscle relaxed, and it may be palpated from the posterior aspect of the greater trochanter to the lateral edge of the ischial tuberosity. As it is a

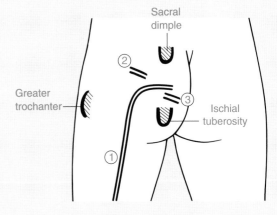

1 = Sciatic nerve
2 = Superior gluteal nerve and artery
3 = Inferior gluteal nerve and artery

Figure 9.19   Surface marking of buttock structures.

lateral rotator of the hip, medially rotating the femur will place the muscle on stretch and make palpation easier. The *piriformis* is located along a line from the greater trochanter to the 2nd, 3rd and 4th sacral segments. If deep manual pressure is used points within the muscles may be chosen. For dry needling, use of points close to the greater trochanter or ischial tuberosity avoids the risk of hitting the sciatic nerve.

The *quadratus lumborum* and *erector spinae* may be palpated along the iliac crest. To facilitate location the patient should be side flexed away from the painful side to place the muscle on stretch. The *multifidus* is large and thick in the lumbar spine and in the area between the PSIS and sacral spines down to a level of S4 (the multifidus triangle), and muscle may be treated for trigger points with either manual therapy or dry needling (Fig. 9.20).

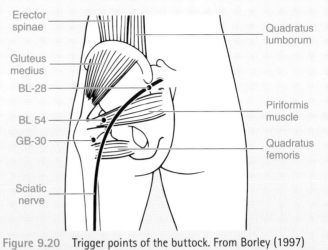

Figure 9.20   Trigger points of the buttock. From Borley (1997) with permission.

Definition

Hip adduction syndrome occurs when athletes stand favouring one leg in a swayback posture. The weight bearing leg drifts into adduction and medial rotation, and the trunk side flexes over the stance leg. The posterior fibres of the gluteus medius muscle become long and weak as a result.

---

medial rotation). Pain and burning occur along the lateral aspect of the hip and thigh, and is worse in the morning after sleeping. Discomfort reduces with activity but increases with fatigue, particularly with prolonged standing.

Restoration of muscle balance is the key to management. Exercises to shorten the PGM are used which combine hip abduction and lateral rotation in side lying (Fig. 6.9c, p. 127). Athletes with this condition should avoid crossing their legs when sitting. When standing they should make a conscious effort to carry their weight evenly over both legs. During prolonged standing they should perform gluteal bracing (20–30 second hold) every 30 minutes.

Hamstring syndrome

Puranen and Orava (1988) described athletes with gluteal pain radiating into the posterior thigh who had no history of trauma. Pain occurred most often in the sitting position, and when stretching the hamstrings. Local tenderness was evident to the ischial tuberosity, neurological examination was normal, and extensive physiotherapy, including electrical modalities stretching and strengthening (no specific details given), failed to remove the symptoms.

At operation, tight fibrotic bands were found from the semitendinosus and biceps femoris, with the thickest actually within the bulk of the biceps. These were located close to the sciatic nerve and in some cases actually adhered to it.

Release of the tight bands gave symptomatic relief to 52 of the 59 patients treated. The authors proposed that excessive stretching may have led to hypercompensation within the muscles, particularly in sprinters and hurdlers.

Keypoint

Fibrotic bands may spread from a hamstring injured at its ischial origin to the sciatic nerve.

HIP PAIN AND THE YOUNG ATHLETE

Pain and limitation of movement in the hip in children should always be treated with caution. The extreme forces placed on the hip by weight bearing, combined with osseous and vascular changes occurring about the joint during adolescence, can lead to a variety of serious orthopaedic conditions.

The blood supply to the femoral head may be compromised in the very young. From birth until the age of 4 years blood reaches the femoral head via the metaphysis. From the age of 8 years, vessels through the ligamentum teres supply the head. Between these two periods the lateral epiphyseal vessels are the only source of blood to the femoral head (Cyriax, 1982). In addition, the upper femoral epiphysis does not fuse with the shaft until about 20 years of age.

Perthes' disease

Persistent hip or groin pain and/or a limp in young males (4–12 years) may be the result of Perthes' disease, an avascular necrosis (osteochondrosis) of the femoral head. The bony nucleus of the epiphysis becomes necrosed. The upper surface of the femoral head flattens and the epiphyseal line widens, altering the biomechanical alignment of the joint. When the bone is revascularized it hardens again, leaving a permanent deformity. Objective examination often reveals slight limitation of all hip movements with protective spasm. The condition may be precipitated by joint effusion at the hip following trauma, or a non-specific synovitis (Apley and Solomon, 1989).

Slipped upper femoral epiphyses

Trauma, or more usually simply weight bearing, in the young athlete (10–20 years) may result in slipping of the upper (capital) femoral epiphysis. The condition is more common in tall adolescents who have shown a rapid increase in height, and in the slightly obese individual. In these two cases hormone imbalance has been suggested, in the first case an excess of growth hormone and in the second an excess of sex hormone (Reid, 1992).

Pain is usually felt in the hip or knee, and may begin simply as a diffuse ache to the knee alone. The epiphyseal junction may soften and, with weight bearing or trauma, may cause the head of the femur to slip on the neck, usually downwards and backwards. If left, the epiphyses will fuse to the femoral neck in the abnormal position. Objective examination often reveals limitation of flexion, abduction and medial rotation (the athlete is unable to touch the abdomen with the thigh). The leg is often rested in lateral rotation, and the gait pattern is antalgic.

Leg shortening up to 2 cm is common, and radiographs reveal widening and a 'woolly' appearance of the epiphyseal plate. On the X-ray, a line traced along the superior aspect of the femoral neck will reveal a step deformity (Fig. 9.21). The line remains superior to the head rather than passing directly through it (Trethowan's sign).

> ### Keypoint
>
> Hip pain in the sporting adolescent must always be taken seriously, and full examination is mandatory. X-rays should be taken if hip movement range is limited with a hard end-feel and the athlete is unable to touch the abdomen with the thigh.

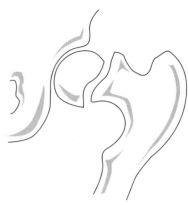

Figure 9.21 Slipped upper femoral epiphysis. The step deformity is apparent on X-ray.

CAPSULAR TIGHTENING

Inflammation within the hip joint leads to the characteristic capsular pattern of marked limitation of flexion and medial rotation with some limitation of abduction. Adduction and lateral rotation are generally full (Cyriax and Cyriax, 1983). Initially, the synovium becomes inflamed, giving synovitis. Pain is from chemical stimulation of sensory nerve endings within the synovium and is often dull and throbbing in nature, being worse at night and at rest. If the synovitis does not resolve, swelling causes capsular pain by mechanically stretching nerve endings between the collagen fibres of the capsule. Eventually, secondary capsular fibrosis occurs, leading to capsular tightening and deformity. When pain and inflammation abate, the capsular tightening and associated loss of muscle stretch and strength leave the patient with hip dysfunction.

Capsular tightening will respond to mobilization procedures and later to stretching exercises. Hip flexion may be stretched using the Thomas test as an exercise. The patient lies supine with the popliteal area of the knees over the couch end. The unaffected leg is straight and hangs below couch level, while the knee and hip of the affected side are flexed to chest level. Hip extension may be promoted with the modified lunge described above.

Treatment note 9.2   Manual therapy techniques to the hip

The hip is a joint which responds well to manual therapy, but as the largest joint in the body, treatment can be difficult. In sports especially it is common to have a very large sportsman such as a rugby player and a very small therapist. The answer is to use leverage and body position and a variety of seatbelt techniques to reduce the stress on the therapist.

QUADRANT TEST
The flexion/adduction or quadrant test (Maitland, 1986) is a useful test to assess the surface of the hip joint. However,

the test requires that the therapist take the weight of the whole leg which, in the case of a large athlete, may be considerable. To make this test more manageable, the therapist should link the fingers over the patient's knee (Fig. 9.22) and rest the far forearm along the patient's calf. The couch should be just below hip level to allow the therapist to lean over the hip as the flexion/adduction force is applied. In this position a longitudinal force (axial compression) may be applied as the therapist flexes the knee slightly, and the body and forearms may be twisted

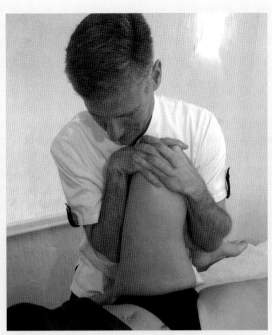

Figure 9.22   Quadrant test using close grip and bodyweight.

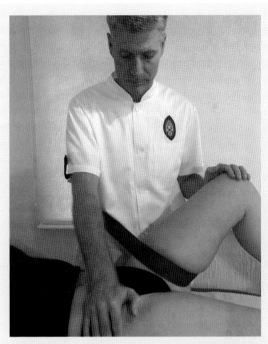

Figure 9.24   Lateral gliding in crook lying using seatbelt.

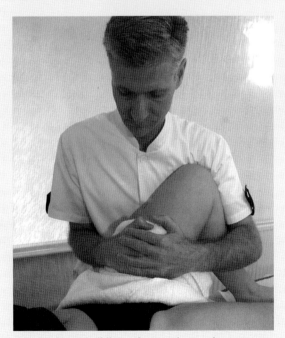

Figure 9.23   Lateral gliding using quadrant grip.

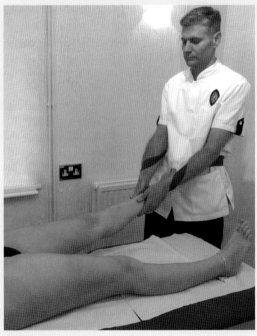

Figure 9.25   Longitudinal distraction in loose pack position using seatbelt.

to medially rotate the joint to increase the contact area of the joint.

LATERAL GLIDING

A lateral gliding (transverse) accessory movement is imposed on the joint by modifying the grip used in the quadrant test (Fig. 9.23). The interlinked hands now grip around the patient's thigh (use a towel to protect the skin) and the side of the patient's femur rests on the therapist's chest. The action is to distract the joint using therapist's body sway

rather than arm strength. The movement should come from a slight softening of the therapist's knees together with trunk movement, rather than trunk movement alone.

Lateral glide using seatbelt

The lateral gliding motion may be increased by using a seatbelt or webbing strap. The patient is in crook (hook) lying and a belt is fastened around the thigh and around the therapist's hip at the level of the ischial tuberosities (Fig. 9.24). The femur

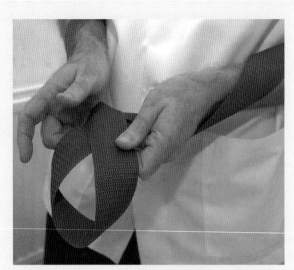

Figure 9.26 Belt position for distraction techniques.

is stabilized by resting it against the therapist's chest and gripping around the knee with the hand. The degree of lateral glide may be assessed by palpating with the right hand. The lateral glide force is produced by the therapist leaning back slightly and softening the knee.

Longitudinal distraction (hip traction)

Hip traction is one of the most relieving mobilizations for the hip joint, where capsular limitation is present. The patient is in supine and the couch positioned below the therapist (Fig. 9.25), and the therapist takes up a stride standing position. A seatbelt is wound around the patient's ankle in a figure of eight – the patient's sock may be left on to protect the skin from abrasion. The belt passes around the therapist's lower waist and the tension is taken up (Fig. 9.26). The hip is positioned in its loose pack position (flexion, abduction, lateral rotation) and the distraction force is imposed by the therapist leaning back. Either an oscillation or continuous traction may be used.

HIP POINTER

The relatively unprotected iliac crest is vulnerable to direct blows from any hard object, be it a hockey ball, boot or another player's head. Contusion is often persistent, especially if the periosteum is affected, and the condition is described as a 'hip pointer'. The pain from the injury is so severe that the trunk is flexed to the affected side. The athlete is often unable to take a breath and may panic.

Following reassurance, the iliac crest is examined and usually reveals dramatic pain but little bruising or swelling. The abdominal muscles are often rigid and the hips pulled into flexion. After 24–48 hours more extensive bruising appears and local tenderness may last for weeks. A raised area may persist for many months. Ice may be used initially to relieve pain, and the area padded when the athlete resumes sport.

CLICKING HIP SYNDROME

Clicking or snapping hip can occur to repeated flexion and extension movements. The condition is common in dancers and young athletes, and is usually painless. However, it is of obvious concern to the athlete as in some cases the sound is loud enough for others to hear.

There are two main types of clicking hip, internal and external (Reid, 1992). Although there have been many proposed causes of this condition, one of the most common causes of internal clicking hip is the suction phenomenon. This can occur during exercises such as sit-ups and requires

reassurance rather than treatment. Alternative causes include tight ligaments and tendons passing over bony prominences.

Definition

The *suction phenomenon* is a result of pressure changes within the synovial fluid of a joint. As a joint moves, positive and negative pressures are created within the fluid. As negative pressure (suction) collapses rapidly, air bubbles are sucked into the fluid giving a soft click.

External clicking hip is usually a result of the gluteus maximus tendon clicking over the greater trochanter, or the iliotibial band clicking over the greater trochanter. Sometimes the click can be reproduced during examination by flexing and extending the hip in adduction, in which case tight abductors are a contributory factor. The Ober manoeuvre is often positive in these cases.

If the condition is painful, treatment designed to reduce local inflammation may be required. In painless instances, stretching of the ITB and hip abductors can help. The athlete begins in a side-lying position with the affected leg uppermost. The upper leg is abducted, and hip hitching is performed to shorten the leg (lateral tilt of the pelvis). The pelvic fixation is maintained as the upper leg is lowered into adduction.

References

Apley, A.G. and Solomon, L. (1989) *Concise System of Orthopaedics and Fractures*, Butterworth-Heinemann, Oxford

Borley, N.R. (1997) *Clinical Surface Anatomy*, Manson Publishing, London

Burkett, L.N. (1970) Causative factors in hamstring strains. *Medicine and Science in Sports and Exercise*, **2**, 39–42

Burkett, L.N. (1975) Investigation into hamstring strains: the case of the hybrid muscle. *American Journal of Sports Medicine*, **3**, 228–231

Burnie, J. and Brodie, D.A. (1986a) Isokinetic measurement in preadolescent males. *International Journal of Sports Medicine*, **7**, 205–209

Burnie, J. and Brodie, D.A. (1986b) Isokinetics in the assessment of rehabilitation: a case report. *Clinical Biomechanics*, **1**, 140–146

Cailliet, R. (1983) *Soft Tissue Pain and Disability*, F.A. Davis, Philadelphia

Cyriax, J. (1982) *Textbook of Orthopaedic Medicine*, 8th edn, Baillière Tindall, London, vol. 1

Cyriax, J.H. and Cyriax, P.J. (1983) *Illustrated Manual of Orthopaedic Medicine*, Butterworth-Heinemann, London

Estwanik, J.J. and McAlister, J.A. (1990) Contusions and the formation of myositis ossificans. *Physician and Sports Medicine*, **18**, (4) 52–64

Grace, J.N., Shives, T.C. and Coventry, M.B. (1989) Wedge resection of the symphysis pubis for the treatment of osteitis pubis. *Journal of Bone and Joint Surgery*, **71A**, 358–364

Gunn, C.C. (1996) *Treatment of Chronic Pain*, Churchill Livingstone, Edinburgh

Gunn, C.C. (2000) *The Gunn Approach to the Treatment of Chronic Pain*, Course notes, Westminster Hospital, London

Jackson, D.W. and Feagin, J.A. (1973) Quadriceps contusions in young athletes: relation of severity of injury to treatment and prognosis. *Journal of Bone and Joint Surgery*, **55A**, (1) 95–105

Kannus, P. (1989) Hamstring/quadriceps strength ratios in knees with medial collateral ligament insufficiency. *Journal of Sports Medicine and Physical Fitness*, **29**, (2) 194–198

Kornberg, C. and Lew, P. (1989) The effect of stretching neural structures on grade one hamstring injuries. *Journal of Orthopaedic and Sports Physical Therapy*, **7**, (2) 481–487

Kurosawa, H., Nakasita, K., Saski, S. and Takeda, S. (1996) Complete avulsion of the hamstring tendons from the ischeal tuberosity: a report of two cases sustained in judo. *British Journal of Sports Medicine*, **30**, 72–74

Lloyd-Smith, T.D., Clement, D.B. and McKenzie, D.C. (1985) A survey of overuse and traumatic hip and pelvic injuries in athletes. *Physician and Sports Medicine*, **13**, 131

Magee, D.J. (2002) *Orthopedic Physical Assessment*, W.B. Saunders, Philadelphia

Maitland, G.D. (1986) *Vertebral Manipulation*, 3rd edn, Butterworth-Heinemann, Oxford

Norkin, C.C. and Levangie, P.K. (1992) *Joint Structure and Function*, 2nd edn, F.A. Davis, Philadelphia

Oravo, S. and Kujala, U.M. (1995) Rupture of the ischeal origin of the hamstring muscles. *American Journal of Sports Medicine*, **23**, 702–705

Palastanga, N., Field, D. and Soames, R. (1994) *Anatomy and Human Movement*, 2nd edn, Butterworth-Heinemann, Oxford

Puranen, J. and Orava, S. (1988) The hamstring syndrome: a new diagnosis of gluteal sciatic pain. *American Journal of Sports Medicine*, **16**, (5) 517–521

Read, M.T. (2000) *A Practical Guide to Sports Injuries*, Butterworth-Heinemann, Oxford

Reid, D.C. (1992) *Sports Injury Assessment and Rehabilitation*, Churchill Livingstone, London

Rold, J.F. and Rold, B.A. (1986) Pubis stress symphysitis in a female distance runner. *Physician and Sports Medicine*, **14**, (June) 61–65

Ruwe, P.A., Gage, J.R., Ozonoff, M.B. and Deluca, P.A. (1992) Clinical determination of femoral anteversion: a comparison of established techniques. *Journal of Bone and Joint Surgery (Am)*, **74**, 820

Sahrmann, S.A. (2002) *Diagnosis and Treatment of Movement Impairment Syndromes*, Mosby, St Louis

Stanton, P. and Purdam, C. (1989) Hamstring injuries in sprinting: the role of eccentric exercise. *Journal of Orthopaedic and Sports Physical Therapy*, **10**, (9) 343–349

Sutton, G. (1984) Hamstrung by hamstring strains: a review of the literature. *Journal of Orthopaedic and Sports Physical Therapy*, **5**, (4) 184–195

Veselko, M. and Smrkolj, V. (1994) Avulsion of the anterior superior iliac spine in athletes: case reports. *Journal of Trauma*, **36**, 444–446

Chapter 10

The knee

CHAPTER CONTENTS

BIOMECHANICS OF THE EXTENSOR MECHANISM

The patella is the largest sesamoid bone in the body. It is attached above to the quadriceps tendon, below to the patellar tendon, and medially and laterally to the patellar retinacula. The breadth of the pelvis and close proximity of the knee creates a valgus angulation to the femur. Coupled with this, the direction of pull of the quadriceps is along the shaft of the femur and that of the patellar tendon is almost vertical (Fig. 10.1). The difference between the two lines of pull is known as the Q angle and is an important determinant of knee health. Normal values for the Q angle are in the region of 15–20°, and knees with an angle greater or less than this can be considered malaligned.

Definition

The *Q angle* is the difference between the direction of pull of the quadriceps along the shaft of the femur, and the direction of pull of the patellar tendon, which is almost vertical.

As the knee flexes and extends, the patella should travel in line with the long axis of the femur. However, the horizontal force vector created as a result of the Q angle tends to pull the patella laterally, a movement which is resisted by the horizontal pull of the lower fibres of vastus medialis. This coupled pull causes the patella to follow a curved path as the knee moves from extension to flexion.

The lower fibres of the vastus medialis can be considered as a functionally separate muscle, the vastus medialis oblique (VMO) (Speakman and Weisberg, 1977). The quadriceps as a whole have been shown to undergo reflex inhibition as the knee swells (de Andrade, Grant and Dixon, 1965; Stokes and Young, 1984). However, the VMO can be inhibited by as little as 10 ml effusion while the vastus lateralis and rectus femoris require as much as 60 ml (Arno, 1990). Minimal effusion occurs frequently with minor trauma and may go unnoticed by the athlete. However, this will be enough to weaken the VMO and alter the biomechanics of the patella.

Patellar contact area

In full extension the patella does not contact the femur, but lies in a lateral position. As flexion progresses, the patella should move medially. If it moves laterally it will butt against the prominent lateral femoral condyle and the lateral edge of the patellar groove of the femur. As flexion progresses, different areas of the patella's undersurface are compressed onto the femur. At 20° flexion the inferior pole of the patella is compressed, and by 45° the middle section is affected. At 90° flexion, compression has moved to the superior aspect of the knee. In a full squatting position, with the knee reaching 135° flexion, only the medial and lateral areas of the patella are compressed (Fig. 10.2). Compression tests of the patella to examine its posterior surface must therefore be performed with the knee flexed to different angles.

Patellofemoral loads may be as high as three or four times body weight as the knee flexes in walking, and nine times body weight when descending stairs (Cox, 1990). While the posterior surface of the patella is compressed, the anterior aspect receives a tensile force when seen in the sagittal plane (Fig. 10.3b). The effect of the Q angle is to create both horizontal and vertical force vectors which tend to compress the lateral aspect of the patella but submit the medial aspect to tensile stress (Fig. 10.3a). Clearly, alterations in Q angle will change the pattern of stress experienced by the patellar cartilage.

Knee angles in the stance phase of walking or running will be altered by foot and hip mechanics through the closed kinetic chain. Excessive foot pronation and hip internal rotation and adduction (causing a 'knock-knee'

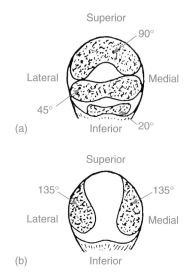

Figure 10.2 Contact areas of the patella at different angles of flexion.

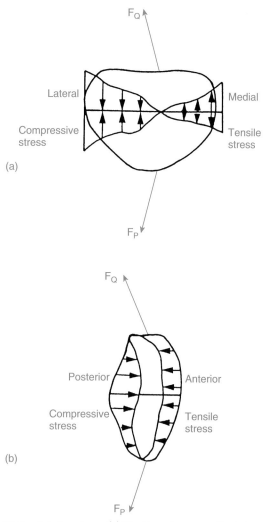

Figure 10.3 Patellar stress. (a) The Q angle causes the lateral edge of the patellar cartilage to be compressed, while the medial aspect is subjected to tensile stress. (b) The posterior surface of the patella is compressed. F_Q, quadriceps pull; F_P, patellar tendon. From Cox (1990), with permission.

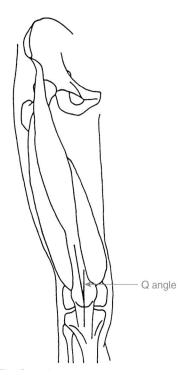

Figure 10.1 The Q angle.

posture) have been linked to patellofemoral pain syndrome (PFPS – see below).

PATELLOFEMORAL PAIN SYNDROME

Pathology

Pain to the undersurface of the patella is variously called anterior knee pain, chondromalacia patellae, patella malalignment syndrome, and patellofemoral pain syndrome (PFPS). The last term is used in this text. It is a condition affecting the posterior surface of the patella, and is sometimes attributed to cartilage damage and, on occasion, incorrectly seen as a direct precursor to osteoarthritis. Since hyaline cartilage is aneural, changes in the patellar cartilage surface itself would not result in PFPS. Furthermore, at arthroscopy cartilage changes are often seen in patients who have no PFPS. If cartilage degeneration does occur with this condition, it is to the ground substance and collagen at deep levels on the lateral edge of the patella. This results in a blistering of the cartilage as it separates from the underlying bone, but the cartilage surface itself is still smooth (Gruber, 1979). In osteoarthritis (OA) the initial changes occur to the cartilage surface of the odd facet (medial) and are followed by fibrillation.

The retinacula supporting the patella may be a major source of pain (Fulkerson, 1982), or the subchondral bone of the odd facet (Hertling and Kessler, 1990). As we have seen, the odd facet is only occasionally compressed in a full squatting position, and so its subchondral bone is less dense and weaker. Lateral movement of the loaded patella could pull the odd facet into rapid contact with the patellar surface of the femur, causing pain.

The complex mechanical relations of the patella make biomechanical assessment of the lower limb a necessity in the treatment of PFPS, and both static and dynamic posture should be analysed.

Muscular factors

Flexibility and strength of the knee tissues and muscles will often reveal asymmetry. The relationship between the hamstrings and quadriceps (HQ ratio) is particularly important and may require isokinetic assessment of peak torque values. Isokinetic testing also demonstrates characteristic changes in the PFPS patient (Fig. 10.4). Eccentric torque production during knee extension is often poor (Bennett and Stauber, 1986) and the torque curve may be irregular (Hoke, Howell and Stack, 1983). Both changes have been suggested to represent a deficiency in motor control, which would explain the often rapid response to quadriceps training that is achieved in these patients. One possibility is that malalignment and patellofemoral (PF) pressure alterations may result partly from subtle shifts in the timing or amount of VMO activity, in particular parts of the movement range (Reid, 1992). The aim of rehabilitation is therefore more a case of motor skill acquisition than pure strength training.

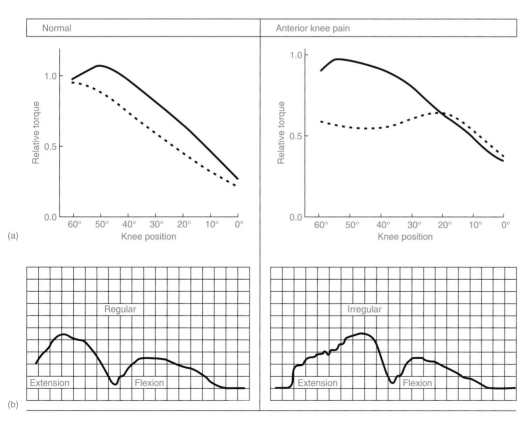

Figure 10.4 Characteristic changes in isokinetic evaluation with anterior knee pain. (a) Relative torque. (b) Shape of torque curve.

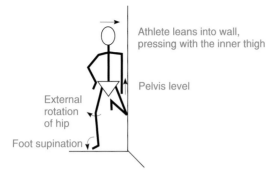

Figure 10.5   Closed chain patellar stability re-education.

> **Keypoint**
>
> In PFPS patella dysfunction may result from a shift in the timing of VMO (vastus medialis obliquus) activity during movement. Retraining depends on re-educating the motor skill involved in knee movement rather than pure strength.

Weakness or malfunction in the VMO will allow the patella to drift laterally as the quadriceps contract. Normally the ratio of VMO to vastus lateralis (VL) is 1:1, and VMO activity is that of a stabilizing muscle in that it is tonic (Reynolds et al., 1983). In the PFPS patient the VMO to VL ratio is less than 1 as the VMO weakens. In addition, its contractile nature becomes phasic, as its endurance capacity is reduced.

Strengthening has traditionally been achieved by the use of short-range quadriceps exercises and straight leg raising exercises. However, these are both open chain movements and as the knee is in closed chain motion during the stance phase of gait, closed chain actions are more likely to carry over into functional activities.

Closed chain VMO re-education may be carried out by performing limited range squats (1/4 squat exercise) or lunges moving the knee from 20–30° flexion to full extension. Step downs from a single stair are useful as they can retrain correct knee motion. The patient should be instructed to keep the knee over the centre of the foot (avoiding adduction and medial rotation) throughout the movement. The use of surface electromyography (sEMG) can help with re-education. The sEMG electrode is placed over the VMO and the patient is taught to activate the muscle in standing and then to maintain this activation throughout the 1/4 squat exercise. The full motor pattern is of foot supination, slight hip abduction and external rotation while maintaining VMO contraction. This may be achieved by standing side on to a wall with the injured leg on the outside (Fig. 10.5). The inner knee and hip are flexed to 45° and this knee presses against the wall, enabling the athlete to hold the trunk vertical while standing on one leg. This body position places significant loading on the gluteus medius of the outer leg to maintain the horizontal pelvic alignment. The foot is supinated, leg turned out and knee slightly flexed to 20°. EMG biofeedback is used over the VMO, and palpation is used to facilitate gluteus medius activity (McConnell, 1994).

In cases where genu recurvatum is present, strengthening of the hamstrings may be required in an attempt to correct the knee hyperextension. In addition to knee musculature, hip strength is particularly important. The hip abductors and lateral rotators warrant special attention as weakness here has been associated with this condition (Beckman, Craig and Lehman, 1989). It is common for young athletes to allow the knee to adduct and medially rotate when descending stairs. This may be due to weakness in the hip abductors, particularly gluteus medius, causing the iliotibial band (ITB) to overwork and tighten. This structure in turn pulls on the patella laterally, displacing or tilting it. Manual muscle testing of the gluteus medius in a side-lying position will often reveal weakness in the affected leg, and tightness in the ITB should be evaluated.

Muscle tightness must be evaluated. The hamstrings, ITB, quadriceps, hip flexors (iliopsoas and rectus femoris), hip rotators and gastrocnemius should all be addressed, as tightness in these structures can alter both knee alignment and gait. Tests, which may also be used as stretching exercises, are shown with average values in Table 10.1. ITB tightness may pull the patella laterally during flexion, while tight hamstrings could result in increased knee flexion and a resultant increase in patellofemoral compression forces. A tight gastrocnemius, in addition to increasing or prolonging knee flexion during gait, will also cause compensatory subtalar pronation.

> **Keypoint**
>
> Soft-tissue assessment and muscle balance tests are a priority in the management of patellar pain.

Foot biomechanics

During normal running gait (see Ch. 8), the subtaloid joint (STJ) is slightly supinated at heel strike. As the foot moves into ground contact, the joint pronates, pulling the lower limb into internal rotation and unlocking the knee. As the gait cycle progresses, the STJ moves into supination, externally rotating the leg as the knee extends (locks) to push the body forward. This biomechanical action is combining mobility and shock absorbtion (STJ pronation and knee flexion) with rigidity and power transmission (STJ supination and knee extension), and shows the intricate link between foot and knee function.

If STJ pronation is excessive or prolonged, external rotation of the lower limb will be delayed. At the beginning of the stance phase, STJ pronation should have finished but if it continues the tibia will remain externally rotated, stopping the knee from locking. The leg must compensate to prevent excessive strain on its structures, and so the femur rotates instead of the tibia and the knee is able to lock once

Table 10.1 Flexibility tests/exercises used in the management of anterior knee pain

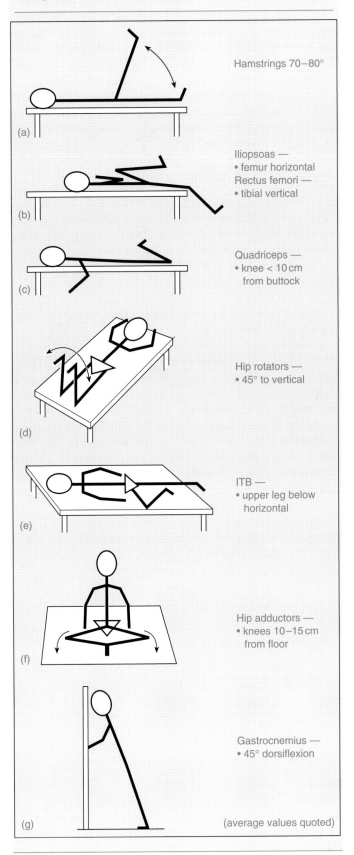

(a) Hamstrings 70–80°

(b) Iliopsoas —
• femur horizontal
Rectus femori —
• tibial vertical

(c) Quadriceps —
• knee < 10 cm from buttock

(d) Hip rotators —
• 45° to vertical

(e) ITB —
• upper leg below horizontal

(f) Hip adductors —
• knees 10–15 cm from floor

(g) Gastrocnemius —
• 45° dorsiflexion

(average values quoted)

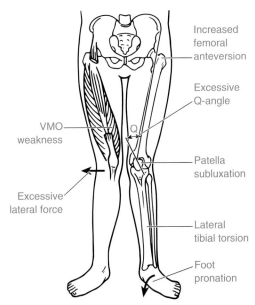

Figure 10.6 Malalignment factors in patellofemoral pain. From Magee (2002), with permission.

more. As the femur rotates internally in this manner, the patella is forced to track laterally.

In certain circumstances the patella can cope with this extra stress, but if additional malalignment factors exist, they are compounded (Fig. 10.6). Anteversion of the femur (internal rotation), VMO weakness and tightness of the lateral retinaculum may all increase the lateral patellar tracking causing symptoms (Tiberio, 1987). For PFPS to be treated effectively therefore, a biomechanical assessment of the lower limb is mandatory. If hyperpronation is present, it must be corrected. This will involve assessment of sports footwear, patient education and orthotic prescription.

> **Keypoint**
>
> Hyperpronation of the foot should be corrected with an orthotic device in cases of patellofemoral pain syndrome.

Patella position

A number of forces are imposed on the patella as a result of active and passive structures (Fig. 10.7). The vastus lateralis pulls at 12–15° to the long axis of the femur, while the vastus medialis longus pulls at 15–18° and the VMO at 50–55° (Lieb and Perry, 1968). The medial and lateral retinacula, if tight, may tilt the patella (Norkin and Levangie, 1992). The ITB attaches to the patella via a small slip from its lower end called the iliopatellar band (Terry, Hughston and Norwook, 1986). The ITB has a connection to the biceps femoris through the lateral intermuscular septum.

Quantifying the position of the patella is important because, as we have seen above, excessive pressure on the odd facet may result if the patella position is at fault.

McConnell (1986) described four different patellar position faults which could be assessed with the patient in the supine position with the quadriceps relaxed. By using the patellar poles as landmarks and comparing their position to the planes of the femur, any malalignment becomes evident. In addition, accessory patellar movements can be assessed with particular emphasis on medial and lateral gliding.

Patellar glide occurs when the patella moves from a neutral position. The distance from the centre of the patella to the medial and lateral femoral condyles is assessed. A difference in the medial distance compared to the lateral of greater than 0.5 cm is significant (Fig. 10.8a). Tightness in the lateral retinaculum, a frequent occurrence in PFPS sufferers, will cause lateralization of the patella. Patellar tilt evaluates the position of the medial and lateral facets of the

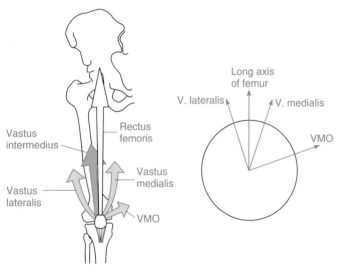

Figure 10.7   Angle of pull of quadriceps onto patella.

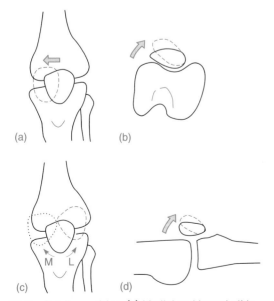

Figure 10.8   Patellar position. (a) Medial and lateral glide. (b) Medial and lateral tilt. (c) Rotation—M: medial, L: lateral. (d) Anteroposterior tilt.

patella, with PF pain patients frequently showing a more prominent medial facet with difficulty actually palpating the lateral and posterior edge of the patella (Fig. 10.8b). Patellar rotation occurs when the inferior pole of the patella deviates from a neutral position. Medial (internal) rotation occurs when the inferior pole of the patella lies medial to the long axis of the femur. Lateral (external) rotation is present when the inferior pole of the patella lies lateral to the long axis of the femur (Fig. 10.8c). Anteroposterior (AP) tilt exists when both the superior and inferior poles are not clear to palpate, indicating that one is lower into the surrounding soft tissue (Fig. 10.8d).

Measurement of patellar position

Arno (1990) attempted to quantify the patellar position clinically with a description of the A angle. This relates patellar orientation to that of the tibial tubercle. The poles of the patella are palpated and a line is drawn bisecting the patella. Another line is drawn from the tibial tubercle to the apex of the inferior pole of the patella and the angle of intersection forms the A angle (Fig. 10.9). The same author argued that an A angle greater than 35° constituted malalignment when the Q angle remained constant.

Radiographic assessment of patellar position is more reliable than clinical measurements (Larsen et al., 1995). Three common measurements are used (Fig. 10.10). Patellofemoral congruence angle (PFCA) is the angle formed between a line bisecting the sulcus angle and a line connecting the apex of the sulcus to the lowest aspect of the patellar ridge. Lateral patellofemoral angle (LPFA) is the angle between lines drawn joining the summits of the femoral condyles and the patellar poles. Lateral patellar displacement (LPD) is the distance between the highest point of the medial femoral condyle and the most medial border of the patella.

Using these measurements, patellar malalignment is considered to exist when the LPD is greater than 1 mm, the PFCA is >+5° or the LPFA equals 1° (Crossley et al., 2000).

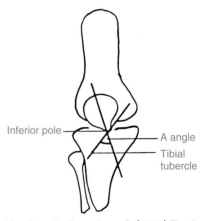

Figure 10.9   The A angle. From Arno, S. (1990) The A angle: a quantitative measurement of patella alignment and realignment. *Journal of Orthopaedic and Sports Physical Therapy*, **12**(6), 237–242. With permission.

Patellar taping

Pain relief may often be provided by temporarily correcting any underlying fault in patella position through taping. Exercising with this taping in place may re-educate correct muscle sequencing to improve patellar alignment (McConnell, 1994). Initially, open web adhesive taping is applied to protect the skin against excessive tape drag. The pull of the final taping is applied using 5-cm zinc oxide tape. Decreased medial glide is corrected by pulling a piece of

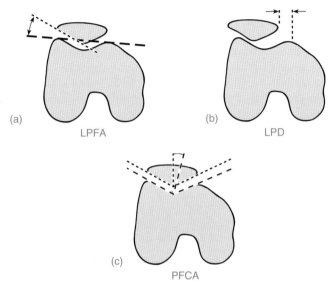

(a) LPFA

(b) LPD

(c) PFCA

Figure 10.10 Radiographic measurements of patellar position. Modified from Crossley et al. (2000) with permission.

tape from the lateral border of the patella (Fig. 10.11a). The soft tissue over the medial femoral condyle is lifted towards the patella to give a skin bunching appearance. Lateral tilt is corrected again by a medially orientated tape. This time, however, the tape covers only the medial half of the patellar face, and again the medial soft tissue is lifted towards the patella (Fig. 10.11b). Rotation is corrected by pulling the patella around its central axis. Internal rotation is corrected by attaching the tape to the upper inner quadrant of the patella. The tape is pulled down medially to rotate the patella clockwise (Fig. 10.11c). External rotation is corrected by placing the tape over the lower inner quadrant of the patella and pulling anti-clockwise. A posterior tilt of the inferior pole should be corrected first to elevate the pole away from the fat pad. The tape is placed over the upper pole of the patella and the patella is taped medially (Fig. 10.11d).

Evidence exists to support the clinical use of patellar taping. Roberts (1989) found a change in LPFA (1.2°) and a reduction in LPD of 1.1 mm in taped knees. Somes et al. (1997) showed a significant improvement in LPFA in weight bearing but none in non-weight bearing with taped knees. Larsen et al. (1995) showed improved PFCA in healthy subjects with taped knees, but this change lessened after 15 minutes of vigorous exercise.

One of the functions of patellar taping is to facilitate selective recruitment of the VMO in the belief that patellar pain patients contract their VMO after the VL (McConnell, 1986). Some studies have supported this hypothesis (Nicholas et al., 1996; Christou and Carlton, 1997; Millar et al., 1999), but others have not (Herrington and Payton, 1997).

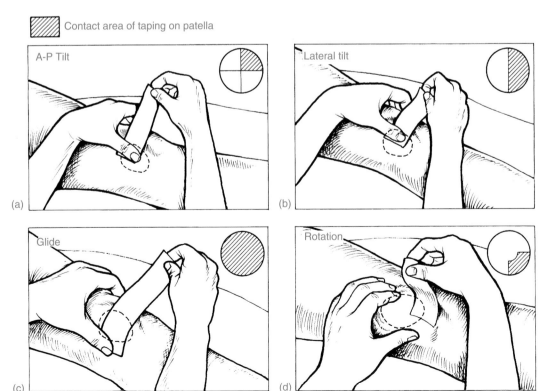

Contact area of taping on patella

(a) A-P Tilt

(b) Lateral tilt

(c) Glide

(d) Rotation

Figure 10.11 Correction of patellar position using tape. After McConnell, J. (1992) McConnell Patellofemoral Course, London. With permission.

Interestingly, patellar taping seems to enhance proprioception, but only in those subjects where proprioception is poor to begin with (Callaghan et al., 2000).

Surgery

Before surgery is considered, conservative management must be attempted. Indeed, Insall (1979) stated that surgery was only indicated when continuous pain limited normal activities for at least 6 months and the condition had not responded to conservative management.

> **Keypoint**
>
> Surgery for patellar pain should only be considered after conservative management has been tried and has failed.

The complex aetiology of the condition has led to a number of different surgical procedures (Fig. 10.12).

Release of tight lateral retinaculum is performed through a small incision or arthroscopy to divide the retinaculum from the lower fibres of the vastus lateralis. Although this technique may be used to decrease a patellar tilt greater than 12° (Zachazewski, Magee and Quillen, 1996), the procedure has been shown to be ineffective at treating subluxation (Post and Fulkerson, 1992) or articular degeneration (Shea and Fulkerson, 1992).

Patellar debridement/shaving has been carried out to remove degenerate articular cartilage on the patella undersurface. Small areas of cartilage may be removed en bloc or larger areas shaved (chondroplasty).

Realignment procedures involve structural transfer to reduce or alter compression forces on the patella. The Maquet operation elevates the tibial tubercle to reduce patella reaction forces and the Hauser manoeuvre uses distal and medial transfer to reduce the valgus vector acting on the patellofemoral joint. The Goldthwait procedure involves release and transfer of part of the patellar tendon. Proximal realignment, by moving the attachment of the vastus medialis, aims at increasing the mechanical advantage of the VMO. This technique is used in the young where alteration of the tibial tuberosity will detrimentally affect

the apophysis. Facetectomy involves excision of all or part of a single patellar facet, and patellectomy entails excision of the whole patella.

PATELLAR FRACTURE

Patellar fractures in sport occur most frequently in adolescent athletes, usually as a result of jumping. Fracture may occur at the pole of the patella, or as transverse, vertical, or comminuted injuries. In the young, the bony fragment may pull off a substantial amount of articular cartilage from the patella undersurface, giving a 'sleeve' fracture. Stress fracture at the distal third of the patella has been reported after sprinting (Jerosch, Castro and Jantea, 1989). Conservative treatment, consisting of immobilizing the limb in a cast for 2–3 weeks, is sufficient in 50–60% of cases (Exler, 1991). Surgical treatment involves internal fixation of the patellar fragments, and hemipatellectomy or total patellectomy in the case of comminuted injuries, combined with immobilization in a cast.

Following immobilization, mobility exercises and quadriceps strengthening is started. Strengthening begins with quadriceps setting (QS) exercises and straight leg raising (see p. 221). An extension lag is common in these patients. The leg is locked from a long sitting position, and as it is raised, the tibia falls 2–3 cm as the patient is unable to maintain locking.

> **Definition**
>
> An *extension lag* occurs when the straight (locked) leg is lifted from a sitting position and the tibia drops slightly. The leg continues to lift but the unlocked position is maintained, because the quadriceps are unable to pull the leg into its final degrees of extension and initiate the screw home effect.

Re-education of the knee-locking mechanism may be achieved in a side-lying (gravity eliminated) position. This is followed by knee bracing with a rolled towel under the knee, the patient being instructed to 'push down' on the towel with the back of the knee and, at the same time, to lift the heel from the couch surface. Short range movements

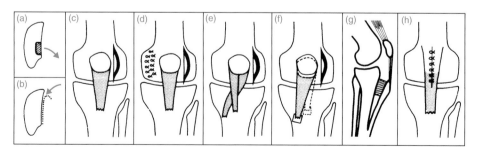

Figure 10.12 Surgical procedures used in anterior knee pain treatment. (a) Excision of diseased area (chondroplasty). (b) Shaving (debridement). (c) Lateral release. (d) lateral release and medial reefing. (e) release and transfer of part of tendon (Goldthwait). (f) Release and transfer of entire extensor insertion (Hauser). (g) Tibial tubercle elevation (Maquet). (h) Patellectomy. From Apley and Solomon (1993), with permission.

over a knee block using a weight bag is the next progression. When 60–90° knee flexion is achieved, light weight training on a universal machine with a relaxation stop, or isokinetic training, is used before closed chain activities.

PATELLAR DISLOCATION

Patellar dislocation may occur traumatically with any athlete, but is more frequently seen in children between the ages of 8 and 15 years and in middle-aged women who are overweight and have poor muscular development of the quadriceps. Biomechanically, individuals are more susceptible to this condition if they demonstrate genu valgum, femoral anteversion or external rotation of the tibia, and if the VMO is weak. Patellar mobility may be assessed by lateral gliding. If the patella is divided into quadrants (Fig. 10.13), reduced mobility occurs when the patella can only glide laterally by 1 quadarant. Increased mobility and therefore susceptibility to dislocation is present when the patella glides by 2 quadrants or more. In this case, more than half of the patellar surface moves over the femoral condyle (Magee, 2002).

The injury usually occurs when the knee is externally rotated and straightened at the same time, such as when the athlete turns to the left while pushing off from the right foot. In this position the tibial attachment of the quadriceps moves laterally in relation to the femur, increasing the lateral force component as the muscle group contracts. The patella almost always dislocates laterally and is accompanied by a ripping sensation and excruciating pain, causing

> **Keypoint**
>
> Patellar dislocation usually occurs when an athlete turns and pushes off at the same time, combining external rotation and extension of the knee.

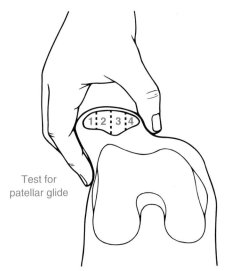

Test for patellar glide

Figure 10.13   Test for patellar glide. From Magee (2002), with permission.

the knee to give way. As the knee straightens, the patella may reduce spontaneously with an audible click.

Swelling is rapid due to the haemarthrosis, causing the skin to become taught and shiny. Bruising forms over the medial retinaculum, and the athlete is normally completely disabled by pain and quadriceps spasm. On occasion the VMO may avulse from the patella, revealing a hollow, and little tissue resistance to palpation, along the medial edge of the patellofemoral joint.

Initial treatment is to immobilize the knee completely and apply the RICE protocol. Aspiration may be required if pain is intense, but usually swelling abates with non-invasive management. Quadriceps re-education plays an important part in the rehabilitation process, with VMO strengthening being particularly important. The medial retinaculum must be allowed to heal fully, and it is a mistake to allow these athletes to mobilize unprotected too soon. Only when 90° knee flexion is achieved and the patient is able to perform a straight leg lift with 30–50% of the power of the uninjured leg are they ready to walk without support.

Early quadriceps exercises

The question of which quadriceps exercise to use at the beginning of rehabilitation is one of considerable debate within physiotherapy. The decision depends on a number of factors including PF reaction forces, the efficiency of an exercise to emphasize the VMO, and the relevance of an exercise movement to functional requirements (see Training specificity, Chapter 5).

The choice is often between open and closed chain movements, and bracing or lifting leg actions. In the gait cycle, the quadriceps are active during leg loading as the opposite leg moves into the swing phase, and to a lesser extent at the beginning of toe-off. In jumping, these muscles create very large concentric and eccentric forces in closed chain format. In a fast kicking action they work in an open chain action, but most of the work is from the two-joint rectus femoris (Richardson and Bullock, 1986). Both open chain and closed chain actions are important, but for early stage rehabilitation closed chain action emphasizing stability is more appropriate.

Comparing the leg extension with the leg press, Steinkamp et al. (1993) found PF joint stress, PF reaction force and quadriceps force to be significantly greater in a leg extension exercise from 0–30°, but significantly greater in a leg press action from 60–90°. These authors concluded that

> **Keypoint**
>
> Closed chain movements reduce patellofemoral (PF) joint forces during inner range of the quadriceps. In addition they are more functional than open chain actions because they simulate the normal weight-bearing activities of daily living.

the leg press was more appropriate because it placed minimal stress on the PF joint in the functional range of motion and simulated normal movement patterns.

It is often argued that QS with isometric hip adduction will increase the recruitment of the VMO because some of the VMO fibres originate from adductor magnus (Reid, 1992). However, Karst and Jewett (1993) compared quadriceps setting (QS), straight leg raising (SLR), SLR with the hip laterally rotated, and SLR with isometric hip adduction with resistance equivalent to 5% bodyweight. These authors found that QS elicited a greater degree of activity than SLR. In addition, SLR with either hip adduction or lateral rotation failed to increase emphasis on the VMO over that of the rest of the quadriceps.

ITB FRICTION SYNDROME

The ITB is a non-elastic collagen cord stretching from the pelvis to below the knee. At the top it is attached to the iliac crest where it blends with the gluteus maximus and tensor fascia lata. As the tract descends down the lateral side of the thigh, its deep fibres attach to the linea aspera of the femur. The superficial fibres continue downwards to attach to the lateral femoral condyle, lateral patellar retinaculum and anterolateral aspect of the tibial condyle (Gerdy's tubercle). A large amount of the lateral retinaculum actually arises from the ITB to form the iliopatellar band having a direct effect on patellar tracking (Zachazewski, Magee and Quillen, 1996).

In standing, the ITB lies posterior to the hip axis and anterior to the knee axis, and therefore helps to maintain hip and knee extension, reducing the muscle work required to sustain an upright stance. As the knee flexes to 30° the ITB passes posterior to the knee joint axis, and in so doing it glides over the lateral femoral condyle. In running, during the swing phase the ITB lies anterior to the greater trochanter and hip flexion/extension axis, reducing the workload required for hip flexion.

Aetiology

Tightness of the ITB can occur in a number of patient groups. The tall, lanky teenager who has recently undergone the adolescent growth spurt may experience pain if soft tissue elongation lags behind long bone development. Tightness in adolescent females is a consistent factor in PFPS, although the relationship between the ITB and the patella has been debated by some authors (Rouse, 1996). The second major group of sufferers are adult athletes, particularly distance runners. A number of factors can contribute to problems within this group. Running on cambered roads and using shoes worn on their lateral edge will increase varus knee angulation and may overstretch a tight ITB. Rapid increases in speed or hill work can place excessive stress on the structure. In addition, imbalances of muscle strength and flexibility around the knee and hip may lead to the gradual onset of symptoms.

Pain normally occurs over either the trochanteric bursa or the lateral femoral condyle (Fig. 10.14). Pain is experienced to palpation, but also to limited range squats or lunges on the affected leg. As the knee flexes and the ITB passes over the lateral femoral condyle, friction may occur, causing pain of increasing intensity. Flexibility tests, particularly the Ober manoeuvre and Thomas test, often reveal pain and a lack of flexibility. In addition, compressing the ITB over the proximal part of the lateral femoral condyle with the knee flexing and extending to 30° may elicit pain

> **Keypoint**
>
> In ITB friction syndrome, tightness in the ITB and tensor fascia lata (ITB/TFL) is usually associated with poor tone and lengthening of the gluteus medius muscle. The ITB/TFL must be stretched and the gluteus retrained in its inner range to shorten it.

Figure 10.14 Iliotibial band friction syndrome.

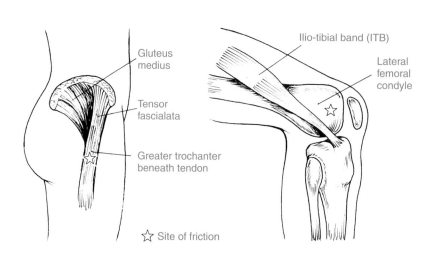
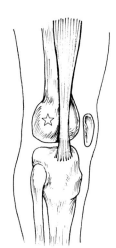

Gluteus medius

Tensor fascialata

Greater trochanter beneath tendon

Ilio-tibial band (ITB)

Lateral femoral condyle

☆ Site of friction

(Noble, 1980). Where the ITB is tight and the tensor fascia lata overactive, the gluteus medius muscle is normally lengthened. Both muscles must therefore be addressed in treatment.

Management

The initial inflammation of this condition responds to anti-inflammatory modalities, but the underlying cause must be addressed. Modifications include alterations of running surface and footwear, and changes to training intensity, frequency, duration and content. Where limited range motion is identified, stretching procedures are called for. Hip flexor and extensor flexibility is regained by using exercises previously described, and the ITB itself is stretched using an adaptation of the Ober manoeuvre.

The ITB insertion at the knee is first heated with hot packs or diathermy. The pelvis is stabilized by the patient flexing and holding the lower knee. The affected upper leg is initially abducted and extended at the hip and flexed at the knee. From this position, hip extension is maintained and the leg is pushed downwards into adduction, and held for 30–60 seconds, with the stretch being repeated four or five times. As adduction commences, the patient's pelvis will tend to tilt and an assistant should press down on the rim of the ilium to stabilize the pelvis and increase the stretch.

Between treatment sessions the patient should attempt this procedure at home. The weight of the leg may be used to press it into adduction, and a weight bag on the knee will assist this. In addition, a training partner or family member can be taught to help maintain lumbopelvic stability.

Weakness in the hip abductors may allow the pelvis to tilt or 'dip' during the stance phase of walking or running. This often gives the impression of a mild Trendelenburg gait, and may be habitual following lower limb injury. Gait re-education and abductor strengthening are called for. The abductors may be strengthened from an open chain or more functional closed chain starting position. Open chain strengthening is performed using a weight bag in a side-lying hip abduction exercise. Closed chain strengthening is carried out with the athlete standing on the affected leg, and keeping it locked. The unaffected leg is flexed at the knee. From this position, the pelvis is allowed to drop towards the unsupported side and pulled back to the horizontal position by hip abductor action (Fig. 10.15).

The gluteus medius muscles, if lengthened, should be worked using combined abduction and lateral rotation of the hip to target the (postural) posterior fibres.

COLLATERAL LIGAMENT INJURIES

The medial collateral ligament (MCL) is a broad flat band about 8 or 9 cm in length. It travels downwards and forwards from the medial epicondyle of the femur to the medial condyle and upper medial shaft of the tibia. The ligament

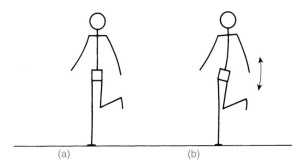

Figure 10.15 Hip abductor strengthening. (a) Athlete stands on affected leg. (b) Allowing the opposite hip to drop and then pulling it up works the abductors of the weight-bearing limb.

has both deep and superficial fibres, with the deep fibres attaching to the medial meniscus, and the superficial fibres extending below the level of the tibial tuberosity. The superficial fibres have anterior, middle and posterior portions.

> **Keypoint**
>
> The medial collateral ligament has both deep and superficial fibres. The deep fibres attach to the medial meniscus. The superficial fibres have anterior, middle and posterior portions which must all be considered in treatment.

When the knee is in full extension, it is in close pack formation. The medial femoral condyle is pushed backwards, and the medial epicondyle lifts away from the tibial plateaux, tightening the posterior part of the MCL. As the knee is flexed, the posterior part of the ligament relaxes, but the anterior and middle parts remain tight. By 80–90° flexion, the middle of the ligament is still tight, but the anterior and posterior portions are lax. In this way, the strong middle section of the ligament remains tight for most of the range of movement. The changing distribution of tension strain in the ligament means that the section which is affected through injury will depend on the knee joint angle when the injury occurred, so an accurate history is extremely helpful.

The lateral collateral ligament (LCL) is a round cord about 5 cm long, which stands clear of the joint capsule. It travels from the lateral epicondyle of the femur to the lateral surface of the head of the fibula. The ligament splits the tendon of biceps femoris, and is separated from the joint capsule by the popliteus muscle, and the lateral genicular vessels and nerve (Palastanga, Field and Soames, 1989). The lower end of the lateral ligament is pulled back in extension, and forwards in flexion of the knee.

Damage to the MCL can result from excessive valgus angulation of the knee coupled with external rotation, while LCL damage is normally through varus strains coupled with internal rotation. MCL damage usually gives pain over the medial epicondyle of the femur, the middle third of the joint line or the tibial insertion of the ligament. With LCL

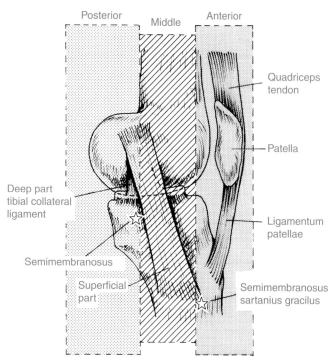

Figure 10.16 Palpation of medial knee structures.

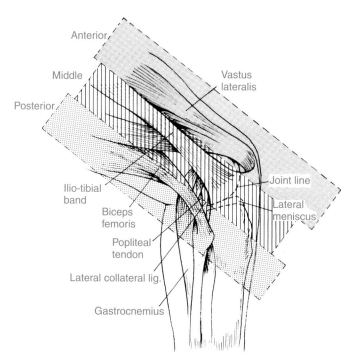

Figure 10.17 Palpation of lateral knee structures. Adapted from Reid (1992), with permission.

damage, pain is normally over the head of the fibula or lateral femoral epicondyle.

Palpating the collateral knee structures

The joint line of the knee can be found by sliding one finger up the patellar tendon and palpating the apex (lower part) of the patella. Rest one finger horizontally across this point and the joint line lies at the lower edge of the finger tip.

> **Keypoint**
>
> To find the knee joint line, slide one finger up the patellar tendon until it touches the lower part of the patella. Rest the finger horizontally across this point and the joint line is felt as a shallow groove at the lower edge of the finger tip.

Palpation of the medial aspect of the knee is made easier by dividing the area into thirds (Fig. 10.16). The anterior third comprises the edge of the patellar tendon and extensor retinaculum and the superficial border of the MCL. Inferior and medial to the tibial tubercle are the insertions of semi-tendinosus, sartorius and gracilis (pes anserine structures). The middle third comprises the MCL and the coronary ligaments. The posterior third comprises the deep part of the MCL and the diverse expansion from the semi-membranosus. Palpation of the lateral aspect of the knee may be similarly divided into thirds (Fig. 10.17). The anterior third consists of the lateral edge of the patellar tendon and the

lateral retinaculum. The middle third is dominated by the ITB and the posterior third consists of the fibular collateral ligament, the tendon of biceps femoris, the lateral head of gastrocnemius and popliteus.

Ligament tests

The integrity of the ligaments is tested by applying a varus and valgus stress to the knee flexed to 30°. Performing the same test with the knee locked is ineffective as this is the close pack position, and nearly 50% of medial and lateral stability is provided by the cruciate ligaments and joint capsule. The easiest way to perform the varus/valgus test is with the patient's hip abducted, thigh supported on the couch and the lower leg over the couch side.

First and second degree injuries are generally treated conservatively. Third degree injuries (complete rupture) have been treated surgically, but some authors argue that stability of the knee is not improved to a greater extent than with non-operative intervention (Keene, 1990). First degree injuries are generally treated partial or full weight bearing with the ligament supported by strapping. Second and third degree injuries are managed non-weight bearing.

Initially, the aim is pain relief, swelling reduction and the start of mobile scar formation. Isometric quadriceps drill is begun and modalities used to reduce pain and swelling (Table 10.2). At night a knee brace may be used to protect the ligament. By the third or fourth day after injury (sometimes earlier with a first degree and later with a third degree injury) gentle mobility exercises are begun, either in a side-lying starting position or in the pool. Gentle transverse

Table 10.2 Guidelines for medial collateral ligament rehabilitation

Phase one (0–7 days)
Immediate post-injury care
  RICE Protocol
  Knee immobilizer (grade II/III injuries) or knee sleeve (grade I injury)
  Modalities to reduce pain and inflammation

2–7 days
Active knee mobility exercises within pain-free range
Progress to static cycle (high saddle)
Deep transverse frictions at multiple joint angles
Avoid valgus stress
Begin hip adductor strengthening with resistance above knee
Begin quadriceps and hamstring strengthening, open and closed chain

Phase two (7–14 days)
Increase resistance on open chain isotonic exercise
Progress closed chain exercise to 1/4 squat (partial weight-bearing if still painful)
Increase range motion using active assisted and automobilization exercises
Begin proprioceptive work

Phase three (14 days onwards*)
Progress all strength exercise
Obtain final degrees of motion range
Progress proprioceptive work
Introduce acceleration/deceleration work
Multi-direction agility skills (sports specific), e.g. zig-zag run, shuttle run, plyometric exercises

(Use aerobic/upper limb activities throughout programme)

* Criterion for progression to phase three: no joint effusion; minimal pain to direct ligament palpation; full or near full painless range of motion; knee stable to hop/hop and turn tests. After Reid (1992), with permission.

frictions are used to encourage mobile scar formation. The sweep should be quite broad and a large section of the ligament treated. Free or light resisted exercises are begun to the knee, hip and calf musculature within the pain-free range. Isokinetics may be used with the aim of restoring the HQ ratio to that of the uninjured limb.

When 90° of pain-free movement is obtained (usually 10–14 days after injury with a grade 3 sprain), the rehabilitation programme can be progressed further to include more vigorous activities, and increased mobility and strength training. An exercise cycle or light jogging may be used, and swimming (not breaststroke) started. Weight training is progressed to use leg machines, and some power training is added. Towards the end of this period, depending on pain levels, shallow jumping, bench stepping, circle running and zig-zagging in the gym are used to gradually introduce rotation, shear and valgus stress to the knee. In addition to improving strength and power, these exercises build confidence and provide an assessment of knee stability.

Occasionally, anteroposterior X-ray will show a bony plaque under the femoral attachment of the MCL (Pellegrini-Stieda disease). The attachment of the adductor magnus onto the adductor tubercle may also be partially avulsed. The condition is normally due to ossification of the haematoma formed at the time of injury (Apley and Solomon, 1993), and MCL injuries which do not improve or get worse with treatment should be examined radiographically to check for this condition. Infrequently it may occur in the absence of apparent trauma. The condition will normally resolve with rest, but where pain is continuous, surgical removal is required.

Definition

Pellegrini-Stieda disease is an ossification of the haematoma formed when the medial collateral ligament (MCL) is injured. The attachment of the adductor magnus onto the adductor tubercle may also be partially avulsed.

CRUCIATE LIGAMENTS

Structure and function

The cruciate ligaments are strong rounded cords within the knee joint capsule, but outside its synovial cavity. The ligament fibres are 90% collagen and 10% elastic, arranged in two types of fasciculi. The first group travels directly between the femur and tibia, as would be expected, but the second set spiral around the length of the ligament. This structure enables the ligament to increase its resistance to tension when loaded. Under light loads only a few of the fasciculi are under tension, but as the load increases, the spiral fibres unwind, bringing more fasciculi into play and effectively increasing the ligament strength.

The anterior cruciate ligament (ACL) is attached from the tibia, anterior to the tibial spine. Here, it blends with the anterior horn of the lateral meniscus and passes beneath the transverse ligament. Its direction is posterior, lateral and proximal to attach to the posterior part of the medial surface of the lateral femoral condyle. As it travels from the tibia to the femur, the ligament twists in a medial spiral. The posterolateral part of the ACL is taut in extension and the anteromedial portion is lax. In flexion, all of the fibres except the anteromedial portion are lax.

The posterior cruciate ligament (PCL) arises from the posterior intercondylar area of the tibia and travels anteriorly, medially and proximally, passing medial to the ACL to insert into the anterior portion of the lateral surface of the medial femoral condyle. The majority of the PCL fibres are taut in flexion, with only the posterior portion being lax, and in extension the posterior fibres are tight but the rest of the ligament is lax.

The ACL provides 86% of the resistance to anterior displacement and 30% to medial displacement, while the PCL provides 94% of the restraint to posterior displacement and 36% to lateral stresses (Palastanga, Field and Soames, 1989).

Injury

Of the two ligaments, the ACL is far more commonly injured in sport, with over 70% of knee injuries with acute haemarthrosis involving ACL damage (Noyes, Bassett and Grood, 1980). The athlete has often participated in either a running/jumping activity or skiing. The history is usually of a non-contact movement such as rapid deceleration, a 'cutting' action in football, or a twisting fall. The combination is frequently one of rotation and abduction, a similar action to that which causes MCL or medial meniscus damage, and the three injuries often coalesce to form an 'unhappy triad'.

Following injury, swelling is usually immediate as a result of haemarthrosis, leaving a hot, tense, inflamed knee within 1 or 2 hours after injury. This contrasts with simple effusion which may take many hours to form (normally overnight). In addition, the athlete often describes 'something going', 'popping' or 'ripping' inside the knee as it gave way. Rapid swelling, a feeling of internal tearing and giving way are essential elements of the history of injury with this condition. The classic anterior draw test is often negative at this stage due to hamstring muscle spasm and effusion. The high strain rates encountered in sports situations cause the majority of injuries to occur to the ligament substance rather than the osseous junction and so X-ray is usually unrevealing.

Manual testing

Diagnosis relies heavily on clinical history and tests for instability, the latter being the subject of some debate. The two most common tests are the anterior draw test and modifications of this, and the pivot shift.

The classic anterior draw test (Fig. 10.18) involves flexing the patient's knee to 90° and stabilizing the foot with the examiner's bodyweight. The proximal tibia is pulled anteriorly and the amount of movement compared to the 'normal' value of the uninjured leg. Various grades of movement may be assessed, grade 1 being up to 5 mm of anterior glide, grade 2, 5–10 mm and grade 3 over 30 mm. The test can, however, give false negatives if haemarthrosis prevents the

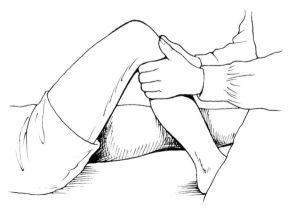

Figure 10.18 Anterior draw test.

knee being flexed to 90°. Movement can also be limited by protective hamstring spasm or if the posterior horn of the medial meniscus wedges against the medial femoral condyle.

Keypoint

The classic anterior draw test can give a false negative result if haemarthrosis prevents the knee being flexed to 90°. Movement can also be limited by protective hamstring muscle spasm.

Lachman test

The Lachman test, a modification of the anterior draw, has been shown to be highly reliable (Donaldson, Warren and Wickiewicz, 1985). The test is performed with the patient lying supine. The examiner holds the patient's knee in 20° flexion, minimizing the effect of hamstring spasm and reducing the likelihood of meniscal wedging. The reduced angle of flexion compared with the anterior draw test is less painful for the patient, and comfort can be further enhanced by placing the knee over a pillow. One hand stabilizes the femur and the other applies an anterior shearing force to the proximal tibia, avoiding medial rotation (Fig. 10.19a).

Clinically, the test may be modified in a number of ways to avoid holding the weight of the whole leg. The therapist may place his or her flexed knee on the couch and rest the patient's leg over it (Fig. 10.19b). Alternatively, the patient's femur may be supported on the couch with the tibia over the couch end. The femur is stabilized with a strap, leaving both of the therapist's hands free to shift the tibia (Fig. 10.19c). If anterior translation of the tibia is felt, the test is positive. The movement is compared to the uninjured knee, both for range and end-feel, an ACL tear giving a characteristically soft end-feel. The same grading system is used as with the anterior draw test.

With the anxious patient who is unable to relax, the reverse Lachman test may be used (Rebman, 1988). Here, the patient is in prone lying with the knee flexed to 20°. The examiner grasps the patient's tibia with the forefingers over the tibial tubercle and the thumbs over the politeal fossa (Fig. 10.19d). Anterior displacement, rather than being felt (as in the classic Lachman test) is actually seen with this modified test.

Pivot shift tests

Another frequently used test is the pivot shift, and its adaptations (Galway, Beaupre and MacIntosh, 1973). These work on the basis that the ACL-deficient knee will allow the lateral tibial plateau to sublux anteriorly (Fig. 10.20). By applying forces to enforce this and then moving the knee, the tibia can be made to reduce rapidly, causing a 'thud'. The pivot shift test starts with the affected leg in full extension. The examiner grasps the ankle of this leg with his or her distal hand and the outside of the ipsilateral knee with his or her proximal hand. The ankle and tibia are forced into maximum internal rotation, subluxing the lateral tibial plateau anteriorly. The knee is slowly flexed as the proximal hand applies a valgus stress. If the test is positive, tension in the ITB will reduce the tibia at 30–40° causing a sudden backward 'shift'. The major disadvantage with this test is that the patient must be relaxed throughout the manoeuvre, a situation often not possible because of pain. Donaldson,

Warren and Wickiewicz (1985) tested over 100 ACL-deficient knees preoperatively and found the pivot shift test to be positive in only 35% of cases. The same examination carried out under anaesthesia (muscles completely relaxed) gave 98% positive results.

> **Keypoint**
>
> The pivot shift test is only accurate if the patient remains relaxed throughout the movement. Accuracy is increased from 35% for the conscious patient to 98% when the test is performed under anaesthetic.

This test is reversed in the jerk test (Table 10.3), while the flexion rotation draw (FRD) test eliminates the need for a valgus force by using gravity to sublux the tibia. A reliability of 62% has been reported for the FRD, rising to 89% with the anaesthetized patient (Jensen, 1990). The Slocum (ii) test (Slocum, James and Larson, 1976) uses a side-lying position to perform a pivot shift and is particularly suitable for heavier patients.

Since the ACL has two functionally separate portions (see above), depending on the knee angle at the time of injury, only one portion may be damaged, resulting in a partial ligament tear. If the anteromedial band is damaged but the posterolateral portion is intact, the Lachman test may be negative but the anterior draw positive. This is because the anteromedial portion is tightened as the knee flexes, and so will be tighter (and therefore instability will be more apparent) with the 90° knee angle of the anterior draw. Similarly, if the posterolateral band is disrupted (the more usual situation), the anterior draw may be negative but the Lachman

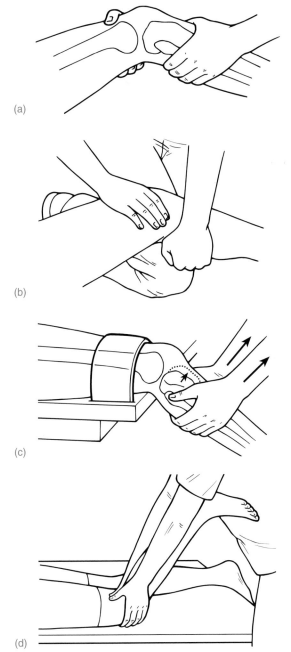

Figure 10.19 The Lachman test and modifications. (a) Standard test. (b) Patient's leg supported over the therapist's knee. (c) Patient's leg over couch end and supported by a strap. (d) Reverse Lachmann's.

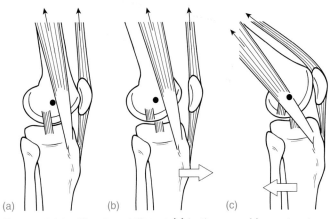

Figure 10.20 The pivot shift test. (a) In the normal knee at rest, anterior pull of the quadriceps and iliotibial band (ITB) is resisted by the intact anterior cruciate ligament (ACL). The ITB lies in front of the knee pivot point. (b) In the ACL-deficient knee the tibia is drawn forwards, pushing the ITB anterior to the pivot point of the knee. (c) In the ACL-deficient knee the pivot point of the knee moves backwards (closer to the ITB) allowing the tibia to reduce with a thud. From Reid (1992) with permission.

Table 10.3   Manual laxity tests of the knee

Anterior draw	Knee flexed to 90°, foot stabilized, tibia drawn forwards
Lachman	Knee flexed to 20°, femur stabilized, tibia drawn forwards
Pivot shift (MacIntosh)	Knee extended, foot/tibia internally rotated, valgus strain on knee as it is flexed
Jerk (reverse pivot shift)	Knee flexed to 90°, valgus stress on knee, internally rotate tibia and extend knee
Flexion/rotation drawer	Leg held by tibia only, knee in 20° flexion posterior force on tibia, then flex knee
Slocum	(i) Knee and hip flexed, anterior drawer test in 30° external rotation. AMRI if medial condyle still moves forwards
	(ii) Patient on uninjured side, pelvis rotated posteriorly. Ankle on couch. Knee flexed to 10°, apply valgus stress and push further into flexion. Tests for ALRI
Losee	Knee flexed to 45°, tibia externally rotated. Knee extended, and valgus force applied, allowing tibia to internally rotate

Adapted from Jensen (1990). Manual laxity tests for anterior cruciate ligament injuries. Journal of Orthopaedic and Sports Physical Therapy, **11**(10), 474–481. With permission.
AMRI–anteromedial rotary instability, ALRI–anterolateral rotary instability.

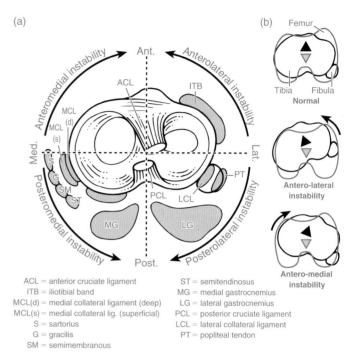

ACL = anterior cruciate ligament
ITB = iliotibial band
MCL(d) = medial collateral ligament (deep)
MCL(s) = medial collateral lig. (superficial)
S = sartorius
G = gracilis
SM = semimembranous

ST = semitendinosus
MG = medial gastrocnemius
LG = lateral gastrocnemius
PCL = posterior cruciate ligament
LCL = lateral collateral ligament
PT = popliteal tendon

Figure 10.21   (a) Structures contributing to combined instabilities of the knee. (b) Movement directions. From Magee (2002), with permission.

positive, as this portion of the ligament becomes tighter as the knee approaches extension.

Partial tears usually remain intact and show good long-term results. However, Noyes et al. (1989) argued that progression to complete deficiency, although unlikely in knees which have sustained injury to one quarter of the ligament, may be expected in 50% of knees with half ligament tears and 86% of those with three-quarter tears.

Combined instabilities

Most ligament tests assess instability in only one plane, but various combinations of instability exist in two or more planes (Fig. 10.21). The two most common instabilities are *anteromedial*, in which the medial tibial plateau moves anteriorly on the femur, and *anterolateral*, where the lateral tibial plateau moves anteriorly. Movement of the lateral tibial plateau posteriorly (posterolateral instability) or the medial tibial plateau posteriorly (posteromedial instability) may also occur. Anteromedial instabilities may be assessed using a modified anterior draw and anterolateral instabilities by the pivot shift (above).

For the modified anterior draw test or Slocum (i), the patient sits with the hip and knee flexed. The test is to perform the anterior draw initially with the tibia in neutral and then with tibial rotation. The degree of anterior movement of the medial tibial condyle is assessed using the standard draw test and then the tibia is externally rotated to 15–30°. The external rotation tenses ('winds up') the anteromedial structures, and if the tibial rotation *fails to reduce the anterior movement of the medial condyle* the test is positive.

Arthrometer testing

An arthrometer measures joint motion. The most commonly reported arthrometer in the literature for assessing knee joint motion is the KT-1000 (Med Metrics Corp. Inc., San Diego, California, USA). To perform anteroposterior testing, patients are placed in the Lachman test position (see above) with the knee flexed to 30°. In this position the patella is engaged in the trochlea, so that it does not move during assessment of tibial movement relative to the femur. The arthrometer unit is placed on the anterior tibia and held in place with Velcro straps around the calf. Leg rotation is avoided by supporting the heel in a shallow rubber cup on the couch.

The arthrometer handle applies a force to the tibia usually of 67 N (15 lb) and 89 N (20 lb). The difference in anterior displacement between the two forces is called the 'compliance index' and is a frequently quoted measure of knee joint stability. Alternatively, maximal manual force may be used and the injured and non-injured legs compared (side-to-side measurement). Tibial translation (to the nearest 0.5 mm) is measured by the change in relative alignment of pads placed on the tibial tuberosity and patella. However, the translation values seen with arthrometry do not represent actual bony motion specifically. When arthrometer readings are compared with stress radiographs, different values are obtained (Staubli and Jakob, 1991), suggesting that an amount of tissue compression is occurring.

Arthrometer measurement has been found to be consistently accurate. Using maximal manual testing and side-to-side measurement, 90% of conscious and 100% of anaesthetized patients with acute ACL tears had measurements greater than 3 mm (Daniel, Malcom and Losse, 1985). Using 141 uninjured subjects, Bach, Warren and Wickiewicz (1990) showed 99% to have side-to-side measurements less than 3 mm using a force of 89 N.

A number of factors can influence measurement consistency and accuracy. First, muscle relaxation must be obtained. Comparing conscious and anaesthetized patients at force values of 67 N and 136 N, Highgenboten, Jackson and Meske (1989) found side-to-side differences greater than 2 mm in 64% and 81% in conscious patients, but 72% and 83% in anaesthetized patients, respectively. Greater muscle relaxation can be obtained as patients become familiar with the testing procedure, and repeated measurements have certainly been shown to be more effective than isolated tests (Wroble et al., 1990). In addition, arthrometer measurement has been found to be operator dependent (Forster and Warren-Smith, 1989). Consistently accurate results will only be obtained with trained testers who have gained significant expertise. Larger testing forces tend to produce better reproducibility, with maximal manual testing giving the most accurate results with all instruments (Torzilli, 1991; Anderson et al., 1992).

Management

First and second degree injuries may be immobilized initially and then subjected to intense rehabilitation to re-strengthen the supporting knee musculature. A de-rotation brace may be used to protect the knee until muscle strength is sufficient. Third degree injuries, with marked instability, may be treated surgically, although some authors argue that rehabilitation alone is the better solution (Garrick and Webb, 1990).

General guidelines of indications for surgery include combined injuries (ACL, MCL and/or meniscus), and high degrees of anterior shear (Feagin et al., 1995). Isolated injuries treated conservatively seem to remain functional. Jackson, Peters and Marczyk (1980) reported a retrospective study with a mean follow-up of 10 years. Of those patients treated non-operatively, 80% of isolated ACL injuries had no functional deficit, compared to only 10% of those with combined injuries. In a later study (Evans et al., 2001), 90% of those with isolated injuries who were treated non-operatively reported that they were satisfied with the result compared to 60% for those with combined injuries.

Patients treated non-operatively are often presumed to be at risk of developing meniscal injury and joint degeneration (Kannus and Jarvinen, 1989). However, X-ray examination and bone scan of patients treated both operatively and non-operatively has shown an increased incidence of degenerative joint disease in the surgically treated group. However, the explanation for this finding is the subject of debate (Woo et al., 1994).

Surgery

Surgery involves repair and reconstruction, most authors agreeing that the latter is more appropriate. Reconstruction techniques may be either extracapsular, intracapsular, or a combination of the two.

Extracapsular reconstruction has been described using the MacIntosh procedure (Wilson, Lewis and Scranton, 1990). A 10×1 cm strip of the ITB is passed beneath the fibular collateral ligament, under the lateral attachment of the gastrocnemius, and then looped back on itself. The knee is flexed to 60° and the leg externally rotated before the ITB is pulled tight and secured with sutures.

Alternatively, a graft may be cut from the middle third of the patellar tendon, to include both non-articular patellar and tibial tubercle bone. This has the advantage that it leaves other structures around the knee intact. Tunnels are then drilled in the tibia and femur, travelling through the attachments of the ACL. The graft is passed through the bone tunnel and attached to the lateral aspect of the lateral femoral condyle and the tibial tubercle. The graft is secured with cancellous screws and sutures. This procedure gives a very strong graft, but may have the complication of patellar pain following surgery. Flexion contraction of 5° or more may be present in almost one quarter of these patients (Sachs et al., 1989), and PF irritability can result. Where contracture is a likelihood, rehabilitation should place a greater emphasis on maintaining full knee extension. A similar technique has been described by Wilson and co-workers (1990) using the semitendinosus tendon instead of the patellar tendon, to avoid patellar complications.

Several structures may be used for grafts, and Noyes, Butler and Grood (1984) showed the patellar tendon graft to have a strength of 168% of the ACL while the semitendinosus had only 70%, gracilis 49%, and the quadriceps/patellar retinaculum only 21%. Synthetic tissues, such as polytetrafluoroethylene (PTFE), are now used more frequently, and mobility may be attained more rapidly following surgery using these materials. However, synthetics are generally only used where intra-articular reconstructions have failed. Bovine substances have been used, but problems have been caused by reactive synovitis following these operations. Allogenic tendon grafts from cadavers and amputation specimens have been used to good effect with patients suffering chronic ACL insufficiency (Shino et al., 1986).

Guidelines for rehabilitation following ACL reconstruction

Rehabilitation will depend very much on the particular surgical procedure which has been performed. As synthetic grafts do not need to redevelop a blood supply, they can be rehabilitated more quickly than autogenous grafts. Intra-articular repairs weaken with revascularization, so the repairing ligament will reach only 25–50% of its ultimate strength by 6–12 weeks following surgery. In contrast, extra-articular grafts regain approximately 75% of their original strength in the same time (Reid, 1992). Tendon grafts often suffer fewer complications and the patello-femoral joint remains mobile, while extracapsular grafts require more restraint on movement. Patellar tendon reconstructions tend to be the strongest grafts but cause greater morbidity due to the anterior surgical approach (Briggs, Sandor and Kenihan, 1995). Arthroscopic repairs will recover more quickly than open repairs as the knee joint is less affected. There is less swelling and a reduced likelihood of complications.

The dichotomy is that immobilization is thought desirable for healing of the graft, but early mobility is required to avoid cartilage degeneration, soft tissue contracture and muscle atrophy. To overcome the combined problem of healing and mobility, the patient is mobilized early, providing the movement used does not overly stress the graft.

The range of motion possible without placing undue tension on the graft must be established, and a protective brace may be used to limit undesirable movements. Sandberg, Nilsson and Westlin (1987) showed the time needed to return to sport to be 5 weeks shorter and range of motion significantly better following the use of a hinged cast allowing knee flexion from 20° to 70°. Noyes, Mangine and Barber (1987) mobilized patients on the second day after surgery and found no adverse effects on the ligament reconstruction. Some authors even begin weight bearing immediately (Shelbourne and Nitz, 1990).

Early rehabilitation (up to 4 days following surgery) focuses on avoiding the standard complications following general surgery, and reducing pain (Table 10.4). Simultaneous contraction of the hamstrings and quadriceps are used to aid the leg muscle pump, but isolated quadriceps exercises and straight leg raising are avoided. Isolated quadriceps bracing has been shown to place considerable

> **Keypoint**
>
> Early mobilization is required to avoid cartilage degeneration, soft tissue contracture and muscle atrophy. However, any movement used must not overly stress the graft.

Table 10.4 Guidelines for ACL rehabilitation

Initial stage (0–4 days)	Speed walking, flat, incline, uneven (not decline)
Modalities to reduce pain/inflammation, and facilitate healing	Step up (not down)
Co-contractions of quadriceps and hamstrings	Side step, backward walk, grapevine speed walk
Prone leg hanging	Flexion mobility exercises
Patellar mobilizations	
	Late stage (6–12 weeks)
Intermediate stage (5–14 days)	Speed walk on varying terrain
Standing single-leg bracing (partial weight-bearing)	Progress weight training
Add trunk flexion to above to increase hamstring work	Jogging
Wall and floor heel slide (ROM)	— flat ground
Shuttle exercise on smooth floor or gym bench	— figure-of-eight
Upper body work for cardiopulmonary fitness	— shuttle run
Ensure terminal extension gained	— zig-zag (slow)
Proprioceptive work (static joint repositioning)	— cutting (slow)
Proprioceptive work (joint stability)	— backward running
— single-leg standing	Box jump (up, not down)
— single-leg stand on trampette	Controlled hopping
Passive (auto-assisted) flexion work	Stair running (up, not down)
	Controlled single hop down (50 cm box) progressing to repetitions
Late stage (15 days–6 weeks)	As above with twist
Static cycle and step machine (holding hand rail)	As above with eyes closed
Leg press	Progress to full range flexion
1/4 squat (partial weight-bearing initially)	
Restore muscle balance (Q/H ratio)	*Pre-competition testing*
Proprioceptive work (joint stability)	Run and sudden stop
— uneven surface walking	Sudden directional change
— balance board	Downhill running
— single-leg standing on trampette, simultaneous arm and contralateral leg actions	Descending stairs (fast walk)
— slide trainer	Repeated jump down from low (50 cm) box
Hop and hold exercises	Sports-specific skill, e.g. dribbling, tackling

After Reid (1992).

stress on the ACL whereas isolated hamstring actions actually reduce strain (Renstrom, Arms and Stanwick, 1986). Prone-lying leg hanging (Fig. 10.22a) is a useful exercise for regaining terminal extension while placing minimal stress on the healing tissues. The patient lies prone, with the thigh supported on a folded towel, leaving the anterior knee free. The weight of the tibia presses the knee into extension. Resistance may be supplied by a small weight bag attached to the heel. The patient then performs eccentric hamstring actions, allowing the tibia to lower as far as pain will allow. A wedge may be used below the tibia as a relaxation stop.

From 5 to 14 days following surgery, co-contraction activities of the quadriceps and hamstrings are performed by using simple closed chain actions. Co-contraction of the hamstrings and quadriceps has been shown to place 15% of the quadriceps tension on the ACL at 5° knee flexion. By the time flexion had increased to a mean angle of 7.4° this force is reduced to zero. As the angle of flexion increases still further, a posterior draw force is imposed (Yasuda and Sasaki, 1987).

Closed chain terminal leg extension is a useful exercise for co-contraction of the quadriceps and hamstrings (Fig. 10.22b). The athlete stands predominantly on the unaffected leg, placing sufficient weight on the injured leg to prevent the foot from moving. An elastic resistance band attached to a wallbar is placed around the mid-thigh, and the action is to extend the hip and knee simultaneously. Adding trunk flexion (Fig. 10.22c) has been shown to increase hamstring activity on surface EMG (Ohkoshi et al., 1991).

The heel slide against a wall or on the floor is useful at this stage (Fig. 10.23a). This exercise may be progressed by performing it against isometric resistance using a large diameter swiss ball or isotonic resistance against rubber tubing. Shuttle exercises may be used on a sliding platform or low friction surface. A declined bench is useful and a linoleum surface or the 'slide trainer' used in popular exercise classes, both provide suitable low friction surfaces. Static cycles and step machines provide useful closed kinetic chain actions in a partial weight-bearing starting position, and will also improve cardiopulmonary fitness.

> **Keypoint**
>
> Closed chain activities using quadriceps/hamstring co-contractions are more functional and place less stress on the graft than isolated muscle contractions.

Muscle imbalance and proprioception in the ACL deficient knee

Excessive hypertrophy of the quadriceps relative to the hamstrings will lead to a muscle imbalance which will alter ACL loading (Fig. 10.24). The normal even distribution of pressure on the femoral articular surface seen with balanced musculature has been shown to change to a focused high pressure point in the absence of opposing hamstring coactivation (Barratta et al., 1988).

However, functional return is not related directly to hamstring strength, but rather to reflex contraction (Seto, Orofino and Morrissey, 1988). Co-contraction of the agonist and antagonist muscles of a joint will enhance stability. As the knee extends, the muscle spindles in the hamstrings will be stretched, leading to mild hamstring contraction (Solomonow, Barratta and D'Ambrosia, 1989). In addition, mechanical stress on the ACL has an inhibitory effect on the quadriceps, but will simultaneously excite the hamstrings (Barratta et al., 1988). A reflex arc from the ACL mechanoreceptors may allow dynamic torque regulation during ligament loading, and mechanoreceptor stimulation from muscles and the joint capsule causes hamstring stimulation to stabilize the knee (Reid, 1992).

Both tension and mechanoreceptors are present in the ACL. Failure of the feedback system from these structures can result in a loss of reflex muscular splinting and the increased likelihood of reinjury (Kennedy, Alexander and Hayes, 1982). Normally there is a minimal, 2%, variation in the threshold to detection of passive movement (TTDPM, see p. 000) between the two knees. With ACL-deficient knees variation values as high as 25% have been found (Kennedy, Alexander and Hayes, 1982). The proprioceptive deficit seems to be increased at near terminal range of

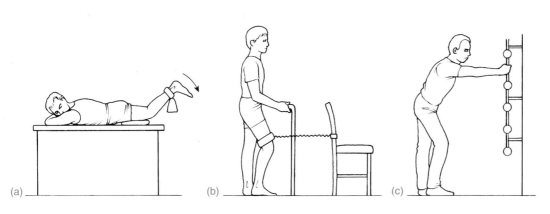

Figure 10.22 Staged anterior cruciate ligament (ACL) exercises. (a) Prone leg hang – to regain terminal extension while working the hamstring muscles. (b) Closed chain co-contraction of quadriceps and hamstrings. (c) Adding trunk flexion increases hamstring muscle work.

(a) (b) (c)

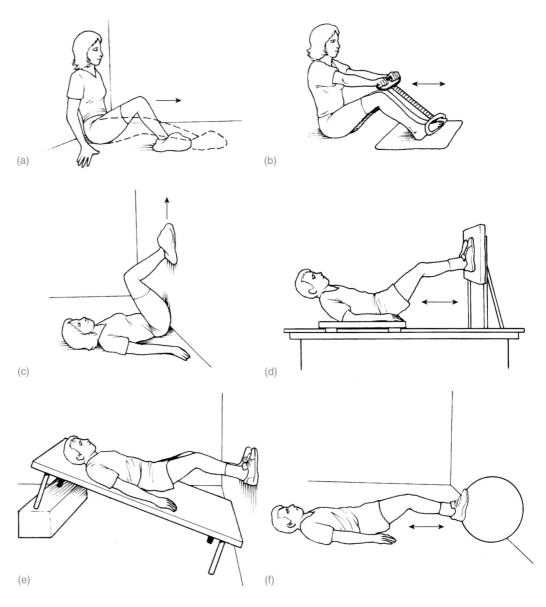

Figure 10.23 Closed kinetic chain action following anterior cruciate ligament (ACL) repair. (a) Floor slide. (b) Slide against resistance tubing. (c) Wall slide. (d) Shuttle. (e) Declined bench. (f) Gym ball pass.

(a)

(b)

(c)

(d)

(e)

(f)

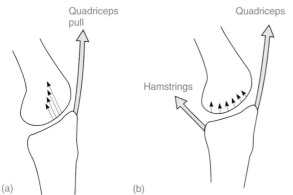

Quadriceps pull

Quadriceps

Hamstrings

(a)

(b)

Figure 10.24 Articular surface pressure distribution with muscle co-activation. (a) Focused high pressure point at the anterior articular surface in the absence of opposing hamstring co-activation. (b) Low, evenly distributed articular surface pressure with hamstring co-activation. After Baratta, R. et al. (1988) Muscular coactivation: the role of the antagonist musculature in maintaining knee stability. *American Journal of Sports Medicine*, **16**, 113–122. With permission.

motion. Lephart and Fu (1995) reported longer TTDPM in the involved knee tested at 15° knee flexion, but no significant difference when tested at 45°.

Hamstring contraction of ACL-deficient patients occurs earlier in the gait cycle and is of longer duration (Kalund et al., 1990; Sinkjaer and Arendt-Nielsen, 1991). Clinically, ACL deficient patients have an increased hamstring contraction latency – the time interval between displacement of the tibia and reflex reaction of the hamstrings (Fig. 10.25). ACL-deficient patients have been found to have a mean contraction latency of 90.4 ms compared to the normal

Definition

Hamstring contraction latency is the time interval between displacement of the tibia and reflex reaction of the hamstrings attempting to stabilize the knee.

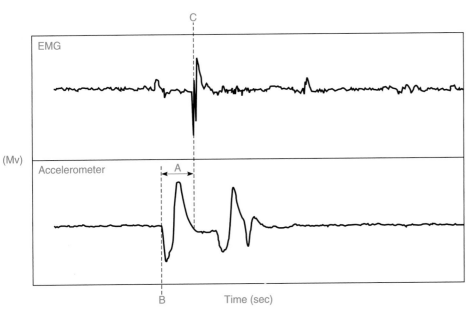

Figure 10.25 Reflex hamstring contraction latency is the time interval between the initial tibial displacement and the first measurable reaction of the hamstrings. A. Reflex hamstring contraction latency. B. First recorded displacement of the tibia (accelerometer). C. First reflex reaction of the hamstrings (EMG). Adapted from Beard et al. (1994) with permission.

uninjured knee with a mean latency of 49.1 ms (Beard et al., 1994).

Quadriceps exercises using short range (from 45° to full extension) should be preceded by isometric hip extension to facilitate hamstring contraction (Seto, Brewster and Lombardo, 1989). Indeed, the use of a standard leg extension regime using a sitting position has been severely criticized (Palmitier et al., 1991). Contraction of the quadriceps from this open chain position places considerable anterior shear on the knee and may stretch the ACL. When performing leg extension on an isokinetic dynamometer, an anti-shear device will greatly reduce shear forces generated with the exercise (Malone, 1986; Timm, 1986). When using weight training, however, closed chain motions such as the squat or leg press movement are more appropriate as they produce co-contraction of the quadriceps and hamstrings to reduce shear.

Proprioceptive exercises for the knee include three components. First, sudden alterations in joint position are employed to retrain reflex stabilization. Secondly, general posture and balance activities are used. Finally, joint-positioning skills form the basis of retraining for automatic motor control.

Definition

Proprioceptive exercises for the knee use: (i) sudden alterations in joint position, (ii) general posture and balance activities, and (iii) joint-positioning skills.

Single-leg standing activities begin the training, progressing from positions with the eyes open to those with eyes closed. These activities may be performed on an uneven surface (thick mat and then mini trampette) and later in combination with trunk and upper limb movements. Reflex

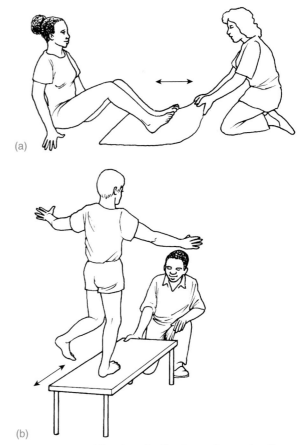

(a)

(b)

Figure 10.26 Rehabilitation of reflex hamstring contraction. (a) Therapist pulls towel suddenly, athlete must rapidly flex knee to stop movement. (b) Therapist minimally displaces stool suddenly, athlete must maintain balance.

hamstring contraction may be performed in crook sitting (Fig. 10.26a). A towel is placed under the patient's heel. The patient must hold the towel in place with a sudden downward pressure (hip extension and knee flexion) as the

Table 10.5 Proprioceptive training to prevent ACL injuries in soccer players

Phase	Exercise
1	Single leg standing for 2.5 mins four times each day
2	Single leg training (1/2 step exercise) on a rocker board for 2.5 mins
3	Single leg training on balance board
4	Single leg training, combined rocker and balance board
5	Single leg training on BAPS board

From Caraffa, A. et al. (1996) Prevention of anterior cruciate ligament injuries in soccer. *Knee Surgery, Sports Traumatology and Arthroscopy*, **4**, 19–21. With permission.

therapist pulls on the towel suddenly. Similar actions may be performed on a low stool (Fig. 10.26b). The patient stands on the affected leg only, eyes closed. The therapist produces a very small but sudden displacement of the stool. Partner activities include single leg standing (eyes closed) with a partner suddenly pushing on the patient's shoulders from any direction. Again, the movement, while rapid, is of small amplitude.

Posture and coordination activities include backward walking, zig-zags, crossover drills of varying complexity and figure-of-eight running. Running on uneven surfaces and lateral step-ups are useful, as is speed walking and uphill walking. Multidirectional running skills based on the functional tests used for the knee (p. 236) also form part of the rehabilitation at this stage.

Accurate static joint repositioning uses cognitive skills and is helpful at various stages of rehabilitation. This may be performed by passive movement on a one-to-one basis with the therapist, or on a dynamometer which shows a display for range of motion. In each case, the patient is encouraged to reposition the joint exactly in the range that the limb rested in before movement began.

A variety of apparatus is useful for proprioceptive rehabilitation. Standard rocker boards and wobble boards, used so frequently for ankle re-education, are also of use for the knee. The 'slide trainer' (Forza Fitness Equipment, London) and 'fitter' machine (Fitter International, Calgary, Canada) are also helpful.

Proprioceptive training using balance boards has also been shown to reduce the incidence of ACL injuries in soccer players. In a study of 600 soccer players, those who included 20 minutes per day of a progressive regime of

Keypoint

Proprioceptive exercises used for ACL rehabilitation have also been shown to reduce the incidence of ACL injuries. They should therefore form a part of a general training programme for 'at risk' sports, and are used to help protect the knee from ACL injury.

five different proprioceptive exercises (Table 10.5) had an incidence of 0.15 ACL injuries per team year compared to 1.15 in the control group (Caraffa et al., 1996).

The early stages of rehabilitation emphasized hamstring activity to reduce shear forces imposed on the knee. Now, any imbalance between the quadriceps and hamstring muscle groups must be corrected with both concentric and eccentric quadriceps training. Again, the emphasis is on closed chain activity, but limited open chain activity may be introduced. With all activities, the shearing stress placed on the knee must be considered (Fig. 10.27), noting that downhill running and resisted isometric quadriceps activity at 20° flexion, for example, produce the greatest ACL elongation (Henning, Lynch and Glick, 1985).

It must be remembered that following knee injury, there is a selective atrophy of type I muscle fibres (see p. 000), so endurance ability must be regained to ensure joint stabilization. Patients have been shown to be able to restore quadriceps strength 6 weeks after surgery (on a leg extension bench) but to still have a 20% deficit in endurance capacity (Costill, Fink and Habansky, 1977).

The squat exercise in knee rehabilitation

The squat is a controversial exercise in both rehabilitation and general training. Generally, the parallel squat (to a point where the femur is horizontal) rather than the full squat (buttock to heel) is recommended (Baechle, 1994), as it is claimed that less stress is placed on the knee using the reduced range of motion. When performing this exercise, less skilled individuals have been shown to produce a large initial drop velocity, to bounce in the low position, and to lean the trunk forwards while pushing the hips back (McLaughlin, Lardner and Dillman, 1979). This trunk angulation increases the leverage forces imposed on the lower back (Norris, 1993). The more skilled individual, by limiting trunk extension, places more stress on the quadriceps and reduces the leverage effect on the lower spine.

The squat has the advantage of being a closed chain activity, but is often said to 'overstretch the knee ligaments' and so is frequently derided. The squat has been shown to work the quadriceps, but significant co-contraction of the hamstrings has been questioned (Gryzlo et al., 1994). Heavy resistance squatting (130–200% bodyweight) used over a 21-week training period has not been shown to increase knee laxity (Panariello, Backus and Parker, 1994). Ligament stability was assessed in 32 professional football players using an arthrometer at 30° and 90° flexion after 12 and 21 weeks.

Keypoint

A squat exercise, *used correctly*, will not overstretch the knee ligaments. It is a functional closed chain movement which, as well as working the knee, rehearses good lifting technique.

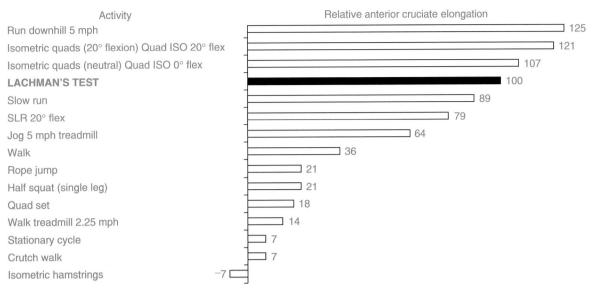

Figure 10.27   Anterior cruciate ligament (ACL) elongation relative to Lachman test (using an 80 lb pull). After Henning, C.E. (1988) Semilunar cartilage of the knee: function and pathology. *Exercise and Sport Sciences Review*, **16**, 67–75. With permission.

Knee stiffness

Knee stiffness is a common problem following ACL surgery. There are a variety of possible causes, including adhesions within the suprapatellar pouch and/or patellofemoral joint, quadriceps contracture and retraction of the alar folds (Reid, 1992). Furthermore, patients have been described with an involvement of the infrapatellar fat pads (p. 250), producing infrapatellar contracture syndrome (Paulos, Rosenberg and Drawbert, 1987).

Initially, stiffness begins with inflammation, immobility and quadriceps weakness. Patients are unable to gain full extension and may complain of excessive pain. Patellar glide is restricted and pain may be located around the patellofemoral joint. Later, fat pad involvement may be noted and the patellar tendon may become rigid. Patellar mobility is virtually eliminated and both active and passive knee motion is severely restricted. Flexion contracture is often present by this time and the patient walks with an apparent 'short leg'.

If progress in regaining knee mobility begins to slow, this must be recognized immediately and acted upon. Intense rehabilitation is the key to preventing development of this condition. Patellofemoral joint mobilization and the restoration of full knee extension is vital.

Posterior cruciate damage

The PCL is the strongest ligament in the knee (Baylis and Rzonca, 1988) and is much less frequently damaged in sport than the ACL. When an injury does occur, it may be the result of a posteriorly directed force onto a flexed knee (typically a road traffic accident), forced hyperextension, or forced flexion where the athlete falls into a kneeling position, pressing the ankle into plantarflexion (Keene, 1990). Unlike ACL injury, the athlete with a damaged PCL can

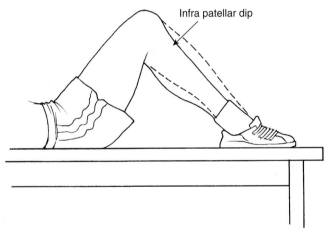

Figure 10.28   Posterior sag with posterior cruciate ligament (PCL) deficient knee.

usually continue playing and may only notice minimal swelling, but there is marked pain on the posterior aspect of the knee.

Posterior subluxation of the tibia often occurs during walking and standing. It may be seen clinically from the side if the knee is flexed to 90° (Fig. 10.28). This may be accentuated if the patient contracts the quadriceps against a resistance provided by the examiner. The patient is asked to 'slide the foot down the couch' (Daniel et al., 1988) as the examiner stabilizes the ankle. If not viewed from the side, the subluxation may be missed and the injury wrongly diagnosed as an ACL tear, the tibia moving forwards to reduce and mimicking an anterior drawer sign.

The posterior shift of the tibia moves the patellar tendon closer to the axis of rotation of the knee, reducing the mechanical advantage of the quadriceps (Fig. 10.29). The change in quadriceps muscle efficiency is reflected in the gait cycle.

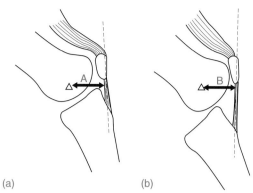

(a)   (b)

Figure 10.29   Alteration in mechanical advantage of the knee following posterior cruciate ligament (PCL) rupture. (a) Normal knee: axis of rotation to patellar tendon distance gives mechanical advantage. (b) PCL deficient knee: tibial shift gives reduced mechanical advantage.

With the PCL deficient knee, athletes demonstrate quadriceps activity before heel strike, in contrast to normal individuals who show this contraction after heel strike (Reid, 1992).

Rehabilitation

As with ACL damage, conservative treatment involving intensive muscle strengthening is tried first. Isolated hamstring contractions will cause posterior shear of the tibia on the femur and so should be avoided. In addition, excessive external rotation of the tibia as the knee approaches full extension will stress the repaired tissue. As with ACL rehabilitation, co-contraction exercises should be favoured.

The PCL is contained within a synovial sheath which enhances its ability to heal in continuity (Fowler and Messieh, 1987). Reconstruction may be attempted using a similar patellar tendon graft to that described above. This time, the graft is positioned lateral to the tibial attachment of the PCL and travels through the femur at the junction of the medial condyle and the intercondylar notch.

The knee with isolated PCL insufficiency producing unidirectional instability generally does well when treated conservatively, but when PCL damage is associated with additional tissue damage which results in multidirectional instability, surgery should be considered (Torg, 1989). In a study investigating the long-term effects of non-operative management of PCL damage, Parolie and Bergfeld (1986) assessed 25 athletes on average 6.2 years after injury. Of these, 84% had returned to their previous sport. Importantly, those who were not satisfied with their knee had less than 100% strength compared to the undamaged knee (measured as mean torque on an isokinetic dynamometer at varying angular velocities), and those who were satisfied had strength values greater than 100%. The importance of maintaining superior muscle strength following PCL injuries is therefore clear.

Of those patients who are symptomatic enough to seek treatment, damage to the medial compartment is more common with chronic injuries, and to the lateral compartment with acute injuries (Geissler and Whipple, 1993). Damage includes meniscal tears and articular cartilage defects.

Functional testing of the cruciate ligament deficient knee

Functional testing may be used to assess stability, pain and confidence in the knee. Tests normally aim to reproduce some key aspect of a sport to enhance specificity. In each case the injured and uninjured sides of the body are compared.

For the crossover test the athlete stands on the affected leg and uses the unaffected leg to step in front and behind the injured one, imparting multiplane stress on the knee (Fig. 10.30). The test may also be performed with the injured leg on a small stool to increase flexion stress on the knee.

The single-leg hop test measures the distance obtained on the injured side and divides this figure by that obtained for the uninjured side to obtain a 'hop ratio' which may be recorded throughout treatment (Reid, 1992). Combining straight hopping with hop-and-turn activities increases and varies the stress imposed on the knee, as does hopping down or up from a low stool.

Figure-of-eight, slalom, and slope/stair running circuits are also useful. The figure-of-eight may be performed with a gradual curve or a sharp one to impose more or less stress on the knee. The knee on the outside of the circle is exposed to a varus stress as the body leans inwards. The slalom or zig-zag run imposes sudden direction changes and shear on the knee. This test is particularly suitable for assessing function in sports which involve 'cutting' actions. Slope/stair running may be performed on an inclined or declined surface, or on a camber. In each case repetitive shearing stress is imposed on the knee.

THE MENISCI

The menisci are fibrocartilage structures which rest on the tibial condyles. They are crescent-shaped when viewed from above, but triangular in cross-section. Their peripheral border is formed from fibrous tissue and attached to the deep surface of the joint capsule. These same fibres attach the menisci to the tibial surface, forming the coronary ligaments. Anteriorly, the two menisci are joined by the transverse ligament, a posterior transverse ligament being present in 20% of the population (Palastanga, Field and Soames, 1989).

The medial meniscus is the larger of the two, semicircular in shape, and broader posteriorly. Its anterior horn is attached to the front of the intercondylar area of the tibia in front of the ACL. The posterior horn attaches to the posterior intercondylar area between the PCL and the lateral meniscus. It has an attachment to the MCL and the oblique popliteal ligament coming from semimembranosus

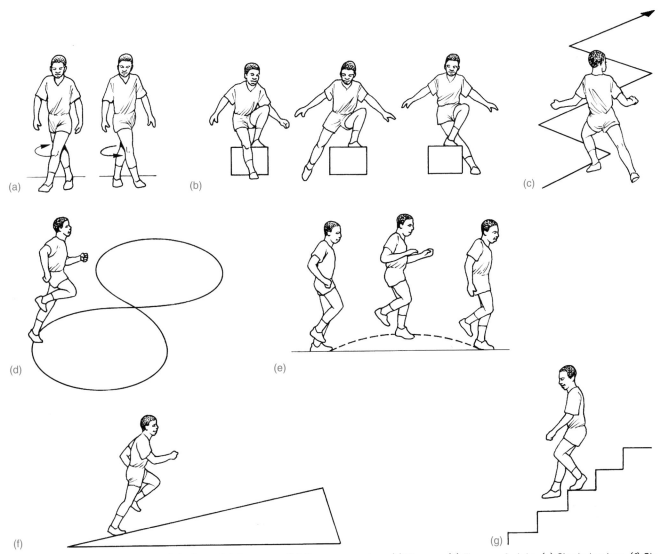

Figure 10.30   Functional testing of the knee. (a) Crossover. (b) Crossover on box. (c) Zig-zag. (d) Figure-of-eight. (e) Single leg hop. (f) Slope running. (g) Ascending and descending stairs.

(Fig. 10.31a). The upper part of the meniscus is firmly attached to the MCL, the fibres here forming the medial meniscofemoral ligament (Fig. 10.31b). The lower part, attached to the coronary ligament, is more lax. This has important functional consequences because the medial meniscus is anchored more firmly to the femur than to the tibia. In flexion/extension the femur is thus able to glide on the tibia, while in rotation, the meniscus can slide over the tibial plateau (Evans, 1986).

The lateral meniscus is more circular, and has a uniform breadth. Its two horns are attached close together, the anterior horn blending with the attachment of the ACL. The posterior horn attaches just anterior to the posterior horn of the medial meniscus. The meniscus has a posterolateral groove which receives the popliteus tendon, and a few fibres from this muscle attach to the meniscus itself. In addition, the tendon of popliteus partially separates the lateral meniscus from the joint capsule, a configuration which makes the lateral meniscus more mobile than its medial counterpart. The posterior part of the lateral meniscus has two ligamentous attachments, the anterior and posterior meniscofemoral ligaments (Fig. 10.32). These divide around the PCL, and in extreme flexion, as the PCL tightens, so do the anterior and posterior meniscofemoral ligaments. The lateral meniscus is thus pulled back and medially.

Keypoint

Because the lateral meniscus attaches through the meniscofemoral ligaments to the posterior cruciate, it is more mobile than the medial meniscus and so less likely to be trapped and torn.

The menisci receive blood flow from the inferior genicular arteries which supply the perimeniscal plexus (Fig. 10.33).

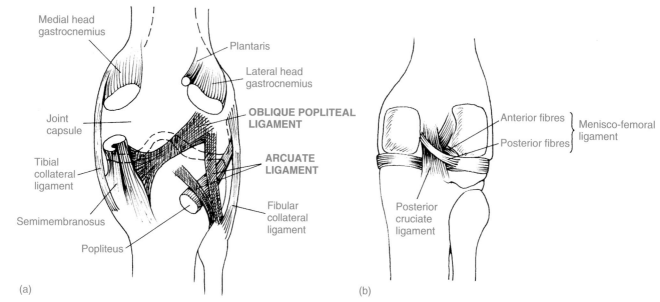

(a)

Figure 10.31   Attachments of the medial menisci.

(b)

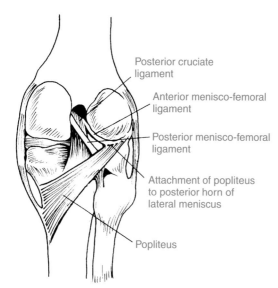

Figure 10.32   Posterior aspect of the left knee.

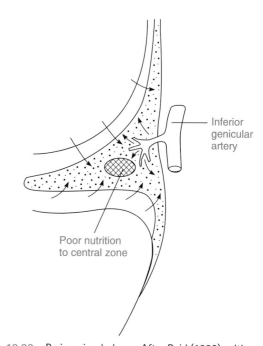

Figure 10.33   Perimeniscal plexus. After Reid (1992), with permission.

Small penetrating branches from this plexus enter the meniscus via the coronary ligaments. Up until the age of about 11 years, the whole meniscus has a blood supply, but in the adult only 10–25% of the periphery of the meniscus is vascular. The anterior and posterior horns are covered by vascular synovium and have a good blood supply (Arnoczky and Warren, 1983). The peripheral vessels are within the deeper cartilage substance, the surface receiving its main nutrition via diffusion from the synovial fluid. A few myelinated and non-myelinated nerve fibres are found in the outer third of the menisci, but no nerve endings.

Because the menisci are held more firmly centrally, they are able to alter their shape and move forwards and backwards over the tibial plateau. The lateral meniscus has a greater amount of movement, and is often 'pulled away from trouble', leaving the medial meniscus to be more commonly injured in association with the MCL and ACL, to which it has attachments.

In flexion, the lateral meniscus is carried backwards, onto the steep posterior slope of the lateral tibial plateau, and with extension, it moves forwards again. In flexion/extension the medial meniscus is held firm until the last 20° of extension when the knee begins to rotate (screw home mechanism). As this happens, the medial meniscus is carried backwards. The lateral meniscus has the greater movement therefore – approximately 11 mm versus only 5 mm for the medial (Reid, 1992). In extension, the menisci are

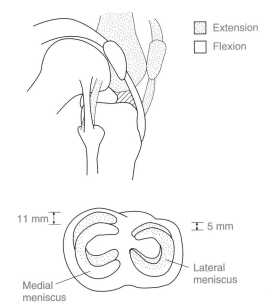

Extension

Flexion

11 mm

5 mm

Medial
meniscus

Lateral
meniscus

Figure 10.34   Movement of the menisci with flexion and extension
of the knee.

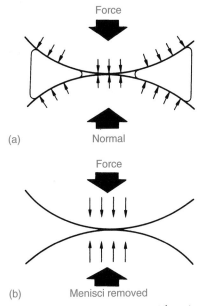

Force

(a)   Normal

Force

(b)   Menisci removed

Figure 10.35   The effect of cartilage removal (meniscectomy) on
the knee. (a) Forces on the normal knee. (b) Menisci removed. The
bones take more jarring strain.

squeezed and elongated in an anteroposterior direction,
and in flexion they become wider (Fig. 10.34).

The menisci enlarge the tibiofemoral contact area, thus
spreading the pressure taken by the subchondral bone (Fig.
10.35). It has been estimated that the menisci disperse
between 30% and 55% of the load across the knee (Kelley,
1990). When only a portion of the meniscus is removed, the
joint surface contact forces may increase by 350% (Seedhom
and Hargreaves, 1979).

The menisci contribute substantially to knee stability.
In the ACL deficient knee, the anterior drawer test may be

> **Keypoint**
>
> When a portion of the meniscus is removed, the joint
> surface contact forces may increase by 350%. Following
> meniscectomy bone adaptation will take time, and
> weightbearing should be progressed slowly. Shock
> absorbing padding should be used in all sports footwear.

positive in only 35% of knees with an intact medial meniscus, but in 83% when the meniscus is removed (Levy,
Torzilli and Warren, 1982). The menisci limit sagittal gliding
of the femur over the tibial plateau, a movement greatly
increased in patients who have undergone meniscectomy.
In addition, they allow a dual movement to occur, normally
only possible in joints which are far more lax. The menisci
also aid joint lubrication by spreading the synovial fluid
over the surface of the articular cartilage.

Injury

It has been estimated that meniscal injury has a frequency of
61 per 100 000 individuals. The condition is three times
more prevalent in males than females, with the medial
meniscus being injured four times as often as the lateral
(Kelley, 1990).

With ageing, degeneration and asymptomatic tearing
occurs. Noble and Hamblen (1975) examined 400 cadaveric
menisci and found 29% to have horizontal cleavage tears,
and 60% to have a significant meniscal lesion of some sort.

In the active athlete, the history of injury is usually one
which combines twisting on a semi-flexed knee with the
foot fixed on the ground. The onset is sudden, and pain is
felt deep within the knee, the patient often saying they 'felt
something go'. Effusion may be extensive after injury, and
haemarthrosis may result if the injury occurs in combination with ACL or MCL damage. Tears may be to the periphery or body of the meniscus, running horizontally or
vertically (Fig. 10.36). A longitudinal tear (bucket handle) of
the medial meniscus may allow its lateral portion to slip
over the dome of the medial femoral condyle causing
blocked extension (true locking). Shakespeare and Rigby
(1983) reviewed 272 patients found to have bucket handle
tears at operation. Of these, 43% presented with true locking. When the knee unlocks, either spontaneously or
through manipulation, anterior extension of the bucket
handle tear, rather than meniscal relocation, may occur
(Reid, 1992).

On examination, effusion is apparent and tenderness is
often found over the joint line, most usually medially.
A capsular pattern may be noticeable (Table 2.7), and terminal extension is often blocked with a springy end-feel if muscle spasm is not present. Various tests are used to assess the
problem, of which the two most common are McMurray's
and Apley's.

McMurray's test (Fig. 10.37a) requires full flexion of the knee and so is not suitable for the acute joint. The medial joint line is palpated and from the fully flexed position the knee is externally rotated and extended, as a slight varus strain is applied. If positive, a painful click or thud is felt over the medial meniscus. The lateral meniscus can be similarly tested by extending the knee with internal rotation and a valgus strain, although the value of lateral testing in this way is questionable (see below). In each case only the middle and posterior portion of the meniscus is tested, and so a negative McMurray's sign does not preclude meniscal damage, but when positive the test is clinically revealing.

The McMurray's test has been shown to be useful only with medial meniscal tears (Evans, Bell and Frank, 1993). In this evaluation the authors found that a thud elicited on the medial joint line was the only significant sign to correlate with meniscal injury. They showed the test to have a positive predictive value of 83% and a specificity of 98%.

Apley's grinding test (Fig. 10.37b) involves placing the patient in a prone-lying position, flexing the knee to 90°, rotating the tibia and compressing it against the femur in an attempt to elicit a popping or snapping sensation. It is important not to force the movements too far, as this may further tear the already damaged meniscus (Garrick and Webb, 1990). The intention with this test is to help differentiate between meniscal and MCL damage at the joint line. Symptoms will be present as the knee is compressed when the meniscus is damaged but not if the MCL alone is injured, because this structure will be relaxed by the compression force (Apley and Solomon, 1989). Conversely, a distraction force stretches the ligament but disengages the meniscus, so giving pain where MCL damage has occurred in isolation.

The results of meniscal tests combined with the clinical history will indicate if damage is likely, in which case arthroscopy is called for to confirm the findings.

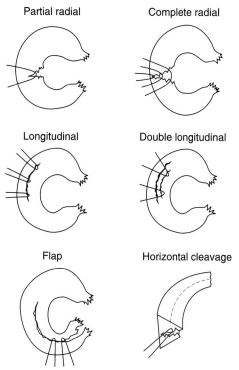

Partial radial   Complete radial

Longitudinal   Double longitudinal

Flap   Horizontal cleavage

Figure 10.36 Common meniscal tears. The longitudinal tear may extend anteriorly to form a bucket-handle tear. From Zuluaga, Briggs and Carlisle (1995), with permission.

Keypoint

For a complete diagnosis, clinical history, meniscal tests and arthroscopy are all required.

Management

If a meniscal tear is present, the choice is either non-operative management or surgical intervention involving removal or repair of the injured meniscus.

Figure 10.37 (a) Apley grinding test. (b) McMurray's test.

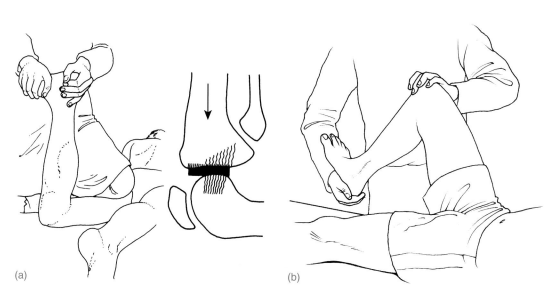

(a)   (b)

Non-operative management

Henning (1988) argued that meniscal tears of less than 10 mm in length and partial thickness injuries involving 50% or less of the vertical height of the meniscus could be treated non-operatively, providing the ACL was undamaged. Weiss et al. (1989) reported that stable vertical longitudinal tears in the vascular outer area of the meniscus had a good potential for healing, whereas stable radial tears did not. They performed a repeat arthroscopy on 32 patients (on average 26 months after the first procedure), and found that 17 longitudinal tears had healed completely. Five radial tears showed no evidence of healing and one had extended. No degenerative changes were found in the adjacent articular cartilage of the stable lesions.

Meniscal repair

The peripheral part of the meniscus has a blood supply sufficient to support healing. Initial healing in this region is by fibrosis with vessels from the capillary plexus and synovial fringe penetrating the area. Fibrous healing may be complete within 10 weeks, and the scar tissue can be remodelled into normal fibrocartilage within several months (Hammesfahr, 1989). The mid-portion of the meniscus is avascular and has been traditionally thought not to heal. However, Arnoczky and Warren (1983) demonstrated healing in canine tissue by cutting an access channel from the peripheral region to the mid-point of the meniscus. The peripheral vessels proliferated through the channel into the lesion, giving fibrovascular scarring throughout both areas.

The peripheral tear may be sutured, and healing improved by abrading the parameniscal synovium. Henning (1988) argued that healing may be further enhanced by injecting an exogenous blood clot into the injury site. Results are good when repair is limited to the vascular area of the meniscus and to vertical tears (Ryu and Dunbar, 1988). Weight bearing or full range motion will deform the menisci and so pull on the scar site. For this reason rehabilitation of the repaired meniscus is much less intense than that of a patient who has undergone meniscectomy. General recommendations for rehabilitation (DeHaven and Bronstein, 1995) include the restriction of weight bearing for 6 weeks, with no flexion allowed for the first 2 weeks. After 2 weeks, 20–70° flexion is allowed, with free motion allowed 4 weeks after surgery. Full weight bearing is allowed, and resistance exercises are progressed. Return to full sports is not permitted for 6 weeks.

For successful repair, DeHaven and Bronstein (1995) produced a number of recommendations. First, that the tear should lie within 3 mm of the meniscosynovial junction and that the overall contour of the meniscus should be normal. In addition, these authors stated that the tear should be at least 7 mm long and making the meniscus unstable. For tears further than 4 mm from the meniscosynovial junction and those with deformity, healing enhancement using fibrin clot was recommended.

DeHaven, Black and Griffiths (1989) reported follow-up results on 80 repaired menisci on average 4.6 years after surgery. Of these, 11% had torn again (only three at the repair zone), and these authors recommended meniscal repair in view of the degenerative changes following meniscectomy.

Meniscectomy

The preceding descriptions of non-operative management and meniscal repair make it apparent that meniscectomy is not the first choice in many cases of meniscal tearing.

Degenerative changes which have been described after total meniscectomy include joint narrowing, ridging and flattening (Fairbank, 1948). Follow-up after meniscectomy (Jorgensen, Sonne-Holm and Lauridsen, 1987) has shown patients to be increasingly dissatisfied with the knee. Incidence of complaint grew from 53% after 4.5 years to 67% after 14.5 years. A positive anterior draw sign was demonstrated in 10% after 4.5 years and 36% after 14.5 years, with 34% of the latter group giving up sport as a result of knee symptoms (Table 10.6).

Where the meniscus is grossly damaged and the knee is unstable, however, a partial or total meniscectomy may be required. The minimum amount of tissue should be removed to reduce the biomechanical impairment to the joint.

The traditional method for meniscectomy (O'Donoghue, 1976) is with the patient supine, knee flexed to 90° over the table end. For a medial meniscectomy a straight incision is often used, starting proximal to the lower pole of the patella

Table 10.6 Follow-up after complete meniscectomy

	4.5 years (n = 131) %	14.5 years (n = 101) %
Symptoms		
Swelling	19	29
Pain		
Weight-bearing	38	30
On stairs	15	23
When first walking	–	23
At rest	12	13
Sensation of instability	20	21
Signs		
Crepitus	18	38
Quadriceps wasting	7	12
Positive anterior drawer	10	36
Joint line tenderness	10	12
Activity		
Unchanged	53	19
Reduced because of knee	12	12
No sport because of knee	15	34

After Jorgensen, U. et al. (1987) Long term follow up of meniscectomy in athletes: a prospective longitudinal study. *Journal of Bone and Joint Surgery*, 69, 80. With permission.

and medial to the patellar tendon, and stretching parallel to the tendon. The retinaculum is split and the joint washed out (lavaged) with warm saline to remove any blood. The whole cartilage may be visible if the knee can be sprung open medially, but usually only palpation with forceps is possible. The bony attachment of the meniscus is dissected and the meniscus itself removed.

Arthroscopic removal of all, or part, of the meniscus is commonplace nowadays. An anterolateral or anteromedial approach may be taken, depending on which compartment of the knee the lesion lies in. The knee is held in 10° flexion and the joint is gapped by applying a valgus or varus stress. The joint is distended with fluid to allow easier inspection of the tissue surfaces. An initial incision is made into the anterior part of the meniscus, and the incision is then extended into the middle and posterior segments. The posterior horn is released, followed by the anterior horn, and the meniscus is removed. In cases where only part of the meniscus is removed, the edge of the remaining tissue is trimmed.

Results of arthroscopic partial meniscectomy are generally good, but are dependent on the amount of tissue damage which occurred at the time of injury. Investigating 67 patients on average 12.2 years after arthroscopic partial meniscectomy, Higuchi, Kimura and Shirakura (2000) found 79% to have a satisfactory outcome (52% excellent, 27% good, 10.5% fair). Osteoarthritic deterioration was noticed in 48% of patients the amount being dependent on the amount of cartilage degeneration noticed at the time of surgery. Of the original group, 39 had normal knee cartilage, and 28 had articular degeneration.

Arthroscopy, although commonplace, is not without risk of complication. The Committee on Complications of Arthroscopy of North America (1985) found a 0.8% complication rate in over 100,000 procedures, while Sherman et al. (1986) reported a complication rate of 8.2%. Neurological injury, poor wound healing, instrument breakage, intra-articular infection, knee ligament injury and pulmonary embolism resulting in death have all occurred. The patient's age and the length of time that a tourniquet is used have been found to be the most significant factors in predicting problems (Sherman et al., 1986).

The use of arthroscopy with local anaesthesia is steadily increasing (Ngo et al., 1985; Besser and Stahl, 1986; Buckley, Hood and Macrae, 1989), and obviously removes the risk inherent in any procedure involving a general anaesthetic. In addition, complication rate is lessened, cost is reduced and the patient is discharged significantly earlier than when general anaesthesia is used. The skin puncture sites are injected with lidocaine (lignocaine) or similar, and the joint is distended with saline and anaesthetic solution. Studying 400 patients in total, Jacobson, Forssblad and Rosenberg (2000) compared results from elective knee arthroscopy using either local, general, or spinal anaesthesia and obtained a 92% success rate using local anaesthesia in 200 of the patients. They concluded that the use of local anaesthesia was superior to either spinal or general anaesthetic in this group.

Following meniscectomy of any type, the initial aim is to limit effusion and pain (Table 10.7). As this is achieved, the leg musculature is progressively built up. Initially, open chain movements are used within the pain-free range, to protect the joint from excessive loading. Range of motion is gradually increased, and as this is achieved, closed chain movements are introduced. Functional activities and power training are used in late stage rehabilitation, with sports specific progressions forming the mainstay of pre-competitive work.

Table 10.7   Guidelines for post-meniscectomy rehabilitation

Initial stage (0–2 weeks)
Quadriceps setting (ensure no extensor lag)
Straight leg raise over block
Standing knee brace (partial weight-bearing)
Ankle exercise
Hip exercise (all ranges)
Begin walking re-education
Active and assisted knee flexion within pain-free range
Cardiopulmonary upper body work
Ensure passive range to patellofemoral joint
Modalities to reduce pain and inflammation

Intermediate stage (2–4 weeks)
Static cycle (high seat)
Aquajogger
General lower limb hydrotherapy
Increasing range of motion for knee
Resisted quadriceps in sitting (open chain)
Leg press to 90° (closed chain)
1/4 squat (partial weight-bearing)
Single (injured) leg standing on rebounder
As above with contralateral leg movements
Bench stepping—up, down, over, introduce slow twist
Ensure full accessory movements present
Modalities to increase circulation and warm tissue
Speed walking/inclined speed walk

Late stage (4–6 weeks)*
Cycling
Increased resistance on weight training
Final range of motion obtained (physiological and accessory)
Increased closed chain work and proprioceptive work
Running—shuttle, zig-zag, stop/start, figure-of-eight, uneven
   surface
Plyometric progressions—jumping, hopping, increasing height, jump
and twist
Full squat (free)
Full leg press (resisted)
Introduce sports-specific skills, e.g. ball dribbling, kicking

Pre-competition testing
Sports-specific skills to repetition
Advanced plyometrics
Endurance work for leg

*Progress to late stage when no/minimal swelling is present and full range motion obtained. After Zuluaga, Briggs and Carlisle (1995) and Reid (1992), with permission.

Meniscal cysts and discoid meniscus

The discoid meniscus (Fig. 10.38) is more usually seen on the lateral side than the medial. Even so, the condition is unusual. Smillie (1974) reported a total of 467 discoid lateral menisci (and only seven medial) in 10 000 meniscectomies. In the fetus, the meniscus is disc shaped rather than semi-lunar. When this shape remains later in life, the discoid meniscus is said to be present.

Definition

The meniscus of the knee in a unborn child is disc shaped rather than moon shaped. When this shape remains later in life, a *discoid meniscus* is present.

Discoid menisci may be classified as complete, incomplete (partial) or Wrisberg type (DeHaven and Bronstein,

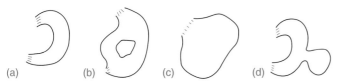

(a)   (b)   (c)   (d)

Figure 10.38   Meniscal abnormalities. (a) Normal. (b) Partial discoid. (c) Complete discoid. (d) Cyst.

1995). In the latter type the posterior osseous attachment of the meniscus is absent, leaving it attached only by the meniscofemoral ligament (Wrisberg's ligament).

The abnormal shape of the meniscus subtly alters both the contact area between the tibia and femur and joint mobility. In the young, the discoid meniscus may be asymptomatic, with 65% of those who present with symptoms being over 18 years old (Reid, 1992). A clunk may be felt in the knee at 110° as it is bent, and at 10° as it is straightened again (Apley and Solomon, 1993). Surgical treatment may be by meniscectomy or repair.

Meniscal cysts (ganglia) are again more common in the lateral meniscus, with the posterior and mid-portion of the meniscus being affected. The cyst is associated with a horizontal tear, and may be the result of infiltration of synovial fluid through the tear, with the edge of the tear acting as a one-way valve (Barrie, 1979). In a series of 18 patients with MRI documented cysts, all were found to have horizontal cleavage tears at arthroscopy (Ryu and Ting, 1993).

The cyst generally begins as a small pedicle and gradually enlarges, the size fluctuating with varying activities. It is more easily seen with the knee flexed to 45°. Arthroscopic repair of the tear site is possible, allowing the cyst to decompress into the joint (DeHaven and Bronstein, 1995). Where no tear is identified, removal of the cyst is attempted. The meniscal rim is scarified and the perimeniscal tissue reattached, leaving the meniscus proper fully intact. Some cysts respond to direct aspiration (Reid, 1992).

Manual therapy techniques for the knee

Manual therapy techniques around the knee can be used either to relieve pain or to mobilize a stiff joint (see Treatment note 1.2, p. 20). The aim is to use either a sustained stretch or a small amplitude oscillation; for manipulation, a high velocity, low amplitude movement is used at end-range.

Abduction/adduction in extension
The patient lies supine with the couch raised to the hip level of the therapist. The therapist grasps the patient's leg tucking the shin beneath their arm and gripping it into the side of their body with the elbow (Fig. 10.39). The leg is then supported with the hands either side of the knee, thumbs resting loosely over the top of the patella, fingers curled over the popliteal area of the knee. The action is to impart an abduction and adduction oscillation with the knee extended or minimally unlocked. The valgus stress to the knee can be increased by drawing the inner hand distally and the outer hand proximally and gapping the joint. Similarly a varus stretch may be applied by moving the inner hand proximally and the outer hand distally.

Abduction/adduction in flexion
The therapist moves close into the couch and grips the patient's ankle with the inner hand and rests the outer hand

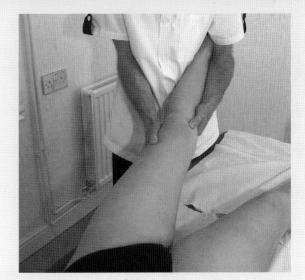

Figure 10.39   Abduction/adduction in extension.

on the lateral aspect of the knee. The movement is one of flexion by pressing the heel towards the buttock (Fig. 10.40). An abduction force is applied by drawing the heel laterally or an adduction force by drawing the heel medially. These

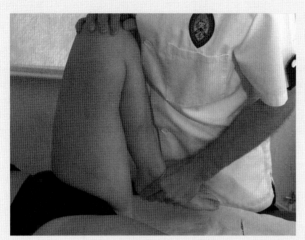

Figure 10.40 Abduction/adduction in flexion.

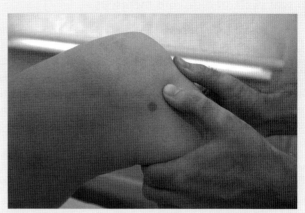

Figure 10.42 Posteroanterior (PA) glide in crook lying.

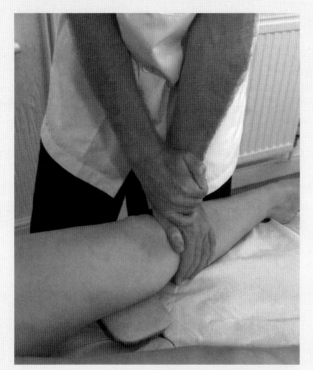

Figure 10.41 Anteroposterior (AP) glide using block.

movements may be combined with either a lateral rotation (abduction) or medial rotation (adduction) by surrounding the calcaneus in the cup of the hand and using the fingers for leverage.

Anteroposterior (AP) glide

The patient's thigh (femur) is placed on a block leaving the tibia free. The therapist lowers the couch below waist height and uses the heel of the hand to impart an AP glide to the tibia while the femur is blocked. For low grade movements both hands may be used surrounding the tibia, for high grade movements the motion is imparted through the straight arm (Fig. 10.41).

Posteroanterior (PA) glide

The patient is supported in crook lying with the knee flexed between 45 and 90°. The therapist lightly sits on the patient's foot to prevent it slipping. The patient's shin is gripped with the heel of the hands on the anterior aspect of the tibia and the fingers curled around the back of the calf (Fig. 10.42). The PA draw is performed by drawing the tibia forwards and may be combined with either external rotation (foot turned out) or internal rotation (foot turned in).

Lateral glide

In the crook lying position, a webbing belt is placed around the patient's tibia and the therapist fixes the belt around his or her own waist standing to the side of the patient. The tibia is supported with one hand and the femur with the other (Fig. 10.43). The lateral glide movement is instigated by the therapist swaying backwards; movement may be monitored using the thumb over the lateral joint line.

Capsular stretch

A joint distraction or capsular stretch to flexion may be imposed using the therapist's forearm as a pivot. The couch is raised above waist level and the patient sits in crook lying. The therapist places his or her arm under the popliteal area of the patient's knee and the distal arm contacts the tibia. The action is to apply flexion against the pivot point of the forearm, in a 'nutcracker' action (Fig. 10.44). The flexion movement may be combined with internal or external rotation simultaneously.

Joint distraction

The couch is raised above waist height and the knee is placed in its open pack position of slight flexion. The patient's shin is fixed beneath the therapist's arm and the action is a distraction movement which is brought on by swaying the body back (Fig. 10.45).

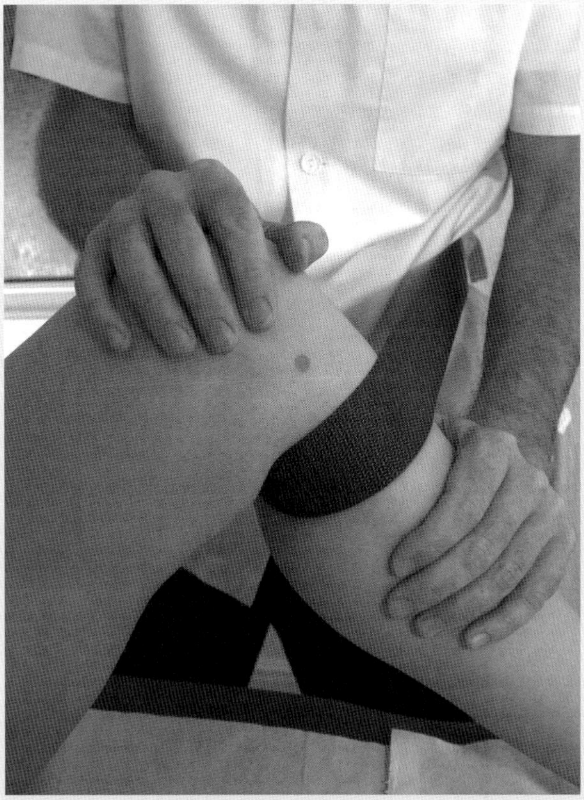

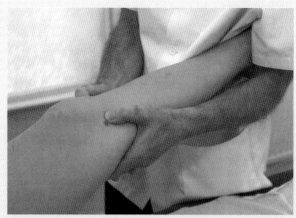

Figure 10.45   Joint distraction gripping patient's tibia beneath arm.

Figure 10.43   Lateral glide using seatbelt.

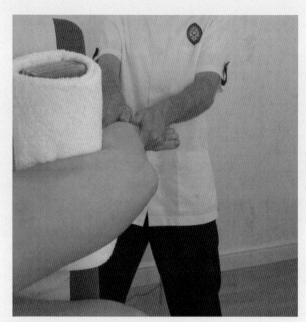

Figure 10.46   Joint distraction using couch headboard.

For higher grade distraction movements, the patient begins side lying with the femur supported against the headboard of the couch. The therapist grasps the patient's ankle and leans back with their full body weight to impart a distraction force (Fig. 10.46). This distraction force may be combined with rotation of the tibia to perform a loose body manipulation of the knee (Cyriax and Cyriax, 1983) muscles.

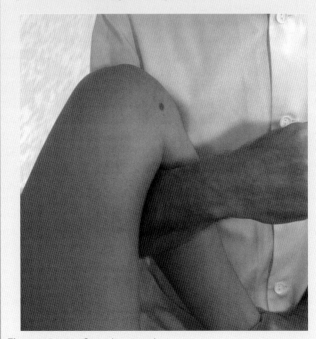

Figure 10.44   Capsular stretch.

JUMPER'S KNEE

Jumper's knee is a patellofemoral pain syndrome (PFPS) affecting the teno-osseous junctions of the quadriceps tendon as it attaches to the superior pole of the patella, and the patellar tendon as it attaches to the inferior pole of the patella and tibial tuberosity. It is, therefore, an insertional tendonopathy resulting in derangement of the bone–tendon unit (Colosimo and Bassett, 1990).

Definition

Jumper's knee is patellar pain affecting the insertion of the patellar tendon into either the patella itself or the tibial tuberosity.

The injury is often described as patellar or quadriceps tendinitis, although these conditions represent an inflammation of the tendon itself rather than isolated damage to the tenoosseous (T/O) junction. In a strict sense the conditions should be considered separately, but they are generally accepted as a single entity. However, it should be remembered that tendinitis does not necessarily mean that the T/O junction is affected, but when the tendon insertion itself is damaged, the tendon will almost always be inflamed.

Jumper's knee occurs more frequently in athletes who regularly impose rapid eccentric loading (traction) on the extensor mechanism of the knee, especially on hard surfaces.

The condition affects the inferior pole of the patella in 80% of cases and is most common at this site in athletes over 40 years of age. The insertion of the quadriceps is more commonly affected in the over 40s, and the tibial tuberosity is the most common sight for jumper's knee in children (David, 1989).

Repetitive stress on the T/O junction causes microtearing over time, and an insidious onset of pain. The condition progresses in a series of stages. Initially, pain is experienced only after intense activity, as a well-localized dull ache without a history of trauma. With time, pain occurs at the onset of activity and disappears when the athlete is warmed up, only to reappear when sport has finished. Eventually, pain is constant, with consequent impairment of performance, and as a final but rare scenario, the tendon may rupture completely.

On examination, quadriceps wasting is apparent in longstanding cases and pain occurs to resisted extension, with slight soreness to full passive flexion. Some swelling may be noticed around the patellar tendon in acute cases, with fluctuance present if the condition is severe. A non-capsular pattern is found.

Palpation is performed with the knee in full extension to relax the patellar tendon. Palpation to the lower pole of the patella is best performed by pressing with the flat of the hand onto the upper surface of the patella to tilt it. This brings the lower pole into prominence and enables the practitioner to reach the part of the T/O junction which lies on the undersurface of the angular lower pole.

Radiographic changes are usually apparent where symptoms have been present for more than 6 months (Colosimo and Bassett, 1990). An elongation of the involved pole of the patella may be seen, with calcification of the affected tendon matrix. Bone scan has indicated increased blood pooling and concentration of radioactive tracer in the inflamed area (Kahn and Wilson, 1987).

Both intrinsic and extrinsic factors have been implicated as possible causes. Intrinsic factors include biomechanical alterations in the extensor mechanism, such as hypermobility, altered Q angle and genu valgum or genu recurvatum. Changes in the HQ ratio and hamstring flexibility may also have a part to play and should be examined. Muscle imbalance, consisting of weakness of the glutei, hamstrings and abdominals, combined with hip flexor shortening, has been noted (Sommer, 1988). In addition, on landing, players who are susceptible to this condition, have a greater tendency to adduct the knee and internally rotate the leg (knock-knee posture).

Extrinsic factors include frequency and intensity of training, training surface and footwear. Ferretti (1986) showed a correlation between jumper's knee and both hardness of playing surface and training frequency. In his study, 37% of players (matched for sport, playing position, and training type) using cement surfaces suffered from the condition, compared to only 5% of those using softer surfaces (Fig. 10.39a). In addition, the percentage number of players affected by the condition escalated as the number of training sessions per week increased. Only 3.2% of those with the condition trained twice each week, whereas nearly 42% trained four times or over (Fig. 10.47b).

As with any overuse syndrome, part of the management of the condition involves avoidance or modification of training. Athletes should be encouraged to warm up adequately, and practise flexibility exercises to both the quadriceps and

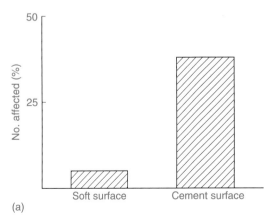
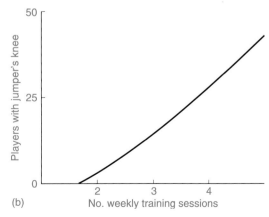

Figure 10.47 Incidence of jumper's knee. Data from Ferretti, A. (1986) Epidemiology of jumper's knee. *Sports Medicine*, **3**, 289–295. With permission.

(a)   (b)

hamstrings. Strength must be developed symmetrically, and footwear should incorporate shock-absorbing materials.

In the early stages of the condition these modifications, combined with ice application when pain is acute, are usually sufficient. Later, transverse frictional massage is the treatment of choice. Frictions to the T/O junction attaching to the patella (infrapatellar tendon) are only effective if the patella is tilted and pressure from the therapist's finger is directed at a 45° angle to the long axis of the femur rather than straight down.

> **Keypoint**
>
> Frictions to the teno-osseous (T/O) junction of the patella tendon are only effective if the patella is tilted. Pressure from the therapist's finger is directed at a 45° angle to the long axis of the femur rather than straight down.

In chronic conditions, where scar tissue has formed at the T/O junctions, limitation in flexion may be apparent. Flexibility exercises will increase the range of movement, but more by stretching the quadriceps than the scar tissue. Where this is the case, a soft tissue manipulation may be required in an attempt to rupture the adherent scarring. If this procedure fails to produce a complete result surgery may be required. Various procedures have been described, some attempting to alter underlying malalignment and others to excise abnormal tissue.

Exercise therapy aims at restoring the shock-attenuating function of the leg musculature and re-educating take-off and landing patterns. Any muscle imbalance must be identified and corrected. Eccentric loading of the leg musculature is increased through progressive closed chain activities, using 'drop and stop' exercises of varying intensities. These are progressed initially to slow concentric-eccentric coupling and eventually to plyometrics.

Stretching and gradual eccentric strengthening of the anterior tibials has been shown to be effective (Reid, 1992). Passive plantarflexion is performed initially to stretch the musculature. Slow concentric activity is then used as the athlete actively dorsiflexes against manual resistance. Eccentric activity follows as the athlete controls the rate of plantarflexion against therapist resistance. The exact mechanism for the effectiveness of this programme is not known, but both infrapatellar ligament stretching, and quadriceps/foreleg strength ratio changes have been suggested (Reid, 1992).

SINDING–LARSEN–JOHANSSON DISEASE

In this condition the secondary ossification centre on the lower border of the patella is affected in adolescents. The epiphysis is tractioned, leading to inflammation and eventual fragmentation. Avascular necrosis is not usually present, but a temporary osteoporosis has been described (Traverso, Baldari and Catalani, 1990) during the adolescent growth spurt. This may weaken the inferior pole of the patella making avulsion more likely.

> **Definition**
>
> *Sinding–Larsen–Johansson disease* affects the secondary ossification centre on the lower border of the patella in adolescents. Inflammation, bone fragmentation and occasionally temporary (transient) osteoporosis may occur.

Sinding–Larsen–Johansson (SLJ) disease can easily be confused with chondromalacia on first inspection as it gives pain to the lower pole of the patella, especially when kneeling. However, on closer examination the differences are soon apparent, and X-ray confirms the bony change. Initially, no abnormalities are seen on X-ray, but after 2–4 weeks, irregular calcification is noted at the inferior pole. The calcifications are seen to coalesce later, and may finally be incorporated into the patella (Medlar and Lyne, 1978).

The condition may exist with Osgood–Schlatter's syndrome (Traverso, Baldari and Catalani, 1990), and the conservative management of the two syndromes is largely the same, involving the use of pain relieving/anti-inflammatory modalities and training modification. Surgical removal of the lower pole of the patella has been recommended in persistent cases (Williams and Sperryn, 1976).

OSGOOD–SCHLATTER'S SYNDROME

This condition affects adolescents, especially males. Most often the patient is an active sportsperson who has recently undergone the adolescent growth spurt. With Osgood–Schlatter's syndrome traction is applied to the tibial tubercle, eventually causing the apophysis of the tubercle to separate from the proximal end of the tibia. Initially, fragmentation appears, but with time the fragments coalesce and further ossification leads to an increase in bone. This gives the characteristic prominent tibial 'bump' often noticeable when the knee silhouette is compared to that of the unaffected side.

The infrapatellar tendon shows increased vascularization and, particularly where radiographic changes are not apparent, soft tissue swelling and infrapatellar fat pad involvement is noted. Pain is highly localized to the tibial tubercle and exacerbated by activities such as running, jumping and descending stairs. The condition may coalesce with patellar malalignment faults such as patella infera and patella alta. Patellar tendon avulsion can occur following this condition, and Levi and Coleman (1976) reported 26% of those seen with this type of fracture to have had a previous history of Osgood–Schlatter's disease.

Initial management is by limiting activity. Pain relief and reduction of inflammation may be obtained by using electrotherapy modalities alone, or iontophoresis with an anti-inflammatory medication and local anaesthetic (Antich and Brewster, 1985). Injection of the tibial tubercle with hydrocortisone has been described (Grass, 1978). The use of local dry needling to the tibial tuberosity and trigger point acupuncture to the rectus femoris has been described (Norris, 2001). An infrapatellar strap to reduce the pull of the quadriceps onto the tibial tubercle has been used with some success (Levine and Kashyap, 1981).

Assessment of the lower limb musculature often reveals hypertrophy and inflexibility of the quadriceps. When passive knee flexion is tested, intense pain precludes the use of quadriceps stretching. However, when pain has subsided, flexibility of this muscle group must be regained. Where prolonged rest has given rise to muscle atrophy, strengthening exercises are indicated. Ice packs may be used to limit pain or inflammation following activity. Restoration of acceleration/deceleration mechanics in jumping and landing (closed chain) is as for jumper's knee (see above).

Synovial plica

The synovial plica is a remnant of the septum which separates the knee into three chambers until the fourth intrauterine month. Three types of plica are seen. The infrapatellar plica (ligamentum mucosum) lies within the intercondylar notch and runs parallel to the anterior cruciate ligament. The suprapatellar plica is found on the medial aspect of the suprapatellar pouch, lying proximal to the superior pole of the patella. The mediopatellar plica extends from the medial suprapatellar pouch over the medial femoral condyle and onto the synovium covering the infrapatellar fat pad (Fig. 10.48). The medio-patellar plica is by far the most important in terms of pathology.

> **Definition**
>
> A *synovial plica* is a remnant of the tissue which separates the knee into three chambers in the unborn child. A *mediopatellar plica* is the most common type to give problems in sport.

A mediopatellar plica may be present in some 20–60% of knees (Amatuzzi, Fazzi and Varella, 1990), but does not necessarily cause symptoms. In a series of 3250 knee disorders, Koshino and Okamoto (1985) found only 32 patients to have the complaint (1%). The structure separates the knee joint into two reservoirs, one above the patella and the other constituting the joint cavity proper. The normal plica is a thin, pink, flexible structure, but when inflamed it becomes thick, fibrosed and swollen, loosing its elasticity and interfering with patellofemoral tracking.

These tissue changes are often initiated by trauma that results in synovitis, and is more common in athletes. Pain is usually intermittent and increases with activity. Discomfort is experienced when descending stairs and may mimic PFPS. However, pain of plical origin normally subsides immediately when the knee is extended. In addition, the 'morning sign' may be present. This is a popping sensation which occurs as the knee is extended, particularly on rising, but disappears throughout the day. The popping may be accompanied by giving way, and is caused by the thickened plica passing over the medial femoral condyle. As the day progresses, joint effusion pushes the plica away from the condyle. This sign may be reproduced with some patients by extending the knee from 90° flexion while internally rotating the tibia and pushing the patella medially. The pop is usually experienced between 45° and 60° flexion.

> **Keypoint**
>
> A popping sensation may be caused as the plica passes over the medial femoral condyle when the knee is extended. This may be reproduced by: (i) extending the knee from 90° flexion while (ii) internally rotating the tibia and (iii) pushing the patella medially.

Conservative treatment has been found to be effective in 60% of cases (Amatuzzi, Fazzi and Varella, 1990) and aims at reducing the compression over the anterior compartment of the knee, by using stretching exercises. The length of the hamstrings, quadriceps and gastrocnemius muscles should be assessed and these muscles stretched if noticeable shortening is found. Where conservative treatment fails and symptoms limit sport or daily living, surgery may be warranted. Koshino and Okamoto (1985) reported pain and symptom relief in 90% of knees treated surgically by plical resection, but did not quote figures for long-term follow-up.

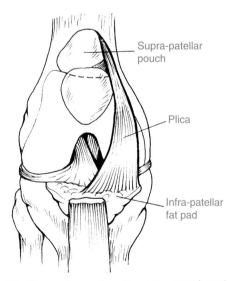

Figure 10.48   The mediopatellar plica. After Reid (1992), with permission.

TENDINITIS

Tendinitis around the knee occurs most commonly within the patellar tendon (jumper's knee, see above), the semimembranosus and the popliteus.

Semimembranosus has a complex insertion consisting of five slips onto the proximal tibia (Williams, 1995), making direct palpation of an inflamed area difficult. The five insertions are:

1. into a small tubercle on the posterior aspect of the medial tibial condyle (the tuberculum tendinis)
2. the medial margin of the tibia immediately behind the medial collateral ligament
3. a fibrous expansion to the fascia covering popliteus
4. a cord-like tendon to the inferior lip of the medial tibial condyle below the MCL
5. the oblique popliteal ligament passing upwards and laterally (Fig. 10.49).

Tendinitis of this muscle gives a persistent ache over the posteromedial aspect of the knee. It occurs as the semimembranosus tendon slides over the medial corner of the medial femoral condyle, and is distinct from semimembranosus bursitis which affects the area of the medial tibial condyle. Pain may occur within the tendon substance itself, or over the teno-osseous junction, when an insertional tendinitis is present. Increased tracer uptake has been noted on bone scan with this latter condition (Ray, Clancy and Lemon, 1988).

Popliteus tendinitis is related to increased pronation of the STJ and excessive internal rotation of the tibia (Brody, 1980). The increased internal rotation causes traction on the popliteus attachment to the lateral femoral condyle. The popliteus acts with the PCL to prevent forward displacement of the femur on the flexed tibia, and so will be overworked with downhill running (Baylis and Rzonca, 1988). On examination, tenderness is revealed over the popliteus just anterior to the fibular collateral ligament. The patient is examined in a supine position with the injured knee in the 'figure of four' position, that is affected hip flexed, abducted and externally rotated, knee bent to 90° and foot placed on the knee of the contralateral leg. The condition is differentiated from ITB friction syndrome by testing resisted tibial internal rotation with the knee flexed, and palpating the popliteus while internal rotation is resisted in extension (Allen and Ray, 1989).

Treatment for tendinitis involves rest, anti-inflammatory modalities and training modification. Flexibility of the knee musculature and the biomechanics of the lower limb should be assessed and corrected as necessary.

BURSITIS

The knee joint has on average 14 bursae (see Table 10.8) in areas where friction is likely to occur, between muscle, tendon, bone and skin. Any of these can become inflamed and give pain when compressed through muscle contraction or direct palpation. Those most commonly injured in sport include the pre-patellar, pes anserine, and semimembranosus.

Pre-patellar bursa

The pre-patellar bursa is usually injured by falling onto the anterior aspect of the knee, or by prolonged kneeling (housemaid's knee). Haemorrhage into the bursa can cause

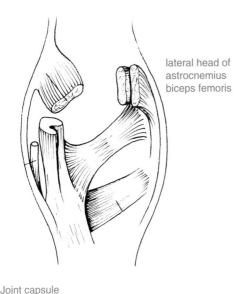

Joint capsule

Figure 10.49 Extensive insertion of semimembranosus.

lateral head of astrocnemius
biceps femoris

Table 10.8 Bursae around the knee

Bursa	Lying between
Subcutaneous prepatellar	Lower patella/skin
Deep infrapatellar	Upper tibia/patellar ligament
Subcutaneous infrapatellar	Lower tibial tuberosity/skin
Suprapatellar	Lower femur/deep surface of quadriceps (communicates with joint)
No specific name	Lateral head of gastrocnemius/capsule
	Lateral collateral ligament/tendon of biceps femoris
	Lateral collateral ligament/popliteus
	Popliteus tendon/lateral condyle of femur
	Medial head gastrocnemius/capsule
	Medial head of gastrocnemius/semimembranosus
Pes anserine	Superficial to medial collateral ligament/sartorius, gracilus, semitendinosus
No specific name	Deep medial collateral ligament/femur, medial meniscus
Semimembranosus	Semimembranosus/medial tibial condyle, gastrocnemius
No specific name	Semimembranosus/semitendinosus

an inflammatory reaction and increased fluid volume. Enlargement is noticeable and the margins of the mass are well defined, differentiating the condition from general knee effusion or subcutaneous haematoma. Knee flexion may be limited, the bursa being compressed as the skin covering the patella tightens.

> **Keypoint**
>
> Falling directly onto the point of the knee may cause housemaid's knee (pre-patellar bursitis). Only the anterior aspect of the knee is swollen, and pain is increased by knee flexion as the bursa is compressed.

Septic bursitis may result by secondary infection if the skin over the bursa is broken by laceration or puncture wound. If the condition becomes chronic, the bursa may collapse and the folded walls of the thickened bursal sac appear as small hardened masses on the anterior aspect of the knee. In these cases, erythema and exquisite tenderness are usually present.

Minor cases normally respond to rest and ice, but more marked swelling requires aspiration. Aspiration is carried out under sterile conditions, and a compression bandage applied.

Semimembranosus and pes anerine bursae

Semimembranosus bursitis gives rise to pain and swelling over the lower posteromedial aspect of the knee. Pain may be made worse by hamstring or gastrocnemius contraction against resistance, and in activities involving intense action of these muscles, such as sprinting and bounding.

Pes anserine bursitis gives pain and swelling over the metaphyseal area of the tibia, sometimes referred to the medial joint line (Baylis and Rzonca, 1988). The bursa may be injured by direct trauma (hitting the knee on a hurdle) or by overuse of the pes anserine tendons.

With both of the latter causes of bursitis, rest and anti-inflammatory modalities are required. Biomechanical assessment of the lower limb and analysis of the athlete's training regime are called for where there is no history of injury.

Baker's cyst

One condition often referred to as 'bursitis' is a Baker's cyst. This is actually a posterior herniation of the synovial membrane into the bursa lying between semimembranosus and the medial head of gastrocnemius (Fig. 10.50).

The mass bulges into the popliteal space, and occurs particularly in rheumatoid arthritis. The posterior knee ligaments weaken and fail to support the joint capsule, allowing the herniation to occur. The cyst can be palpated over the medial side of the popliteal space beneath the medial head of gastrocnemius.

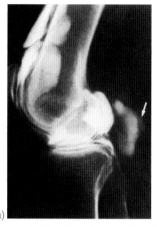 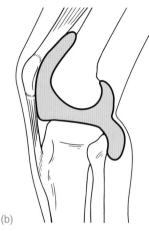

(a)   (b)

Figure 10.50   Baker's cyst. From Reilly, B.M. (1991) *Practical Strategies in Outpatient Medicine*. W.B. Saunders, Philadelphia. With permission.

> **Definition**
>
> A *Baker's cyst* is a bulging (herniation) of the synovial membrane backwards into the bursa lying between semimembranosus and the medial head of gastrocnemius.

When painless, the condition may be managed conservatively, but where the enlargement compromises venous return or causes severe pain, aspiration or excision of the mass is called for.

FAT PADS

Fat pads consist of fat cells (adipose tissue) packed closely together and separated from other tissues by fibrous septa. They have an abundant blood supply, and are well innervated. Most significant to the knee is the infrapatellar fat pad, lying beneath the patellar tendon, and in front of the femoral condyles. The fat pad is intracapsular but extra-synovial, and a piece of synovial membrane (ligamentum mucosum, see above) may pass from the pad to the intra-condylar notch of the femur. When the knee is fully flexed, the infrapatellar fat pad fills the anterior aspect of the inter-condylar notch. As the knee extends, the fat pad covers the trochlear surface of the femur within the patellar groove (Hertling and Kessler, 1990).

The usual pathology of the infrapatellar fat pad is an enlargement causing increased pressure with resultant pain (Hoffa's disease). Direct trauma can cause haemorrhage and local oedema, and swelling may also occur as a result of premenstrual water retention. Space occupying lesions, such as osteochondrotic fragments, may also cause enlargement, and Smillie (1974) described a case where a displaced bucket handle tear of the medial meniscus was forced into the infrapatellar fat pad of the knee.

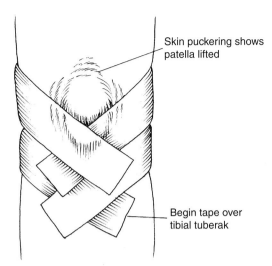

Skin puckering shows
patella lifted

Begin tape over
tibial tuberak

Figure 10.51 Fat pad unloading using taping.

fatty tissue with fibrinoid material. Complete fibrosis was later seen. Silver and Campbell (1985) described persistent inflammation of the knee fat pads as a cause of delayed recovery in dancers with knee injuries. Surgical removal of the pad resulted in restoration of full range motion at the knee. Tsirbas, Paterson and Keene (1990) described excision of the fat pad tip to relieve patellofemoral pain. Patients presented with a history of pain inferomedial, and sometimes inferolateral, to the patella. On examination, impingement pain occurred deep to the inferior pole of the patella at 20° flexion with resisted quadriceps contraction.

Relief of mild compression pain may be achieved with taping (McConnell, 1992). Taping begins over the tibial tubercle and extends laterally and medially in a 'V' shape. The tape is placed under traction to lift the patella in a cephalic direction. This effectively forms a sling to prevent the patella pressing into the fat pad (Fig. 10.51).

Enlargement and entrapment of the patellar fat pad has been described by Finsterbush, Frankl and Mann (1989). The entrapped pad was shown to be in various stages of tissue degeneration, including fat necrosis and replacement of the

References

Allen, M.E. and Ray, G. (1989) Popliteus tendinitis, a new perspective. *Sports Training and Medical Rehabilitation*, **1**, 219–226

Amatuzzi, M.M., Fazzi, A. and Varella, M.H. (1990) Pathologic synovial plica of the knee. *American Journal of Sports Medicine*, **18**, (5) 466–469

Anderson, A.F., Snyder, R.B., Federspiel, C.F. and Lipscomb, A.B. (1992) Instrumented evaluation of knee laxity: a comparison of five arthrometers. *American Journal of Sports Medicine*, **20**, 135–140

Antich, T.J. and Brewster, C.E. (1985) Osgood-Schlatter disease: review of literature and physical therapy management. *Journal of Orthopaedic and Sports Physical Therapy*, **7**, (1) 5–10

Apley, A.G. and Solomon, L. (1989) *Concise System of Orthopaedics and Fractures*, Butterworth-Heinemann, Oxford

Apley, A.G. and Solomon, L. (1993) *Apley's System of Orthopaedics and Fractures*, 7th edn, Butterworth-Heinemann, Oxford

Arno, S. (1990) The A angle: a quantitative measurement of patella alignment and realignment. *Journal of Orthopaedic and Sports Physical Therapy*, **12**, (6) 237–242

Arnoczky, S. and Warren, R. (1983) Microstructure of the human meniscus. *American Journal of Sports Medicine*, **11**, (3) 131–140

Bach, B.R., Warren, R.F. and Wickiewicz, T.L. (1990) Arthrometric evaluation of knees that have a torn anterior cruciate ligament. *Journal of Bone and Joint Surgery*, **72A**, 1299

Baechle, T.R. (1994) *Essentials of Strength Training and Conditioning*, Human Kinetics, Champaign, Illinois

Baratta, R., Solomonow, M., Zhou, B.H., Letson, D., Chuinard, R. and D'Ambrosia, R. (1988) Muscular coactivation: the role of the antagonist musculature in maintaining knee stability. *American Journal of Sports Medicine*, **16**, 113–122

Barrie, H.J. (1979) The pathogenesis and significance of meniscal cysts. *Journal of Bone and Joint Surgery*, **61B**, 184

Baylis, W.J. and Rzonca, E.C. (1988) Common sports injuries to the knee. *Clinics in Podiatric Medicine and Surgery*, **5**, 3

Beard, D.J., Kyberd, P.J., O'Connor, J.J., Fergusson, C.M. and Dodd, C.A.F. (1994) Reflex hamstring contraction latency in anterior cruciate ligament deficiency. *Journal of Orthopaedic Research*, **12**, (2) 219–227

Beckman, M., Craig, R. and Lehman, R.C. (1989) Rehabilitation of patellofemoral dysfunction in the athlete. *Clinics in Sports Medicine*, **8**, (4) 841–860

Bennett, J.G. and Stauber, W.T. (1986) Evaluation of PFPS using eccentric exercise. *Medicine and Science in Sports and Exercise*, **18**, 520

Besser, M.I.B. and Stahl, S. (1986) Arthroscopic surgery performed under local anesthesia as an outpatient procedure. *Archives of Orthopaedic Trauma and Surgery*, **105**, 296–297

Briggs, C., Sandor, S.M. and Kenihan, M.A.R. (1995) The knee. In *Sports Physiotherapy* (ed. M. Zuluaga), Churchill Livingstone, London

Brody, D.M. (1980). Running injuries. *Clinical Symposia*, **32**, (4), Ciba Pharmaceutical Company

Buckley, J.R., Hood, G.M. and Macrae, W. (1989) Arthroscopy under local anaesthesia. *Journal of Bone and Joint Surgery*, **71B**, 126–127

Callaghan, M.J., Selfe, J., Bagley, P.J. and Oldham, J.A. (2000) Effects of patellar taping on knee joint proprioception. *Physiotherapy*, **86**, (11) 590

Caraffa, A., Cerulli, G., Projetti, M. and Aisa, G. (1996) Prevention of anterior cruciate ligament injuries in soccer. *Knee Surgery, Sports Traumatology and Arthroscopy*, **4**, 19–21

Christou, E.A. and Carlton, L.G. (1997) The effect of knee taping on the EMG activity of the vastus medialis and vastus leteralis muscles. *Medicine and Science in Sports and Exercise*, **29**, (Suppl.)(5) s211

Colosimo, A.J. and Bassett, F.H. (1990) Jumper's knee: diagnosis and treatment. *Orthopaedic Review*, **19**, 2

Committee on Complications of Arthroscopy Association of North America (1985) Complications of arthroscopy and arthroscopic surgery: results of a national survey. *Arthroscopy*, **1**, 214–220

Costill, D.L., Fink, W.J. and Habansky, A.J. (1977) Muscle rehabilitation after knee surgery. *Physician and Sports Medicine*, **7**, 71

Cox, A.J. (1990) Biomechanics of the patello-femoral joint. *Clinical Biomechanics*, **5**, 123–130

Crossley, K., Cowan, S.M., Bennell, K. and McConnell, J. (2000) Patellar taping: is clinical success supported by scientific evidence? *Manual Therapy*, **5**, (3) 142–150

Cyriax, J.H. and Cyriax, P.J. (1983) *Illustrated Manual of Orthopaedic Medicine*, Butterworths, London

Daniel, D.M., Malcom, L.L. and Losse, G. (1985) Instrumented measurement of anterior knee laxity in patients with acute anterior cruciate ligament disruption. *American Journal of Sports Medicine*, **13**, 401

Daniel, D.M., Stone, M.L., Barnett, P. and Sachs, R. (1988) Use of the quadriceps active test to diagnose posterior cruciate ligament disruption and measure posterior laxity of the knee. *Journal of Bone and Joint Surgery*, **70A**, 386–391

David, J.M. (1989) Jumper's knee. *Journal of Orthopaedic and Sports Physical Therapy*, **11**, (4) 137–141

de Andrade, J.R., Grant, C. and Dixon, A. (1965) Joint distention and reflex muscle inhibition in the knee. *Journal of Bone and Joint Surgery*, **47A**, 313–322

DeHaven, K.E., Black, K.P. and Griffiths, H.J. (1989) Open meniscus repair: technique and two to nine year results. *American Journal of Sports Medicine*, **17**, 788–795

DeHaven, K.E. and Bronstein, R.D. (1995) Injuries to the menisci of the knee. In *The Lower Extremity and Spine in Sports Medicine*, 2nd edn (eds J.A. Nicholas and E.B. Hershman), C.V. Mosby, St Louis

Donaldson, W.F., Warren, R.F. and Wickiewicz, T. (1985) A comparison of acute anterior cruciate ligament examinations. *American Journal of Sports Medicine*, **13**, 5–10

Evans, P. (1986) *The Knee Joint: A Clinical Guide*, Churchill Livingstone, London

Evans, P.J., Bell, G.D. and Frank, C. (1993) Prospective evaluation of the McMurray test. *American Journal of Sports Medicine*, **21**, 604–608

Evans, N.A., Hall, F., Chew, W.D. and Stanish, M.D. (2001) The natural history and tailored treatment of ACL injury. *Physician and Sportsmedicine*, **29**, (9) 70–84

Exler, Y. (1991) Patella fracture: review of the literature and five case presentations. *Journal of Orthopaedic and Sports Physical Therapy*, **13**, (4) 177–183

Fairbank, T.J. (1948). Knee joint changes after meniscectomy. *Journal of Bone and Joint Surgery*, **30B**, (4) 664–670

Feagin, J.A., Levy, A.S., Lintner, S.A. and Zorilla, P.A. (1995) Current concepts in anterior cruciate ligament surgery. *Sports Exercise and Injury*, **1**, (4) 176–182

Ferretti, A. (1986) Epidemiology of jumper's knee. *Sports Medicine*, **3**, 289–295

Finsterbush, A., Frankl, U. and Mann, G. (1989) Fat pad adhesion to partially torn anterior cruciate ligament: a cause of knee locking. *American Journal of Sports Medicine*, **17**, (1) 62–69

Forster, I.W. and Warren-Smith, C.D. (1989) Is the KT-1000 knee ligament arthrometer reliable? *Journal of Bone and Joint Surgery*, **71B**, 843

Fowler, P.J. and Messieh, S.S. (1987) Isolated posterior cruciate ligament injuries in athletes. *American Journal of Sports Medicine*, **15**, 553–557

Fulkerson, J.P. (1982) Awareness of the retinaculum in evaluating patello-femoral pain. *American Journal of Sports Medicine*, **10**, 147–149

Galway, R.D., Beaupre, A. and MacIntosh, D.L. (1973) Pivot shift: a clinical sign of symptomatic anterior cruciate ligament insufficiency. *Journal of Bone and Joint Surgery*, **54B**, 763

Garrick, J.G. and Webb, D.R. (1990). *Sports Injuries: Diagnosis and Management*, W.B. Saunders, London

Geissler, W.B. and Whipple, T.L. (1993) Intraarticular abnormalities in association with posterior cruciate ligament injuries. *American Journal of Sports Medicine*, **21**, 846–849

Grass, A.L. (1978) Treatment of Osgood-Schlatter injury. *Journal of the American Medical Association*, **240**, 212–213

Gruber, M.A. (1979) The conservative treatment of chondromalacia patellae. *Orthopedic Clinics of North America*, **10**, (1) 105–115

Gryzlo, S.M., Patek, R.M., Pink, M. and Perry, J. (1994) Electromyographic analysis of knee rehabilitation exercises. *Journal of Orthopaedic and Sports Physical Therapy*, **20**, 36–43

Hammesfahr, R. (1989) Surgery of the knee. In *Orthopaedic Physical Therapy* (eds R. Donatelli and M.J. Wooden), Churchill Livingstone, London

Henning, C.E. (1988) Semilunar cartilage of the knee: function and pathology. *Exercise and Sports Science Review*, **16**, 67–75

Henning, C.E., Lynch, M.A. and Glick, K.R. (1985) An in vivo strain gauge study of elongation of the ACL. *American Journal of Sports Medicine*, **13**, 34–39

Herrington, L. and Payton, S. (1997) Effects of corrective taping of the patella on patients with patellofemoral pain. *Physiotherapy*, **83**, (11) 566–572

Hertling, D. and Kessler, R.M. (1990) *Management of Common Musculoskeletal Disorders*, J.B. Lippincott, Philadelphia

Highgenboten, C.L., Jackson, A. and Meske, N.B. (1989) Genucom, KT-1000, and Stryker knee laxity measuring device comparisons: device responsibility and interdevice comparison in asymptomatic subjects. *American Journal of Sports Medicine*, **17**, 743

Higuchi, H., Kimura, M. and Shirakura, K. (2000) Factors affecting long term results after arthroscopic partial meniscectomy. *Clinical Orthopedics*, **377**, 161–168

Hoke, B., Howell, D. and Stack, M. (1983) The relationship between isokinetic testing and dynamic patellofemoral compression. *Journal of Orthopaedic and Sports Physical Therapy*, **4**, 150

Insall, J. (1979) Chondromalacia patellae: patellar malalignment syndrome. *Orthopaedic Clinics of North America*, **10**, 117–127

Jackson, R.W., Peters, R.I. and Marczyk, R.I. (1980) Late results of untreated anterior cruciate ligament rupture. *Journal of Bone and Joint Surgery*, **62B**, 127

Jacobson, E., Forssblad, M. and Rosenberg, J. (2000) Can local anesthesia be recommended for routine use in elective knee arthroscopy? *Arthroscopy*, **16**, 183–190

Jensen, K. (1990) Manual laxity tests for anterior cruciate ligament injuries. *Journal of Orthopaedic and Sports Physical Therapy*, **11**, (10) 474–481

Jerosch, J.G., Castro, W.H.M. and Jantea, C. (1989) Stress fracture of the patella. *American Journal of Sports Medicine*, **17**, 4

Jorgensen, U., Sonne-Holm, S. and Lauridsen, E. (1987) Long term follow up of meniscectomy in athletes: a prospective longitudinal study. *Journal of Bone and Joint Surgery*, **69**, 80

Kahn, D. and Wilson, M. (1987) Bone scintigraphic findings in patellar tendinitis. *Journal of Nuclear Medicine*, **28**, 1768–1770

Kalund, S., Sinkjaer, T., Arendt-Nielsen, L. and Simonsen, O. (1990) Altered timing of hamstring muscle action in anterior cruciate ligament deficient patients. *American Journal of Sports Medicine*, **18**, 245–248

Kannus, P. and Jarvinen, M. (1989) Post-traumatic anterior cruciate ligament insufficiency as a cause of osteoarthritis in a knee joint. *Journal of Rheumatology*, **18**, 251–260

Karst, G.M. and Jewett, P.D. (1993) Electromyographic analysis of exercises proposed for differential activation of medial and lateral quadriceps femoris muscle components. *Physical Therapy*, **73**, 286–299

Keene, J.S. (1990) Ligament and muscle tendon unit injuries. In *Orthopaedic and Sports Physical Therapy*, 2nd edn (ed. J.A. Gould), C.V. Mosby, St Louis, pp. 137–165

Kelley, M.J. (1990) Meniscal trauma (of the knee) and surgical intervention. *Journal of Sports Medicine and Physical Fitness*, **30**, (3) 297–306

Kennedy, J.C., Alexander, I.J. and Hayes, K.C. (1982) Nerve supply of the human knee and its functional importance. *American Journal of Sports Medicine*, **10**, 329

Koshino, T. and Okamoto, R. (1985) Resection of painful shelf (Plica synovialis mediopatellaris) under arthroscopy. *Arthroscopy*, **1**, 136–141

Larsen, B., Adreasen, E., Urfer, A. and Mickelson, M.R. (1995) Patellar taping: a radiographic examination of the medial glide technique. *American Journal of Sports Medicine*, **23**, (4) 465–471

Lephart, S.M. and Fu, F.H. (1995) The role of proprioception in the treatment of sports injuries. *Sports Exercise and Injury*, **1**, (2) 96–102

Levi, J.H. and Coleman, C.R. (1976) Fractures of the tibial tubercle. *American Journal of Sports Medicine*, **4**, 253–263

Levine, J. and Kashyap, S. (1981). A new conservative treatment of Osgood-Schlatter's disease. *Clinical Orthopaedics and Related Research*, **158**, 126–128

Levy, I.M., Torzilli, P.A. and Warren, R.F. (1982) The effect of medial meniscectomy on anterior-posterior motion of the knee. *Journal of Bone and Joint Surgery*, **64**, 883–888

Lieb, F.J. and Perry, J. (1968) Quadriceps function: an anatomical and mechanical study using amputated limbs. *Journal of Bone and Joint Surgery*, **50A**, 1535–1548

McConnell, J. (1986) The management of chondromalacia patella: a long term solution. *Australian Journal of Physiotherapy*, **31**, 214–223

McConnell, J. (1992) McConnell Patellofemoral Course, London

McConnell, J. (1994) McConnell Patello-femoral Course, London

McLaughlin, T.M., Lardner, T.J. and Dillman, C.J. (1979) Kinetics of the parallel squat. *Research Quarterly*, **49**, (2) 175–189

Magee, D.J. (2002) *Orthopedic Physical Assessment*, 4th edn, W.B. Saunders, Philadelphia

Malone, T. (1986) Clinical use of the Johnson anti-shear device: how and why to use it. *Journal of Orthopaedic and Sports Physical Therapy*, **7**, 304–309

Medlar, R.C. and Lyne, D. (1978) Sinding-Larsen-Johansson disease: its etiology and natural history. *Journal of Bone and Joint Surgery*, **60A**, 1113

Millar, A.L., Berglund, K., Blake, B. and Amstra, C. (1999) Effects of patellofemoral taping on knee pain and EMG activity of the quadriceps. *Medicine and Science in Sports and Exercise*, **31**, (Suppl.)(5) s207

Ngo, I.U., Hamilton, W.G., Wichern, W.A. and Andree, R.A. (1985) Local anesthesia with sedation for arthroscopic surgery of the knee: a report of 100 consecutive cases. *Arthroscopy*, **1**, 237–241

Noble, C.A. (1980) Iliotibial band friction syndrome in runners. *American Journal of Sports Medicine*, **9**, 232

Noble, J. and Hamblen, D.L. (1975) The pathology of the degenerate meniscal lesion. *Journal of Bone and Joint Surgery*, **57**, 180

Norkin, C.C. and Levangie, P.K. (1992) *Joint Structure and Function: A Comprehensive Analysis*, 2nd edn, F.A. Davis, Philadelphia

Norris, C.M. (1993) *Weight Training: Principles and Practice*, A. and C. Black, London

Norris, C.M (2001) *Acupuncture: Treatment of Musculoskeletal Conditions*, Butterworth-Heinemann, Oxford

Noyes, F.R., Bassett, R.W. and Grood, E.S. (1980) Arthroscopy in acute traumatic hemarthrosis of the knee. *Journal of Bone and Joint Surgery*, **62A**, 687

Noyes, F.R., Butler, D.L. and Grood, E.S. (1984) Biomechanical analysis of human ligament grafts used in knee ligament repairs and reconstructions. *Journal of Bone and Joint Surgery*, **66A**, 344

Noyes, F.R., Mangine, R.E. and Barber, S. (1987) Early motion after open and arthroscopic anterior cruciate ligament reconstruction. *American Journal of Sports Medicine*, **15**, 149–160

Noyes, F.R., Mooar, L.A., Moorman, C.T. and McGinniss, G.H. (1989) Partial tears of the anterior cruciate ligament: progression to complete ligament deficiency. *Journal of Bone and Joint Surgery*, **71B**, 825–833

O'Donoghue, D.H. (1976) *Treatment of Injuries to Athletes*, W.B. Saunders, Philadelphia

Ohkoshi, Y., Yasuda, K., Kaneda, K., Wada, T. and Yamanaka, M. (1991) Biomechanical analysis of rehabilitation in the standing position. *American Journal of Sports Medicine*, **19**, 605–611

Palastanga, N., Field, D. and Soames, R. (1989) *Anatomy and Human Movement*, Butterworth-Heinemann, Oxford

Palmitier, R.A., An, K., Scott, S.G. and Chao, E.Y.S. (1991) Kinetic chain exercise in knee rehabilitation. *Sports Medicine*, **11**, (6) 402–413

Panariello, R.A., Backus, S.I. and Parker, J.W. (1994) The effect of the squat exercise on anterior-posterior knee translation in professional football players. *American Journal of Sports Medicine*, **22**, 768–773

Parolie, J.M. and Bergfeld, J.A. (1986) Long term results of nonoperative treatment of isolated posterior cruciate ligament injuries in the athlete. *American Journal of Sports Medicine*, **14**, 53–58

Paulos, L.E., Rosenberg, T.D. and Drawbert, C.W. (1987) Infrapatellar contraction syndrome: an unrecognised cause of knee stiffness with patellar entrapment and patella infera. *American Journal of Sports Medicine*, **15**, 331

Post, W., and Fulkerson, J. (1992) Distal realignment of the patellofemoral joint. *Orthopaedic Clinics of North America*, **23**, 6–11

Ray, J.M., Clancy, W.G. and Lemon, R.A. (1988) Semimembranosus tendinitis: an overlooked cause of medial knee pain. *American Journal of Sports Medicine*, **16**, 4

Rebman, L.W. (1988) Lachman's test: an alternative method. *Journal of Orthopedic and Sports Physical Therapy*, **9**, (11) 381–382

Reid, D.C. (1992) *Sports Injury Assessment and Rehabilitation*, Churchill Livingstone, London

Reilly, B.M. (1991) *Practical Strategies in Outpatient Medicine*, 2nd edn, W.B. Saunders, Philadelphia

Renstrom, P., Arms, S.W. and Stanwick, R.J. (1986) Strain within the anterior cruciate ligament during hamstring and quadriceps activity. *American Journal of Sports Medicine*, **14**, 83–87

Reynolds, L., Levin, T., Medeiros, J., Adler, N. and Hallum, A. (1983) EMG activity of the vastus medialis oblique and vastus lateralis and their role in patellar alignment. *American Journal of Physical Medicine*, **62**, (2) 61–71

Richardson, C. and Bullock, M.I. (1986) Changes in muscle activity during fast, alternating flexion-extension movements of the knee. *Scandinavian Journal of Rehabilitation Medicine*, **18**, 51–58

Roberts, J.M. (1989) The effect of taping on patellofemoral alignment: a radiological pilot study. Manipulative Therapists Association of Australia Conference, Adelaide, pp. 146–151

Rouse, S.J. (1996) The role of the iliotibial tract in patello-femoral pain and iliotibial band friction syndromes. *Physiotherapy*, **82**, (3) 199–202

Ryu, R.K.N. and Dunbar, W.H. (1988) Arthroscopic meniscal repair with two-year follow-up: a clinical review. *Arthroscopy*, **4**, 168–173

Ryu, R.K.N. and Ting, A.J. (1993) Arthroscopic treatment of meniscal cysts. *Arthroscopy*, **9**, 591–595

Sachs, R.A., Daniel, D.M., Stone, M.L. and Garfein, R.F. (1989). Patellofemoral problems after anterior cruciate ligament reconstruction. *American Journal of Sports Medicine*, **17**, 760–765

Sandberg, R., Nilsson, B. and Westlin, N. (1987) Hinged cast after knee ligament surgery. *American Journal of Sports Medicine*, **15**, 270–274

Seedhom, B.B. and Hargreaves, D.J. (1979) Transmission of the load in the knee joint with special reference to the role of the menisci. Part II: Experimental results, discussion and conclusions. *Engineering Medicine*, **8**, 220–228

Seto, J.L., Brewster, C.E. and Lombardo, J. (1989) Rehabilitation of the knee after anterior cruciate ligament reconstruction. *Journal of Orthopaedic and Sports Physical Therapy*, **10**, 8

Seto, J.L., Orofino, A.S. and Morrissey, M.C. (1988) Assessment of quadriceps/hamstring strength, knee ligament stability, functional and sports activity levels five years after anterior cruciate ligament reconstruction. *American Journal of Sports Medicine*, **16**, 170–180

Shakespeare, D.T. and Rigby, H.S. (1983) The bucket handle tear of the meniscus: a clinical and arthrographic study. *Journal of Bone and Joint Surgery*, **65**, 383

Shea, K. and Fulkerson, J. (1992) Pre-operative computed tomography scanning and arthroscopy in predicting outcome after lateral release. *Arthroscopy*, **8**, 327–334

Shelbourne, K.D. and Nitz, P. (1990) Accelerated rehabilitation after cruciate ligament reconstruction. *American Journal of Sports Medicine*, **18**, 292–299

Sherman, O.H., Fox, J.M., Snyder, S.J. et al. (1986) Arthroscopy - 'No problem surgery'. An analysis of complications in two thousand six hundred and forty cases. *Journal of Bone and Joint Surgery*, **68A**, 256–265

Shino, K., Kimura, T., Hirose, H., Inoue, M. and Ono, K. (1986) Reconstruction of the anterior cruciate ligament by allogenic tendon graft: an operation for chronic ligamentous insufficiency. *Journal of Bone and Joint Surgery*, **68B**, 739–746

Silver, D.M. and Campbell, P. (1985) Arthroscopic assessment and treatment of dancer's knee injuries. *Physician and Sports Medicine*, **13**, (11) 74–82

Sinkjaer, T. and Arendt-Nielsen, L. (1991) Knee stability and muscle coordination in patients with anterior cruciate ligament injuries: an electromyographic approach. *Journal of Electromyography and Kinesiology*, **1**, 209–217

Slocum, D.B., James, S.L. and Larson, R.L. (1976) Clinical test for anteriolateral rotatory instability of the knee. *Clinical Orthopaedics and Related Research*, **118**, 63

Smillie, I.S. (1974) *Diseases of the Knee Joint*, Churchill Livingstone, London

Solomonow, M., Barratta, R. and D'Ambrosia, R. (1989) The role of the hamstrings in the rehabilitation of the anterior cruciate ligament deficient knee in athletes. *Sports Medicine*, **7**, 42

Somes, S., Worrell, T.W., Corey, B. and Ingersol, C.D. (1997) Effects of patellar taping on patellar position in the open and closed kinetic chain: a preliminary study. *Journal of Sports Rehabilitation*, **6**, 299–308

Sommer, H.M. (1988) Patellar chondropathy and apicitis and muscle imbalances of the lower extremities in competitive sports. *Sports Medicine*, **5**, 386

Speakman, H.G.B. and Weisberg, J. (1977) The vastus medialis controversy. *Physiotherapy*, **63**, (8) 249–254

Staubli, H-U. and Jakob, R.P. (1991) Anterior knee motion analysis: measurement and simultaneous radiography. *American Journal of Sports Medicine*, **19**, 172

Steinkamp, L.A., Dillingham, M.F., Markel, M.D., Hill, J.A. and Kaufman, K.R. (1993) Biomechanical considerations in patellofemoral joint rehabilitation. *American Journal of Sports Medicine*, **21**, 438–444

Stokes, M. and Young, A. (1984) The contribution of reflex inhibition to arthrogenous muscle weakness. *Clinical Science*, **67**, 7–14

Terry, G.C., Hughston, J.C. and Norwook, L.A. (1986) Anatomy of the iliopatellar band and iliotibial tract. *American Journal of Sports Medicine*, **14**, 39–45

Tiberio, D. (1987) The effect of excessive subtalar joint pronation on patellofemoral mechanics: a theoretical model. *Journal of Orthopaedic and Sports Physical Therapy*, **9**, 4

Timm, K.E. (1986) Validation of the Johnson anti-shear accessory as an accurate and effective clinical isokinetic instrument. *Journal of Orthopaedic and Sports Physical Therapy*, **7**, 298–303

Torg, J.S. (1989) In *Year Book of Sports Medicine* (eds R.J. Shephard, J.L. Anderson, E.R. Eichner et al.), Yearbook Medical Publishers, Chicago, p. 186

Torzilli, P.A. (1991) Measurement reproducibility of two commercial knee test devices. *Journal of Orthopaedic Research*, **9**, 730

Traverso, A., Baldari, A. and Catalani, F. (1990) The coexistence of Osgood-Schlatter's disease with Sinding-Larsen-Johansson's disease. *Journal of Sports Medicine and Physical Fitness*, **30**, (3) 331–333

Tsirbas, A., Paterson, R.S. and Keene, G.C.R. (1990) Fat pad impingement: a missed cause of patello-femoral pain? *Australian Journal of Science and Medicine in Sport*, December, 24–26

Weiss, C.B., Lundberg, M., Hamberg, P., DeHaven, K.E. and Gillquist, J. (1989) Non-operative treatment of meniscal tears. *Journal of Bone and Joint Surgery*, **71A**, 811–822

Williams, P.L. (1995) *Gray's Anatomy*, 38th edn, Churchill Livingstone, Edinburgh

Williams, J.G.P. and Sperryn, P.N. (1976) *Sports Medicine*, Edward Arnold, London

Wilson, W.J., Lewis, F. and Scranton, P.E. (1990) Combined reconstruction of the anterior cruciate ligament in competitive athletes. *Journal of Bone and Joint Surgery*, **72A**, (5) 742–748

Woo, S.L-Y., Ohno, K., Weaver, C.M., Pomaybo, A.S. and Xerogeanes, J.W. (1994) Non-operative treatment of knee ligament injuries. *Sports Exercise and Injury*, **1**, (1) 2–13

Wroble, R.R., Van Ginkel, L.A., Grood, E.S. et al. (1990) Repeatability of the KT-1000 arthrometer in a normal population. *American Journal of Sports Medicine*, **18**, 396

Yasuda, K. and Sasaki, T. (1987) Muscle exercise after anterior cruciate ligament reconstruction: biomechanics of the simultaneous isometric contraction method of the quadriceps and hamstrings. *Clinical Orthopaedics and Related Research*, **220**, 266–274

Zachazewski, J.E., Magee, D.J. and Quillen, W.S. (1996) *Athletic Injuries and Rehabilitation*, Saunders, Philadelphia

Zuluaga, M., Briggs, C. and Carlisle, J. (1995) *Sports Physiotherapy*, Churchill Livingstone, Edinburgh

Chapter 11

The shin

The term 'shin splints' is often used as a blanket description of any persistent pain occurring between the knee and ankle in an athlete. A more accurate description comes with the various 'compartment syndromes' which identify the anatomical structures affected. The anterior compartment contains the tibialis anterior, extensor hallucis longus, extensor digitorum longus, and the anterior tibial artery and vein. The lateral compartment contains the peronei, and the superficial peroneal nerve. The superficial posterior compartment contains the gastrocnemius and soleus and the deep posterior compartment contains the tibialis posterior, flexor digitorum longus, flexor hallucis longus, the peroneal artery and vein, and the posterior tibial artery and vein (Fig. 11.1). The deep and superficial posterior compartments are separated by the deep transverse fascia of the leg.

ANTERIOR COMPARTMENT SYNDROME

Anterior compartment syndrome involves pain in the anterior lower leg (Fig. 11.2a), which is increased in resisted dorsiflexion. There is usually a history of a sudden increase in training intensity, frequently involving jumping or running on a hard surface. The anterior compartment muscles swell, and in some cases hypertrophy occurs. The fascia covering

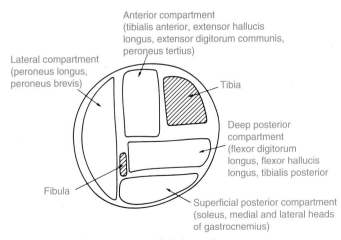

Figure 11.1   Compartments of the lower leg.

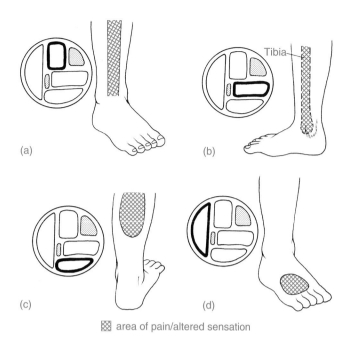

(a)

(b) Tibia

(c)

(d)

▨ area of pain/altered sensation

Figure 11.2 Anterior compartment syndrome. Pain on the anterolateral aspect of the lower leg. (b) Deep posterior compartment syndrome (medial tibial stress syndrome). Pain over distal third of tibia (see also Fig. 11.3). (c) Superficial posterior compartment syndrome. Pain within the calf bulk. (d) Lateral compartment syndrome. Loss of sensation over the dorsum of the foot.

the muscles may be too tight and inflexible to accommodate the increase in size. As a consequence, when the muscles relax, their intramuscular pressure remains high and fresh blood is unable to perfuse the tissues freely. This decrease in blood flow leads to ischaemia with associated pain and impairment of muscle function.

Usually, when a muscle contracts, its blood flow is temporarily stopped. Arterial inflow occurs once more between the muscle contractions as the intramuscular pressure falls. Normal resting pressure within the tibialis anterior in the supine subject is about 5–10 mmHg, increasing to as much as 150–250 mmHg with muscle contraction. Muscle relaxation pressure, that which occurs between repeated contractions, is between 15 and 25 mmHg in the normal subject, but in athletes with anterior compartment syndrome pressures may rise to 30–35 mmHg and take up to 15 minutes to return to normal values (Styf, 1989).

> **Keypoint**
>
> In anterior compartment syndrome the resting pressure within the tibialis anterior can be 50% greater than normal.

The exact cause of the condition is not known. Hypertrophy may be one factor, as the condition occurs frequently when training intensity is increased. However, bodybuilders rarely suffer from the condition, so the rate rather than the amount of muscle hypertrophy may be important. Microtrauma and excessive stress to the blood capillaries and lymphatics may give rise to inflammation and in some cases myositis in the area (Styf, 1989).

LATERAL COMPARTMENT AND SUPERFICIAL PERONEAL NERVE

This is an unusual cause of shin pain and occurs when the peronei muscles are affected, usually by hyperpronation (Brody, 1980). The condition may have existed for some time but is brought to the fore when running begins. Again, there is ischaemia and pain, but in addition the superficial peroneal nerve may be compressed as it emerges from the lateral compartment.

The nerve lies deep to the peroneus longus and then passes forwards and downwards between the peronei and the extensor digitorum longus. It pierces the fascia in the distal third of the leg where it divides into medial and lateral branches to enter the foot. Entrapment may occur if muscle herniation or fascial defect exist. In addition, ankle sprain, fasciotomy, and an anomalous course of the nerve have been suggested as contributory factors (Styf, 1989). Clinically, the patient presents with loss of sensation over the dorsum of the foot, especially the second to fourth toes (Fig. 11.2d). Certain resting positions may compress the nerve and bring on the symptoms. To test the nerve, it is compressed over the anterior intermuscular septum 8–15 cm proximal to the lateral malleolus while the patient actively dorsiflexes and everts the foot. Tinel's sign, involving local percussion over the compression site, may be positive.

> **Keypoint**
>
> With lateral compartment syndrome the superficial peroneal nerve may be compressed, giving loss of sensation over the dorsum of the 2nd, 3rd and 4th toes. To test the nerve, compress it 8–15 cm proximal to the lateral malleolus while the patient actively dorsiflexes and everts the foot.

POSTERIOR COMPARTMENT

The superficial compartment contains the soleus and gastrocnemius. These muscles are usually affected by trauma rather than ischaemia, and are dealt with separately below. Pain occurs within the calf bulk (Fig. 11.2c) and is increased with resisted plantarflexion.

The deep posterior compartment contains tibialis posterior, flexor digitorum longus and flexor hallucis longus, and is the most common site for shin pain. Pain in this region is usually experienced over the distal third of the medial tibia (Fig. 11.2b) and represents *medial tibial stress syndrome* (Mubarak et al., 1982). The exact site of pain will

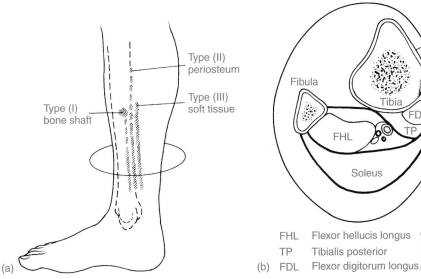

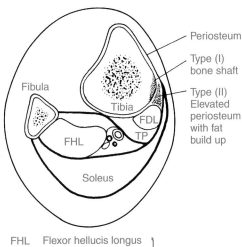

FHL   Flexor hellucis longus
TP   Tibialis posterior   } Type (III)
FDL   Flexor digitorum longus

(a)   (b)

Figure 11.3   Medial tibial stress syndrome. (a) Painful areas of palpation. (b) Cross-section of structures affected. After Detmer, D.E. (1986) Chronic shin splints: classification and management of medial tibial stress syndrome. *Sports Medicine*, 3, 436–444. With permission.

vary depending on the specific structures affected, and Detmer (1986) described a system of classification involving three types of chronic condition (Fig. 11.3).

Definition

Medial tibial stress syndrome is pain over the distal third of the inner aspect of the tibia. The disorder may affect the bone, periosteum (bone membrane), fascia, or muscles.

Type I involves microfractures or stress fracture of the bone itself. The patient is usually a runner who has recently increased his or her mileage. The stress imposed by the sport exceeds the ability of the bone to adapt and remodel. The condition may present as a stress fracture showing a concentrated positive uptake in a single area on bone scan and point tenderness to palpation (type IA), or as a diffuse area along the medial edge of the tibia giving more generalized pain (type IB). In chronic conditions which have existed for some time, the tibial edge may be uneven due to new bone formation.

Type II medial tibial stress syndrome involves the junction of the periosteum and fascia, and occurs particularly in sprinters and those involved in jumping activities. Pain is maximal just posterior to the bone, and has often persisted for a number of years. Initially, pain occurs only with activity, but as the condition progresses discomfort is felt with walking and even at rest. In this condition compartment pressures may not be elevated, and the periosteum is unchanged. One explanation is that the periosteum is traumatically avulsed from the bone by the action of soleus through its attachment to the fascia. During the chronic stage of this condition, adipose tissue has been found, during surgery, between the periosteum and underlying bone

(Detmer, 1986). In the early stages of the condition the periosteum may heal back with rest, but when the condition becomes chronic, it is unable to heal, and continues to cause pain when stressed by activity.

The type III condition involves ischaemia of the distal deep posterior compartment and presents as a dull aching over the posterior soft tissues brought on by exercise. Intramuscular pressures are elevated as with anterior compartment syndrome (see above), and remain elevated after exercise.

MANAGEMENT

Initial management of shin pain involves a reduction of the stresses which caused the condition in the first place. This involves accurately identifying the structures affected and taking a thorough history of causal factors, particularly stresses imposed during training. Biomechanical assessment of the lower limb is mandatory and prescription of orthotics should be made where necessary. Initially, rest and anti-inflammatory modalities are used to allow the acute inflammation to settle, but external compression and elevation of the limb may exacerbate the problem (Di Manna and Buck, 1990). If training stresses can be modified, and the condition has been identified early enough, this may be all that is required.

In chronic conditions in which conservative management has failed, decompression by fasciotomy may be called for. Here, the fascia of the affected compartment is surgically split along its length. The procedure is often performed on

---

Definition

Fasciotomy is surgical splitting (cutting) of the fascia along its length to reduce pressure within the fascial compartment.

Treatment note 11.1   Manual therapy for shin pain

Trigger point massage

Trigger point (TrP) massage for anterior compartment syndrome focuses on the tibialis anterior and the extensor digitorum longus. The TrP for the tibialis anterior is located approximately one-third of the way distally from the knee and to the lateral side of the tibia. A muscle stripping technique can be used starting from half-way down the tibia progressing up towards the knee in a slow movement gradually progressing in depth (Fig. 11.4). The thickness of the muscle means that both thumbs must be used simultaneously or a pressure tool where ischaemic compression is used. The elbow is the tool of choice, direct compression is given and maintained for 3–10 seconds or until pain subsides.

Ice massage may be used over the same point, beginning from the knee and extending down the length of the tibia; a progressive stretch of plantarflexion and inversion is then used.

The long toe extensors (extensor digitorum longus (EDL) and extensor hallucis longus (EHL)) may be similarly treated. The EDL TrP is located approximately 8 cm distal and slightly anterior to the head of the fibula. The EHL is located at the junction of the middle of the distal thirds of the lower leg (Fig. 11.5). Home stretching may again be used, this time forcing the foot into plantarflexion and the distal toes into flexion.

For lateral compartment syndrome, the peroneus longus and peroneus brevis muscles are targeted. The TrP for peroneus longus is approximately 2–4 cm distal to the fibular head, close to the shaft of the fibular itself, while that of the peroneus brevis is located at the junction of the middle and distal third of the lower leg.

Ischaemic compression may be used with the thumbs and ice stretch may again be given, this time stretching the foot into plantarflexion and inversion (Fig. 11.6).

Posterior compartment syndrome and medial tibial stress syndrome require treatment of the flexor digitorum longus (FDL) and tibialis posterior along the lower third of the posterior edge of the tibia. Where the muscle itself is stressed, the TrP is targeted on the medial border of the upper tibia. The patient lies in crook side lying and the palpation point is between the medial edge of the tibia and the gastrocnemius muscles (Fig. 11.7). The gastrocnemius is pushed posteriorly and the pressure is then applied downward and then laterally. For the flexor hallucis longus (FHL), the patient may be treated in prone and this time the thumb is positioned lateral to the mid-line, pressing on the edge of the soleus at the junction between the middle and lower thirds of the lower leg.

Self-help trigger point methods

The athlete may be taught to use trigger point therapy as a self-treatment to relieve pain as it occurs. For the tibialis anterior, the easiest method is to use the heel of the opposite foot (Fig. 11.8). The movement is on the lateral edge of the tibia and begins at mid-shin level, the pressure being in a continuous sweep towards the lateral edge of the knee.

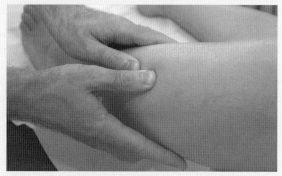

Figure 11.4   Muscle stripping technique for tibialis anterior trigger point.

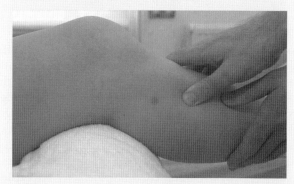

Figure 11.6   Trigger points of the lateral compartment muscles.

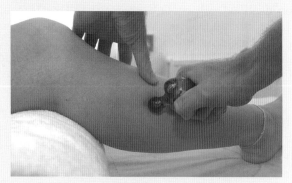

Figure 11.5   Trigger points of the long toe extensors.

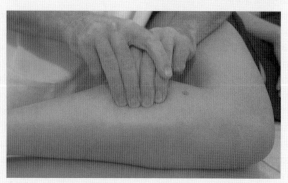

Figure 11.7   Trigger points of the posterior compartment.

For the peroneal muscles, pressure may be given by the index finger, supported by the middle finger or by a single flexed knuckle (Fig. 11.9). For the flexor digitorum longus and tibialis posterior, one or two fingers may suffice. Alternatively, hands may wrap around the shin and both thumbs may be used to apply to the peroneus longus.

Where pressure on the trigger points is too tiring for the hands, apparatus such as the 'backnobber' (Physiomed, Manchester, UK) can be used to create more force (Fig. 11.10).

Dry needling techniques for trigger point therapy

For anterior tibial syndrome, traditional acupuncture points on the stomach meridian may be used. Point ST. 36 located three finger breadths below the lateral aspect of the knee and point ST. 40 located midway between the lateral maleolus and the knee joint line may be used. Lateral compartment syndrome responds to needling along the gall-bladder meridian. GB 34 located distal and lateral to the head of the fibula and GB 39 located three finger breadths above the apex of the lateral maleolus on the edge of the tibia may be used.

For medial tibial stress syndrome, the point Sp. 6 may be used; located 3 finger breadths above the apex of the medial maleolus on the edge of the tibia, this point is directly opposite to GB 39 (Fig. 11.11). See Norris (2001) for specific details.

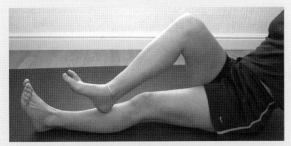

Figure 11.8   Self-treatment of the tibialis anterior using the heel.

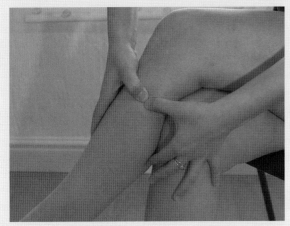

Figure 11.9   Self-treatment of the peroneus longus using both hands.

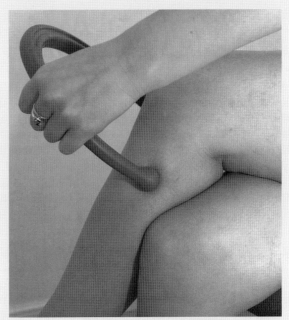

Figure 11.10   Creating more force by using the 'backnobber' apparatus. Pressure Positive Co., with permission.

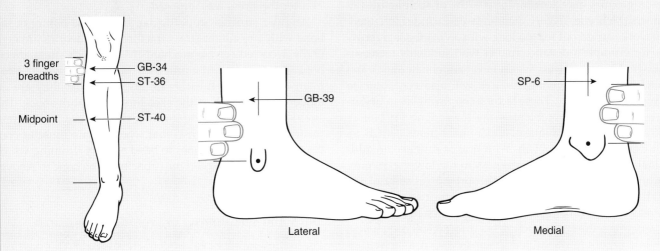

Figure 11.11   Traditional acupuncture points used in the treatment of shin pain.

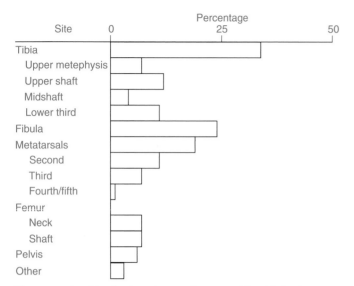

Figure 11.12 Distribution of stress fractures. After McBryde (1985), with permission.

an out-patient basis, with two incisions being made, at the junction of the proximal and middle third of the leg and the middle and distal third. Athletes mobilize early and are often able to resume running after 3 weeks.

If fasciotomy is not successful, it may be the case that the epimysium over the tibialis posterior has been missed at surgery. Hannaford (1988) argued that the tibialis posterior should be classified as a condition independent from that affecting the other deep posterior muscles.

STRESS FRACTURES

Over 50% of all stress fractures occur to the tibia and fibula (McBryde, 1985) with the remaining sites being mostly to the lower limb (Fig. 11.12). Stress fractures are usually the end point in a sequence of overuse. A number of causal factors usually coexist to begin the development of the condition. Training errors may account for 60–75% of such injuries in runners (McBryde, 1985). Common faults include high intensity work carried out for too long with an inadequate recovery, for example a distance runner who suddenly increases mileage. Faulty footwear which fails to attenuate shock and exercising on unforgiving surfaces will also contribute to lower limb pathology. These factors, coupled with an underlying malalignment problem of the lower limb (or biomechanical faults in technique of upper limb actions, see Ch. 6), will exacerbate the problem. With novice runners, an additional factor is muscular weakness in the lower extremity leading to a reduction in shock-absorbing capacity of the soft tissues. In each case, the overload on the tissues exceeds the elastic limit, causing a plastic deformation of bone (p. 8).

Very often, the stress fracture is a direct result of a change of some type – in the athletes themselves, in the environment in which they train, or in the activity (Garrick and Webb, 1990). In terms of the athlete, stress fractures often emerge following the onset of a growth spurt or at the menopause as a result of to the large body adaptations occurring at these times. Similarly, following illness, the body must be allowed time to readapt to training demands. Environmental changes, such as new clothing (shoes) or a new playing surface, will also require time to allow tissue adaptation, and failure to allow for this may lead to tissue breakdown, of which stress fractures are one type. Finally, alterations in the quality or quantity of a training programme itself will require a period of adaptation.

Far from being inert, bone is a dynamic tissue which is continually remodelling in response to mechanical stress. A balance usually exists between bone proliferation and reabsorption, which maintains the bone integrity. The result of athletic activity is normally that bone strengthens, but if unbalanced stresses cause bone reabsorption to exceed proliferation, the bone weakens.

> **Keypoint**
>
> Exercise (loading) normally causes microscopic damage within bone, and the body responds by producing stronger bone material. If the amount of damage caused by loading is greater than the ability of the bone to restrengthen, stress fracture occurs.

Examining excessive running and jumping in rabbits, Li et al. (1985) demonstrated that osteoblastic activity occurred from 7–9 days later than osteoclastic activity. Remodelling began on day 2, with the haversian blood vessels dilating, and by day 7 osteoclastic activity was noted in the bone cortex. New bone formation began in the periosteum by the 14th day of excessive stress. The adaptation to this excessive stress was reabsorption which occurred for some time before the formation of new cortical bone, thus weakening the bone structure. Abnormal X-rays were not found until day 21 after the stress was imposed.

Angular stresses, in particular, may cause failure of the bone with a resultant stress fracture. Two theories are generally accepted for the mechanisms by which stress affects bone. The first (fatigue) proposes that training which is too intense causes the muscles to fatigue so that they are no longer able to support the skeleton and absorb shock. The strain passes to the bone, causing the fracture. The second theory (overload) suggests that when certain muscles contract, they cause the bones to bend slightly. Training which is too intense will exceed the capacity of the bone to recover from this stress.

Signs and symptoms

The main symptom of a stress fracture is pain. This has been categorized into four types, depending on its characteristic (Puffer and Zachazewski, 1988). With type I pain, the athlete

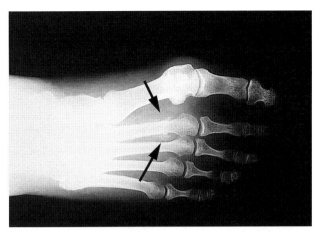

Figure 11.13 X-ray of stress fracture. From Read (2000) with permission.

Table 11.1 Pain classification

Classification	Characteristics	Action
Type I	Pain only after activity	↓ workload by 25%
Type II	Pain during activity but not restricting performance	↓ workload by 50%
Type III	Pain during activity restricting performance	Total rest
Type IV	Chronic unremitting pain at rest	Splint/cast Medical investigation

After Puffer, J.C. and Zachazewski, J.E. (1988) Management of overuse injuries. *American Family Physician*, **38**(3), 225–232. With permission.

only feels discomfort after activity. With type II and III pain, discomfort is felt while training, but with type II this does not restrict activity. Type IV pain is chronic and unremitting in nature. Further symptoms include warmth and tenderness over the injured area, made worse with sporting activity and better with rest. Swelling may be evident in the later stages of the condition if the bony surface is superficial. Accuracy of palpation when assessing bone pain is vital. The tenderness of a stress fracture is usually well localized, whereas that of compartment syndrome is more diffuse. Initially radiographs are usually negative, it taking at least 2 weeks for X-ray changes to be apparent (Li et al., 1985; Rzonca and Baylis, 1988). Local periosteal reaction and new bone growth may be seen after 6 weeks in long bone (Markey, 1987) and compressive stress fractures in cancellous bone are sometimes visible after 24 hours (Puddu et al., 1994). Taunton and Clement (1981) found radiographs to be positive in only 47.2% of their cases, while bone scan was accurate in 95.8%. Bone scan is normally revealing at the onset of symptoms and is generally more reliable. Phosphate labelled with technetium-99m is incorporated into osteoblasts and a hot spot appears over the active area, 6–72 hours after the onset of pain (Puddu et al., 1994).

Pain may be produced over the superficial fracture site by vibration. This may be produced from a tuning fork or ultrasound unit (Lowden, 1986), and is generally of more use in low risk areas, such as the foot and shin. Where there is a risk of complication through displacement (such as in the neck of the femur, see p. 194) bone scan with possible surgical intervention may be more appropriate. (Fig. 11.13).

Treatment

Treatment of a stress fracture is primarily that of rest. As a general guide, with type I or II pain the workload should be reduced by 25% and 50%, respectively. Total rest is called for where type III pain is experienced, and type IV pain requires immediate medical investigation (Table 11.1). In the more severe conditions, rest should be total, because even allowing an athlete to train the upper body will often result in 'just trying the leg out' in the gym. Training should not resume until the athlete has been totally pain free for 10 days. It should be emphasized to the athlete that this means at the end of each day he or she should go to bed having felt no pain over the injured area during that day.

The timescale of healing will vary depending on the site of injury. With reduced activity, fibular stress fractures will normally heal in 4–6 weeks, tibial stress fractures in 8–10 weeks and femoral neck stress fractures in 12–16 weeks (Reid, 1992).

When activity is resumed, the athlete should be closely monitored, and activities stopped if any pain occurs. Return to sport should be progressive and varied. Different speed, running surfaces, and activities should all be used to spread the emphasis of training. Alternative training should be used, to reduce the weight bearing on the limb. Swimming and cycling may be utilized to restore cardiopulmonary fitness, for example.

TENNIS LEG

Of the sural muscles, it is the gastrocnemius which is usually injured. The soleus is infrequently affected by trauma being a single-joint muscle, but is more usually the victim of temporary ischaemia, giving rise to superficial posterior compartment syndrome.

Tennis leg is a strain of the gastrocnemius, normally involving the medial head at its musculotendinous junction with the Achilles tendon. The history of injury is usually a sudden propulsive action, such as a lunge or jump as the athlete pushes off from the mark. Women are more commonly affected, and the athlete is usually over 30 years of age

> **Keypoint**
>
> Calf muscle strain usually effect the gastrocnemius muscle rather than the soleus. The medial head of the muscle is more commonly affected, at the junction of the middle and proximal third.

(Garrick and Webb, 1990). The condition is often described as a rupture of the plantaris, more by tradition than anything else, because this muscle is rarely the cause of symptoms.

The athlete often feels something 'go' in the back of the leg, as though he or she were hit from behind. Pain and spasm occur rapidly, preventing the athlete from putting the heel to the ground. Later, swelling and bruising develop distal to the injury site, peaking at 48 hours after injury. There is local tenderness over the medial head of gastrocnemius at the junction between the middle and proximal third of the calf. Pain to passive stretch is worse with the knee straight than with it flexed.

Initial treatment is to immobilize the calf to prevent further tissue damage. Some authorities recommend a plantarflexed position with a 2–4 cm heel lift (Cyriax, 1982), while others claim that a 90° neutral ankle position gives a better result by preventing contraction and tightening the fascia to limit the spread of bruising (Garrick and Webb, 1990). Pain and the amount of tissue damage is usually the deciding factor. Partial ruptures are best immobilized non-weight bearing in plantarflexion to approximate the tissue, whereas less serious injuries can be prevented from shortening by adopting a neutral resting position.

Compression from an elastic bandage limits the formation of swelling, and strength and flexibility is maintained by starting rehabilitation early. Massage involving calf kneading and transverse frictions ensures adequate broadening of the muscle fibres. Stretching to the gastrocnemius begins in the long sitting position. A towel or band is placed over the foot and the athlete gently pulls the foot into dorsiflexion. Stretching with the toes on a block in a partial, and later full weight-bearing position is the exercise progression. Strength is regained by utilizing a comparable long sitting position but substituting an elastic band for the strap. The foot is pressed into plantarflexion against the resistance of the band. Heel raises are performed in a standing position, initially from the floor and later with the heel on a 2–3 cm block.

Gait re-education is used to encourage equal stride length and the adoption of a normal heel-toe rhythm avoiding external rotation of the leg. When the calf is pain free, strength activities give way to power movements, to build up the fast twitch nature of the muscle (Ng and Richardson, 1990). Gentle jogging, jumping and skipping are used and progressed to plyometrics. The athlete should be instructed to jump and land correctly. The toes should be the last point to leave the floor in a jump and the first to contact the floor on landing. Toe contact is followed by progressive lowering through the foot with the knee and hip flexing as the heel touches the floor to minimize shock. Flat foot landing and remaining on the toes must be avoided (Fig. 11.14). Slow squats raising up onto the toes at the top point give way to toe springing actions with and without weight resistance (dumb-bells or a weighted jacket). Leg drives from a mark are useful, as are 'side hops' and 'hop and twist' actions over a bar.

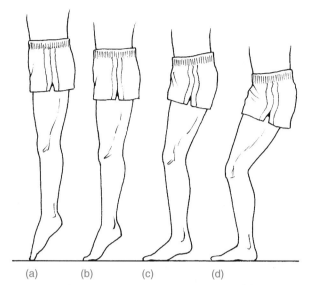

(a)   (b)   (c)   (d)

Figure 11.14   Correct landing action from a jump. (a) Toe contacts floor first. (b) Foot flexes to absorb shock. (c,d) Knee and hip flex ('give') as heel touches ground.

ACHILLES TENDON

Achilles tendon pain (achillodynia) is a common condition in sport, with the incidence in runners being as high as 9% (Lysholm and Wiklander, 1987). Interestingly, the condition was relatively uncommon until the 1950s and is still very rarely seen in China (40 Achilles tendon ruptures among 2.5 million people over a 5-year period) (Jozsa, Kvist and Balint, 1989). The increased incidence of Achilles tendon rupture may be a result of the increasingly sedentary lifestyles seen in the Western industrialized countries (Kvist, 1994).

The Achilles tendon is the largest tendon in the body, being some 15 cm long and about 2 cm thick. It is able to sustain loads of up to 17 times bodyweight while utilizing only 13% of the oxygen supply of a muscle (Khan and Maffulli 1998). The tendon consists of connective tissue containing fibroblasts (tenoblasts) in a ground substance. The main extracellular component (80% of the dry weight of the tendon) is collagen, predominently type 1, with a small amount of type III.

Definition

Type I collagen is white and glistening and consists of large diameter fibres. It is found predominantly in skin and tendon. *Type III collagen* forms a delicate supporting network and is more common in young and repairing tissue. It is found commonly in skin and blood vessel walls.

Analysis of normal and ruptured Achilles tendon has shown that ruptured tendon has a greater percentage of type III collagen, making the tendon less resistant to tensile

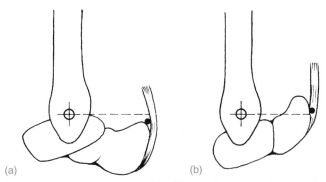

Figure 11.15 Contact point of Achilles tendon moves downwards as plantarflexion increases.

forces and increasing the risk of rupture (Maffulli, Ewen and Waterston, 2000).

The tendon originates from the musculotendinous junction of the calf muscles, the soleus inserting lower down on the deep surface of the tendon. The Achilles tendon gradually becomes more rounded as it travels distally, and flares out to insert into the posterior aspect of the calcaneum. The tendon is separated from the calcaneum by the retrocalcaneal bursa and from the skin by the subcutaneous calcaneal bursa.

> **Keypoint**
>
> The retrocalcaneal bursa separates the Achilles tendon from the calcaneum (heel bone). The subcutaneous calcaneal bursa separates the tendon from the skin.

The force from the Achilles tendon is delivered not through its insertion into the calcaneum, but via the point of contact on the posterior aspect of the calcaneum over the retrocalcaneal bursa (Reid, 1992). With increasing plantarflexion, the tendon 'unrolls' in such a way that this contact point moves lower down. In this way, the lever arm is maintained throughout the range of motion (Fig. 11.15).

The whole tendon rotates through 90° as it descends, so that the medial fibres become posterior by the time the tendon attaches to the calcaneum. This rotation is thought in part to account for the elastic properties of the tendon, giving it an elastic recoil when stretched. In the running action, as the lower limb moves from heel strike to mid-stance, the Achilles tendon is stretched, storing elastic energy. At toe off, the tendon recoils, releasing its stored energy and reducing the work required from the calf muscles to propel the body forwards.

The Achilles tendon is surrounded by a soft membranous paratenon which is continuous proximally with the muscle fascia and distally with the calcaneal periosteum. On the medial and lateral aspects of the dorsal surface there are thin spaces between the tendon and skin. These spaces are filled with thin gliding membranes covered in lubricating mucopolysaccharides. The membranes move freely over each other and greatly reduce friction. On the ventral side of the tendon there is fatty areolar tissue and connective tissue containing blood vessels.

The blood supply to the tendon is from either end and from the paratenon itself, but a relatively avascular zone exists between 2 and 6 cm proximal to the tendon insertion. Under normal circumstances, blood vessels do not travel from the paratenon to the tendon substance, and removal of the paratenon does not seem to compromise the blood supply (Williams, 1986). Tendon tissue in general has a low metabolic rate, and this, coupled with the poor blood supply to the tendon, means that the structure has a slow rate of healing.

Injuries to the Achilles tendon fall broadly into one of two categories. First, those which affect the tendon substance (partial or complete rupture), and, secondly, injury to the surface of the tendon and its covering (tendinitis or peritendinitis).

Tendinitis

Tendinitis presents as a swelling of the Achilles tendon of gradual onset. The main change is a disruption of the ground substance causing the tendon fibres to separate, which in turn leads to degeneration.

In peritendinitis the paratenon is inflamed and thickened, and there is local oedema and crepitus. Kager's triangle (the space between the inner surface of the Achilles tendon, the deep flexors and the calcaneus) is obliterated. Hard scarred bands appear within the paratenon and adhesions develop between the Achilles tendon and surrounding tissue. Kvist et al. (1988) showed that the fatty tissue surrounding the tendon was still thickened and swollen, after nearly 2 years in subjects with paratenonitis (peritendinitis). Connective tissue had increased, and local blood vessels had degenerated or been obliterated, suggesting the presence of immature scar tissue.

Initial management of tendinitis or peritendinitis aims at reducing local oedema. Rest and ice are used in conjunction with electrotherapy modalities aimed at reducing pain and resolving inflammation. Transverse friction massage has been used extensively (Cyriax and Cyriax, 1983), for both the teno-osseous (T/O) junction and tendon itself. The T/O junction may be frictioned with the patient prone and the foot plantarflexed (Fig. 11.16a). The therapist uses the side of his flexed forefingers to impart the friction, pulling the hands distally against the curved insertion of the Achilles tendon into the calcaneum. The musculotendinous junction is frictioned with the foot dorsiflexed, and the tendon gripped from above between the finger and thumb. The movement is perpendicular to the tendon fibres (Fig. 11.16b). The tendon sheath may be treated by placing the length of the finger alongside the tendon and pressing inwards. The forearm is pronated/supinated to impart the friction (Fig. 11.16c).

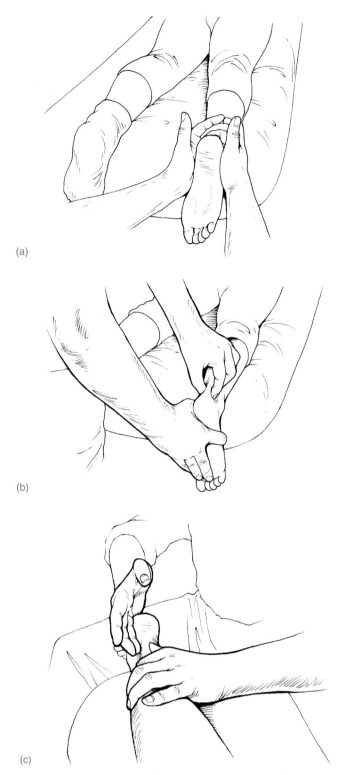

(a)

(b)

(c)

Figure 11.16   Transverse frictional massage for the Achilles tendon. (a) Teno-osseous junction. (b) Musculotendinous junction. (c) Tendon sheath/underside.

A heel raise is used to reduce the stretch on the tendon, and the calf may be strapped in plantarflexion (Fig. 5.3). If pain is intense the patient should initially be non-weight bearing.

Eccentric exercise in the management of tendinitis

The use of eccentric loading in the treatment of Achilles tendinitis was popularized in the late 1980s. The aim is to increase the tensile strength of the tendon by subjecting it to active lengthening and high tensile forces. Eccentric exercise also prepares the tendon for rapid unloading which has been associated with injury. The sudden release of force has been suggested to break interfibrillar connections within the tendon (Curwin, 1994) (see Ch. 1).

In a study of 200 Achilles tendinitis patients treated by eccentric loading, 44% had complete pain relief and 43% showed a marked decrease in their symptoms (Stanish, Robinovich and Curwin, 1986). Comparing concentric to eccentric protocols, Niesen-Vertommen et al. (1992) showed better subjective pain scale scores for the eccentric group. Heavy eccentric loading has also been shown to be superior to surgery. The eccentric group achieved full function in 12 weeks compared to the surgery group timescale of 24 weeks, and pain response and strength deficit were better in the eccentric group (Alfredson et al., 1998).

Eccentric training may be given by performing a heel raise, rising on the uninjured leg and lowering on the injured side. Progression may be made to eccentric drops and hopping. Recommendations of 3 × 20 repetitions of eccentric lowering with a straight leg and the same volume with a bent knee have been made, varying the speed and resistance as progression (Hunter, 2000).

Tendon substance

Focal degeneration (tendonosis) may occur in the tendon with athletes in their early 30s. The onset is usually gradual, giving highly localized pain. Microscopically there is proliferation of capillary cells and lacunae along the tendon fibres giving a loss of the normal wavy alignment of collagen. This is a non-inflammatory condition resulting in haphazard collagen fibre orientation and relative absence of tenocytes, increased interfibrillar glycoaminoglycans (GAG), and scattered vascular in-growth. Collagen fibres fray and thin, losing their orientation and the quantity of type III collagen increases. There may be a reduction in fibre cross-linkage, reducing the tensile properties of the tendon (Movin et al., 1997; Hunter, 2000).

Tendon rupture generally occurs later in an athlete's life, being more common from the late 30s to mid-40s. With partial rupture, a few fibres or nearly all of the tendon may be affected. The characteristic history is one of sudden onset. There is swelling, pain on resisted movement, and the patient is unable to support his or her weight through the toes of the affected foot.

In complete rupture there is usually a single incident where the patient feels a sudden sharp 'give' in the tendon as though he or she had been struck from behind. Immediately afterwards there may be little pain but gross weakness. The

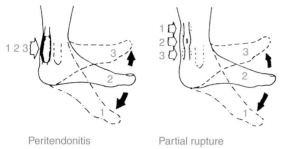

Peritendonitis   Partial rupture

Figure 11.17   The 'painful arc' in diagnosis of Achilles tendon pain. If the lesion is in the tendon, the point of maximum tenderness moves with excursion into dorsiflexion or plantarflexion. In peritendinitis it remains fixed. From Williams, J.G.P. (1986) Achilles tendon lesions in sport. *Sports Medicine*, **3**, 114–135. With permission.

patient is again unable to take the weight through the toes. Active plantarflexion is minimal, being accomplished by the peronei and posterior tibial muscles only. With the patient in a prone position, Simmond's test may be performed. The calf is squeezed, and the foot fails to plantarflex. Closer examination reveals a depression (the Toygar angle) visible in the normal smooth contour of the Achilles tendon. If the athlete is not seen for a number of days, this hollow will have been bridged by haematoma and scar tissue, giving a raised fibrous area unless the tendon ends have retracted. Without surgery, the tendon will heal, but very slowly. Granulation tissue forms poorly, partly due to repeated use, and partly as a result of the anticoagulant effect of synovial fluid contained by the unruptured paratenon (Williams, 1986).

Lesions of the tendon may be differentiated from those of the paratenon by using the 'painful arc' sign (Williams, 1986). The point of maximum tenderness is palpated as the foot is dorsiflexed and plantarflexed. When the tendon alone is affected, the painful area will move up and down as the tendon moves. However, when the paratenon is affected, as the tendon slides within its sheath, the area of maximum pain remains fixed (Fig. 11.17).

When examining the patient it must be remembered that the Achilles tendon is painful to palpation normally, so the intensity of discomfort must always be compared with that of the contralateral limb.

Surgical management

Surgical management of Achilles tendon injuries carries a high rate of complication. Williams (1986) described complications in 64 out of 461 surgical procedures (13.9%), and Paavola, Orava and Leppilahti (2000) reported a similar percentage of 46 out of 432 patients (11%). These included mainly wound dehiscence (bursting), scar hypertrophy, wound infection and nerve irritation. Surgery may be called for where conservative management has failed and symptoms have persisted for more than 3 months.

Achilles tendon repair is the subject of considerable debate. Many authors claim that conservative treatment does not allow direct realignment of the torn tendon fibres and so the repair is less secure. In addition, they claim that re-rupture of surgically treated injuries is less likely (Turco and Spinella, 1987). Others argue that the risk of surgical complications is too great, and that the sophistication of rehabilitation is as important to the eventual outcome of the condition as whether the surgical or non-surgical route was chosen (Garrick and Webb, 1990). A number of repair methods have been described, including direct suture, reinforcement with plantaris or peroneus brevis tendon, and reconstruction using carbon fibre or polypropylene mesh.

Whatever the surgical method used, following immobilization the main problem is initially lack of flexibility to the Achilles tendon, ankle and subtaloid joint in particular. Intense rehabilitation of the foot, ankle and leg is needed to regain full function.

Rehabilitation following surgery

Early mobility following Achilles tendon repair is a vital factor to the success of the procedure. A typical rehabilitation period normally includes an equinus plaster for 8 weeks followed by a heel raise for a further 6 weeks (Apley and Solomon, 1993). However, Saw et al. (1993) showed improved mobility and strength and a reduction in complications using total immobilization in an equinus plaster for 1 week only. Following this, the plaster was removed and active dorsiflexion was practised in sitting. The plaster was replaced between therapy sessions. Sutures were removed after 2 weeks and the foot placed in a lower leg walker. Solveborn and Moberg (1994) showed similar results using a patellar tendon bearing cast with a metal frame attached for 6 weeks. The cast allowed pain-free motion of the foot while taking full bodyweight for walking. No complications were seen, with a reduction of skin/tendon adhesions and a rapid return to normal strength values.

On removal of the cast, stretching procedures are begun non-weight bearing, hooking a towel over the forefoot and gently pulling into dorsiflexion being sufficient. Partial weight-bearing activities in sitting are used to begin the closed kinetic chain exercises, with the athlete gently pressing into dorsiflexion using varying foot angles. The same starting positions are chosen for early static and later dynamic strength training using straps and elastic bands. Isokinetics is used for the calf specifically and the lower limb in general.

Walking re-education using parallel bars or sticks introduces functional movements and introduces skill work. When full weight-bearing activities are begun, the flexibility and strength work is progressed and augmented with skill training involving balance and coordination exercises (see ankle rehabilitation, Ch. 12) and further walking re-education.

Both static and dynamic flexibility training is used from the earliest stages, and eccentric actions are begun as soon as possible (often in the pool to limit weight bearing) to mimic the true function of the Achilles tendon. When function has improved sufficiently, walking pace is increased and speed walking introduced, followed by on-the-spot and, later, small-step jogging. Straight running, zig-zags, and circle running are all used. Thick-heeled training shoes are used, and gradually the heel is lowered. Toe walking progresses to jogging on the toes.

General fitness is maintained throughout the programme by cardiopulmonary activities in the pool (assuming good healing of the scar) and, later, static cycle riding, until the intensity of rehabilitation itself is sufficient to challenge aerobic fitness. Pain is the rate limiting factor for both exercise intensity and progression.

Assuming the surgery has been totally successful, the final stages of training must include the use of plyometric exercise to develop elastic strength. Poor results can be expected if the rehabilitation programme is stopped at the stage of heavy isotonic exercise and not progressed in terms of speed. Hopping and jumping actions are used on forgiving surfaces with progression to bounding.

Aetiology

A number of factors may combine to cause Achilles tendon pain, including training alterations, footwear and flexibility. Alterations in training type or intensity, such as a sudden increase in the distance run over a holiday period, or more intensive training in the lead up to a competition, can both produce problems. Only in recreational athletes is trauma the predominant cause. In the competitive athlete, as many as 90% of Achilles tendon injuries result from overuse in the form of microtrauma established over months, or, in some cases, many years (Kvist, 1994).

Footwear is an important factor to the development of this condition. Inadequate shock-absorbing properties stress the Achilles tendon during eccentric loading, a situation aggravated when an athlete has a rigid cavus foot. Good shock absorption of the shoe heel is important for athletes who exercise on a hard surface. In addition to reducing the impact at heel strike, the height of the heel will also reduce the stretch on the Achilles tendon. A rigid sole lengthens the ankle to forefoot lever arm, affecting Achilles tendon mechanics, but may be necessary to protect the first toe (see below). If the heel counter of a sports shoe is hard, it can abrade the Achilles tendon as the foot plantarflexes at toe off. A negative heel counter, or a soft tab, is to be encouraged.

Lack of flexibility in the calf and Achilles tendon may contribute greatly to injury. When flexibility is limited, the tendon loses some of its elastic recoil, making it more susceptible to damage through rapid eccentric loading of the calf in mid-stance. Flexibility exercises should be used for prevention and management of the subacute injury. Stretching may be performed with the forefoot on an angled block. The heel is kept on the ground and the hip is pressed forward, bringing the knee over the forefoot and increasing dorsiflexion. The exercise is first performed with the knee locked to stretch the gastrocnemius, and then with the knee flexed to 20° to stress the Achilles tendon and soleus. A static stretch is used and held for 20–30 seconds. The range of motion is generally greater when the tendon is warm, after a hot shower or bath for example.

Malalignment of the lower limb is probably a contributory factor to Achilles tendon pain, although, as such faults have generally been present for some time before the Achilles tendon condition started, it is unlikely to be the sole cause. Increased pronation of the foot stresses the medial aspect of the Achilles tendon. A 30° increase in rearfoot position has been shown to lengthen these fibres by 10% (Nichols, 1989). In addition, excessive tibial rotation caused by hyperpronation will twist the Achilles tendon fibres together, 'wringing them out'. This will close any blood vessels between the tendon fibres, temporarily reducing an already poor blood supply.

Viewing the athlete's foot and lower limb from behind can be revealing. In an optimal alignment the Achilles tendon should appear vertical and the medial longitudinal arch be present. The gap between the floor and the navicular bone should be approximately one finger breadth. Excessive pronation (Fig. 11.18b) causes the Achilles to curve and deviate outwards with the medial longitudinal arch flatter (pes planus). Using a medial calcaneal wedge to control pronation at the subtalar joint (Fig. 11.18c) realigns the Achilles.

In an interesting survey of 109 runners with Achilles tendon problems, Clement, Taunton and Smart (1984) found 75% showed training errors, 56% demonstrated hyperpronation, 39% suffered inflexibility of the calf and 10% wore improper footwear.

Corticosteroid injections may affect ligament failure. Inhibition of collagen synthesis, reduction in the speed of tendon repair, lower elastic limit and fatty degeneration have all been described (Nichols, 1989). Various studies have shown an increased likelihood of Achilles tendon rupture after injection (Chechick et al., 1982; Kleinman and Gross, 1983; Urban, 1989). Cyriax (1982) argued that Achilles tendon rupture only occurred when an incorrect injection technique was used, the corticosteroid being introduced into the

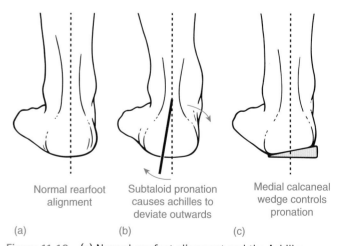

Normal rearfoot alignment

Subtaloid pronation causes achilles to deviate outwards

Medial calcaneal wedge controls pronation

(a)   (b)   (c)

Figure 11.18   (a) Normal rearfoot alignment and the Achilles. (b) Subtaloid pronation causes Achilles to deviate outwards. (c) Medial calcaneal wedge controls pronation.

tendon substance rather than along its surface. However, Williams (1986) claimed that both techniques had been shown to precipitate rupture, and further argued that the benefits of such injections were relatively short-lived. In addition, he contested that in acute peritendinitis, similar results could be obtained using a local anaesthetic and hyaluronidase.

> **Keypoint**
>
> In the competitive athlete, 90% of Achilles tendon injuries result from microtrauma due to overuse. Inadequate shock-absorbtion in shoes, training type and volume, lack of flexibility in the calf and Achilles, and lower limb malalignment are all factors to consider.

RETROCALCANEAL PAIN

Sever's disease

Calcaneal apophysitis (Sever's disease) may occur in adolescents during the rapid growth spurt, sometimes in association with Achilles tendon pain itself. The condition is more common in boys than girls, and occurs between the ages of 11 and 15 years. The posterior aspect of the calcaneum develops independently of the main body and is separated by an epiphyseal plate. The plate lies vertically and is therefore subjected to shearing stress from the pull of the Achilles tendon and through jarring stress in jumping. Pain frequently occurs during deceleration from running as well as take off and landing from a jump. Sever's is inappropriately named as it is not a true disease entity, but rather a traction injury similar in many respects to Osgood–Schlatter's disease in the adolescent knee.

On examination, there is tenderness to medial and lateral heel compression, but no noticeable skin changes. Radiographically, sclerosis and irregularity of the calcaneal apophysis is seen as a result of avascular necrosis (Caspi, Ezra and Horoszowski, 1989). Associated Achilles tendon tightness has been described, with the affected side showing 4–5° less passive dorsiflexion than the unaffected side (Mitcheli and Ireland, 1987). In addition, excessive foot pronation is also common in this patient group.

Initially, total rest is called for to allow the condition to settle. Later, any sporting activity which exacerbates the pain is avoided, and shock-absorbing heel pads are used in all shoes. Achilles tendon stretching is taught to restore dorsiflexion range, and foot position is corrected.

> **Keypoint**
>
> In Sever's disease consider: (i) calf-Achilles stretching, (ii) shock-absorbing heel pads in all footwear, and (iii) orthotic prescription.

HAGLUND'S SYNDROME

Haglund's syndrome is present when an exostosis is found over the posterior lateral aspect of the calcaneum. Radiographically, a spur of bone is seen coming from the calcaneal insertion of the Achilles tendon, showing as a prominence of the posterior superior calcaneal angle (Wooten and Chandler, 1990). Assessment of radiographs may be made by comparing 'parallel pitch lines' (Pavlov et al., 1982). The first line joins the anterior and posterior calcaneal tubercles. A second line is drawn parallel to the first, but this time starting from the posterior lip of the talar articulation (Fig. 11.19). If the posterior superior calcaneal angle stands prominent to this second line, the diagnosis is positive.

In addition to the bony changes, a painful soft tissue swelling (pump bump) is noted at the insertion of the Achilles tendon. This swelling can vary in size and shape depending on the stage of the condition. Haglund's syndrome commonly exists in association with retrocalcaneal bursitis, the inflamed bursa becoming visible on X-ray when low penetrating radiation is used (Rossi et al., 1987).

Contributing factors to the formation of Haglund's syndrome include a hard edge to the posterior aspect of the shoe (heel tab) and a rearfoot varus. As the foot is plantarflexed,

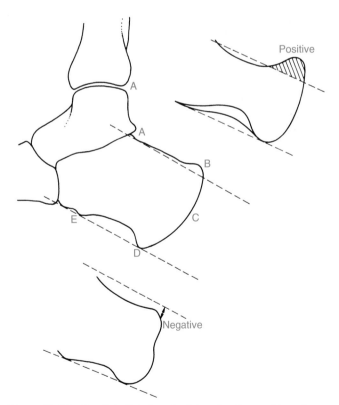

Figure 11.19 Parallel pitch lines to determine the position of the posterior superior calcaneal angle. A, Posterior lip of talar articulation. B, Posterior superior calcaneal angle. C, Posterior calcaneal tuberosity. D, Medial calcaneal tuberosity. E, Anterior calcaneal tuberosity. From Rossi, F. et al. (1987) The Haglund syndrome: clinical and radiological features and sports medicine aspects. *Journal of Sports Medicine*, **27**, 258–265. With permission.

the hard heel tab will abrade the posterior aspect of the calcaneum. If a rearfoot varus exists, compensatory pronation will cause the heel to twist in the shoe and soft tissue pressure occurs over the posterior calcaneum. Although soft tissue changes could be expected from abrasion of this type, bony changes are less likely. The bony change itself could be the result of a secondary ossification centre in the calcaneus (Horn and Subotnick, 1989).

Management of retrocalcaneal pain is by pain relief until the condition settles. A horseshoe pad made from non-compressible rubber is placed over the painful calcaneal area, and held in place by an ankle sock. A heel raise may be used to reduce stress through the tendon onto the calcaneus, and gentle tendon stretching is taught. Electrotherapy modalities are used to alleviate pain and reduce inflammation.

Surgery includes bursectomy and resection of the superoposterior portion of the calcaneus, as far as the insertion of the Achilles tendon. Return to sport is relatively protracted, with athletes taking 3–5 months to begin full competition (Ghiggio, Nobile and Bronzo, 1993). With restoration of sport, athletes should still be advised to wear soft-back shoes to avoid local abrasion.

References

Alfredson, H., Pietila, T., Johnsson, P. and Lorentzon, R. (1988) Heavy load eccentric calf muscle training for the treatment of chronic Achilles tendonitis. *American Journal of Sports Medicine*, **26**, (3) 360–366

Apley, A.G. and Solomon, L. (1993) *Apley's System of Orthopaedics and Fractures*, 7th edn, Butterworth-Heinemann, Oxford

Brody, D.M. (1980) Running injuries. *Clinical Symposia*, **32**, (4), Ciba Pharmaceutical Company, New Jersey

Caspi, I., Ezra, E. and Horoszowski, H. (1989) Partial apophysectomy in Sever's disease. *Journal of Orthopaedic and Sports Physical Therapy*, **10**, (9) 370–373

Chechick, A., Amit, Y., Israli, A. and Horoszowski, H. (1982) Recurrent rupture of the Achilles tendon induced by corticosteroid injection. *British Journal of Sports Medicine*, **16**, 89–90

Clement, D.B., Taunton, J.E. and Smart, G.W. (1984) Achilles tendinitis and peritendinitis: aetiology and treatment. *American Journal of Sports Medicine*, **12**, (3) 179–184

Curwin, S.L. (1994) The aetiology and treatment of tendinitis. In *Oxford Textbook of Sports Medicine* (eds M. Harries, C. Williams, W.D. Stanish and L.J. Micheli), Oxford University Press, Oxford

Cyriax, J. (1982) *Textbook of Orthopaedic Medicine*, 8th edn, Baillière Tindall, London, vol. 1

Cyriax, J.H. and Cyriax, P.J. (1983) *Illustrated Manual of Orthopaedic Medicine*, Butterworth, London

Detmer, D.E. (1986) Chronic shin splints: classification and management of medial tibial stress syndrome. *Sports Medicine*, **3**, 436–446

Di Manna, D.L. and Buck, P.G. (1990) Chronic compartment syndrome in athletes: recognition and treatment. *Athletic Training*, **25**, 1

Garrick, J.G. and Webb, D.R. (1990) *Sports Injuries: Diagnosis and Management*, W.B. Saunders, Philadelphia

Ghiggio, P., Nobile, G. and Bronzo, P. (1993) Haglund's disease in athletes. *Journal of Sports Traumatology*, **15**, 89–96

Hannaford, P.G.H. (1988) Shin splints re-visited. *Excel*, **4**, (4) 16–19

Horn, L.M. and Subotnick, S.I. (1989) Surgical intervention. In *Sports Medicine of the Lower Extremity* (ed. S.I. Subotnick), Churchill Livingstone, Edinburgh, pp. 461–566

Hunter, G (2000) The conservative management of Achilles tendinopathy. *Physical Therapy in Sport*, **1**, (1) 6–14

Jozsa, L., Kvist, M. and Balint, B.J. (1989) The role of recreational sports activity in Achilles tendon rupture: a clinical, pathoanatomical, and sociological study of 292 cases. *American Journal of Sports Medicine*, **17**, 338–343

Kahn, K.M. and Maffulli, N (1998) Tendinopathy: an Achilles heel for athletes and clinicians. *Clinical Journal of Sports Medicine*, **8**, (3) 151–154

Kleinman, M. and Gross, A.E. (1983) Achilles tendon rupture following steroid injection: report of three cases. *Journal of Bone and Joint Surgery*, **65A**, 1345–1346

Kvist, M. (1994) Achilles tendon injuries in athletes. *Sports Medicine*, **18**, 173–201

Kvist, M.H., Lehto, M.U.K., Jozsa, L., Jarvinen, M. and Kvist, H.T. (1988) Chronic Achilles paratenonitis. *American Journal of Sports Medicine*, **16**, (6) 616–622

Li, G., Zhang, S., Chen, G., Chen, H. and Wang, A. (1985) Radiographic and histological analysis of stress fracture in rabbit tibias. *American Journal of Sports Medicine*, **13**, 285–294

Lowden, A. (1986) Application of ultrasound to assess stress fractures. *Physiotherapy*, **72**, (3) 160–161

Lysholm, J. and Wiklander, J. (1987) Injuries in runners. *American Journal of Sports Medicine*, **15**, 168–171

Maffulli, N., Ewen, S.W. and Waterston, S. (2000) Tenocytes from ruptured and tendinopathic Achilles tendons produce greater quantities of type III collagen than tenocytes from normal Achilles tendons: an in vitro model of human tendon healing. *American Journal of Sports Medicine*, **28**, 499–505

Markey, K.L. (1987) Stress fractures. *Clinics in Sports Medicine*, **6**, 405–425

McBryde, A.M. (1985) Stress fractures in runners. *Clinics in Sports Medicine*, **4**, (4), October, 737–752

Mitcheli, L.J. and Ireland, M.L. (1987) Prevention and management of calcaneal apophysitis in children: an overuse syndrome. *Journal of Paediatric Orthopaedics*, **7**, 34–38

Movin, T., Gad, A., Reinholt, F.P. and Rolf, C. (1997) Tendon pathology in long standing achillodynia: biopsy findings in 40 patients. *Acta Orthopaedica Scandinavica*, **68**, (2) 170–175

Mubarak, S.J., Gould, R.N., Lee, Y.F. and Schmidt, D.A. (1982) The medial tibial stress syndrome. *American Journal of Sports Medicine*, **10**, 201–205

Ng, G. and Richardson, C.A. (1990) The effects of training triceps surae using progressive speed loading. *Physiotherapy Practice*, **6**, 77–84

Nichols, A.W. (1989) Achilles tendinitis in running athletes. Journal of the *American Board of Family Practice*, 2, (3) 196–203

Niesen-Vertommen, S.L., Taunton, J.E., Clement, D.B. and Mosher, R.E. (1992) The effect of eccentric versus concentric exercise in the management of Achilles tendonitis. *Clinical Journal of Sports Medicine*, **2**, (2) 109–113

Norris, C.M. (2001) *Acupuncture: Treatment of Musculoskeletal Conditions*, Butterworth-Heinemann, Oxford

Paavola, M., Orava, S. and Leppilahti, J. (2000). Chronic Achilles tendon overuse injuries: complications after surgical treatment. *American Journal of Sports Medicine*, **28**, (3) 77–82

Pavlov, H., Henegan, M., Hersch, A., Goldman, A. and Vigorita, V. (1982) The Haglund syndrome: initial and differential diagnosis. *Radiology*, **144**, 83–88

Puddu, G., Cerullo, G., Selvanetti, A. and De Paulis, F. (1994) Stress fractures. In *Oxford Textbook of Sports Medicine* (eds M. Harries, C. Williams, W.D. Stanish and L.J. Micheli), Oxford University Press, Oxford

Puffer, J.C. and Zachazewski, J.E. (1988) Management of overuse injuries. *American Family Physician*, **38**, (3) 225–232

Read, M.T. (2000) *A Practical Guide to Sports Injuries*, Butterworth-Heinemann, Oxford

Reid, D.C. (1992) *Sports Injury Assessment and Rehabilitation*, Churchill Livingstone, London

Rossi, F., La Cava, F., Amato, F. and Pincelli, G. (1987) The Haglund syndrome: clinical and radiological features and sports medicine aspects. *Journal of Sports Medicine*, **27**, 258–265

Rzonca, E.C. and Baylis, W. J. (1988) Common sports injuries to the foot and leg. *Clinics in Podiatric Medicine and Surgery*, **5**, (3), July, 591–612

Saw, Y., Baltzopoulos, V., Lim, A., Rostron, P.K.M., Bolton-Maggs, B.G. and Calver, R.F. (1993) Early mobilisation after operative repair of ruptured Achilles tendon. *Injury*, **24**, 479–484

Solveborn, S-A., and Moberg, A. (1994) Immediate free ankle motion after repair of acute Achilles tendon ruptures. *American Journal of Sports Medicine*, **22**, 607–610

Stanish, D.W., Robinovich, R.M. and Curwin, S. (1986) Eccentric exercise in chronic tendinitis. *Clinical Orthopedics and Related Research*, **208**, (7) 65–68

Styf, J. (1989) Chronic exercise-induced pain in the anterior aspect of the lower leg. *Sports Medicine*, **7**, 331–339

Taunton, J.E. and Clement, D.B. (1981) Lower extremity stress fractures in athletes. *Physician and Sports Medicine*, **9**, 77–86

Turco, V.J. and Spinella, A.J. (1987) Achilles tendon ruptures: peroneus brevis transfer. *Foot and Ankle*, **7**, 253–259

Urban, K. (1989) Partial rupture of the Achilles tendon in athletes. *Acta Chirurgiae Orthopaedicae et Traumatologiae Cechoslovaca*, **56**, (1) 30–38

Williams, J.G.P. (1986) Achilles tendon lesions in sport. *Sports Medicine*, **3**, 114–135

Wooten, B. and Chandler, J. (1990) Use of an orthotic device in the treatment of posterior heel pain. *Journal of Orthopaedic and Sports Physical Therapy*, **11**, (9) 410–413

Chapter 12

The ankle

CHAPTER CONTENTS

Approximately 14% of all sports injuries are sprains to the ankle, representing one ankle injury each season for every 17 participants. In high risk sports, such as jumping and running, this percentage is even higher, at 25% of all lost-time injuries (Reid, 1992). Ankle sprain has been shown to be 2.4 times more common in the dominant leg, and to have a high (73.5%) prevalence of recurrence (Yeung et al., 1994).

The joint mechanics of the ankle and foot have been described in Chapter 8. The ankle joint is the articulation between the trochlear surface of the talus and the distal ends of the tibia and fibula. The fibula may support 15–20% of the body weight (Lambert, 1971), with the fibula moving downwards and laterally during the stance phase of running to deepen the ankle mortice and enhance stability. This fibular motion creates tension in the interosseous membrane and tibiofibular ligament to provide some shock attenuation. Loss of this mechanism through tibiofibular disruption greatly affects the ankle joint, with a 1–2 mm lateral shift of the fibula increasing joint forces by as much as 40% (Reid, 1992).

Keypoint

The fibula can support up to 1/5 of the bodyweight and moves during the stance phase of running to deepen the ankle mortice and enhance ankle stability.

The ankle is subjected to considerable compression forces during sport (Fig. 12.1). Compression forces as high as five times body weight have been calculated during walking and up to 13 times body weight during running (Burdett, 1982).

COLLATERAL LIGAMENTS

The joint is strengthened by a variety of ligaments, the collaterals being the most important from the point of view of injury. Both medial and lateral collateral ligaments travel from the malleoli, and have bands attaching to the calcaneus and talus.

The medial (deltoid) ligament (Fig. 12.2a) is triangular in shape. Its deep portion may be divided into anterior and

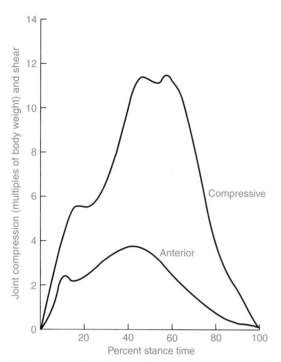

Figure 12.1 Compression forces on the talus during running. From Burdett, R.G. (1982) Forces predicted at the ankle during running. *Medicine and Science in Sports and Exercise*, **14**, 308. With permission.

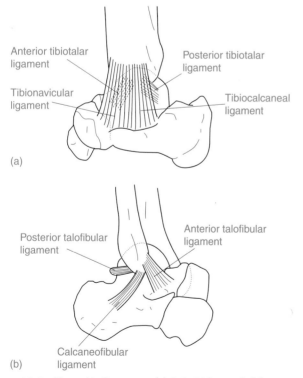

Figure 12.2 The ankle ligaments. (a) Deltoid (medial). (b) Lateral.

posterior tibiotalar bands. The more superficial part is split into tibionavicular and tibiocalcaneal portions, which attach in turn to the spring ligament. The lateral ligament (Fig. 12.2b) is composed of three separate components, and is

Table 12.1 Role of the collateral ligaments in ankle stability

Movement	Controlled by
Abduction of talus	Tibiocalcaneal and tibionavicular bands
Adduction of talus	Calcaneofibular ligament
Plantarflexion	ATF ligament and anterior tibiotalar band
Dorsiflexion	Posterior tibiotalar band and PTF ligament
External rotation of talus	Anterior tibiotalar and tibionavicular bands
Internal rotation of talus	As above with ATF ligament

Adapted from Palastanga, Field and Soames (1989).

somewhat weaker than its medial counterpart. The anterior talofibular (ATF) ligament is a flat band 2–5 mm thick and 10–12 mm long which travels from the anterior tip of the lateral malleolus to the neck of the talus, and may be considered the primary stabilizer of the ankle joint (Palastanga, Field and Soames, 1989). The posterior talofibular (PTF) ligament travels almost horizontally from the fossa on the bottom of the lateral malleolus to the posterior surface of the talus. Lying between the ATF and PTF ligaments is the calcaneofibular ligament, arising from the front of the lateral malleolus to pass down and back to attach onto the lateral surface of the calcaneum. The role of the collateral ligaments in maintaining talocrural stability is summarized in Table 12.1.

INJURY

The most common injury to the ankle is damage to the ATF ligament with or without involvement of the peroneus brevis. The subtaloid and mid-tarsal joints may be involved, but will be dealt with separately for clarity. The typical history of ankle injury is one of inversion, sometimes coupled with plantarflexion. The athlete 'goes over' on the ankle, usually on an uneven surface. One of three grades of ligament injury may occur (p. 51).

Keypoint

The anterior talofibular (ATF) ligament is 2–5 mm thick and 10–12 mm long, approximately the width of the index finger. Its fibres run roughly parallel to the sole of the foot. Injury to the ATF is the most common sports injury affecting the ankle.

There is usually an egg-shaped swelling in front of, and around, the lateral malleolus. When viewed from behind, the definition of the Achilles tendon is a good indicator of severity of injury (Reid, 1992). With more severe injuries (grade III) the definition of the Achilles tendon is lost due to excessive bleeding into the joint (Fig. 12.3).

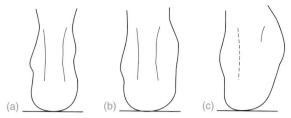

Figure 12.3 Assessing severity of ankle injury from swelling. (a) Normal joint. Contour of Achilles tendon well defined. (b) Grade I/II injury. Clear swelling but Achilles tendon outline still visible. (c) Grade III injury. Profuse swelling obscures outline of Achilles tendon.

The lateral malleolus should be gently palpated to assess if bone pain is present; if it is, an X-ray may be required. If palpation reveals tenderness below, rather than over, the lateral malleolus and the athlete is able to bear weight, there is a 97% probability of soft tissue injury alone (Vargish and Clarke, 1983). Any fracture that is missed by this type of close palpation is likely to be an avulsion or non-displaced hairline type that will respond favourably to management as a sprain (Garrick and Webb, 1990).

Stress tests to the ankle are useful to assess the degree of instability in the subacute phase, and to give a differential diagnosis. Acute injuries may be exacerbated by full range motion with overpressure. The capsule of the ankle joint itself is assessed by passive dorsiflexion and plantarflexion only, the capsular pattern presenting as a greater limitation of plantarflexion. However, as the ankle ligaments span the subtaloid and mid-tarsal joints, inversion/eversion and adduction/abduction are also included in ankle joint examination.

The ATF ligament is placed on maximum stretch by passive inversion, plantarflexion, and adduction. The heel is held with the cupped hand and the subtaloid joint inverted. The opposite hand grasps the forefoot from above and swings it into plantarflexion and adduction. In addition, anterior glide of the talus on the tibia should be assessed with the foot in a neutral position. The heel is again held in the cupped hand, but this time the palm of the opposite hand is over the anterior aspect of the lower tibia. The calcaneus and talus are pulled forward as the tibia is pushed back. Movements are compared with that of the uninjured side for range and quality.

Keypoint

The ATF ligament is tested by passive inversion, plantarflexion, and adduction. The athlete's heel is held with the cupped hand and the heel is twisted inwards. The opposite hand grasps the forefoot from above and draws down and in.

The calcaneocuboid ligament is stressed by combined supination/adduction and the calcaneofibular ligament by inversion in a neutral position. The medial collateral ligament is stressed by combined plantarflexion/eversion/abduction (anterior fibres) or eversion alone (middle fibres). Resisted eversion will not be painful unless the peronei are affected (see below).

Following severe ankle sprain or fracture, a bony link may form between the tibia and fibula (tibiofibular synostosis). Typically, pain occurs after an injury, and increases during vigorous activity, mimicking stress fracture. Pain is most severe during the push-off action of running and jumping, and dorsiflexion is often limited to 90°, mimicking impingement pain (see below). The synostosis is revealed by X-ray and removed surgically (Flandry and Sanders, 1987).

MANAGEMENT OF AN ANKLE SPRAIN

Immediate management consists of the RICE protocol, with electrotherapy modalities as appropriate. Intermittent pneumatic compression (IPC) used in conjunction with cooling is effective. In the subacute phase, massage, especially finger kneading around the malleolus is of value in preventing the development of pitting oedema. Transverse frictions may be used to encourage the development of a mobile scar, and as a prelude to manipulation for scar tissue rupture in a chronic injury. Grade II and III injuries present with marked swelling and are protected non-weight bearing (severe injury) or preferably partial weight bearing with a compression bandage. Where minimal swelling indicates a grade I injury, an eversion strapping may be applied to protect the ligament from inversion stresses and to shorten it. A felt wedge is used beneath the heel to evert the subtaloid joint, and a U-shaped pad is placed over the submalleolar depressions to prevent pockets of oedema forming and to apply even compression when the ankle is strapped. Adhesive strapping is applied after skin preparation or underwrap, initially to lock the subtaloid joint and then to passively evert the foot. The athlete can then walk partial weight bearing in a well-supporting shoe.

Early mobility is essential to increase ligament strength and restore function. For grade I and II injuries, early mobilization has been shown to be more effective than immobilization. In a group of 82 patients with these grades of injury, 87% who were immobilized with a plastercast for 10 days still had pain after 3 weeks. This compared to 57% of those who received early mobilization in the form of an elastic strap for 2 days followed by a functional brace for 8 days (Eiff, Smith and Smith, 1994).

Non-weight-bearing ankle exercise is instigated within the pain-free range, and fitness is maintained by general exercise. Strapping is replaced by a tubular elastic bandage as pain subsides.

REHABILITATION OF THE INJURED ANKLE

As with any joint, rehabilitation of the ankle aims at restoring mobility, strength and function (Table 12.2). With the ankle, however, of particular concern is the restoration of normal proprioception.

Table 12.2 Guidelines for rehabilitation of ankle sprain

Immediate post-injury management
RICE protocol
Consider use of intermittent pneumatic compression (IPC) with ice
Other modalities to reduce pain and inflammation
Careful assessment of possible bony injury
Athlete non-weight-bearing

Initial rehabilitation (2–5 days after injury)
Massage, especially finger kneading around malleolus
Range of motion exercise, inversion to pain tolerance only
Tranverse frictions to encourage mobile scar formation
Partial weight-bearing with eversion taping and felt padding or
  ankle orthosis
Walking re-education
Begin resisted exercise (elastic bands)
Active stretch into inversion and plantarflexion
Begin accessory mobilizations of surrounding joints

Intermediate rehabilitation (6–14 days)
Progress resisted exercise of ankle in all directions
Passive stretching into inversion and plantarflexion
Proprioceptive work (single-leg standing, eyes closed)
Gradually introduce balance board and trampette work
Ensure full range dorsiflexion
Uphill treadhill work progressing to speed walk and slow run
Side step and zig-zag speed walking–building endurance
Introduce varied terrain–slopes, rough ground, sand
Ensure cuboid mobility

Final rahabilitation (2–6 weeks)
Build to maximum resisted eversion
General weight training for lower limb
Running drills–figure-of-eight, circle run, zig-zag
Introduce low hop and progress to hop and hold, side hop, and hop
  and twist–building power and speed
Sport specific work including ball kicking and varying terrain

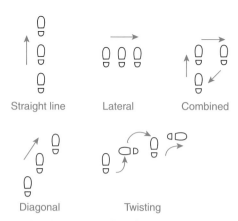

Figure 12.4 Hopping patterns in ankle rehabilitation.

Resisted exercise using rubber powerbands is used for inversion, eversion, dorsiflexion and plantarflexion, together with combinations of these movements. Maximum repetitions are used to restore muscle endurance, while strength is developed using maximal resistance. Eversion movements are performed with the band placed over both forefeet. For other movements, one end of the band is placed around a table leg, and the other over the foot. Various thicknesses of band are used as the exercises are progressed.

Static stretching exercises include calf and Achilles tendon stretching (see above), and inversion/eversion movements applied manually by the athlete. The starting position for these latter movements is sitting with the injured leg crossed over the contralateral limb. The exercise mimics the stability test for the ligaments outlined above.

Partial, and then full weight-bearing exercises are used to develop strength in a closed kinetic chain position and to restore proprioception. In single leg standing (wall-bar support) trunk movements are performed to throw stress onto the ankle; in addition, exercises such as heel raising, toe lifts

and inversion/eversion are performed. A balance beam (flamingo balance) is used, and again trunk and hip movements of the contralateral limb throw stress onto the injured ankle. The foot may be placed along the beam, or with the beam travelling transversely and only the toes supported. Intense muscle activity is seen around the ankle as the athlete attempts to maintain his or her balance. By varying the athlete's footwear and performing the exercises in bare feet, the stresses imposed are altered.

A balance board with a single transverse rib is used for sagittal movements, and a longitudinal rib for frontal plane actions. A board with a domed central raise (wobble board or ankle disc) is used to combine movements for circumduction. In addition to trunk movements, actions such as throwing and catching while standing on the balance board are helpful as these take the athlete's attention away from the ankle, and so are a progression in terms of skill. Performing balance board exercises blindfolded, and therefore eliminating visual input, has been shown to be effective at improving proprioception in the ankle (De Carlo and Talbot, 1986).

Running, hopping and jumping activities are all used, on varying surfaces including sand, grass and a mini-trampoline. Hopping direction is varied to alter the stress on the joint. Straight line hopping places an anteroposterior stress on the joint while lateral hopping imposes a mediolateral stress. Combined directions, diagonal hopping, and twisting when hopping are all used to impose multiple stresses on the joint (Fig. 12.4). Running in a circle, figure-of-eight and on hills/cambers all change the stress on the ankle, and hopping and jumping develop power rather than strength.

Proprioception in the unstable ankle

The importance of proprioceptive training to prevent the development of chronic instability (giving way in normal usage) is of great importance. Freeman, Dean and Hanham (1965) compared ligament injuries to the foot and ankle treated by immobilization, 'conventional' physiotherapy, and proprioceptive training, which consisted of balance board exercises. After treatment, 7% of the proprioceptive group showed instability compared to 46% of those treated by other means. Balance ability was measured using a modified Rhomberg test, which assesses the ability to maintain single leg standing while the eyes are closed. Lentell, Katzman and Walters (1990) assessed the strength of the ankle musculature in 33 subjects with instability and found that there was no significant difference between the injured and uninjured sides. However, when balance ability was measured, the majority of subjects exhibited a deficit between the two extremities. Konradsen and Ravn (1990) measured the time taken for peroneal contraction to occur in response to a sudden inversion stress in chronically unstable ankles. Their results showed the peroneal reaction time to be prolonged with injured ankles (82 ms) compared to the uninjured side (65 ms), indicating a proprioceptive deficit. Karlsson and Andersson (1992) found similar results, quoting 84.5 ms and 81.6 ms for peroneus longus and peroneus brevis, respectively, for involved limbs compared to 68.8 and 69.2 for uninvolved.

Glencross and Thornton (1981) assessed joint position sense to plantarflexion and found significantly greater errors in the replication of the test position for injured ankles compared to uninjured controls. Lentell et al. (1995) measured the threshold of the detection of passive motion (see p. 000) and found a significant difference (greater amount of inversion) between injured and uninjured sides.

Definition

Peroneal reaction time is the difference between the onset of a rapid inversion force acting on the ankle (mechanical joint displacement) and the initiation of peroneal muscle contraction to try to resist this force (physiological muscle splinting).

Although reflex control of the ankle through peroneal reaction time may be important, central nervous system (CNS) factors have also been shown to act. Konradsen, Voight and Hojsgaard (1997) showed that inversion stress sufficient to cause ligament damage occurred within 100 ms. Although the peroneal muscles may begin their contraction rapidly in response to such a stress (within 50–60 ms), it takes time for sufficient tension to build up to overcome the force of bodyweight. Such a force has been shown to require 170–180 ms to build to sufficient intensity, showing that the ankle musculature cannot react fast enough to protect the ankle from injury due to sudden inversion stress (Caulfield, 2000).

In the trunk, it has been shown that patients with chronic low back pain have lost the ability to anticipate the need for stability (Hodges and Richardson, 1996) and it seems that this anticipatory function may also be important in ankle stability. Dyhre-Poulsen, Simonsen and Voight (1991) measured EMG activity in the soleus and tibialis anterior in jumping activities and found that these muscles contracted before landing, and similar results have been found with the peroneal muscles in jumping tasks (Caulfield, 2000).

As the ankle ligaments and capsule are torn, articular nerve fibres are also likely to be damaged, leading to a partial deafferentiation of the joint. This, in turn, will decrease the athlete's motor control and inhibit reflex stabilization of the foot and ankle. In addition, joint swelling has been shown to affect muscle control in the knee (Stokes and Young, 1984) and ankle (Petrik et al., 1996), and alteration in the motor programme provided by the CNS may occur (Caulfield, 2000). Proprioceptive training should, therefore, be incorporated into general rehabilitation training. Where chronic instability is seen, the modified Rhomberg test should be used to assess the degree of proprioceptive deficit.

Definition

In the Rhomberg test, the patient is assessed by noting body sway and loss of balance. The traditional test is used to assess general balance ability, and the subject stands with the feet together, arms by the sides. The modified test assesses balance sense as a result of ankle proprioception. It consists of *single leg standing* with the eyes closed.

ANKLE TAPING

Ankle taping may be used to reduce excessive inversion–eversion stress in the previously injured athlete, or as a preventive measure. Taping itself has traditionally been used, but semi-rigid orthoses are becoming increasingly popular. These allow dorsiflexion–plantarflexion but limit inversion–eversion and so should have a less detrimental effect on overall lower limb mechanics.

Orthoses have been shown to be as effective as taping at reducing inversion–eversion movement, but have the advantage that this support is more effectively maintained throughout training. Greene and Hillman (1990) compared several ankle orthotics with taping and found that after 20 minutes of exercise the taping revealed maximal losses of restriction while the orthoses demonstrated no mechanical failure. Rovere et al. (1988) showed ankle stabilizers to be more effective than taping at reducing ankle injuries. Surve et al. (1994) showed a lower incidence of ankle sprain and a reduced severity of injury in soccer players with a previous history of ankle injury who wore a semi-rigid ankle orthosis. No change in incidence of injury was seen in those without a previous history of injury.

In addition to support characteristics, the effect on lower limb mechanics is important. Taping has been shown to throw stress onto the forefoot as the foot compensates for the reduction of dorsiflexion in mid-stance in walking subjects (Carmines, Nunley and McElhaney, 1988). Where an ankle orthosis allows normal dorsiflexion, the forefoot is likely to receive less compensatory stress.

The combination of forefoot stress and loss of restriction capabilities may make the use of ankle orthoses preferable to taping in certain circumstances. The contribution of taping to proprioception, providing an increased skin stimulation to movement, may also be of importance. Restoration of full ankle function with a combination of strength and balance activities must always be the main consideration, with ankle supports used as an interim measure wherever possible.

IMPINGEMENT SYNDROMES

Repeated forced dorsiflexion, such as occurs with dismounts in gymnastics, may cause *anterior impingement* of the talus on the tibia. The synovium may be repeatedly trapped, becoming chronically swollen and hypertrophied. Pain occurs over the front of the ankle, and is exacerbated by dorsiflexion with overpressure. Radiographs may reveal talar osteophytes, but these do not usually contribute to the impingement. Forced plantarflexion, for example repeated karate kicks or football, may cause *posterior impingement* giving pain over the back of the ankle without tenderness to the Achilles tendon.

Both conditions show slight swelling, and represent a repeated impaction of the joint surfaces leading to compression of the articular cartilage and subchondral bone. These structures do not show great sensitivity, and will not be the primary source of pain. Instead, pain must come from the periosteum, the joint capsule or, more likely, from chemical irritation and mechanical stress caused by the inflammatory response itself. Impingement syndromes respond to rest, anti-inflammatory modalities and training modification.

If the impingement force persists, an exostosis may form on the back or front of the lower tibia, depending on the type of stress involved.

Definition
An *exostosis* is a benign (non-harmful) growth of bone which occurs at the edge of a joint. It may occur through mechanical stimulation of the bone membrane (periosteum) through repeated microtrauma.

The exostosis may be up to 1 cm long in some cases (O'Donoghue, 1976), and should this break off, it will float in the joint as a loose body. In cases where the exostosis causes symptoms, it should be surgically removed.

Rapid, forceful dorsiflexion, such as may occur in a fall onto the feet, can force the talus up with enough force to stress the distal tibiofibular ligament. The joint is tender to palpation within the sulcus between the tibia and fibula, and pain is elicited to passive dorsiflexion but not inversion or eversion. Treatment involves strapping the foot to limit dorsiflexion, and using a heel raise.

On the posterior aspect of the talus, the flexor hallucis longus travels in a small groove. If the bone lateral to this point is extended, it is called *Stieda's process*. When this piece occurs as a separate bone (ossicle) attached to the talus by fibrous tissue, it is known as the *os trigonum*. Between 8 and 13% of the population have one of these bony configurations (Brodsky and Khalil, 1987) (Fig. 12.5). Three mechanisms have been proposed for the development of the os trigonum (Reid, 1992). The secondary ossification centre in the region may fail to fuse, or repeated trauma (impingement) may cause a stress fracture. An acute fracture may also ensue following forced plantarflexion with or without avulsion of the posterior band of the lateral ligament (Cedell, 1974).

Repeated plantarflexion may compress the os trigonum and give impingement pain, palpable over the posterolateral talus between the Achilles tendon and the peroneal tendons. If symptoms fail to settle with conservative management, surgical removal of the ossicle may be called for. This is often performed with release of the adjacent tendon sheath of flexor hallucis longus.

TENDINITIS IN ASSOCIATION WITH THE MALLEOLI

Peroneal muscles

The tendons of peroneus longus and brevis pass around the lateral malleolus, while those of tibialis posterior, flexor digitorum longus and flexor hallucis longus pass around the medial malleolus (Fig. 12.6). Any of the tendons, their sheaths, or their retaining retinacula may be inflamed or injured.

One complication of ankle sprain is a strain or avulsion of the peroneus brevis as it attaches to the base of the fifth metatarsal. There may be local bruising, and pain is reproduced by resisted eversion. Point tenderness, proximal to the base of the fifth metatarsal, indicates the tendon, while bone pain may indicate avulsion. Radiographs are required to differentiate avulsion from a fracture to the fifth metatarsal itself (Jones fracture). Treatment is similar to that of an ankle injury, with frictions performed to the tendon while the foot is inverted and exercises to restore strength and flexibility of the peroneus brevis. Where swelling has occurred over the peroneus brevis insertion, it may spread to the joints formed by the cuboid bone, and mobilization of this bone may be required.

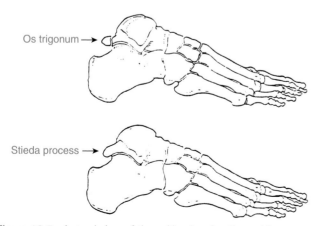

Os trigonum →

Stieda process →

Figure 12.5   Lateral view of the ankle, showing the os trigonum and Stieda's process. From Brodsky, A.E. and Khalil, M.A. (1987) Talar compression syndrome. *Foot and Ankle*, **7**, 338–344. With permission.

> **Keypoint**
>
> Following ankle sprain, the peroneus brevis muscle and its attachment to the base of the 5th metatarsal should be examined. In addition, the mobility of the cuboid bone should be checked, to exclude involvement of either of these structures.

Peroneal tendon dislocation may occur if the tip of the lateral malleolus is fractured with forced dorsiflexion (skiing) or a direct blow (soccer). Occasionally, severe inversion injury may rupture the peroneal retinaculum and allow the tendons to sublux or dislocate forwards over the fibula with resisted dorsiflexion and eversion. Local pain is present, and a 'snapping' sensation is felt as the tendons move over the bone. Surgical management is required, with several procedures being performed to re-establish the anatomy of the region. Re-attachment of the retinaculum, deepening of the peroneal groove, and placing the peroneal tendons under the calcaneofibular ligament have been variously described (Martens, Noyez and Mulier, 1986; Apley and Solomon, 1993).

Flexor hallucis longus

The flexor hallucis longus (FHL) passes behind the medial malleolus in a separate tendon sheath, which runs along the anterior aspect of the talus. The sheath passes between the medial and lateral tubercles of the talus, under the sustentaculum tali, and beneath the flexor retinaculum. The fibro-osseous tunnel so formed predisposes the tendon to mechanical irritation.

Pain may occur to resisted hallux flexion, with tenderness lying medial to the Achilles tendon. Pain is usually noticeable during the push-off phase of walking and running. A fusiform swelling and thickening of the tendon may occur in dancers with repeated point work. Eventually, the thickening may interfere with the movement of the tendon within its sheath giving rise to 'trigger toe' (Sammarco and Miller, 1979).

Tibialis posterior

The tibialis posterior tendon passes in a groove around and beneath the medial malleolus, the latter structure acting as a pulley. During pronation, the tendon is pressed onto the underlying bone of the groove, and in athletes who hyperpronate during the stance phase, tendon or tendon sheath pathology may occur. Tenderness, swelling and/or crepitus is noted in the local area along the tendon sheath. Resisted plantarflexion and inversion may cause pain and will cause the tendon to stand out making palpation easier.

TARSAL TUNNEL SYNDROME

The tarsal tunnel is formed by the medial malleolus, calcaneus and talus on one side and the flexor retinaculum and medial collateral (deltoid) ligament on the other (Fig. 12.7). It begins approximately 2–3 cm proximal to the medial malleolus, and through it travels the posterior tibial nerve. The tunnel ends where the medial and lateral plantar nerves enter the abductor hallucis.

The tunnel may be restricted anatomically by tightness in the fascia and retinacula which normally result from trauma or overuse and the build up of scar tissue. Increased pronation and a valgus (outwardly tilted) heel will tighten the flexor retinaculum and make the condition more likely.

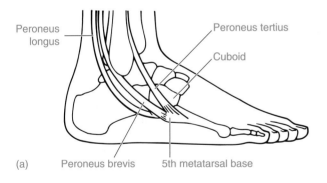

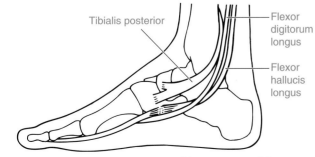

Figure 12.6   Tendons near the malleoli. (a) Lateral view. (b) Medial view.

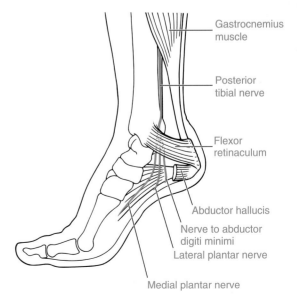

Figure 12.7   The tarsal tunnel. From Magee (2002), with permission.

Following fracture of the calcaneum, tarsal tunnel syndrome may occur in as many as 10% of cases, as a result of either bony impingement or tightness of the cast (Reid, 1992). On occasion, irritation of training shoes may also give a similar clinical picture.

The most common symptom is burning and loss of sensation in the plantar aspect of the foot which is worse with activity and better for rest. The big toe is the most common area of complaint. Nerve conduction tests to the abductor hallucis (and abductor digiti minimi) confirm the diagnosis (Fu, Delisa and Kraft, 1980).

Treatment is by correction of excessive pronation and rearfoot valgus together with modification of footwear. Soft tissue mobilization and stretching may also be needed. Resistant cases may require surgical decompression.

SUBTALOID JOINT

The subtaloid joint (STJ) (Fig. 12.8) has a thin capsule strengthened by the medial, posterior and lateral talocalcaneal ligaments. The joint cavity is isolated from that of the ankle and mid-tarsal joints, and its stability is largely maintained by the interosseous talocalcanean ligament running from the sinus tarsi to the talus.

Subtaloid mobility is often reduced following ankle sprain or fracture of the calcaneus from a fall onto the heel.

Movement may also be reduced by impaction when jumping on a hard surface in inadequate footwear. The lack of mobility sometimes goes unnoticed, unless the patient is assessed by a physiotherapist.

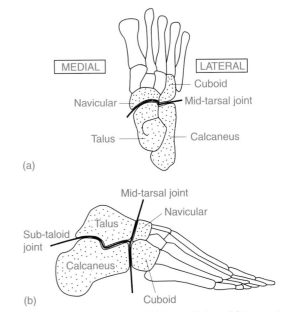

Figure 12.8   The subtaloid and mid-tarsal joints. (a) From above. (b) Lateral view.

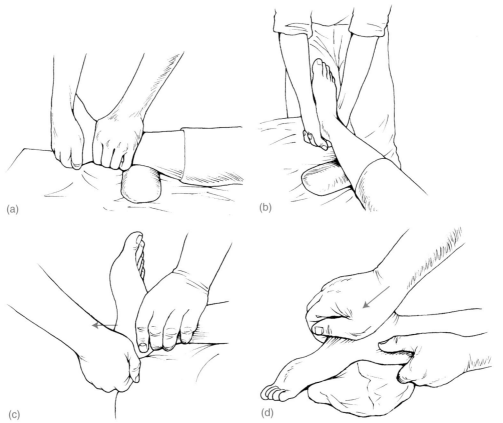

Figure 12.9   Manual therapy of the subtaloid joint. (a) Stabilize lower leg and move talus. (b) Gross subtalar movement. (c, d) Distraction and gliding.

Manual assessment and mobilization of accessory movements may be performed with the patient in a supine-lying position, with the heel over the couch end. Initially, the therapist grips around the distal part of the patient's leg with one hand pressing the leg onto the couch. The therapist's forefingers grip the talus and the calcaneum is cupped in the opposite hand (Fig. 12.9a). The calcaneum is then moved on the fixed talus. Releasing the talus, both talus and calcaneum are moved together on the fixed lower leg. Gross subtaloid joint movement may be performed by cupping the heel in both hands and performing forceful inversion/eversion actions (Fig. 12.9b).

Some distraction may be given to the STJ in supine with one hand cupping the calcaneum laterally and applying a caudal force while the other hand stabilizes the dorsomedial aspect of the mid-foot (Fig. 12.9c). In the prone position, with the patient's foot slightly plantarflexed, and the toes over the couch end, a distraction force may be imparted by pushing caudally with the heel of the hand onto the posterior aspect of the calcaneus near the Achilles tendon insertion (Fig. 12.9d). Following injury, rearfoot position should be assessed as posting may be required.

MID-TARSAL JOINT

The mid-tarsal joint (see Fig. 12.8) is composed of the calcaneal cuboid joint (lateral), and the talocalcaneonavicular joint (medial). Four ligaments are important from the perspective of sports injuries. The *plantar calcaneonavicular* (spring) ligament is a dense fibroelastic structure running from the sustentaculum tali to the navicular behind its tuberosity. The *plantar calcaneocuboid* ligament passes from the anterior inferior aspect of the calcaneus to the plantar surface of cuboid behind the peroneal groove. The *long plantar* ligament stretches the whole length of the lateral aspect of the foot. It arises from between the tubercles of the calcaneus and passes forwards, giving off a short attachment to the cuboid, and so forming a roof over the tendon of peroneus longus. The ligament then attaches to the bases of the lateral four metatarsal bones. The *bifurcate* ligament is in two parts, and travels from a deep hollow on the upper surface of the calcaneus to the cuboid and navicular.

The calcaneocuboid joint takes the full bodyweight as it forms part of the lateral longitudinal arch of the foot. Stability is provided by the plantar calcaneocuboid and long plantar ligaments, reinforced by the tendon of peroneus longus. The talocalcaneonavicular joint is stabilized by the plantar calcaneonavicular and bifurcate ligaments together with the tendon of tibialis posterior.

The calcaneocuboid ligament may be injured at the same time as the ATF. Pain is reproduced by fixing the rearfoot in dorsiflexion and eversion, and inverting and adducting the forefoot. Often the condition goes unnoticed at the time of injury as the AFT sprain is the dominant pain. Chronic pain results, and transverse frictions and scar tissue rupture may be required, with temporary forefoot posting. Mobilization of the cuboid or navicular may be called for (see p. 207).

References

Apley, A.G. and Solomon, L. (1993) *Apley's System of Orthopaedics and Fractures*, 7th edn, Butterworth-Heinemann, Oxford

Brodsky, A.E. and Khalil, M.A. (1987) Talar compression syndrome. *Foot and Ankle*, **7**, 338–344

Burdett, R.G. (1982) Forces predicted at the ankle during running. *Medicine and Science in Sports and Exercise*, **14**, 308

Caulfield, B. (2000) Functional instability of the ankle joint. *Physiotherapy*, **86**, (8) 401–411

Carmines, D.V., Nunley, J.A. and McElhaney, J.H. (1988) Effects of ankle taping on the motion and loading pattern of the foot for walking subjects. *Journal of Orthopaedic Research*, **6**, 223–229

Cedell, C.A. (1974) Rupture of the posterior talotibial ligament with avulsion of a bone fragment from the talus. *Acta Orthopaedica Scandinavica*, **45**, 454

De Carlo, M.S. and Talbot, R.W. (1986) Evaluation of ankle joint proprioception following injection of the anterior talofibular ligament. *Journal of Orthopaedic and Sports Physical Therapy*, **8**, (2) 70–76

Dyhre-Poulsen, P., Simonsen, E. and Voight, M. (1991) Dynamic control of muscle stiffness and H-reflex modulation during hopping and jumping in man. *Journal of Physiology*, **437**, 287–304

Eiff, M.P., Smith, A.T. and Smith, G.E. (1994) Early mobilisation versus immobilisation in the treatment of lateral ankle sprains. *American Journal of Sports Medicine*, **22**, 83–88

Flandry, F. and Sanders, R.A. (1987) Tibiofibular synostosis: an unusual cause of shin splint-like pain. *American Journal of Sports Medicine*, **15**, 280–284

Freeman, M.A.R., Dean, M.R.E. and Hanham, I.W.F. (1965) The etiology and prevention of functional instability of the foot. *Journal of Bone and Joint Surgery*, **47B**, (4) 678–685

Fu, R., Delisa, J.A. and Kraft, G.H. (1980) Motor nerve latencies through the tarsal tunnel in normal adults. *Archives of Physical Medicine and Rehabilitation*, **61**, 243

Garrick, J.G. and Webb, D.R. (1990) *Sports Injuries: Diagnosis and Management*, W.B. Saunders, London

Glencross, D. and Thornton, E. (1981) Position sense following joint injury. *Journal of Sports Medicine*, **5**, 241–242

Greene, T.A. and Hillman, S.K. (1990) Comparison of support provided by a semirigid orthosis and adhesive ankle taping before, during, and after exercise. *American Journal of Sports Medicine*, **18**, (5) 498–506

Hodges, P.W. and Richardson, C.A. (1996) Contraction of transversus abdominis invariably precedes movement of the upper and lower limb. In *Proceedings of the 6th International Conference of the International Federation of Orthopaedic Manipulative Therapists*, Lillehammer, Norway

Karlsson, J. and Andersson, G. (1992) The effect of external ankle support in chronic lateral ankle joint instability. *American Journal of Sports Medicine*, **20**, 257–261

Konradsen, L. and Ravn, J.B. (1990) Ankle instability caused by prolonged peroneal reaction time. *Acta Orthopaedica Scaninavica*, **61**, (5) 388–390

Konradsen, L., Voight, M. and Hojsgaard, C. (1997) Ankle inversion injuries: the role of the dynamic defence mechanism. *American Journal of Sports Medicine*, **25**, 54–58

Lambert, K. (1971) The weight bearing function of the fibula. *Journal of Bone and Joint Surgery*, **53A**, 507

Lentell, G., Bass, B., Lopez, D., McGuire, L. and Sarrels, M. (1995) The contributions of proprioceptive deficits, muscle function, and anatomic laxity to functional instability of the ankle joint. *Journal of Orthopedic and Sports Physical Therapy*, **21**, 206–215

Lentell, G.L., Katzman, L.L. and Walters, M.R. (1990) The relationship between muscle function and ankle stability. *Journal of Orthopaedic and Sports Physical Therapy*, **11**, (12) 605–611

Magee, D.J. (2002) *Orthopedic Physical Assessment, 4th edn*, Saunders, Philadelphia

Martens, M.A., Noyez, J.F. and Mulier, J.C. (1986) Recurrent dislocation of the peroneal tendons: results of rerouting the tendons under the calcaneofibular ligament. *American Journal of Sports Medicine*, **14**, 148–150

O'Donoghue, D.H. (1976) *Treatment of Injuries to Athletes*, W.B. Saunders, Philadelphia

Palastanga, N., Field, D. and Soames, R. (1989) *Anatomy and Human Movement*, Heinemann Medical, Oxford

Petrik, J., Mabey, M.A., Rampersaud, R.J. and Amendola, A. (1996) The effects of isolated ankle effusion on H reflex amplitude, viscoelasticity, and postural control of the ankle. *Proceedings of the American Academy of Orthopedic Surgeons*, (**12**, (2) 81–86)

Reid, D.C. (1992) *Sports Injury Assessment and Rehabilitation*, Churchill Livingstone, London

Rovere, G.D., Clarke, T.J., Yates, C.S. and Burley, K. (1988) Retrospective comparison of taping and ankle stabilizers in preventing ankle injuries. *American Journal of Sports Medicine*, **16**, 228–233

Sammarco, G.J. and Miller, E.H. (1979) Partial rupture of the flexor hallucis longus in classical ballet dancers. *Journal of Bone and Joint Surgery*, **61A**, 440

Stokes, M. and Young, A. (1984) The contribution of reflex inhibition to arthrogenous muscle weakness. *Clinical Science*, **67**, 7–14

Surve, I., Schwellnus, M.P., Noakes, T. and Lombard, C. (1994) A fivefold reduction in the incidence of recurrent ankle sprains in soccer players using the sport-stirrup orthosis. *American Journal of Sports Medicine*, **22**, 601–606

Vargish, T. and Clarke, W.R. (1983) The ankle injury: indications for the selective use of X-rays. *Injury*, **14**, 507–512

Yeung, M.S., Chan, K-M., MPhil, C.H.S. and Yuan, W.Y (1994) An epidemiological survey on ankle sprain. *British Journal of Sports Medicine*, **28**, 112–116

Chapter 13

The foot

The foot is the athlete's main contact area with the ground – an obvious point, but one which helps account for the very high number of conditions affecting this area in sport. An athlete's foot may have to withstand forces two or three times greater than bodyweight, and this may be repeated more than 5000 times every hour when running. Most sports involve some sort of running or jumping, and so the foot is continually called upon to provide both stability and shock attenuation.

THE FIRST METATARSOPHALANGEAL JOINT

The first metatarsal bone joins proximally to the first cuneiform to form the first ray complex (p. 182). Distally, the bone forms the first metatarsophalangeal (MP) joint with the proximal phalanx of the hallux. The first MP joint is reinforced over its plantar aspect by an area of fibrocartilage known as the volar plate (plantar accessory ligament). This is formed from the deep transverse metatarsal ligament, and the tendons of flexor hallucis brevis, adductor hallucis, and abductor hallucis. It has within it two sesamoid bones which serve as weight-bearing points for the metatarsal head (Fig. 13.1).

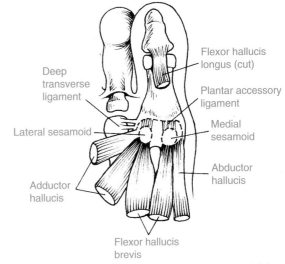

Figure 13.1   Structure of the first metatarsophalangeal joint.

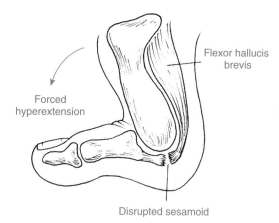

Figure 13.2   Forced hyperextension causes soft tissue damage and possible sesamoid disruption – 'turf toe'.

Movement of the joint is carried out by flexor hallucis longus, flexor hallucis brevis, extensor hallucis longus, the medial tendon of extensor digitorum brevis, and abductor and adductor hallucis. This fairly complex structure is often taken for granted but does give rise to a number of important conditions.

Turf toe

Turf toe is a sprain involving the plantar aspect of the capsule of the first MP joint. It is most often seen in athletes who play regularly on synthetic surfaces, and results from forced hyperextension (dorsiflexion) of the first MP joint. Normally this joint has a range of 50–60°, but with trauma the range may be forced to over 100°. The condition is quite common, with studies of American football players showing that 45% of athletes had suffered from turf toe at some stage (Rodeo et al., 1989a).

Forced hyperextension of the first MP joint causes capsular tearing, collateral ligament damage and damage to the plantar accessory ligament. Sometimes force is so great that disruption of the medial sesamoid occurs (Fig. 13.2). Examination reveals a hyperaemic swollen joint with tenderness over the plantar surface of the metatarsal head. Local bruising may develop within 24 hours. Differential diagnosis must be made from sesamoid stress fracture (insidious onset) and metatarsal or phalangeal fractures (site of pain and radiograph).

Treatment aims at reducing pain and inflammation and supporting the joint by taping (Fig. 13.3). An oval piece of felt or foam with a hole in the middle is placed beneath the toe, the hole corresponding to the metatarsal head. The first MP joint is held in neutral position and anchors are applied around the first phalanx and mid-foot. Strips of 2.5 cm inelastic tape are applied as stirrups between the anchors on the dorsal and plantar aspects of the toe. In each case the tape starts at the toe and is pulled towards the mid-foot, covering the first MP joint. The mid-foot and phalanx strips are finished with fixing strips.

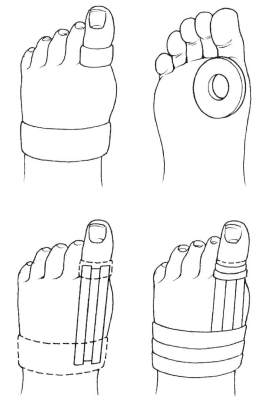

Figure 13.3   Turf toe taping.

A number of factors may predispose the athlete to turf toe. The condition is more common with artificial playing surfaces than with grass (Bowers and Martin, 1976). Artificial turf is less shock-absorbing, and so transmits more force directly to the first MP joint. Sports shoes also have an important part to play. Lighter shoes tend to be used with artificial playing surfaces. These shoes are more flexible around the distal forefoot, and allow the MP joint to hyperextend. In addition, shoes which are fitted by length size alone, rather than width, may cause problems for athletes with wider feet. This person must buy shoes which are too long to accommodate his or her foot width. Such a shoe increases the leverage forces acting on the toe joints and allows the foot to slide forwards in the shoe, increasing the speed of movement at the joint.

Preventive measures include wearing shoes with more rigid soles to avoid hyperextension of the injured joint. In addition, semi-rigid (spring steel or heat-sensitive plastic) insoles may be used. Some authors recommend the use of rigid insoles as a preventive measure when playing on all-weather surfaces, for all athletes with less than 60° dorsiflexion at the first MP joint (Clanton, Butler and Eggert, 1986).

An increased range of ankle dorsiflexion has been suggested as a risk factor which may predispose an athlete to turf toe (Rodeo et al., 1989b). However, in walking subjects, when the ankle is strapped to reduce dorsiflexion, the heel actually lifts up earlier in the gait cycle, causing the range of motion at the metatarsal heads to increase (Carmines,

Nunley and McElhaney, 1988). This increased range may once again predispose the athlete to turf toe (George, 1989), so the amount of dorsiflexion per se may not be that important. If injury has recently changed the range, the athlete may not have had time to fully adapt to the altered movement pattern, and the altered foot/ankle mechanics in total may be the problem.

As with many soft tissue injuries, if incorrectly managed the condition may predispose the athlete to arthritic changes in later life. In the case of turf toe, this may occur as calcification of the soft tissues around the injury site, presenting as hallux valgus or hallux rigidus.

HALLUS VALGUS

Hallux valgus usually occurs when the first MP joint is hypermobile, and the first ray is shorter than the second (Morton foot structure). When this is the case, the second metatarsal head takes more pressure than in a non-Morton foot (Rodgers and Cavanagh, 1989) (Fig. 13.4). In addition, hallux valgus is more common in athletes who hyperpronate.

As the first MP joint dorsiflexes during the propulsive phase of running, the instability allows the hallux to deviate from its normal plane. Adduction and axial rotation occur, and the long flexors which normally stabilize the joint now themselves become deforming influences, causing bowstring effect. As the first metatarsal head adducts, the sesamoids sublux and eventually erode the plantar aspect of the first metatarsal head – this is one source of pain. Compensatory stress is placed on the joints proximal and distal to the first MP and further pain arises through synovial inflammation and capsular distraction. Eventually, secondary osteoarthritis occurs in the first MP joint and sesamoids.

Hallux valgus may occur in one of two types. *Congrous hallux valgus* is an exaggeration of the normal angulation between the metatarsal and the phalax of the 1st toe. Importantly the joint surfaces remain in opposition and the condition does not progress. The normal angulation of the 1st MPJ (measured between the long axis of the metatarsal and that of the proximal phalanx) is 8–20°; in congrous hallux valgus this angle may increase to 20–30° (Fig. 13.5a). Once the angle increases above 30°, the joint surfaces move out of congruity and may evenutally sublux. This condition is now classified as *pathological hallux valgus*, and may progress, with the angulation increasing to as much as 60° (Magee, 2002).

Bunion formation to the side of the first metatarsal head is common. The bursa over the medial aspect of the MPJ thickens and a callus develops. In time an exostosis is seen on the metatarsal head and the three structures combined lead to the cosmetic change which is noticeable (Fig. 13.5b).

Management of this condition is initially to stabilize the first MP joint by correcting faulty foot mechanics (especially hyperpronation) and advising on correct athletic footwear. If conservative management fails, surgery may be required. If the deformity is purely soft tissue in nature, the bunion may be removed, and the dynamic structures around the

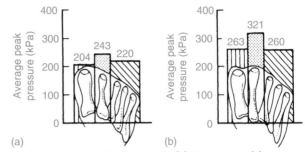

Figure 13.4 Pressure distribution in (a) Morton and (b) non-Morton feet. From Rodgers, M.M. and Cavanagh, P.R. (1989) Pressure distribution in Morton's foot structure. *Medicine and Science in Sports and Exercise*, **21**, 23–28. With permission.

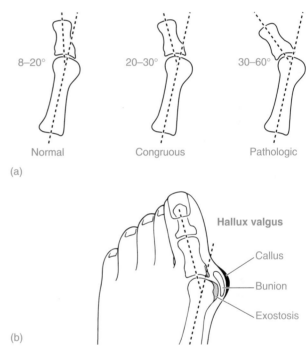

Figure 13.5 Hallux valgus. (a) Metatarsophalangeal angle and (b) appearance. After Magee (2002) with permission.

first toe realigned. If bony deformity is present, osteotomy or arthroplasty may be necessary.

Hallux limitus/rigidus

A reduction in movement of the first MP joint, *hallus limitus*, may progress to complete immobility or *hallux rigidus*. The condition is more common when the first metatarsal is longer than the second. Pain is generally worse during sporting activities, and occurs especially when pushing off. On examination, the joint end feel is usually firm, and limitation of movement is noted to dorsiflexion. To differentiate between a tight flexor hallucis longus and joint structures, the foot is assessed both with the foot dorsiflexed and everted (tendon on stretch) and then plantarflexed and inverted (tendon relaxed).

> **Keypoint**
>
> In hallux limitus, movement may be restricted by either a tight flexor hallucis longus (FHL) or joint structures. To differentiate between the two, movement range is assessed both with the tendon on stretch (FHL limits) and with the tendon relaxed (joint limits).

Limitation of motion through muscle tightness responds well to stretching procedures, while joint limitation which is soft tissue in nature is treated by joint mobilization. Distal distraction and gliding mobilizations with the metatarsal head stabilized are particularly useful (Cibulka, 1990). Where bony deformity is present, surgery is indicated. A number of surgical procedures are available for hallux conditions, and the interested reader is referred to Horn and Subotnick (1989) for an excellent review.

PLANTAR FASCIITIS

The plantar fascia (plantar aponeurosis) is the thickest fascia in the body. It attaches from a point just behind the medial tubercle of calcaneus and runs anteriorly as five slips. As the slips approach the metatarsal heads, they split into superficial and deep layers (Fig. 13.6a). The superficial layer attaches to superficial fascia beneath the skin, while the deep layer divides into medial and lateral portions to allow the passage of the flexor tendons. Each of the five portions attaches to the base of a proximal phalanx and to the deep transverse ligament. As the toes dorsiflex the fascia is wound around the metatarsal head (windlass effect). In so doing the fascia is tightened and the longitudinal arch elevated (Fig. 13.6b).

Inflammation of the plantar fascia is common in sports which involve repeated jumping, and with hill running. Overuse may cause microtears and inflammation of the fascial insertion, and nodules from the fascial granuloma can occasionally be felt (Tanner and Harvey, 1988).

Normally, during mid-stance the foot is flattened, stretching the plantar fascia and enabling it to store elastic energy to be released at toe off. However, a variety of malalignment faults may increase stress on the fascia. Excessive rearfoot pronation will lower the arch and overstretch the fascia, and a reduction in mobility of the first metatarsal may also contribute to the condition (Creighton and Olson, 1987). In addition, weak peronei, often the result of incomplete rehabilitation following ankle sprains, will reduce the support on the arch, thus stressing the plantar fascia. Congenital problems such as pes cavus will also leave an athlete more susceptible to plantar fasciitis.

As the foot is plantarflexed with the toes on the ground, the fascia is stretched over the metatarsal heads, raising the longitudinal arch and making the foot more rigid. Plantar fasciitis is therefore exacerbated if the Achilles tendon is tight, or if high-heeled shoes are worn. Pain is often worse

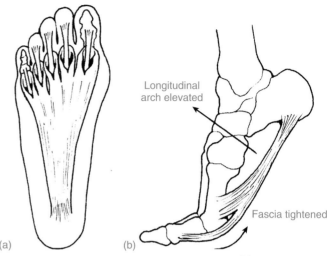

Figure 13.6 Plantar fascia structure and action. (a) Normal tension in fascia. (b) Raising onto the toes tightens the plantar fascia and raises the longitudinal arch.

when taking the first few steps in the morning until the Achilles tendon is stretched.

Sports shoes play an important part in the course of this condition. Inadequate rearfoot control may fail to eliminate hyperpronation, and a poorly fitting heel counter will allow the calcaneal fat pad to spread at heel strike, transmitting extra impact force to the calcaneus and plantar fascia. On a hard surface, the shock-absorbing qualities of the shoe are important, and a patient's footwear should always be examined.

Pain is usually over the calcaneal attachment of the fascia or its medial edge. Pain may be localized to the heel as though the athlete is 'stepping on a stone', or may present as a burning pain over the arch. The problem must be differentiated from rheumatoid conditions which often give bilateral pain, and Sever's disease which gives pain to the insertion of the Achilles tendon.

Treatment

Taping the foot (Fig. 13.7) may often give surprisingly rapid relief. The foot is locked in neutral position (p. 181) and an anchor strap placed just behind the metatarsal heads. Three strips of tape (medial, lateral and central) are then passed from the anchor over the heel to stop on the posterior aspect of the calcaneum. A horseshoe-shaped fixing strip secures the tape behind the heel. Additional strips may be placed transversely across the foot from the metatarsal heads to the calcaneal tubercle.

Trigger point therapy for the plantar muscles (especially quadratus plantae and flexor hallucis) may give excellent results even long term. The thickness of the tissues in this area means that a massage tool should be used to save the therapist's fingers. The athlete sits with the therapist sitting towards the end. Ischaemic pressure is placed onto the muscles and fascia in the sole of the foot and the tissues are

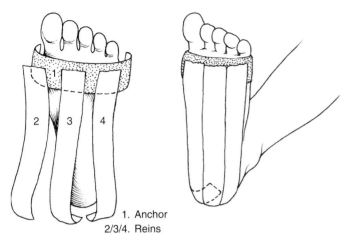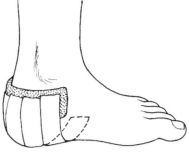

Figure 13.8 Taping for heel pad.

1. Anchor
2/3/4. Reins

Figure 13.7 Plantar fascia taping.

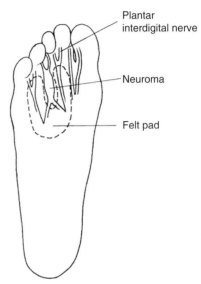

Figure 13.9 Padding for interdigital neuroma.

gradually tightened as pain allows by plantarflexion the foot and flexing the toes (windlass effect). The athlete can be taught self-management by pressing the sole of the foot down onto a hard ball (marble or snooker ball) or crossing the legs and pressing directly into the sole with the thumbs. See also Treatment note 13.1.

More permanent management may require rearfoot posting to control excessive pronation. In addition, strengthening the intrinsic foot musculature is important. Although the plantar fascia is inert, stress on the structure may be increased when the intrinsic foot musculature is weak. The role of foot strengthening, including actively increasing the arch height, and 'gripping' the floor with the toes, may have a re-education effect on plantar proprioception.

HEEL PAD

The calcaneus is covered by elastic adipose tissue in the same way as the finger tips. The fat cells are arranged in columns made from fibrous septa which lie vertically. As weight is taken, the walls of the columns bulge and spring back as the weight is released. With age the septa lose elasticity and the thickness of the heel pad reduces.

Athletes who wear poorly padded sports shoes and those who land heavily on the heel when jumping may bruise this area. In more severe cases rupture of the fibrous septa may occur causing spillage of the enclosed fat cells (Reid, 1992). In turn, the loss of the heel pad shock-absorbing mechanism places excessive compression stress onto the calcaneum.

Pain is increased when walking barefoot. Typically, athletes complain of pain first thing in the morning when getting out of bed. The first few steps are exquisitely tender, later subsiding to a dull ache. Pain is brought on by prolonged standing and walking.

Management is by additional padding, and preventing the heel pad from spreading. Non-bottoming shock-absorbing materials are useful, and taping to surround the heel and prevent spread of the pad is effective in the short term

(Fig. 13.8). Activity modification is required during the acute stage of the condition.

MORTON'S NEUROMA

Morton's neuroma affects the plantar interdigital nerve between the third and fourth metatarsal heads. Symptoms may occur spontaneously and are often described as feeling like 'electric shocks' along the sensory nerve distribution. The condition is more common with runners (particularly when sprinting and running uphill) and dancers, and is often aggravated by wearing narrow high-heeled shoes. The sustained dorsiflexed position of these activities stretches the digital nerve causing inflammation. Once swollen, the nerve is open to entrapment between the metatarsal heads, and eventually the nerve is scarred and permanently enlarged to form a neuroma.

The patient's pain may be reproduced by direct pressure over the neuroma while compressing the forefoot medially and laterally. If the condition is caught in its oedematous stage, alteration of footwear (larger toe box and lower heel), ice application and ultrasound are effective. Injection with corticosteroid and local anaesthetic is also used. Padding the area with orthopaedic felt (Fig. 13.9) to take some of the bodyweight off the neuroma can give temporary relief. The arms of the pad rest on the adjacent metatarsals, leaving the area of the neuroma free.

Once the neuroma has formed, surgical excision under local anaesthesia is frequently required, with studies showing improvement in 80% of patients (Mann and Reynolds, 1983). There may be a permanent loss of sensation over the plantar aspect of the foot supplied by the digital nerve, but in some cases regeneration occurs between 8 and 12 months after surgery.

METATARSALGIA

The term 'metatarsalgia' is often used to describe any pain in the forefoot. Such pain may come from a variety of conditions, including those affecting the hallux, a digital neuroma, or even stress fractures. However, in this description we will limit the term to 'functional metatarsalgia', where altered foot function causes abnormal mechanical stress in the forefoot, which is symptomatic.

The transverse arch of the foot is supported at the level of the cuneiforms by peroneus longus, which pulls the medial and lateral edges of the foot together (Palastanga, Field and Soames, 1989). More distally, the arch is formed by the metatarsal heads, the highest point or 'keystone' being the second metatarsal.

> **Keypoint**
>
> The transverse arch of the foot is supported by peroneus longus. Distally, the arch is formed by the metatarsal heads, the highest point or 'keystone' being the second metatarsal.

In mid-stance, the arch flattens and the five metatarsal heads come to lie in the same transverse plane to take the bodyweight. The first metatarsal takes weight through its sesamoid bones, and it and the fifth metatarsal are more mobile than the other three. Stability to the metatarsal heads is provided both passively, by the transverse metatarsal ligament, and actively, by adductor hallucis and, to a lesser extent, the intrinsics. Normally, these structures keep the metatarsals together. However, in cases of hypermobility such as excessive pronation or hallux valgus, the metatarsal heads may splay apart, effectively increasing the width of the forefoot, and allowing the central metatarsal heads to take too much weight.

Hypermobility may cause abnormal shearing forces, especially in an ill-fitting shoe, giving plantar keratosis. As the metatarsal heads splay, the transverse ligament and intrinsic muscles are subjected to tensile stress, giving pain. Rigidity of the foot may also cause problems. If any of the metatarsals are fixed, or if the toes are 'clawed', plantar compression will occur, again giving keratoma (Neale and Adams, 1989).

Clearly, successful management of the condition relies to a large extent on the identification of any underlying biomechanical abnormality in the foot. Short-term relief may be obtained by using anti-inflammatory modalities, and padding and strapping to relieve the stress on the forefoot tissues. An adhesive plantar metatarsal pad (PMP), made from orthopaedic felt, is contoured to cover the heads and upper shafts of the three central metatarsals, lifting them above ground level on weight bearing (Fig. 13.10). The pad is cut around the head of the first metatarsal to avoid excessive pressure at this point. To prevent metatarsal splaying, inelastic strapping is placed around the forefoot, encircling the metatarsals just beneath the first and fifth metatarsal heads. If the metatarsals are immobile, a metatarsal bar may be built into the shoe. This has the effect of transferring the bodyweight to the metatarsal shafts and away from the painful metatarsal head.

Coupled with strapping and padding, strengthening the intrinsic muscles is essential. Simple exercises, such as gripping the floor with the toes in bare feet, are effective at building isometric strength and endurance of the intrinsics. Eccentric strength is similarly developed by initially tensing the intrinsic muscles of the foot and increasing the arch with the leg non-weight bearing. The bodyweight is then taken onto the foot and gradually the arch is allowed to flatten under control.

CUBOID SYNDROME

Pain over the lateral aspect of the foot may represent subluxation of the cuboid. This is more common in dancers, where 17% of foot and ankle injuries have been found to be cuboid-related (Marshall and Hamilton, 1992). The condition is also seen following ankle sprain. At the time of injury, the ligamentous support of the calcaneocuboid joint and the metatarsal cuboid joint may be disrupted. When this occurs in an athlete with a markedly pronated foot, the peroneus longus, travelling through the groove of the cuboid, may pull the medial edge of the cuboid down.

Dull pain is experienced over the lateral aspect of the foot and along the course of peroneus longus tendon. Pain is

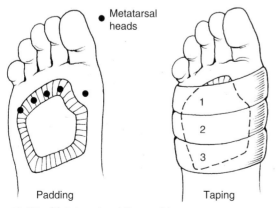

Metatarsal heads

Padding   Taping

Figure 13.10   Metatarsal padding and tape.

increased with prolonged standing and exercise on unforgiving surfaces and/or in poor athletic footwear. Typically, the pain is worse for the first few steps in the morning and is lessened when non-weight bearing, and when walking on the toes (foot supinated).

The subluxation may be reduced by manual therapy. Two methods are typically used (Marshall and Hamilton, 1992). In the first, the patient is supine and the therapist distracts the cuboid fourth metatarsal joint by placing traction through the fourth metatarsal shaft. At the same time the foot is plantarflexed and relocation of the cuboid is spontaneous. Where this technique fails, manipulation may succeed. The patient is prone and the therapist grasps the patient's foot, placing his or her thumbs over the plantar surface of the cuboid. A high velocity, low amplitude thrust is then performed, forcing the foot into plantarflexion, while the reduction pressure is maintained over the base of the cuboid. Once reduced, the cuboid position is maintained with a felt pad and tape.

ACCESSORY MOVEMENTS OF THE FOOT

In many conditions affecting the foot and ankle, accessory movements of the joints of the mid-foot and forefoot may be reduced. Mobilization procedures require accurate fixation of one segment while mobilization of an adjacent segment is carried out. Kaltenborn (1989) described a logical series of movements of use for examination and manual treatment.

On the lateral side of the foot a number of movements focus on the cuboid. Initially, the cuboid is moved on the fixed calcaneum. The navicular and lateral cuneiform are fixed and the cuboid is then moved upon them. Finally the cuboid itself is fixed and the fourth and fifth metatarsals are moved.

On the medial side of the foot, movements are around the navicular and cuneiforms. The navicular is fixed and the cuboid and then the cuneiforms are moved. The navicular itself is moved on the talus. Finally, the cuneiforms are fixed and the second and third metatarsals moved (Fig. 13.11). See also Treatment note 13.1.

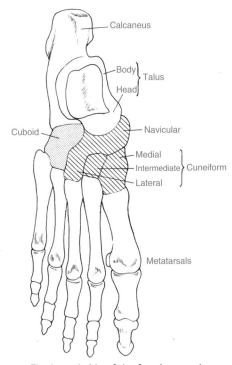

Figure 13.11   The lateral side of the foot is moved around the cuboid, the medial side around the navicular cuneiforms.

Treatment note 13.1   Manual therapy techniques for the foot

Mobilization of the cuboid bone
The cuboid may become stiff due to lateral ligament sprain where inflammation has been caused to the peroneus brevis tendon connected to the tubercler of the 5th metatarsal. Swelling may then spread on to the cuboid articulations.

To locate the cuboid, find the tubercle on the 5th metatarsal. The cuboid is the flat block-like bone which lies immediately superior to this. Grip the cuboid with the thumb and forefinger of one hand and fix the calcaneous with the other. Move the cuboid on the fixed calcaneous (Fig. 13.12). Secondly, fix the cuboid with the thumb and forefinger of one hand and move the 4th and 5th metatarsals on this fixed point.

Mobilization of the tarsometatarsal (TM) joint of the first toe
To find the first TM joint, palpate the ball of the large toe and follow the metatarsal along its length, tracing it with the knife edge of the thumb. The thumb comes to rest in a

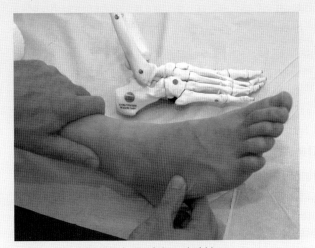

Figure 13.12   Mobilizations of the cuboid bone.

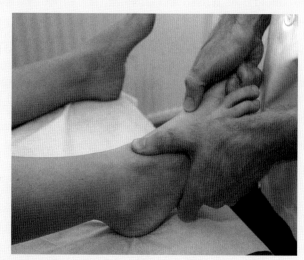

Figure 13.13   Longitudinal mobilization of the first ray.

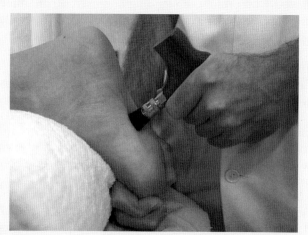

Figure 13.14   Ischaemic pressure using a 'plunger' for the plantarfascia.

shallow hollow between the base of the first metatarsal and the medial cuneiform bone. Stabilize the metatarsal with the thumb and forefinger of one hand while mobilizing the medial cuneiform with the thumb and forefinger of the opposite hand.

Longitudinal mobilization traction of the first ray

Longitudinal mobilization to the first metatarsal phalangeal (MP) joint and the tarsometatarso (TM) joint of the first toe can be extremely relieving in cases of halux rigidus. Support the shaft of the first metatarsal with one hand while surrounding the proximal phalanx of the great toe with the fingers of the opposite hand (Fig. 13.13). The movement is a distraction force for first MP joint. While maintaining the stabilization on the shaft of the first metatarsal bone, abduction and adduction may be imposed on the first MP joint.

Trigger point massage of the quadratus plantae and the flexor digitorum

These muscles (quadratus plantae is also known as flexor accessorius) become tight and painful in cases of plantarfasciitis and respond well to ischaemic compression. Because of the thickness of the sole of the foot it is difficult to provide sufficient pressure using the practitioner's thumb.

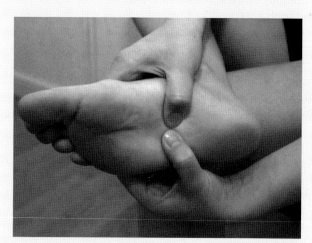

Figure 13.15   Self-treatment in cross leg sitting using thumbs.

For this reason, a plunger is used. Pressure is initially applied with the foot slightly plantarflexed and the toes flexed to release the muscle (Fig. 13.14). As pain eases, the plantarfascia itself is stretched by plantarflexion and flexion of the first toe to use the windlass effect. The patient may be taught this technique, using a small marble or ball on the floor and moving the foot up and down over it. Alternatively, massage into the sole of the foot by crossing one leg over the other and using the ball of the thumb (Fig. 13.15).

SKIN AND NAIL LESIONS

Subungual haematoma

In this condition, a haematoma forms directly below the nail plate as a result of direct trauma. Pressure builds up in the space between the nail and nail bed, causing acute pain and throbbing. In some cases the pressure may be great enough to loosen the nail from its bed. Subungual haematoma is often referred to as 'black toe' or 'runner's toe'. Ill-fitting shoes are a common cause; if the toe box is too small the nail may rub, especially when running downhill.

When the problem is acute, the haematoma is often decompressed by the athlete penetrating the nail with a red-hot needle or paperclip to release the blood (Subotnick, 1989). A less hazardous approach is for the therapist to use a sterile needle. The best treatment for chronic haemorrhage is to remove the cause, and buy shoes which allow enough room for the toes to spread on weight-bearing and expand with warmth. When standing, a sports shoe should allow one thumb's breadth between the end of the shoe and the athlete's longest toe.

Ingrown toenail (onychocryptosis)

Onychocryptosis, or ingrown toenail, is particularly common in the hallux of athletes, especially males. It may occur secondarily to ill-fitting sports shoes, or to incorrect toenail cutting. Shoes are often too narrow, leading to lateral pressure on the hallux, and athletes often cut the toenails too short, causing the underlying soft tissues to protrude. Cutting across the corners of the nail is another common fault in foot care, allowing the nail to embed itself into the nail grooves. Frequently, excessive sweating (hyperhidrosis) causes skin softening, a condition exacerbated by prolonged hot bathing.

A splinter of nail grows into the subcutaneous tissue, and with time, acute inflammation occurs, possibly with infection (paronychia). The skin becomes red, tight and shiny, and the toe swells. There is throbbing pain and acute tenderness to palpation. Normal healing will not take place as long as the nail splinter remains, and so hypergranulation occurs. The combination of granulation tissue and the swollen nailfold overlaps the nail plate itself.

When the condition occurs without infection, the nail splinter may be removed with a scalpel (size 15), avoiding further damage to the sulcus. The edge of the nail is smoothed and the area washed with saline. The nail edge is then packed with cotton wool, allowing some to rest under the nail plate itself. The area is protected with a sterile dressing, and regularly inspected.

When the condition is accompanied by infection, a local anaesthetic is used, injecting at the base of the toe away from the infected area. Oral antibiotics may be used and/or an antiseptic dressing applied. Hypergranulation tissue is excised. If this procedure is ineffective, nail surgery involving partial or complete nail avulsion is required (Neale and Adams, 1989).

Prevention of the problem relies on the use of correctly fitting sports shoes, and on cutting the nails to the shape of the end of the toe while avoiding splintering the nail sides. It is good practice to address basic foot care at the beginning of the season, especially with athletes new to the squad.

Nailbed infection (onychia)

Nailbed infection (onychia) and inflammation of the lateral aspect of the nail (paronychia) is common with the nail of the first toe. The condition occurs through poor foot hygiene and nail management, repetitive trauma, and as a reaction to soaps and nail varnish etc. The infection is usually due to staphylococcus or streptococcus, or as a secondary effect of a fungal infection (see below). There is intense pain, redness and pus formation (suppuration) which may also be accompanied by changes in the appearance of the nail itself.

Management is by antiseptic soaks three times a day with the application of a topical antiseptic cream together with general foot hygiene (clean, breathable socks and disinfect normal footwear which has been worn without socks). Persistent cases may require antibiotics, nail debridement or even nail excision.

Blisters

Blisters occur as a result of compression or shearing on the skin. A narrow toe box may cause blisters over the medial aspect of the fifth toe, and between the first and second toes in the case of hallux valgus. Blisters over the plantar aspect of the foot are common when sports shoes are loose. Shoes should be fitted correctly and friction reduced wherever possible. Petroleum jelly or plastic backed moist gel squares used between the toes are helpful. Proper foot hygiene, which may include powder or astringents to dry the foot, should be observed.

Acute blisters may be drained through a puncture hole. A sterile needle is used and enters the blister at the side, the needle being held parallel to the skin. This will leave a skin flap intact for protection. The underlying cause of the blister should be addressed.

Athlete's foot

Tinea pedis or 'athlete's foot' is the most common fungal infection of the feet, and is particularly rampant in communal washing areas within sport and where standards of hygiene are poor. Sports shoes create moisture and warmth between the toes, conditions in which the complaint thrives. Three types of tinea pedis are generally seen. First, the lateral toe spaces become macerated due to three organisms: *Trichophyton rubrum*, *Trichophyton interdigitale* and *Epidermophyton floccosum*. Secondly, the condition may spread to the soles of the feet where vesiculation occurs as a result of *T. interdigitale* and *E. floccosum*, and finally a diffuse 'moccasin type' scaling appears, usually due to *T. rubrum*. The condition may also spread to the nails and hands in some cases.

Treatment is initially aimed at removing the scaling tissue by the application of surgical spirit. When the scaling has cleared, antifungal dusting powders, such as tolnaftate, are used. Sprays containing clotrimazole and dusting powders are used by the athlete, and socks and footwear should be changed daily and preferably disinfected. While the infection remains, athletes should not go barefoot in public areas (changing rooms and swimming baths), and should not share towels, socks or footwear.

Callus formation (hyperkeratosis)

Keratinization is a normal physiological process which turns the stratum corneum of the skin into a hard protective cover. The process becomes overactive if the skin is continually subjected to mechanical stress, for example on the hands of heavy manual workers or the feet of athletes. Hyperaemia occurs, stimulating a proliferation of epidermal cells, and at the same time the rate of desquamation reduces. This type of keratoma or callus on the foot has a protective function, and providing it is asymptomatic it should be left in place. However, when the bulk of such tissues becomes excessive and causes pain or deformity, treatment is required.

The size and shape of the hyperkeratosis is largely dictated by the stress imposed on the skin. A callus is a diffuse area of thickened skin resulting from stress over a fairly wide area, while a corn is a smaller concentrated area which has formed into a nucleus.

Definition

A callus is a diffuse area of thickened skin resulting from stress over a fairly wide area, while a corn is a smaller concentrated area which has formed into a nucleus.

Corns typically seen in sports medicine are either soft or hard, although vascular and neurovascular types do exist. Soft corns are common in the cleft between the fourth and fifth toes, and appear macerated due to sweat retention. The corn nucleus is generally ring-shaped and the centre of the lesion is very thin. Hard corns occur on the plantar aspect of the foot beneath the metatarsal heads, or on the dorsum of the interphalangeal joints. They develop because of concentrated pressure due to bodyweight and ground reaction forces. The corn nucleus is often associated with surrounding callus due to shearing stress.

The corn or callus may be removed with a scalpel by a therapist and the corn nucleus eradicated. Antiseptic agents such as cetrimide and chlorhexidine are then applied. Moist skin is treated with salicylic acid or aluminium chlorohydrate, and excessively dry skin managed with an emollient containing urea, or soft white paraffin. It is important to remove the underlying cause of the keratoma so that it does not simply return. Examination of foot biomechanics and sports footwear is therefore essential.

Verruca

Verruca pedis is a lesion caused by one of the human papilloma viruses (HPV), of which about 15 have been identified. A benign epithelial tumour which is self-limiting is produced in the plantar skin. The wart is covered by hyperkeratotic tissue, and contains brown or black specks caused by intravascular thromboses within its dilated capillaries. Where the wart is over a weight-bearing site, it is forced into the dermis leaving just the hyperkeratotic area on the surface. For this reason athletes often assume a verruca is simply a corn or callus. However, close inspection will usually reveal the papillary appearance of the verruca. A number of other factors differentiate the two. A wart has a far more rapid onset than an area of callus, and may occur in an area of skin not associated with mechanical stress. In addition, bleeding can occur if the verruca is cut because of capillary dilatation, whereas a callus is avascular.

Keypoint

Differentiation of a verruca from a corn: (i) a verruca forms more quickly than corn; (ii) a verruca is found on skin which is not associated with mechanical stress; (iii) a verruca will bleed if cut, but a corn will not.

The virus normally enters the body through broken skin in the foot, especially if the foot has been wet and the skin macerated. Unfortunately, the virus spreads quickly through a population before the plantar wart becomes obvious. The aim of treatment is to destroy all the cells within the lesion by chemical cautery or cryosurgery. Various preparations are used. The skin surrounding the area is protected, and a liquid or paste of salicylic acid (or monochloroacetic acid) is applied. An aseptic necrosis is produced, and destroyed tissue is removed 1 week later.

Cryosurgery aims at freezing the verruca with carbon dioxide snow, nitrous oxide or liquid nitrogen applied through a probe. Tissue necrosis with blister formation occurs when the skin is cooled to $-20°C$ and bluish coloration results. The rapid cooling causes ice crystals to form in the body cells and interstitial fluids, which in turn ruptures the cells. Liquid nitrogen is perhaps the most common of the cryosurgery techniques, applied by dipping a cotton-tipped stick into the liquid. This is applied to the verruca for about 30–60 seconds. The lesion is protected by a cavity pad if it is over a weight-bearing area.

If the verruca is not painful, treatment may not be required as the lesion will regress naturally in some months (Neale and Adams, 1989). However, cross-infection must still be guarded against by the use of plastic waterproof socks in public areas.

THE SPORTS SHOE

The design of sports shoes has received a great deal of attention over the last three decades. This interest has to a large extent been market-led due to the massive increase in the number of people jogging. Manufacturers vie with each other to produce a shoe feature which can act as a 'unique selling point' to give them an increased market share.

There is little doubt that shoe design has improved, and that athletes have benefited from this. However, many developments are simply variations on the same theme and give little substantial improvement to overall shoe design. In addition, the mounting cost of sports shoes makes it imperative that athletes receive the right advice concerning the shoe which will best suit their foot and be appropriate to their sport.

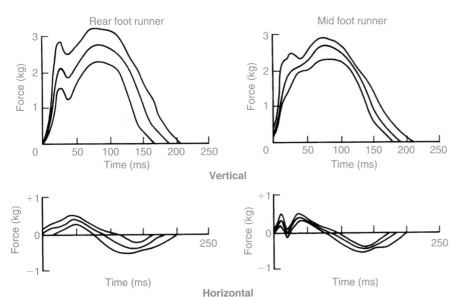

Vertical

Horizontal

Figure 13.16   Ground reaction forces in rearfoot and mid-foot runners. From Segesser and Pforringer (1989).

As most sports involve running, more emphasis will be given to the features of running shoes, as many of these features are carried over into other sports footwear.

Forces acting on the foot

During the stance phase of running, the foot must accommodate to three phases, heel strike, mid-stance and toe off, during which the biomechanics of the foot change considerably. At heel strike the single force of the foot moving downwards and forwards may be resolved into two components. The first is an impact stress acting vertically, and the second a horizontal shearing force, creating friction. Not all athletes strike the ground with the heel when running. For some 80% the initial contact point is at the heel (Frederick, Clarke and Hamill, 1984). The ground reaction force curve in this case shows an initial (passive) peak at heel strike of about half bodyweight, occurring 20–30 ms after heel strike. A secondary (active) peak occurs approximately 100 ms after heel contact as the centre of pressure moves over the ball of the foot prior to toe off (Fig. 13.16).

Other runners show a centre of pressure over the midfoot or rearfoot (Fig. 13.17). The magnitude of the force acting on the foot can be as much as three times bodyweight.

The rearfoot runner strikes the ground with the knee locked, and consequently will require more shock attenuation from the sports shoe. The mid-foot or forefoot striker has the knee slightly flexed, and so part of the contact shock is absorbed by the elasticity of the knee structures.

Keypoint

A *rearfoot* runner strikes the ground with the knee locked, and will require more shock absorbtion from a sports shoe. *Mid-foot* or *forefoot* strikers have the knees slightly flexed, and so some shock is absorbed by the knee.

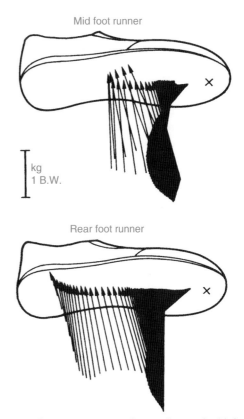

Figure 13.17   Force vector curves for rearfoot and mid-foot runners. From Segesser and Pforringer (1989), with permission.

In some cases, the heel does not touch the ground at all, leaving the stance phase under the control of the posterior leg muscles. With this type of runner, the shock-absorbing function of a heel wedge will be under-utilized.

During mid-stance there can be 5° of abduction of the foot, causing friction between the shoe and running surface. This creates a torsion force which tends to rotate the upper part of the shoe in relation to the sole (Cavanagh, 1989).

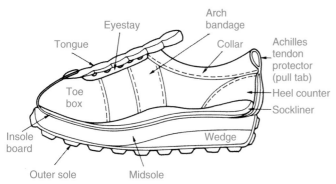

Figure 13.18 Parts of the sports shoe.

Components of a running shoe

The outer sole (Fig. 13.18) of a shoe is generally a carbon rubber material with treads or studs cut in. The outer sole must provide a combination of four features: grip (traction), durability, flexibility and light weight. Studs provide better cross-country grip while bars are more durable on hard surfaces and so better suited to road shoes. However, the thicker studs or cleats of a cross-country or fell-running shoe will also add weight, so faster road-racing shoes tend to have thin, smoother soles.

Beneath the sole is the mid-sole, extending the full length of the shoe, and the wedge which begins behind the metatarsal heads and extends back to the heel. These take the place of the wooden 'shank' of the traditional street shoe. Both the mid-sole and wedge are designed for cushioning, giving good elastic recoil, but they must also maintain good foot control. They are usually two or three layers of different foam materials, such as ethyl vinyl acetate (EVA), or more expensive polyurethane. Thicker materials tend to give better cushioning, but they will also raise the foot off the ground, creating greater leverage forces if the foot contacts the ground at the side of the sole.

On top of the mid-sole is the insole board, again running the whole length of the shoe. This semi-rigid board stops the foot from twisting and so provides stability. The edge of the shoe upper is usually fastened below the insole board, and the board itself may be chemically treated to resist deterioration from moisture or micro-organism growth.

The heel counter provides rearfoot stability, helping to prevent overpronation and is usually a hard thermoplastic, which will keep its rigidity. Poorer quality shoes may have cardboard heel counters which will feel stiff when the shoe is new, but quickly soften and allow excessive rearfoot motion. Often the heel counter itself will have an additional support.

The shoe upper is contoured to the foot, and made from three sections. The 'vamp' covers the forefoot, and the midfoot and hindfoot are covered by the medial and lateral quarters, respectively. The nylon upper provides lightness and breatheability, and is supported by the eyestay and arch bandage. The eyestay will normally have eyelets for lacing, and the arch bandage is positioned at the highest point of the longitudinal arch of the foot.

The foot rests within the shoe, directly on top of the sock liner. This should be removable for washing and can also have further padding, such as gel or air sacks, incorporated into it. The liner is designed primarily to reduce friction and absorb sweat, and may be removed when an orthotic device is placed into the shoe.

The ankle collar should be heavily padded and soft, and the heel tab (pull tab) should be notched to prevent friction on the Achilles tendon during toe off. Some older designs of sports shoes still have so-called 'Achilles tendon protectors'. Unfortunately, the effect of these is usually to injure rather than protect. As the foot is plantarflexed, the Achilles tendon tab will press onto the Achilles tendon causing friction, one cause of Haglund's syndrome (see p. 267). Shoes of this type may be modified by cutting a slot down each side of the tab or simply cutting the tab off, providing neither of these solutions interferes with the overall shoe structure.

Many shoes have variable lacing systems to accommodate different foot widths and ensure that the shoe fits the foot snugly. With reference to shoe width, it is important to encourage athletes to stand and walk around/jog in sports shoes before they buy them. Obviously the foot spreads with weight bearing, so if the shoe is tried on when sitting it will not give an accurate impression of fit.

Shoe function

Cushioning effects of shoes have been shown to reduce initial impact at heel strike by as much as 50% (Light, McLellan and Klenerman, 1980; Subotnick, 1989). The aim is to reduce or 'attenuate' the peak forces to levels which are well tolerated by the human body, and which do not result either in trauma or overuse injury. At the same time, the forces produced at toe off have to be conserved to maintain running efficiency.

Heel materials which are too soft will compress or 'bottom out', while those which are too hard reduce cushioning. In addition, the construction of the shoe will also affect shock absorption. A stiff insole board, for example, cemented to a soft mid-sole, will give the shoe a functional hardness usually found only with much firmer mid-sole materials (Frederick, 1989).

The overhand or 'flare' of the sole of a running shoe creates leverage force which exaggerates pronation and foot slap (Fig. 13.19). When running barefoot, the subtalar joint axis lies over the ground contact point as does the ankle joint axis (Fig. 13.19a). Wearing a typical running shoe, the leverage force created by the heel flare places the ground contact point further away from the subtalar joint axis, thus increasing the leverage effect by a factor of three (Fig. 13.19b). In the sagittal plane, the heel flare moves the ground contact point back, further from the ankle joint, thus increasing the leverage effect. To compensate, the anterior tibial muscles have to work harder. By altering the heel to a

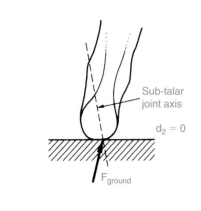

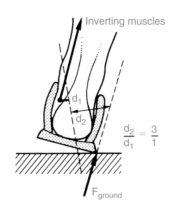

Figure 13.19   Effect of leverage in running shoes. (a) Running barefoot, the subtalar joint axis lies over the ground contact point, as does the ankle joint. (b) The 'overhang' of the shoes moves the ground contact point further from the subtaloid and ankle joints, increasing the leverage effect. Muscle action is required to compensate. From Subotnick (1989).

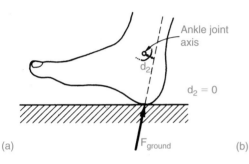

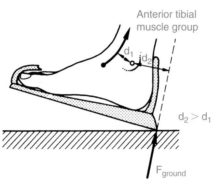

(a)   (b)

more rounded design, and using a shoe with a dual density mid-sole, overpronation can be limited.

The sole of a sports shoe should bend at a point just proximal to the metatarsal heads, to an angle of about 30°. Bending a stiffer sole may increase energy expenditure, and could therefore lead to local muscle fatigue. A lighter shoe is more energy conserving. Frederick (1985) showed that carrying 100 g excess weight on the foot increased energy expenditure by 1%; enough, he claimed, to add 1 or 2 minutes onto the time of a competitive marathon runner. Similarly, softer soled shoes are more energy conserving. The same author showed a 2.8% reduction in energy expenditure for subjects wearing soft-soled shoes while running a marathon.

The ideal combination of features in a running shoe is unfortunately not possible. There is always a compromise because many of the attributes are contradictory. Cushioning conflicts with qualities of stability and flexibility. Decreasing the hardness of the sole can increase pronation, so to get adequate cushioning, a thicker more shock-absorbing sole is chosen rather than a softer one.

By combining data from various sources, Frederick (1989) analysed the relationship between heel height, maximum pronation, and hardness of a sole to find an 'ideal' combination. He concluded that optimum cushioning and rearfoot control are obtained in a shoe with a heel height of 25–35 mm with cushioning values of 40–55 shore A. Hardness is quantified by measuring the resistance of a material to the penetration of a defined object. The shore A scale runs from 0 (softest) to 100 (hardest).

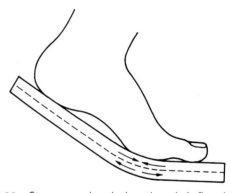

Figure 13.20   Stresses produced when the sole is flexed. The bottom layers are in tension, while the top layers are compressed. From Segesser and Pforringer (1989), with permission.

This combination would, however, give a reduction in sole flexibility, as highly flexible soles are usually soft and thin. Fig. 13.20 demonstrates the stresses produced when a sole is bent. The top of the sole is compressed, and the bottom tensioned. To make the sole more flexible, while still maintaining its cushioning effect, a bar of softer material is placed in the top layer of the sole just behind the metatarsal heads. In addition, grooves are cut in the bottom of the sole at the point of bending.

Fitting a running shoe

The correct fit of a running shoe is vital. Most individuals have one foot slightly larger than the other, so both shoes

Table 13.1   Fitting a running shoe

Try to buy shoes at the end of the day when the feet are largest
Take your own running socks with you to the shop
Fit the shoes weight bearing and then run around the shop in them
Shoes should allow the toes to extend fully
Feet must not bulge over the seams of the shoe
Heel flare should not extend beyond apex of malleoli
Palpate: (i) longest toe (ii) broadest part of forefoot (iii) highest part of midfoot
Shoes should not be expected to stretch with wear or 'run in' – they must fit immediately
Buy specific shoes for a specific sport

After Zachazewski, Magee and Quillen (1996) with permission.

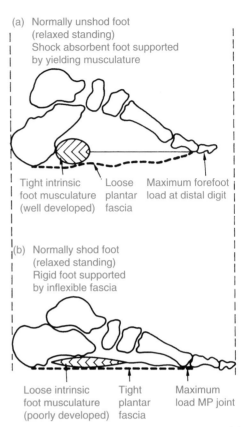

Figure 13.21   Function of intrinsic musculature in the (a) unshod and (b) shod foot. From Robbins, S.E. and Gouw, G.J. (1990) Athletic footwear and chronic overloading. *Sports Medicine*, 9(2), 76–85. With permission.

must be tried on. Fit the shoe to the larger foot, and use extra padding for the smaller foot. If the shoe is too narrow, extra stress may be placed on the longitudinal arch (Zachazewski, Magee and Quillen, 1996) and callus formation over the metatarsal heads is more likely. To test for correct shoe width, take all of the bodyweight through the shoe and ensure that firstly the shoe does not bulge over the sole (too small) and secondly that creases do not form in the shoe upper (too big).

The toe box must be long enough and wide enough to allow the toes to spread and to enable them to fully extend (flatten out). In general the end of the shoe should be about 1.0 cm longer than the end of the longest toe. It is often easier simply to take the insole out of the shoe and rest the foot on this to assess correct length. Palpate the longest toe when the shoe is on the foot, and also palpate the forefoot at its widest part (first MP joint) to ensure than the toe is not being pushed into a valgus position. Ensure that the highest point of the mid-foot fits well into the shoe.

For running, the shoe should flex at the first MP joint, and this can be assessed simply by holding the main shoe in one hand and pressing the sole with the other. Excessive flare of a shoe heel will introduce dangerous leverage forces on the foot and broadly speaking the flare should not extend beyond the apex of the malleoli.

The shape of the shoe 'footprint' is called the last, and this may be straight or curved. A straight last is usually more stable and a curved last less stable. Athletes with a very flexible (pronating) foot will need more control in a shoe and should therefore chose a straight lasted shoe. Several points are summarized in Table 13.1.

Is a running shoe necessary?

Robbins and Hanna (1987) argued that habitually unshod humans are not susceptible to chronic overloading of the foot. Locomotion in barefoot adapted subjects (those who regularly run unshod) differs considerably from that of normal shod subjects. When walking, unshod subjects attempt to grip the ground with their toes, and when run-

ning the medial longitudinal arch flattens completely during mid-stance. Foot flattening when running unshod is probably a result of eccentric muscle action and elastic deformation of the intrinsic foot musculature and plantar fascia. Robbins and Gouw (1990) claimed that this response is behaviourly induced in the barefoot adapted runner. They argued that the subject was attempting to minimize discomfort by transferring forefoot load from the metatarsal phalangeal joints to the distal digits. This process, they claimed, results in hypertrophy of the intrinsic musculature, and relaxes the plantar fascia (Fig. 13.21).

Robbins and Gouw (1990) argued that this shock moderating behaviour of the foot is related to plantar sensibility. The subject attempts to minimize discomfort by increasing the activity of the intrinsic muscles. However, a running shoe with a thick soft sole, will mask sensation to the plantar surface of the foot, and so the subject will not use the intrinsic muscles to their full extent.

The above authors therefore recommended that runners run barefoot, after a progressive period of adaptation. Where a runner is not able to do this each day, or where safety factors prevent it, Robbins and Gouw advised a less yielding shoe which provides adequate sensory feedback.

When assessing proprioceptive function of the foot, foot position error has been shown to be 107.5% poorer with subjects wearing athletic footwear than those who were barefoot. In addition, those who wore footwear were unable to distinguish between a flat surface and a 20° slope angle when blindfolded (Robbins, Waked and Rappel, 1995). These authors argued that the use of footwear was largely responsible for ankle injury, in that it reduced the input from plantar cutaneous mechanoreceptors.

Athletic footwear has also been shown to contribute to falling frequency (Robbins et al., 1994). Using balance beam walking, these authors found that mid-sole hardness was positively related to stability, while mid-sole thickness was negatively related. The authors concluded that shoes with thick, soft soles acted to destabilize an individual whereas thin, hard-soled shoes provided superior stability. Waddington and Adams (2000) compared barefoot conditions, athletic shoes and textured insoles within athletic shoes to determine the effect on ankle movement discrimination. They found that athletic shoes gave significantly worse movement discrimination scores compared to barefoot levels, confirming the work previously quoted. However, the addition of a textured insole improved movement discrimination back to barefoot levels, through enhanced cutaneous feedback on the sole of the foot.

> **Keypoint**
>
> The foot itself has active shock-absorbing mechanisms. In addition, sensory feedback from the plantar surface of the foot is vital for movement discrimination. Protected barefoot activities should be encouraged to enhance both of these features.

The court shoe

In running, foot movements occur cyclically, but in court games such as tennis, squash and badminton the movements are more varied, both in direction and speed. The casual tennis player makes contact mostly with the heel and less with the ball of the foot. However, when a player is under pressure the situation is reversed. Now contact is more frequently made with the ball of the foot than the heel, and contact with the medial and lateral edges of the foot is increased (Nigg, Luthi and Bahlsen, 1989).

Movement most commonly occurs in the forward direction, but when under pressure, the tennis player moves laterally more frequently. This movement is often combined with contact on the forefoot.

A court shoe must allow all of these movements. The same heel–toe mechanism found in a running shoe is required, but in addition, force attenuation from forefoot contact is needed. The frictional characteristics of the shoe to surface are important. Both translational and rotational movements are needed, translation less so in surfaces which permit some degree of sliding, such as indoor courts or sand/granules.

Because the demands placed on the foot when playing court games are so different to those encountered in road running, athletes must be discouraged from wearing the same shoes for both sports unless they use specifically designed 'cross training' footwear. During lateral movements in particular, the leverage involved with the higher (flared) heel of the running shoe makes injury much more likely. Similarly, tennis shoes do not give adequate rearfoot control or shock attenuation for running.

The soccer boot

In football, the ball may reach velocities of 140 km/h (Masson and Hess, 1989). This speed, combined with the weight of the ball, especially when wet, leads to deformation of both the boot and foot with kicking. Forces generated may lead to microtrauma to the foot and ankle. Soccer footwear must therefore be as light as possible to minimize any excessive forces created by kicking. At the same time, the shoe must provide both support and protection for the foot.

Combinations of rotation and flexion with the foot fixed to the ground are particularly taxing on the knee structures. Most boots unfortunately compound this problem by the use of cleats or studs, which, although improving grip on a wet surface, will also increase rotation forces by reducing 'give'. Indoor surfaces in some cases offer greater grip with similar problems, and shoes need a sole with a greater number of smaller studs to compensate for this.

Shoes must allow the increased range of movement required in soccer, and be flexible enough to accommodate forefoot rocking. Any studs must be placed to avoid pressure irritation to the plantar aspect of the foot. Studs on the heel are placed towards the outside of the shoe to avoid rocking or buckling on weight-bearing.

References

Bowers, K.D. and Martin, R.B. (1976) Turf toe: a shoe-surface related football injury. *Medicine and Science in Sports and Exercise*, **8**, 81–83

Carmines, D.V., Nunley, J.A. and McElhaney, J.H. (1988) Effects of ankle taping on the motion and loading pattern of the foot for walking subjects. *Journal of Orthopaedic Research*, **6**, 223–229

Cavanagh, P.R. (1989) The biomechanics of running and running shoe problems. In *The Shoe in Sport* (eds B. Segesser and W. Pforringer), Year Book Medical Publishers, Wolfe, London

Cibulka, M.T. (1990) Management of a patient with forefoot pain: a case report. *Physical Therapy*, **70**, (1) 55–58

Clanton, T.O., Butler, J.E. and Eggert, A. (1986) Injuries to the metatarsophalangeal joints in athletes. *Foot and Ankle*, **7**, 162–176

Creighton, D.S. and Olson, V.L. (1987). Evaluation of range of motion of the first metatarsophalangeal joint in runners with plantar fasciitis. *Journal of Orthopaedic and Sports Physical Therapy*, **8**, 357–361

Frederick, E.C. (1985) The energy cost of load carriage on the feet during running. In *Biomechanics IX* (eds D.A. Winter et al.), Human Kinetics Publishers, Champaign, Illinois

Frederick, E.C. (1989) The running shoe: dilemmas and dichotomies in design. In *The Shoe in Sport* (eds B. Segesser and W. Pforringer), Year Book Medical Publishers, Wolfe, London

Frederick, E.C., Clarke, T.E. and Hamill, C.L. (1984) The effect of running shoe design on shock attenuation. In *Sports Shoes and Playing Surfaces* (ed. E.C. Frederick), Human Kinetics Publishers, Champaign, Illinois, pp. 190–198

George, F.J. (1989). In *Year Book of Sports Medicine* (ed. R.J. Shephard), Year Book Medical Publishers, Chicago, p. 75

Horn, L.M. and Subotnick, S.I. (1989) Surgical intervention. In *Sports Medicine of the Lower Extremity* (ed. S.I. Subotnick), Churchill Livingstone, London

Kaltenborn, F.M. (1989) *Manual Mobilisation of the Extremity Joints*, 4th edn, Olaf Norlis Bokhandel, Norway

Light, L.H., McLellan, G.E. and Klenerman, K. (1980) Skeletal transients on heel strike in normal walking with different footwear. *Journal of Biomechanics*, **13**, 477

Magee, D.J. (2002) *Orthopedic Physical Assessment*, 4th edn, Saunders, Philadelphia

Mann, R.A. and Reynolds, J.C. (1983) Interdigital neuroma: a critical analysis. *Journal of Foot and Ankle Surgery*, **3**, 238

Marshal, P. and Hamilton, W.G. (1992) Cuboid subluxation in ballet dancers. *American Journal of Sports Medicine*, **20**, 169–175

Masson, M. and Hess, H. (1989) Typical soccer injuries their effects on the design of the athletic shoe. In *The Shoe in Sport* (eds B. Segesser and W. Pforringer), Year Book Medical Publishers, Wolfe, London

Neale, D. and Adams, I.M. (1989) *Common Foot Disorders*, Churchill Livingstone, London

Nigg, B.M., Luthi, S.M. and Bahlsen, H.A. (1989) The tennis shoe: biomechanical design criteria. In *The Shoe in Sport* (eds B. Segesser and W. Pforringer), Year Book Medical Publishers, Wolfe, London

Palastanga, N., Field, D. and Soames, R. (1989) *Anatomy and Human Movement*, Heinemann Medical, Oxford

Reid, D.C. (1992) *Sports Injury Assessment and Rehabilitation*, Churchill Livingstone, London

Robbins, S.E. and Gouw, G.J. (1990) Athletic footwear and chronic overloading. *Sports Medicine*, **9**, (2), 76–85

Robbins, S.E. and Hanna, A.M. (1987) Running related injury prevention through barefoot adaptations. *Medicine and Science in Sports and Exercise*, **19**, 148–156

Robbins, S., Waked, E., Gouw, G.J. and McClaran, J. (1994) Athletic footwear affects balance in men. *British Journal of Sports Medicine*, **28**, 117–122

Robbins, S., Waked, E. and Rappel, R. (1995) Ankle taping improves proprioception before and after exercise in young men. *British Journal of Sports Medicine*, **29**, (4), 242–247

Rodeo, S.A., O'Brian, S.J. and Warren, R.F. (1989a) Turf toe: an analysis of metatarsophalangeal joint sprains in professional football players. *American Journal of Sports Medicine*, **17**, (4) 125–131

Rodeo, S.A., O'Brian, S.J., Warren, R.F., Barnes, R. and Wickiewicz, T.L. (1989b) Turf toe: diagnosis and treatment. *Physician and Sports Medicine*, **17**, (4) 132–147

Rodgers, M.M. and Cavanagh, P.R. (1989) Pressure distribution in Morton's foot structure. *Medicine and Science in Sports and Exercise*, **21**, 23–28

Segesser, B. and Pforringer, W. (1989) (eds) *The Shoe in Sport*, Wolfe, London

Subotnick, S.I. (1989) *Sports Medicine of the Lower Extremity*, Churchill Livingstone, London

Tanner, S.M. and Harvey, J.S. (1988) How we manage plantar fasciitis. *Physician and Sports Medicine*, **16**, (8) 39–47

Waddington, G., and Adams, R. (2000) Textured insole effects on ankle movement discrimination while wearing athletic shoes. *Physical Therapy in Sport*, **1**, (4) 119–128

Zachazewski, J.E., Magee, D.J. and Quillen, W.S. (1996) *Athletic Injuries and Rehabilitation*, Saunders, Philadelphia

Chapter 14

The lumbar spine

Spinal problems are among the most common conditions encountered by the physiotherapist or physical medicine practitioner. More working days are lost because of back pain than any other single condition, and sport does not escape this epidemic. It is estimated that 80% of the population will suffer at least one disabling episode of low back pain during their lives, and at any one time as many as 35% of people will be suffering from backache of some sort (Fryomoyer and Cats-Baril, 1991). This commands an immense cost to the country, to the National Health Service, and to each individual in terms of personal suffering (Table 14.1).

In sport, the frequency of back pain suffering presents a similar challenge. Exercise itself has a positive effect on the low back both in terms of injury prevention and rehabilitation. Those with an activity level of at least 3 hours per week have a generally lower lifetime risk of low back pain (Harreby et al., 1997). After an injury has occurred, exercise therapy has been shown to be effective at returning patients to their daily activities and to work (Van Tulder et al., 2000), and has been recommended as the mainstay of treatment for this region (Waddell, Feder and Lewis, 1997).

Although exercise is beneficial to the low back, the varied activities within sport subject the spine to significant stress which often results in injury. In terms of percentage, 10–20%

Table 14.1 Low back pain – the scope of the problem

80% of individuals suffer at least one disabling episode of LBP during their lifetime

At any one time 35% of the population is suffering some form of LBP

£3.8 billion lost to UK each year as a result of LBP

£480 cost annually to NHS

7% of workload of GPs due to LBP

20% of individuals do not recover within 6 weeks

60% of sufferers will experience a second bout of LBP within 1 year

LBP – low back pain; NHS – National Health Service; GP – general practitioner; UK – United Kingdom.
After Fryomoyer and Cats-Baril (1991), and Clinical Standards Advisory Group (1994) *Reports on Back Pain*. HMSO, London. With permission.

Table 14.2   Back pain in specific sports

Sport	Effect
Canoeing	22.5% suffer from lumbago
Cross-country skiing	64% suffer from back pain
Cycling	Incidence of back pain as high at 73.2%
Golf	Lifetime incidence as high as 63%
Gymnastics	86% of rhythmic gymnasts report low back pain. 63% of Olympic female gymnasts have MRI abnormalities
Rowing	Mechanical back pain most common type
Squash	51.8% of competitive players report back injury
Swimming	37% suffer back pain especially with breaststroke and butterfly
Triathlon	32% suffer low back pain
Windsurfing	Low back pain most common ailment
Yachting	Lumbosacral sprain most common injury (29%)

From Thompson, B. (2002) How should athletes with chronic low back pain be managed in primary care? In *Evidence Based Sports Medicine* (eds D. MacAuley and T. Best). BMJ Books, London. With permission.

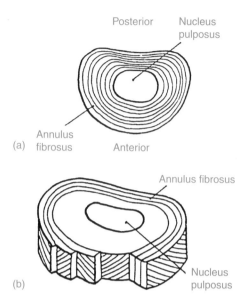

Figure 14.1   (a) Concentric band of annular fibres. (b) Horizontal section through a disc. From Oliver and Middleditch (1991) with permission.

of all sports injuries involve the spine (Thompson, 2002), but this percentage differs between sports (Table 14.2).

A detailed study of back pain is outside the scope of this book, but it is necessary to look at a number of features of spinal injury which are important within the context of sport. Much of the material for the initial parts of this section is modified from Norris (1995), and the reader is referred to that article series and Norris (2000) for a more in-depth review.

STRUCTURE

The spinal disc

There are 24 intervertebral discs lying between successive vertebrae, making the spine an alternately rigid then elastic column. The amount of flexibility present in a particular spinal segment will be determined by the size and shape of the disc, and the resistance to motion of the soft tissue support to the spinal joints. The discs increase in size as they descend the column, the lumbar discs having an average thickness of 10 mm, twice that of the cervical discs. The disc shapes are accommodated to the curvatures of the spine, and the shapes of the vertebrae. The greater anterior widths of the discs in the cervical and lumbar regions reflect the curvatures of these areas. Each disc is made up of three

> **Keypoint**
>
> Discs increase in size going down the spine, with the lumbar (low back) discs having a thickness of about 1 cm, twice that of the cervical discs. In the cervical and lumbar areas discs are wider anteriorly, creating the spinal curves.

closely related components: the annulus fibrosis, nucleus pulposus and cartilage end plates.

The annulus is composed of layers of fibrous tissue arranged in concentric bands (Fig. 14.1). Each band has fibres arranged in parallel, and the various bands are in turn angled at 45° to each other. The bands are more closely packed anteriorly and posteriorly than they are laterally, and those innermost are the thinnest. Each disc has about 20 bands in all, and fibre orientation, although partially determined at birth, is influenced by torsional stresses in the adult (Palastanga, Field and Soames, 1989). The postero-lateral regions have a more irregular make-up, and this may be one reason why they become weaker with age, predisposing them to injury.

The annular fibres pass over the edge of the cartilage end plate of the disc, and are anchored to the bony rim of the vertebra and to its periosteum and body. The attaching fibres are actually interwoven with the fibres of the bony trabeculae of the vertebral body. The outer layer of fibres blend with the posterior longitudinal ligament, but the anterior longitudinal ligament has no such attachment (Vernon-Roberts, 1987).

The hyaline cartilage end plate rests on the surface of the vertebra. This is approximately 1 mm thick at its outer edge and becomes thinner towards its centre. The central portion of the end plate acts as a semi-permeable membrane to facilitate fluid exchange between the vertebral body and disc. In addition, it protects the body from excessive pressure. In early life the end plate is penetrated by canals from the vertebral body, but these disappear after the age of 20–30 years. After this period the end plate starts to ossify and become more brittle, the central portion thinning and in some cases being completely destroyed.

The nucleus pulposus is a soft hydrophilic (water attracting) substance taking up about 25% of the total disc area. It is continuous with the annulus, but the nuclear fibres are far less dense. The spaces between the collagen fibres are filled with proteoglycan, giving the nucleus its water-retaining capacity, and making it a mechanically plastic material. The area between the nucleus and annulus is metabolically very active and sensitive to physical force and chemical and hormonal influence (Palastanga, Field and Soames, 1989). The proteoglycan content of the nucleus decreases with age, but the collagen volume remains unchanged. As a consequence, the water content of the nucleus reduces. In early life the water content may be as high as 80–90%, but this decreases to about 70% by middle age.

> ### Keypoint
>
> With age: (i) the back wall of the disc becomes weaker, (ii) the end plate at the top and bottom of the disc becomes brittle, and (iii) the disc dries up, reducing its water content from 90% (child) to 70% (middle age).

The lumbar discs are the largest avascular structures in the body. The nucleus itself is dependent upon fluid exchange by passive diffusion from the margins of the vertebral body and across the cartilage end plate. Diffusion takes place particularly across the centre of the cartilage end plate which is more permeable than the periphery. There is intense anaerobic activity within the nucleus (Holm et al., 1981), which could lead to lactate build up and a low oxygen tension, placing the nuclear cells at risk. Inadequate adenosine triphosphate (ATP) supplies could lead to cell death.

The facet joint

The facet (zygapophyseal) joints are synovial joints formed between the inferior articular process of one vertebra and the superior articular process of its neighbour. As with all typical synovial joints, they have articular cartilage, a synovial membrane and a joint capsule. However, the zygapophyseal joints do have a number of unique features (Bogduk and Twomey, 1991).

The capsule is a lax structure which enables the joint to hold about 2 ml of fluid. It is replaced anteriorly by the ligamentum flavum, and posteriorly it is reinforced by the deep fibres of multifidus. The joint leaves a small gap at its superior and inferior poles creating the subscapular pockets (Fig. 14.2). These are filled with fat, contained within the

> ### Keypoint
>
> The facet joint has a loose capsule reinforced by the ligamentum flavum at the front and the multifidus muscle at the back. The capsule has small pockets at its top and bottom which contain fat globules which travel in and out of the joint as it moves.

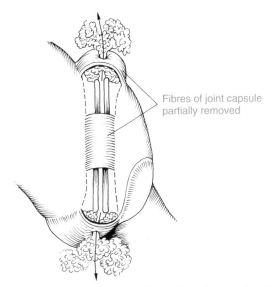

Figure 14.2 Lumbar zygapophyseal joint viewed from behind. Fat in the subscapular pockets moves through foramina in the superior and inferior capsules. From Bogduk and Twomey (1991), with permission.

Fibres of joint capsule partially removed

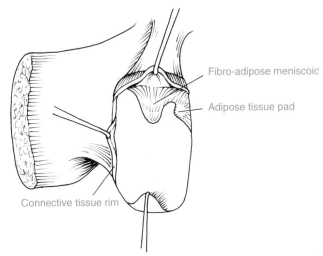

Fibro-adipose meniscoid

Adipose tissue pad

Connective tissue rim

Figure 14.3 Intra-articular structures of the lumbar zygapophyseal joints. From Bogduk and Twomey (1991), with permission.

synovial membrane. Within the subscapular pocket lies a small foramen for passage of the fat in and out of the joint as the spine moves.

Intracapsularly there are three structures of interest (Fig. 14.3). The first is the connective tissue rim, a thickened wedge-shaped area which makes up for the curved shape of the articular cartilage in much the same way as the menisci of the knee do. The second structure is an adipose tissue pad, a 2 mm fold of synovium filled with fat and blood vessels. The third structure is the fibroadipose meniscoid, a 5 mm leaf-like fold which projects from the inner surfaces of the superior and inferior capsules. These latter two structures have a protective function. During flexion, the movement of the articular facets leaves some of their cartilage exposed. Both the adipose tissue pad and the fibroadipose meniscoid are able to cover these exposed regions (Bogduk and Engel, 1984).

With ageing, the cartilage of the zygapophyseal joint can split parallel to the joint surface, pulling a portion of joint capsule with it. The split of cartilage with its attached piece of capsule forms a false intra-articular meniscoid (Taylor and Twomey, 1986). Normally, the fibroadipose meniscus itself is drawn out from the joint on flexion, and should move back in with extension. However, if the meniscoid fails to move back, it will buckle and remain under the capsule, causing pain and acute locking (Bogduk and Jull, 1985). A mobilization or manipulation which combines flexion and rotation may allow the meniscoid to reduce and so relieve pain.

The facet has an overlapping neural supply, with ascending, local and descending facet branches coming from the posterior primary ramus. The nerve endings in the facet joint capsules are similar to those in the annulus of the disc, and although the disc is more sensitive, the facet joints can be a source of referred pain to the lower limb (Hirsch, Ingelmark and Miller, 1963), but not neurological deficit (Mooney and Robertson, 1976).

> **Keypoint**
>
> A facet joint can be a source of referred pain, but not neurological deficit (weakness, paraesthesia, or altered reflexes).

SPINAL LOADING

Vertebral body

Within the vertebra itself, compressive force is transmitted by both the cancellous bone of the vertebral body and the cortical bone shell. Up to the age of 40, the cancellous bone contributes between 25% and 55% of the strength of the vertebra. After this age the cortical bone shell carries a greater proportion of load as the strength and stiffness of the cancellous bone reduces with decreasing bone density due to ageing (Rockoff, Sweet and Bleustein, 1969). As the vertebral body is compressed, blood flows from it into the subchondral post-capillary venous network (Crock and Yoshizawa, 1976). This process reduces the bone volume and dissipates energy (Roaf, 1960). The blood returns slowly as the force is reduced, leaving a latent period after the initial compression, during which the shock-absorbing properties of the bone will be less effective. Exercises which involve prolonged

> **Keypoint**
>
> As the spine is compressed 'spring' is provided by blood flowing out of the spinal bone. As the compression is released, the blood flows back in again. If the spine is not allowed to recover from a single compression force before another is imposed, the spinal bone will be excessively stressed.

periods of repeated shock to the spine, such as jumping on a hard surface, are therefore more likely to damage the vertebrae than those which load the spine for short periods and allow recovery of the vertebral blood-flow before repeating a movement.

Intervertebral disc

Weight is transmitted between adjacent vertebrae by the lumbar intervertebral disc. The annulus fibrosis of a disc, when healthy, has a certain bulk and will resist buckling. When loads are applied briefly to the spine, even if the nucleus pulposus of a disc has been removed, the annulus alone exhibits a similar load-bearing capacity to that of the fully intact disc (Markolf and Morris, 1974). When exposed to prolonged loading, however, the collagen lamellae of the annulus will eventually buckle.

The application of an axial load will compress the fluid nucleus of the disc causing it to expand laterally. This lateral expansion stretches the annular fibres, preventing them from buckling. A 100 kg axial load has been shown to compress the disc by 1.4 mm and cause a lateral expansion of 0.75 mm (Hirsch and Nachemson, 1954). The stretch in the annular fibres will store energy which is released when the compression stress is removed. The stored energy gives the disc a certain springiness which helps to offset any deformation which occurred in the nucleus. A force applied rapidly will not be lessened by this mechanism, but its rate of application will be slowed, giving the spinal tissues time to adapt.

Deformation of the disc occurs more rapidly at the onset of axial load application. Within 10 minutes of applying an axial load the disc may deform by 1.5 mm. Following this, deformation slows to a rate of 1 mm per hour (Markolf and Morris, 1974), accounting for a subject's loss of height throughout the day. Under constant loading the discs exhibit creep, meaning that they continue to deform even though the load they are exposed to is not increasing. Compression causes a pressure rise, leading to fluid loss from both the nucleus and annulus. About 10% of the water within the disc can be squeezed out by this method (Kraemer, Kolditz and Gowin, 1985), the exact amount being dependent on the size of the applied force and the duration of its application. The fluid is absorbed back through pores in the cartilage end plates of the vertebra when the compressive force is reduced.

> **Keypoint**
>
> The disc will compress and deform most within the first 10 minutes of a force being applied. Deformation may be as much as 1.5 mm loss in height initially, and then slows until 10% of the total water content of the disc has been lost.

Exercises which axially load the spine have been shown to result in a reduction in subject height through discal compression. Compression loads of 6–10 times bodyweight have been shown to occur in the L3–L4 segment during a squat exercise in weight training for example (Cappozzo et al., 1985). Average height losses of 5.4 mm over a 25-minute period of general weight training, and 3.25 mm after a 6 km run have also been shown (Leatt, Reilly and Troup, 1986). Static axial loading of the spine with a 40 kg barbell over a 20-minute period can reduce subject height by as much as 11.2 mm (Tyrrell, Reilly and Troup, 1985). Clearly, exercises which involve this degree of spinal loading are unsuitable for individuals with discal pathology (Table 14.3).

The vertebral end plates of the discs are compressed centrally, and are able to undergo less deformation than either the annulus or the cancellous bone. The end plates are, therefore, likely to fail (fracture) under high compression (Norkin and Levangie, 1992). Discs subjected to very high compressive loads show permanent deformation but not herniation (Farfan et al., 1970; Markolf and Morris, 1974). However, such compression forces may lead to Schmorl's node formation (Bernhardt et al., 1992). Bending and torsional stresses on the spine, when combined with compression, are more damaging than compression alone, and degenerated discs are particularly at risk. Average failure torques for normal discs are 25% higher than for degenerative discs (Farfan et al., 1970). Degenerative discs also demonstrate poorer viscoelastic properties and therefore a reduced ability to attenuate shock.

The disc's reaction to a compressive stress changes with age, because the ability of the nucleus to transmit load relies on its high water content. The hydrophilic nature of the nucleus is the result of the proteoglycan it contains, and as this changes from about 65% in early life to 30% by middle age (Bogduk and Twomey, 1987), the nuclear load-bearing capacity of the disc reduces. When the proteoglycan content of the disc is high, up to the age of 30 years in most subjects, the nucleus pulposus acts as a gelatinous mass, producing a uniform fluid pressure. After this age, the lower water content of the disc means that the nucleus is unable to build as much fluid pressure. As a result, less central pressure is produced and the load is distributed more peripherally, eventually causing the annular fibres to become fibrillated and to crack (Hirsch and Schajowicz, 1952).

As a result of these age-related changes the disc is more susceptible to injury later in life. This, combined with the reduction in general fitness of an individual and changes in movement patterns of the trunk related to the activities of daily living, greatly increases the risk of injury to this population. Individuals over the age of 40, if previously inactive, should therefore be encouraged to exercise the trunk under the supervision of a physiotherapist before attending fitness classes run for the general public.

MOVEMENTS OF THE SPINE

Flexion

During flexion movements the anterior annulus of the lumbar discs will be compressed while the posterior fibres are stretched. Similarly, the nucleus pulposus of the disc will be compressed anteriorly while pressure is relieved over its posterior surface. As the total volume of the disc remains unchanged, its pressure should not increase. The increases in pressure seen with alteration of posture are therefore due not to the bending motion of the bones within the vertebral joint itself but to the soft tissue tension created to control the bending.

Discal pressure changes

If the pressure at the L3 disc for a 70 kg standing subject is said to be 100%, supine lying reduces this pressure to 25%. The pressure variations increase dramatically as soon as the lumbar spine is flexed and tissue tension increases (Fig. 14.4). The sitting posture increases intradiscal pressure to 140%, while sitting and leaning forward with a 10 kg weight in each

Table 14.3	Effect of exercise on the spinal disc

Disc deforms by 1.5 mm within 10 minutes of compression
10% of water squeezed out of disc when loaded
Forces 6–10 times bodyweight produced in discs by a squat exercise
Height loss of 5.4 mm after 25 mins of weight training
Height loss of 3.25 mm after 6 km run
Holding 40 kg barbell for 20 mins reduces height by 11.2 mm

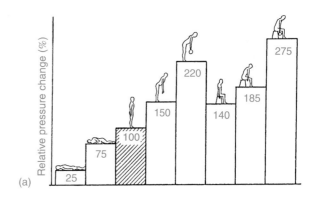
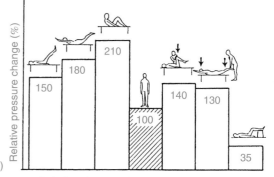

Figure 14.4 Relative pressure changes in the third lumbar disc. (a) In various positions. (b) In various muscle strengthening exercises. From Nachemson (1976).

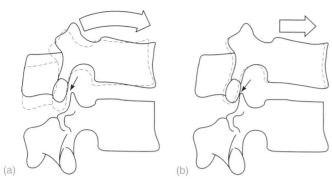

Figure 14.5   Vertebral movement during flexion. Flexion of the lumbar spine involves a combination of anterior sagittal rotation and anterior translation. As sagittal rotation occurs, the articular facets move apart (a), permitting the translation movement to occur (b). Translation is limited by impaction of the inferior facet of one vertebra on the superior facet of the vertebra below. From Bogduk and Twomey (1987), with permission.

hand increases pressure to 275% (Nachemson, 1987). The selection of an appropriate starting position for trunk exercise is therefore of great importance. Superimposing spinal movements from a slumped sitting posture, for example, would place considerably more stress on the spinal discs than the same movement beginning from crook lying.

Keypoint

The highest discal pressures are seen in loaded slumped sitting, that is sitting with the lumbar lordosis reversed (flexed) while holding a weighted object. This type of posture must be avoided in sport, especially during weight training exercises such as seated shoulder press.

During flexion, the posterior annulus is stretched and the nucleus is compressed onto the posterior wall. The posterior portion of the annulus is the thinnest part, and the combination of stretch and pressure to this area may result in discal bulging or herniation (see p. 304).

As the lumbar spine flexes, the lordosis flattens and then reverses at its upper levels. Reversal of lordosis does not occur at L5–S1 (Pearcy, Portek and Shepherd, 1984). Flexion of the lumbar spine involves a combination of anterior sagittal rotation and anterior translation. As sagittal rotation occurs, the articular facets move apart, permitting the translation movement to occur. Translation is limited by impaction of the inferior facet of one vertebra on the superior facet of the vertebra below (Fig. 14.5). As flexion increases, or if the spine is angled forward on the hip, the surface of the vertebral body will face more vertically increasing the shearing force due to gravity. The forces involved in facet impaction will therefore increase to limit translation of the vertebra and stabilize the lumbar spine. Because the zygapophyseal joint has a curved articular facet, the load will not be concentrated evenly across the whole surface, but will be focused on the anteromedial portion of the facets.

The sagittal rotation movement of the zygapophyseal joint causes the joint to open and is therefore limited by the stretch of the joint capsule. Additionally, the posteriorly placed spinal ligaments will also be tightened. Analysis of the contribution to limitation of sagittal rotation within the lumbar spine, through mathematical modelling, has shown that the disc limits movement by 29%, the supraspinous and interspinous ligaments by 19% and the zygapophyseal joint capsules by 39% (Adams, Hutton and Stott, 1980).

Extension

During extension the anterior structures are under tension while the posterior structures are first unloaded and then compressed, depending on the range of motion. With extension movements the vertebral bodies will be subjected to posterior sagittal rotation. The inferior articular processes move downwards causing them to impact against the lamina of the vertebra below. Once the bony block has occurred, if further load is applied the upper vertebra will axially rotate by pivoting on the impacted inferior articular process. The inferior articular process will move backwards, overstretching, and possibly damaging, the joint capsule (Yang and King, 1984). With repeated movements of this type, eventual erosion of the laminal periosteum may occur (Oliver and Middleditch, 1991). At the site of impaction, the joint capsule may catch between the opposing bones giving another cause of pain (Adams and Hutton, 1983). Structural abnormalities can alter the axis or rotation of the vertebra, so considerable variation between subjects exists (Klein and Hukins, 1983).

Rotation

During rotation, torsional stiffness is provided by the outer layers of the annulus, by the orientation of the zygapophyseal joints, and by the cortical bone shell of the vertebral bodies themselves. In rotation movements, the annular fibres of the disc will be stretched according to their direction. As the two alternating sets of fibres are angled obliquely to each other, some of the fibres will be stretched while others relax. A maximum range of 3° of rotation can occur before the annular fibres will be microscopically damaged, and a maximum of 12° before tissue failure (Bogduk and Twomey, 1987). As rotation occurs, the spinous processes separate, stretching the supraspinous and interspinous ligaments. Impaction occurs between the opposing articular facets on one side causing the articular cartilage to compress by 0.5 mm for each 1° of rotation, providing a substantial buffer mechanism (Bogduk and Twomey, 1987). If rotation continues beyond this point, the vertebra pivots around the impacted zygapophyseal joint causing posterior and lateral movement (Fig. 14.6). The combination of movements and forces which occur will stress the impacted zygapophyseal joint by compression, the spinal disc by torsion and shear,

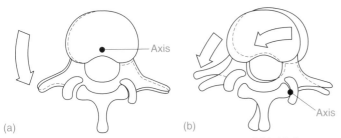

Figure 14.6   Vertebral movement during rotation. (a) Initially rotation occurs around an axis within the vertebral body. (b) The zygapophyseal joints impact and further rotation causes the vertebra to pivot around a new axis at the point of impaction. From Bogduk and Twomey (1987), with permission.

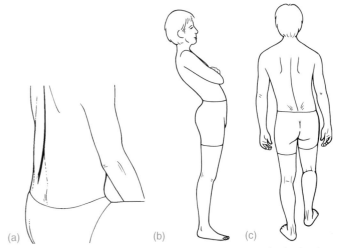

Figure 14.7   Directional patterns of end-range stress in the lumbar spine. (a) Flexion. (b) Extension. (c) Lateral shifting. After O'Sullivan (2000), with permission.

and the capsule of the opposite zygapophyseal joint by traction. The disc provides only 35% of the total resistance (Farfan et al., 1970).

Lateral flexion

When the lumbar spine is laterally flexed, the annular fibres towards the concavity of the curve are compressed and will bulge, while those on the convexity of the curve will be stretched. The contralateral fibres of the outer annulus and the contralateral intertransverse ligaments help to resist extremes of motion (Norkin and Levangie, 1992). Lateral flexion and rotation occur as coupled movements. Rotation of the upper four lumbar segments is accompanied by lateral flexion to the opposite site. Rotation of the L5–S1 joint occurs with lateral flexion to the same side.

Movement of the zygapophyseal joints on the concavity of lateral flexion is by the inferior facet of the upper vertebra sliding downwards on the superior facet of the vertebra below. The area of the intervertebral foramen on this side is therefore reduced. On the convexity of the laterally flexed spine the inferior facet slides upwards on the superior facet of the vertebra below, increasing the diameter of the intervertebral foramen.

END-RANGE SPINAL STRESS IN SPORT

If the trunk is moving slowly, tissue tension will be felt at end-range and a subject is able to stop a movement short of full end-range and protect the spinal tissues from overstretch. However, rapid movements of the trunk will build up large amounts of momentum. When the subject reaches near end-range and tissue tension builds up, the momentum of the rapidly moving trunk will push the spine to full end-range, stressing the spinal tissues. In many popular sports, exercises often used in a warm-up are rapid and ballistic in nature and performed for a high number of repetitions. These can lead to excessive flexibility and a reduction in passive stability of the spine.

In addition, end-range stress can be experienced with postural changes and an alteration in the control of movement

within the lumbar spine. Clinically, a number of directional patterns have been described (O'Sullivan, 2000). Flexion of the lumbar spine is seen with a gross reduction in the depth of the lumbar lordosis (Fig. 14.7). The athlete suffers pain when semi-flexed postures are maintained, and with prolonged sitting activities. When put in a four point kneeling position (p. 321), the lumbar spine remains flexed. Extension of the lumbar spine is seen in the lordotic posture with the pelvis anteriorly tilted. In standing, and especially during extension movements of the whole spine or hip, the lumbar spine appears to 'hinge' as a single level rather than extend through its whole length. Lateral flexion movements are seen with tightness to the lateral flexors (quadratus lumborum and lateral external oblique). This is brought to the fore with single leg standing activities. Here, the patient, instead of transferring bodyweight with the pelvis, laterally flexes the spine and a noticeable scoliosis is apparent.

DISCAL INJURY

During flexion, extension and lateral flexion, one side of the disc is compressed and the other stretched. In flexion, the axis of motion passes through the nucleus, but with extension the axis moves forwards (Klein and Hukins, 1981). This fact, coupled with the increased range of motion during flexion, makes it the more dangerous movement. Combinations of torsion and flexion place the disc at particular risk from plastic deformation, which stretches the annular fibres irreversibly, and may cause fibre damage.

A single movement of flexion will stretch and thin the posterior annulus, but it is repeated flexion, especially under load, which is likely to give the most serious pathological consequences. Discal injury occurs frequently through repeated flexion movements, and when a flexion/rotation strain is placed on the spine during lifting.

When hyperflexion takes place, the supraspinous and interspinous ligaments will overstretch, reducing the support to the lumbar spine. Circumferential tearing will occur to the disc annulus posterolaterally, usually at the junction between the disc lamina and end plate (Oliver and Middleditch, 1991). The outer annular fibres are innervated, a possible cause of the 'dull ache' in the lumbar spine which often precedes disc prolapse. Rotation strain will increase the likelihood of these injuries. Although rotation is limited in the lumbar spine, it is increased significantly as a result of facet joint degeneration and during flexion as the facets are separated.

Posterolateral radial fissuring occurs later, and connects the disc nucleus to the circumferential tear, allowing the passage of nuclear material towards the outer edge of the disc. This type of injury has been produced experimentally during discal compression in a combined flexed and laterally flexed posture (Adams and Hutton, 1982). An annular protrusion can occur when the pressure of the displaced nuclear material causes the annulus to bulge. Eventually, nuclear material is extruded (herniated) through the ruptured annular wall (Fig. 14.8).

The discal injury may occur gradually as a result of repeated bending, giving symptoms of gradually worsening pain. Pain occurs initially in the lower back, and with time the symptoms are peripheralized into the buttock and lower limbs.

> **Keypoint**
>
> Repeated bending may give gradually worsening low back pain. With time the symptoms peripheralize (travel outwards) into the buttocks and legs.

Sudden pain may occur from a seemingly trivial injury which acts as the 'last straw' to cause the disc herniation. Loads of sufficient intensity may give rise to an abrupt massive disc herniation. The stress is usually one of weight combined with leverage during a lifting action. Hyperflexion of the spine occurs, due in part to overstretching of the posterior lumbar ligaments.

Radiographic investigations of discal movement have been made by inserting metal pins into the lumbar nucleus pulposus and asymmetrically loading the disc (reported in McKenzie, 1990). These have shown that the disc migrates towards the area of least load. When the asymmetrical load

was removed, the nucleus remained displaced, but its relocation was accelerated by compression in the opposite direction or by traction.

A number of studies have investigated the phenomenon of discal nuclear movement within the lumbar discs. Beattie, Brooks and Rothstein (1994) showed movement during extension with healthy discs but not with degenerative discs, and Edmondston, Song and Bricknell (2000) demonstrated 6.7% anterior displacement between flexion and extension in L1/2, L2/3 and L5/S1. Fennell, Jones and Hukins (1996) used MRI scanning to demonstrate anterior movement during extension.

SPINAL LIGAMENTS

A number of spinal ligaments are of concern to the biomechanics of the lumbar spinal segment: the anterior and posterior longitudinal ligaments, the intertransverse ligament, the ligamentum flavum, the interspinous and supraspinous ligaments and the capsular ligaments of the facet joint (Fig. 14.9). A general reduction in energy absorption of all the ligaments has been found with age (Tkaczuk, 1968). The stiffest is the posterior longitudinal ligament and the most

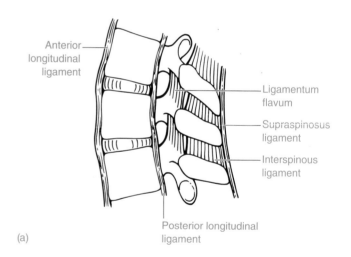

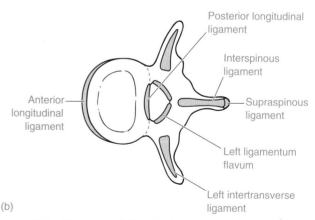

Figure 14.9 Ligaments of the spinal segment. (a) Side view. (b) Superior view. Reprinted by permission from Norris, C.M. (2000) *Back Stability*. Human Kinetics, Champaign, Illinois.

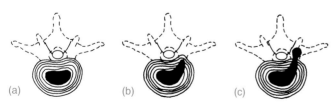

Figure 14.8 Stages of disc herniation. (a) Normal disc. (b) Nuclear bulge with annulus intact. (c) Ruptured annulus, nuclear protrusion onto nerve root.

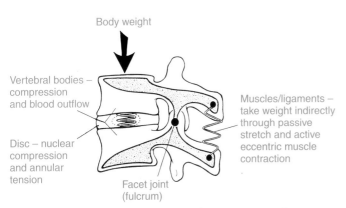

Figure 14.10 The spinal segment as a leverage system. From Kapandji (1974), with permission.

Image labels:
Body weight
Vertebral bodies – compression and blood outflow
Disc – nuclear compression and annular tension
Facet joint (fulcrum)
Muscles/ligaments – take weight indirectly through passive stretch and active eccentric muscle contraction

flexible the supraspinous (Panjabi, Jorneus and Greenstein, 1984). The ligamentum flavum in the lumbar spine is pre-tensioned (resting tension) when the spine is in its neutral position, a situation which compresses the disc. This ligament has the highest percentage of elastic fibres of any tissue in the body (Nachemson and Evans, 1968), and contains nearly twice as much elastin as collagen. The anterior longitudinal ligament and joint capsules have been found to be the strongest, while the interspinous and posterior longitudinal ligaments are the weakest (Panjabi, Hult and White, 1987).

The ligaments act rather like rubber bands, resisting tensile forces but buckling under compressive loads (Fig. 14.10). They must allow adequate motion and fixed postures between vertebrae, enabling a minimum amount of muscle energy to be used. In addition, they protect the spine by restricting motion and in particular protect the spinal cord in traumatic situations, where high loads are applied at rapid speeds. In this situation, the ligaments absorb large amounts of energy.

The longitudinal ligaments are viscoelastic, being stiffer when loaded rapidly, and they exhibit hysteresis as they do not store the energy used to stretch them.

> **Definition**
>
> *Viscoelasticity* is the ability of a material to store and dissipate energy during mechanical deformation. The deformation is dependent on the rate of loading. *Hysteresis* occurs when a material is stressed and does not immediately return to its previous shape when the stress is released.

When loaded repeatedly, they become stiffer, and the hysteresis is less marked, making the longitudinal ligaments more prone to fatigue failure (Hukins, 1987). The supraspinous and interspinous ligaments are further from the flexion axis, and therefore need to stretch more than the posterior longitudinal ligament when they resist flexion.

LOW BACK PAIN

The exact structure which is affected in low back pain is open to discussion, and often it is virtually impossible to identify precisely which tissue is causing a patient's symptoms (Spitzer, LeBlanc and Dupuis, 1987). To a large extent the precise anatomical location becomes irrelevant as long as the patient is made better. The situation is made considerably easier if, instead of focusing attention on the injured structure, we attend to the loss of function and our need to restore this.

To this end, the approach taken by McKenzie (1981) is extremely useful. Back pain may be classified as *mechanical*, or *chemical* (non-mechanical) in origin. Mechanical pain is produced by deformation of structures containing nociceptive nerve endings, and there is a clear correlation between certain body positions and the patient's symptoms.

Non-mechanical pain, on the other hand, is of a constant nature. This may be exacerbated by movement or position, but importantly, no position will be found which completely relieves the symptoms. This category encompasses both inflammatory and infective processes.

> **Keypoint**
>
> *Mechanical* pain is produced by deformation of sensitive structures. There is a definite correlation between body positions and the patient's symptoms. *Non-mechanical* pain is constant, and no position can be found which completely relieves the symptoms.

Inflammation will occur following trauma, and the accumulation of chemical irritant substances will affect the nociceptive fibres and give pain. This type of pain will continue for as long as the nociceptor irritation continues. With rest, irritation will settle and healing progress. Part of this healing process is scar formation, so the type of pain will change from a constant chemical pain to a mechanical pain developed through adaptive shortening of the affected tissues. Non-mechanical conditions also include those which refer pain to the spine, such as vascular or visceral damage and carcinoma. Clearly, it is essential to differentiate between mechanical and non-mechanical pain in the lower back. When no movement can be found which reduces the patient's symptoms and if a period of rest does not allow the symptoms to subside, the patient requires medical investigation.

EXAMINATION OF THE BACK

Screening examination

Examination of the lumbar spine can be either very complex or relatively simple, depending on the approach taken. The reliability and reproducibility of tests for the spine increases when the information to be gained from the tests is kept to a minimum (Nelson et al., 1979). For this reason, the work of Cyriax (1982) and McKenzie (1981) is valuable as it provides enough information to treat the majority of patients. In addition, the tests tell the practitioner when further investigation is necessary.

Observation deals particularly with posture while standing and sitting, and the appearance of the spine at rest. Scoliosis and loss of normal lordosis are of particular note, as is the level of the iliac crests. Flexion, extension and lateral flexion are tested initially as single movements to obtain information about range of motion, end feel and presence of a painful arc. Flexion and extension are then repeated to see if these movements change the intensity or site of pain, bearing in mind the centralization phenomenon and dysfunction stretch. Side-gliding movements are also tested to repetition. Flexion and extension may be further assessed in a lying position to obtain information about nerve root adhesion (flexion) and greater range of extension. This initial examination then indicates whether neurological testing of sensation, power, reflexes and further nerve stretch is required. In addition, the history, signs and symptoms will indicate whether the pelvis and sacroiliac joints warrant further attention, or if resisted tests should be included.

Diagnostic triage

Diagnostic triage extends the screening examination by categorizing low back pain into three types: simple backache, nerve root pain and serious pathology (Table 14.4). With simple backache the patient is generally young to middle age (20–55 years), and the pain is restricted to the low back and buttocks or thighs. The pain is mechanical in nature because it changes with movement, being eased or aggrevated by specific actions which are repeatable. The patient is generally in good health and there is no history of weight loss, nausea or fever. Often there is a history of injury or overuse.

Nerve root pain is normally unilateral and the leg pain may be worse than the pain in the low back. Pain may radiate into the foot, and numbness or paraesthesia (altered sensation) may be present. This type of pain may require further investigation if it does not show signs of significant improvement within 4 weeks of onset.

Where examination reveals non-mechanical pain in a young (under 20) or older (over 55) athlete, specialist investigation is required. This is especially the case where there is a previous history of an associated medical condition, or if the patient has been unwell, shows an obvious structural deformity of the spine or demonstrates gait disturbance. Where altered sensation is present in the 'saddle' area (perineum and genitals) further investigation is required as this indicates possible disc protrusion of the lower sacral nerve roots. Where this is present with difficulty in passing urine, an inability to retain urine and/or a lack of sensation when the bowels are opened, there is a possibility of compression of the cauda equina and immediate emergency referral is required (Kesson and Atkins, 1998; Magee, 2002).

Table 14.4 Diagnostic triage

Simple backache: *specialist referral not required*
Patient aged 20–55 years
Pain restricted to lumbosacral region, buttocks or thighs
Pain is 'mechanical' (i.e. pain changes with, and can be relieved by, movement)
Patient otherwise in good health (no temperature, nausea/dizziness, weight loss, etc.)

Nerve root pain: *specialist referral not generally required within first 4 weeks, if the pain is resolving*
Unilateral (one side of the body) leg pain that is worse than low back pain
Pain radiates into the foot or toes
Numbness and paraesthesia (altered feeling) in the same area as pain
Localized neurological signs (such as reduced tendon jerk and positive nerve tests)

Red flags (caution) for possibly serious spinal pathology: *refer promptly to specialist*
Patient under 20 or over 55 years of age
Non-mechanical pain (i.e. pain does not improve with movement)
Thoracic pain
Past history of carcinoma, steroid drugs, or HIV
Patient unwell or has lost weight
Widespread neurological signs
Obvious structural deformity (such as bone displacement after an accident, or a lump which has appeared recently)
Sphincter disturbance (unable to pass water or incontinent)
Gait disturbance (unable to walk correctly)
Saddle anaesthesia (no feeling in crotch area between legs)
Cauda equina syndrome (bladder and bowel paralysis in addition to saddle anaesthesia) – *refer to specialist immediately*

After Waddell, G., Feder, G. and Lewis, M. (1997) Systematic reviews of bed rest and advice to stay active for acute low back pain. *British Journal of General Practice*, 47, 647–652, with permission and Norris (2000).

Definition

The *cauda equina* is a bundle of lumbar and sacral nerve roots at the end of the spine. The spinal cord finishes at the level of the 1st lumbar vertebra (L1) and the cauda equina nerves extend from this point down to the sacrum.

The straight leg raise

The straight leg raise (SLR) or Lasegue's sign is a widely used test to assess the sciatic nerve in cases of back pain. The test also places stretch on the hamstrings, buttock tissues, sacroiliac joint, posterior lumbar ligaments and facet joints in addition to lengthening the spinal canal (Urban, 1986). Confirmation that the nerve root is the source of pain may be made by raising the leg to the point of pain and then lowering it a few degrees. The neuromeningeal structures are then further stretched either from below by dorsiflexing the foot, or applying firm pressure to the popliteal fossa over

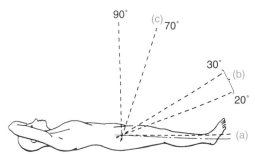

Figure 14.11 Effects of straight leg raising. (a) Movement of sciatic nerve begins at the greater sciatic notch. (b) Movement of roots begins at the intervertebral foramen. (c) Minimal movement only, but increase in tension. From Oliver and Middleditch (1991), with permission.

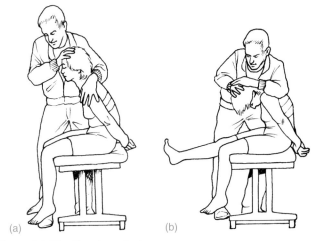

Figure 14.12 The slump test.

the posterior tibial nerve. Pressure from above is produced by flexing the cervical spine. When performing the SLR, as the leg is raised the knee should not be allowed to bend and the pelvis should stay on the couch.

The dura within the spinal canal is firmly attached to the foramen magnum above and the filum terminale below. Trunk flexion causes the spinal canal to lengthen and therefore stretches the dura, whereas extension, by shortening the canal, induces dural relaxation allowing the sheath to fold. The neuromeningeal pathway is elastic, so tension imparted at one point will spread throughout the whole length of the spine. As the SLR is performed, the initial motion is of the nerve at the greater sciatic notch. As hip flexion goes through 35°, movement occurs proximal to the ala of the sacrum, and during the next 35° the movement is at the intervertebral foramen itself. The last degrees of the SLR do not produce further nerve movement, but simply increase the tension over the whole course of the nerve (Grieve, 1970) (Fig. 14.11).

Testing the unaffected leg (crossed SLR or 'well leg' test) may also give symptoms. This manoeuvre pulls the nerve root and dura distally and medially, but increases the pressure on the nerve complex by less than half that of the standard SLR test. When the ipsilateral SLR causes pain, it simply means that one of the tissues connected to the nerve pathway is sensitized. Because the crossed SLR stretches the neural structures less, the resting tension of these tissues must be higher to cause pain. The crossed SLR may therefore be a more reliable predictor of large disc protrusions than the ipsilateral SLR (Urban, 1986).

Keypoint

The well leg test is a more reliable predictor of a large disc protrusion than the standard straight leg raise (SLR).

Slump test

The slump test is used to assess tension in the pain-sensitive structures around the vertebral canal or intervertebral foramen, and to ensure that these structures are able to stretch properly (Maitland, 1986; Butler, 1991). To perform the manoeuvre the patient sits unsupported over the couch side with the knees together and flexed to 90°. The posterior thigh is in contact with the couch. The patient is then instructed to relax the spine completely and 'slump' forward, keeping the cervical spine in its neutral position ('look forwards, not down'). The therapist (standing at the side of the patient) places overpressure onto the patient's shoulders to increase the movement, attempting to bow the spine rather than increase hip flexion (Fig. 14.12a).

From this position the patient is asked to flex the neck ('chin to chest') and then straighten the leg on the unaffected side first (Fig. 14.12b). In each case the examiner places overpressure on the area and assesses the result. The athlete is then asked to dorsiflex the ankle ('pull your toes up'). Neck flexion is slowly released, and the response monitored. The opposite leg is then tested. A normal test result is one where there is a pain-free lack of knee extension by about 30° and slight central pain over T9/10 (Maitland, 1986).

MECHANICAL THERAPY

Three mechanical conditions are recognized in the lower back: the postural syndrome, dysfunction and derangement (McKenzie, 1981).

Postural syndrome

The postural syndrome occurs when certain postures or body positions place pain sensitive soft tissues around the lumbar spine under prolonged stress. Pain is intermittent, and only occurs when the particular posture is taken up, and ceases when the offending posture is changed. This can be frustrating for the patient because they can find nothing wrong. There is no deformity, vigorous activity is frequently painless as the stresses it imposes on the tissues are continually changing. The fault usually lies with poor sitting posture which places the lumbar spine in flexion. After sport, the patient is warm and relaxed and so sits in a slumped position, perhaps in the bar after a game of squash. Discomfort occurs after some time and this gradually changes to pain. The patient often has the idea that sport makes the pain worse, but this is not the case. The poor sitting posture used when relaxing after sport is the true problem.

> **Keypoint**
>
> With the postural syndrome, pain occurs through tension on pain-sensitive soft tissues in the back. Particular body positions cause pain, and when these are released the pain subsides.

Pain may also occur in sport from extreme positions. Hyperflexion when lifting a weight from the ground or performing stretching exercises, hyperextension when pressing a weight overhead, or performing a back walkover in gymnastics are common examples.

The most important part of management with the postural syndrome is patient education. To this end, the slouch-overcorrect procedure for correcting sitting posture is useful (McKenzie, 1981). The patient sits on a stool, and is allowed to slouch into an incorrect sitting posture for some time until back pain ensues. He or she is then taught a position of maximum lordosis, and learns how to change rapidly and at will, from the incorrect slouch to this overcorrect maximum lordosis. Once the patient has seen the relationship between poor sitting posture and pain, he or she is taught a correct sitting posture mid-way between the two extreme movement ranges. The use of a lumbar pad or roll is helpful to maintain the lordosis in sitting.

Where hyperflexion or hyperextension is the cause of postural pain, video is particularly useful in enabling athletes to appreciate the strain they are placing on the lumbar spine. Re-education of movement and skill training, with emphasis on the position of the spine and hips, are helped by video playback. Body landmarks over the pelvis and spine are marked first using white adhesive dots. Biofeedback is also useful, especially when trying to correct hyperflexion. In its simplest form, strips of prestretched elastic tape are placed at either side of the lumbar spine. When the athlete flexes, the tape 'drags' on the skin and acts as a reminder to avoid the flexed position.

Dysfunction

Dysfunction pain is caused by overstretching adaptively shortened structures within the lumbar spine. The previously damaged structures have shortened due to prolonged disuse, or scar tissue formation. When the normal range of motion is attempted at the affected segment, the shortened soft tissues are stretched prematurely. The essential feature with dysfunction is pain at the end of movement range which disappears as soon as the end-range stretch is released.

The position is self-perpetuating because the pain which occurs with stretching causes the patient to avoid the full range motion and so the adaptive shortening is compounded.

Dysfunction may occur secondary to trauma, or as a result of the postural syndrome. Typically, the patient is stiff first thing in the morning and the back 'works loose' through the day, so the patient is generally better with activity. Loss of extension leads to a reduced lordosis, and loss of flexion becomes apparent when the patient tries to touch the toes. Frequently, the patient will deviate to the side of the dysfunction. Once dysfunction has been detected, (static) stretching is required and/or joint mobilization procedures. Although mobilizations at grades III and IV are useful to help restore range of movement, this passive treatment must be coupled with active stretching procedures which the patient can practice at home to help regain lost physiological range.

Accessory movements cannot usually be practised by the patient, and are perhaps a more appropriate form of manual therapy where physiological stretching causes excessive pain. It is important that stretching be practised little and often, to allow the patient to recover from the soreness which follows the lengthening of contracted tissues. The patient must be instructed to press gently into the painful end-range point in an attempt to increase the range of motion. There is always a tendency to try and avoid the painful position with back pain, but with dysfunction this is precisely the position we want to work in.

> **Keypoint**
>
> Dysfunction pain is caused by overstretching adaptively shortened structures within the lumbar spine. The most common form is an extension dysfunction where the lumbar curve (lordosis) appears flat and lumbar extension range is limited.

The most common dysfunction following low back pain is loss of extension (McKenzie, 1981). The extension loss may be regained by a combination of mobilization, manipulation and mechanical therapy. The classic mechanical therapy procedure is extension in lying (EIL), either with or without belt fixation. The patient lies prone on the treatment table, with the lumbar spine held by a webbing fixation belt. This is placed around both the lower spine and treatment table at a point just below the spinal segment which is blocked to extension. From this position, the patient performs a modified press-up exercise, trying to fully extend the arms while keeping the hips in contact with the couch surface (Fig. 14.13). At home the patient should continue the exercise at regular intervals throughout the day. Various modifications may be used to apply the pressure – EIL with the patient lying on a ironing board using a thick belt, or positioning the spine under a low piece of furniture, or manual pressure from a spouse or the weight of a small child.

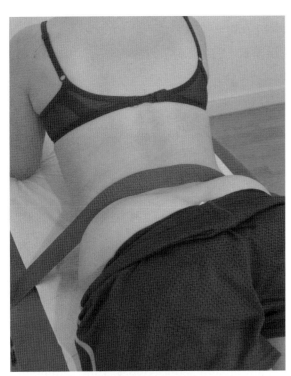

Figure 14.13   Extension in lying (EIL) procedure.

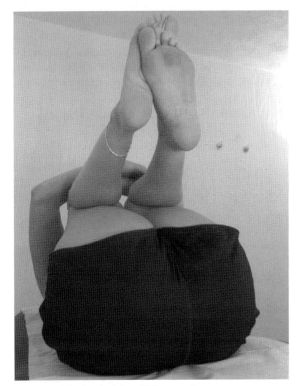

Figure 14.14   Flexion in lying (FIL) procedure.

Loss of flexion may be similarly regained, but this time the mechanical therapy technique is flexion in lying (FIL), or flexion in standing (FIS). Initially the patient uses FIL. The movement begins in a crook-lying position. From this position the patient pulls the knees to the chest. As maximum

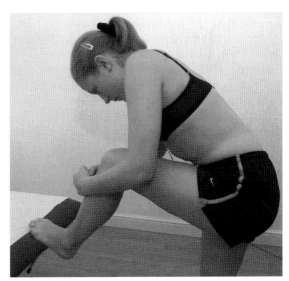

Figure 14.15   Flexion in step standing (FIS).

hip flexion is reached, further movement occurs initially by flexion of the lower lumbar and lumbosacral segments, and then the upper lumbar area (Fig. 14.14). FIS is simply a toe-touching exercise performed very slowly. Gravitation effects place greater stress on the lumbar discs, so the exercise must proceed with caution. The differences between FIS and FIL are two-fold. First, with FIS the legs are straight, and so the nerve roots are stretched, a particularly useful effect when dealing with nerve root adhesion. Secondly, the sequence of flexion is reversed, with the upper lumbar areas moving before the lower lumbar and lumbosacral areas. Where there was a deviation in flexion at the initial examination, flexion in step standing may be used (Fig. 14.15). Here, one leg is placed on a stool and the patient pulls the chest downwards onto the flexed knee. In so doing, flexion is combined with slight lateral bending. Other dysfunctions such as loss of lateral flexion, side-gliding, or rotation may occur but they are less common. In addition, it must be remembered when assessing symmetry of bilateral movements that most people are slightly asymmetrical anyway. We must be certain that any asymmetry that exists is relevant to the patient's present symptoms before we spend time correcting it.

Derangement

Derangement occurs when the nucleus or annulus of the disc is distorted or damaged, altering the normal resting position of two adjacent vertebrae. Pain is usually constant and movement loss is apparent, so much so in some cases that the condition is completely disabling. Derangement of the lumbar disc is a common cause of low back pain, and Cyriax (1982) claimed there are eight ways in which a damaged disc can move, and classified these according to discal position (Table 14.5). McKenzie (1981) described seven types, classified according to symptoms, as derangements 1 to 7. The McKenzie classifications were later simplified (McKenzie and May, 2003), derangements now being classified as

Table 14.5   Cyriax classification of disc lesions

Gradual small posterior displacement
Pain brought on by stooping or lifting and relieved by standing or resting. Articular signs only, sometimes with painful arc, SLR is full

Swift large posterior displacement
Severe low back pain of traumatic origin, or from overuse following prolonged stooping. Constant ache with intermittent twinges. Articular signs of flexion deformity, dural signs of limited SLR and lumbar pain in full neck flexion

Massive posterior protrusion
Posterior longitudinal ligaments may rupture, compression sciatic nerve roots and giving sympathetic signs. Perineal pain and bilateral symptoms, limited SLR with root palsy. Saddle analgesia with bladder weakness

Posterolateral protrusion
Previous history of general backache, changing to unilateral pain, pins and needles or numbness, aggravated by coughing. Limitation of trunk flexion and SLR. Pain often increased by neck flexion

Anterior protrusion in the elderly
Backache and/or unilateral pain with pins and needles in the feet, often mimicking claudication. Symptoms are present only when the patient has been upright for some time and relieved by sitting or lying. Flexion reduces symptoms. SLR full, no neurological deficit

Anterior protrusion in adolescents
Osteochondrosis giving pressure erosion of the vertebral body, and kyphotic posture. Associated with excessive weightbearing

Vertical protrusion
Schmorl's node formation. No pain, but radiographic appearance confirms abnormality. T10 most commonly affected. Alternatively, biconcave disc phenomenon with osteoporosis

Circular protrusion
Compression causes uniform discal bulging, with traction to the periosteum and subsequent osteophyte formation. Limited spinal mobility

Adapted from Cyriax (1982), with permission.

Table 14.6   McKenzie symptom patterns

Pattern	Previous derangement classification
Central (symmetrical)	1, 2, 7
Unilateral (asymmetrical) ± pain to knee	3, 4, 7
Unilateral (asymmetrical), pain below knee	5, 6

After McKenzie and May (2003), with permission.

either central (symmetrical) or unilateral (asymmetrical), with or without pain to the knee (Table 14.6).

Deformities of scoliosis and kyphosis are common, with local or referred pain over the lumbar and sacral dermatomes depending on the severity of injury. Again, management may be by manual or mechanical therapy or a combination of the two. Mechanical therapy aims at centralizing the pain and reversing the sequence of pain development which occurred as the disc lesion progressed. The aim is to transfer pain which is felt laterally in the spine or in the leg to a more central position. It is perfectly acceptable for the intensity of the pain to increase providing its position is altered to a more central one.

The movements used are those which reduced the patient's symptoms in the initial examination. Where a scoliosis exists, initially the most effective movement is usually side-gliding in standing (SGIS). The therapist stands at the side of the patient holding the patient's hips. The therapist then gently presses the patient's shoulders towards the convexity of the scoliosis aiming to obtain a sliding rather than laterally flexing movement. The patient may continue this by placing the hand on a wall (arm abducted to 90°) and shifting the hips towards the wall (Fig. 14.16). Once the pain moves into a more central position, the EIL exercise begins with the aim of centralizing the pain further. Although these movements are frequently very effective for posterolateral protrusions, it must be emphasized that it is the movement which reduces the symptoms which is practised, and this may vary tremendously between patients.

MANUAL THERAPY OF THE LUMBAR SPINE

The point at which manual therapy is used will vary depending on both the condition and the practitioner using the therapy. Some practitioners rarely use manual therapy, claiming that to do so could make a patient dependent upon this type of care, while others use only mobilization and manipulation, claiming that it gives a more rapid response. The true picture probably lies somewhere between the two extremes. There are certainly patients for whom mechanical therapy is too painful initially. These patients usually respond to mobilization to relieve pain and then to increase mobility, and this treatment may be followed by mechanical therapy and exercise therapy at a later date. Equally, there are patients who look upon manual treatment as a panacea which will always cure them, and so they feel they have no need to care for their own spine. For these patients, clearly mechanical therapy must be emphasized.

Mobilization techniques for the lumbar spine

The principles of joint mobilization were outlined in Treatment note 1.2, page 20. For the lumbar spine, there are two techniques (of literally thousands) which are especially valuable and will be briefly described. The first is the rotation movement (Fig. 14.17a). This is performed in the

---

Keypoint

Derangement occurs when a spinal disc is distorted, altering the resting position of the vertebrae. Pain is usually constant and movement loss is seen. The aim is to centralize the pain, taking it from the leg or buttock back into the spine, and finally reducing it altogether.

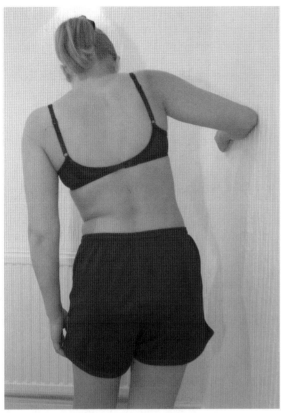

Figure 14.16 Side gliding in standing (SGIS).

side-lying starting position, with the painful side uppermost, so that the pelvis is rotated away from the painful side. Both knees and hips and bent (crook-side lying) with the upper leg bending slightly more than the lower. The therapist stands behind the patient and imparts a grade I or II mobilization by rhythmically pushing on the patient's pelvis, allowing the thorax to rock freely. With grades III and IV, the patient's underneath arm is pulled through to rotate the thorax so that the chest faces more towards the ceiling. The upper leg bends slightly further so that the knee clears the couch side, and the lower leg is straighter to act as a pivot (increasing the flexion of the lower leg will flex the lumbar spine further). Therapist pressure is now over the pelvis and humeral head. This movement may be taken further to apply a manipulation. A lower couch position is used, and the end-range point of spinal rotation is maintained by the therapist pushing down on the patient's pelvis and shoulder through straight arms, and in so doing applying slight traction. As the patient exhales, a high velocity, low amplitude thrust is applied. A tremendous number of variations exist to allow for alterations in range of motion, direction of rotation, and combined movements. These procedures are described in detail by Maitland (1986) and Cyriax and Cyriax (1983).

Extension movements in their simplest form may be produced by using posteroanterior pressures and derivatives of this technique (Fig. 14.17b). Posteroanterior central vertebral pressure (Maitland, 1986) may be performed with the

Figure 14.17 Lumbar mobilization. (a) Rotation. (b) Extension.

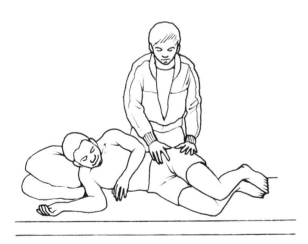

(a)   Grades I and II   Grades III and IV

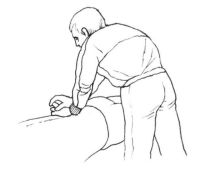

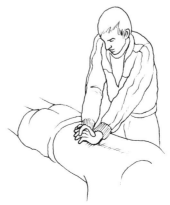

(b)

patient prone. The pressure may be imparted with the pads of the thumbs, or the ulnar border of the hand (pisiform/hamate) pressing over the spinous processes. Movement is gradually taken up as the therapist moves his or her weight directly over the patient's spine and an oscillation is begun. Variations include combined movements, unilateral pressures, bilateral pressure over the transverse processes, and the addition of hip extension among others.

NAGS AND SNAGS

Many patients who have disc lesions seem to respond well to techniques aimed at the facet joints. The connection between these seemingly dissociated conditions is a biomechanical one. As the disc bulges posteriorly, it causes the vertebrae to flex with a loss of lordosis. For this to happen, the facet joints must be mobile enough to open fully. However, in many cases, these joints are far from mobile, and the soft tissue surrounding them is placed on stretch, giving pain, which can be reduced using mobilization procedures.

> **Keypoint**
>
> A bulging disc will cause the vertebrae to flex and the facet joints to open. This will stress the soft tissues surrounding the joint giving pain which will respond to facet based mobilization techniques.

Mulligan (1989) described a number of procedures which combine manual and mechanical therapy, taking into account the planes of movement at the facet joints. In the lumbar spine, movement may be assisted using a sustained natural apophyseal glide (SNAG procedure) by applying therapist pressure over the spinous processes or articular pillars of the lumbar spine as the patient moves. SNAGs are weight-bearing mobilizations which are applied at end of range. They are applied simultaneously with movement, in line with the treatment plane (orientation of the articular surfaces) of the facet joint.

Flexion, extension or lateral flexion may be used either in sitting or standing. Either pisiform or thumb contact is used, and the direction of pressure is vertical in an attempt to separate, or at least assist separation of, the facets.

The starting position is with the patient sitting over the couch side (or standing) with the therapist behind. A belt is placed around the patient's waist over the anterior superior iliac spines (this area may be padded with a towel if necessary). The patient is asked to flex forwards to the point of pain. They then back off slightly and the therapist applies the SNAG as the patient flexes again (Fig. 14.18a). If the correct level has been identified, the movement should be pain-free and of greater range. If pain persists, the level to be treated is changed, or a unilateral SNAG is performed over the articular pillar of the more painful side. For extension, the patient is in the same starting position, but the couch is raised to afford the therapist a better mechanical advantage. The therapist stands slightly to one side in order to be clear of the patient as he or she extends back. The action must be lumbar extension, with the patient extending over the therapist's hand, rather than extension of the whole spine on the hip with the patient pressing the whole bodyweight against the therapist's hand (Fig. 14.18b). Rotation is performed with the patient stride sitting over the couch to fix the pelvis. The therapist grips around the patient's trunk just above the painful level. Again, the overpressure is given with the ulnar border of the hand in the treatment plane (Fig. 14.18c).

The direction of motion and level of pressure application is decided both by the movement which is limited and the action which relieves the patient's symptoms. As the patient moves, the vertical pressure is applied until end-range is obtained. Pressure is continued until the patient resumes the neutral position once more.

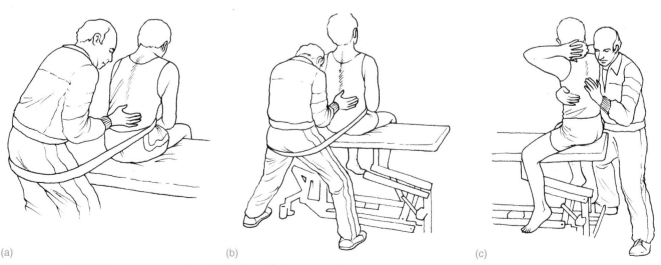

(a) (b) (c)

Figure 14.18   'SNAGS' for the lumbar spine. (a) Flexion. (b) Extension. (c) Rotation.

THE SACROILIAC JOINT

Structure and function

The three bones of the pelvis, the two innominates and the sacrum, form a closed ring. Anteriorly, the innominates join together at the pubic symphysis and posteriorly they join the sacrum via the sacroiliac joints (SIJ). Disorders of the pubic symphysis will often have repercussions on the SIJ, so examination should take place in both joints.

The sacral articular surface is shaped like a letter 'L' lying on its side, and is covered by hyaline cartilage, while the corresponding surface on the ilium is covered by fibrocartilage. The SIJ is a synovial joint, but its posterior surface is firmly secured by the interosseous ligament and so the joint may be considered as fibrous. There is great variation between individuals, in terms of the size, shape and number of articular surfaces, with 30% of subjects having accessory articulations between the sacrum and ilium (Grieve, 1976). With increasing age the joint becomes fibrosed and may eventually show partial bony fusion.

The normal SIJ does move. As the trunk is flexed, the sacral base moves forwards between the ilia, and with trunk extension in standing, the sacrum moves back again. The movement is usually only about 5 mm, but ranges up to 26 mm have been recorded (Frigerio, Stowe and Howe, 1974).

Sacral motion is described as *nutation* and *counter-nutation* (Table 14.7). Nutation of the SIJ is an anterior tilting of the sacrum on the fixed pelvic (innominate or iliac) bones. The sacral base (top, flat area) moves down and forwards and the apex (point) moves up increasing the pelvic outlet. Nutation occurs as the lumbar lordosis increases and the iliac bones are pulled together impacting the SIJ. With counter-nutation the opposite movement occurs. It is a posterior tilting of the sacrum, with the base moving back and the apex (normally facing backwards) moving forwards and down. The pelvic outlet reduces and the pelvic bones move apart,

distracting the SIJ. Counter-nutation occurs in non-weight-bearing position and as the lumbar lordosis flattens.

> **Definition**
>
> As the sacrum is a triangle pointed downwards, the *sacral base* is the large flat upper surface and the *sacral apex* the pointed lower portion. The sacrum and pelvic bones are joined together in a circle. The *pelvic inlet* is the space between the upper part of the bones and the *pelvic outlet* the space between the lower parts.

Postural asymmetry of the pelvis is common, and is evident when there is torsion of one ilium in relation to the other. On examination, one anterior superior iliac spine may be higher and one posterior superior iliac spine may be lower, for example. Unequal leg lengths, although normally asymptomatic, may cause the SIJ to become 'blocked', with a consequent alteration in gluteal muscle tone (Grieve, 1976). When shortening is more than 1–2 cm, torsion of the pelvis occurs with the ilium and sacral base on the side of the longer leg moving backwards and the pubis moving upwards. The degree of postural compensation between individuals will differ and so the pelvic position in reaction to altered leg length is variable.

Hormonal changes in pregnancy and, to a lesser extent, menstruation and menopause will also influence the SIJ. The general softening and relaxation of the pelvis leads to an increased range of motion which may remain for up to 12 weeks following childbirth. Local irritation of the SIJ leads to pain on gapping tests and limited hip abduction on the painful side. In addition, the lower PSIS is usually on the painful side.

Stability

The sacrum is inserted like the keystone of an arch, but seemingly the wrong way round, tending to be displaced rather than forced inwards with pressure. However, as the body-weight is taken, the tension developed in the interosseous sacroiliac ligaments pulls the two halves of the pelvic ring together producing *form closure* (Fig. 14.19). In the sagittal plane the body weight falls ventral to the axis of rotation of the SIJ. This alignment would tend to rotate the sacrum forwards into a nutated position. During nutation the sacrotuberous ligament and the large interosseous ligament of the SIJ are tensioned, drawing the posterior part of the innominate bones together in a mechanism called self-locking. Counter-nutation disengages self-locking and so may lead to SIJ instability. Interestingly, because self-locking is disengaged during forward flexion of the trunk without a pelvic tilt (Lee, 1994), a stoop lift may dislodge the joint and is often a mechanism in SIJ pathology.

Although no strong muscles cross the SIJ, the joint may be actively stabilized by a combination of forces acting over

Table 14.7 Movement of the sacroiliac joint (SIJ)

Nutation	Counternutation
• Anterior tilting of sacrum	• Posterior tilting of sacrum
• Sacral base moves down and forward, apex moves up	• Sacral base moves up and back, apex moves down
• Size of pelvic outlet increased, pelvic inlet decreased	• Pelvic inlet increased, outlet reduced
• Occurs in standing position such as lying	• Occurs in non-weight-bearing
• Increased as lumbar lordosis increased	• Increased as lumbar lordosis decreased (flatback posture)
• Iliac bones pulled together, SIJ impacted	• Iliac bones move apart, SIJ distracted
• Superior aspect of pubis compressed	• Inferior aspect of pubis compressed

From Norris (2000), with permission.

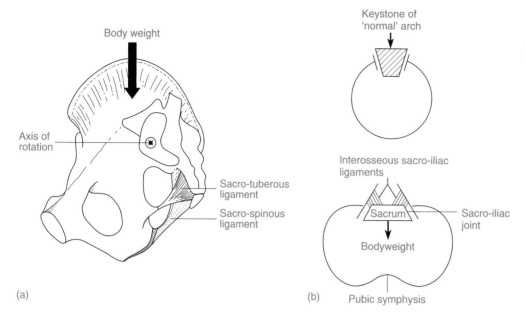

Figure 14.19 The sacroiliac joint. (a) Position. (b) Action in pelvic arch. After Taylor and Twomey (1994), with permission.

the joint, a process called *force closure*. The sacrotuberous ligament (sacrum to ischial tuberosity) and the long dorsal sacroiliac ligament (sacral segments 4/5 to posterior inferior iliac spine) blend to form an expansion measuring 20 mm wide by 60 mm long. This expansion attaches to the posterior layer of the thoracolumbar fascia (TLF) and to the aponeurosis of the erector spinae, and a number of other muscles have important tensioning effects in this area (Vleeming et al., 1995; Vleeming et al., 1997). Five stabilizing systems are described involving trunk and lower limb muscles coupling with lumbosacral fascia and ligaments (Fig. 14.20). These muscle–fascial couplings give the therapist the opportunity to use muscle re-education to stabilize the SIJ during rehabilitation (see Treatment note 14.1, p. 321).

Examination

Subjective examination usually reveals a unilateral distribution of symptoms, perhaps spreading to the buttock, lower abdomen, groin or thigh, although pain may be referred to the foot. The traumatic history is frequently one of a fall, landing on the ischial tuberosity, with patients unable to walk distances without marked pain. The footballer in a mistimed sliding tackle or the youngster who falls while ice-skating are prime examples. In any sport where the range of motion required at the hip is great or repetitive unilateral leg movements are performed, SIJ irritation may be encountered. Tensile forces are increased with jumping activities onto both legs, while shear forces are raised with single leg activities, such as running and hopping. Dancers, gymnasts and high-jumpers are particularly prone to SIJ involvement, but any athlete may suffer trauma to the joint leading to local inflammation or mechanical disturbance.

Objective examination of the pelvis and SIJ is made initially with the patient standing. The general bony alignment and muscle contour is noted. The patient may be reluctant to take weight through the affected leg, and may walk with a limp. Loss of gluteal and abdominal muscle bulk has also been reported (Wells, 1986). The level of the gluteal folds and gluteal cleft is noted, as is that of the iliac crests and iliac spines.

Motion (kinetic) tests

Motion tests of the SIJ are used to assess the side of the body with the predominent dysfunction, and therefore the side to treat (Turner, 2002). They assess the contribution of the SIJ to general pelvic motion and are used before and after a treatment technique to determine effectiveness. Importantly, motion tests cannot accurately by themselves be used to determine the nature of a dysfunction or to imply that an altered motion test is a cause of pain. In addition, they cannot indicate whether a joint is 'stiff' or 'locked'.

Two motion tests of the SIJ are more useful than most in sport (Fig. 14.21). For the first, *hip flexion in standing*, the examiner places his or her thumbs over S2/3 and the PSIS. From the standing position the patient flexes one hip, and movement of the PSIS is noted. Normally, with hip flexion the PSIS moves caudally (drops) and as the leg is brought back to the ground it moves cephalically (lifts). For the second test, *forward flexion in standing*, both PSIS are palpated as the patient flexes the spine. Ideally both PSIS should move equally. If dysfunctional, one joint may move earlier or further up as the patient flexes (Piedallu's sign). It is as though the PSIS is being dragged along by the sacrum. These tests may be used to guide manual therapy techniques but should not be used in isolation diagnostically (see below).

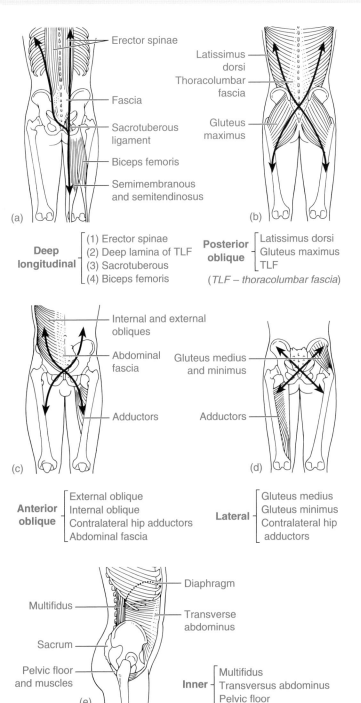

(1) Erector spinae
Deep longitudinal { (2) Deep lamina of TLF
(3) Sacrotuberous
(4) Biceps femoris

Posterior oblique { Latissimus dorsi
Gluteus maximus
TLF

(TLF – thoracolumbar fascia)

Anterior oblique { External oblique
Internal oblique
Contralateral hip adductors
Abdominal fascia

Lateral { Gluteus medius
Gluteus minimus
Contralateral hip adductors

Inner { Multifidus
Transversus abdominus
Pelvic floor

Figure 14.20   Sacroiliac joint stabilization – muscle/fascia coupling. (a) Deep longitudinal muscle system, (b) posterior oblique, (c) anterior oblique, (d) lateral, (e) inner. From Magee (2002), with permission.

Palpation

Motion tests of the SIJ which rely on palpation have been shown to be unreliable (Laslett, 1997) and are only of real clinical use when used in parallel with other forms of objective examination. In a study of 45 patients using experienced manual therapists to assess six commonly used palpation tests, the maximum reliability was only fair, and in some tests the reliability was worse than that obtained

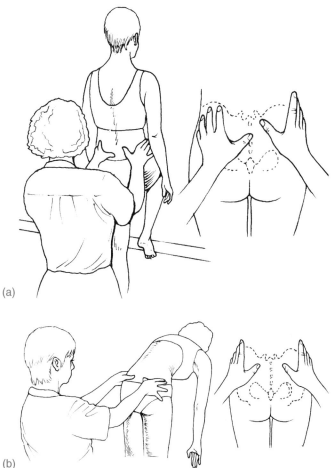

Figure 14.21   Motion tests of the sacroiliac joints. (a) The right PSIS should move caudally as the leg is lowered back to the ground. (b) Joint asymmetry. If one joint is lower, as the patient flexes it will move cephalically (Piedallu's sign).

through chance (van Duersen et al., 1990). Dreyfuss et al. (1992) found that as many as 20% of asymptomatic individuals gave a false positive on the standing or seated flexion tests, and Potter and Rothstein (1985) used experienced manual therapists to test 13 palpatory tests and found that simple agreement on the tests was less than 70% on most of the procedures.

Pain provocation tests are, however, more reliable. Laslett and Williams (1994) assessed 51 patients with six SIJ tests and found that interexaminer agreement was over 94% for the femoral thrust, and 88% for pelvic torsion (Gaenslen's test), distraction and compression tests. These four tests are shown in Fig. 14.22.

With persistent bilateral SIJ pain, the possibility of ankylosing spondylitis should be considered. The range of motion, especially lateral flexion, of the lumbar spine is limited, and muscle spasm may be evident. Where costovertebral involvement is present, chest expansion will be affected – often an early sign. The use of radiographs, erythrocyte sedimentation rate (ESR), and the presence of lumbar antigen HLA B27 aid the diagnosis.

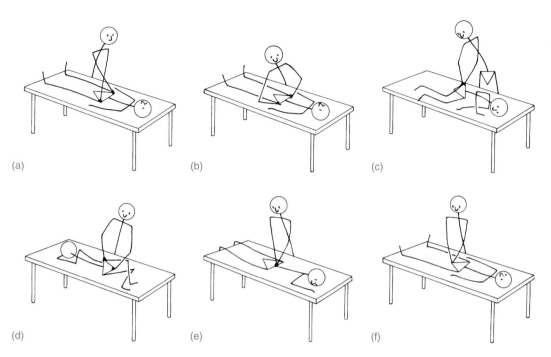

Figure 14.22 Sacroiliac joint pain provocation tests.

(a)   (b)   (c)

(d)   (e)   (f)

Change in leg length as SIJ assessment

A change in leg length may be used as an assessment of SIJ dysfunction (Don Tigny, 1985). The leg length change occurs because altered position of the innominate bones will also change the resting position of the acetabulum, placing it more proximal or distal and consequently altering leg length. The tests are used to identify a reduction in self-locking of the SIJ through nutation (anterior rotation) of the sacrum on the innominates.

Initially patients are positioned in crook lying and they are instructed to form a bridge and to place the hips back onto the couch. The therapist then passively extends the legs and compares leg length by palpating the undersurface the malleoli with the edge of the thumbs. The patient then performs a straight leg sit-up action (they may assist themselves by pulling on the couch with their hands) and the leg length is again assessed. If the leg gets longer (lying to sitting) it indicates a posterior innominate on the side of the longer leg, and if the leg gets shorter the indication is of an anterior innominate (Fig. 14.23).

Treatment is aimed at the more painful side. Where anterior rotation occurs (leg shorter) the treatment is to posteriorly rotate the innominate (see below). Where anterior rotation has occurred (leg longer) it is thought that an upslip has occurred and this should be treated using leg traction (Turner, 2002).

Keypoint

During a sit-up test, if the leg gets shorter the treatment is to posteriorly rotate the innominate (pelvic bone). If the leg gets longer, leg traction should be used.

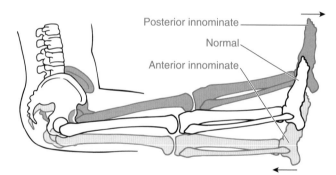

Figure 14.23 Leg length assessment of sacroiliac joint. From Magee (2002) with permission.

Positional faults of the innominates

Three main positional faults occur in the SIJ, *anterior innominate* (common) *upslip* (common) and *posterior innominate* (less common) (Fig. 14.24). A variety of other appearances occur but they are not as frequently seen in day-to-day clinical practice. The reader is referred to Lee (1994) for further information.

With an anterior innominate the anterior superior iliac spine (ASIS) appears higher and the posterior superior iliac spine (PSIS) lower. With a posterior innominate the reverse occurs with the ASIS higher and the PSIS lower. An upslip sees the whole innominate bone higher on that side with both the ASIS and PSIS higher and the pelvic rim itself appearing higher on the affected side. A variety of muscle energy techniques (MET) may be used to treat positional faults.

An anterior innominate is treated with passive hip flexion. The patient is supine and the therapist places one hand

Definition

Muscle energy technique (MET) uses the patient's muscle contraction force (energy) to assist in joint mobilization. MET generally involves gentle isometric contraction followed by relaxation to reduce muscle tone. During this relaxed phase the joint is mobilized.

beneath the ischial tuberosity of the near leg. The other arm grips the femur of the near leg. The action is to resist hip extension and as the muscles relax, to impart a posterior pelvic tilting force by rocking the arms and pulling the ischial tuberosity upwards (Fig. 14.25).

A posterior innominate is treated with a posteroanterior (PA) mobilization on the PSIS. The patient lies prone and the therapist grasps the inside of the near knee. Resisted hip flexion is used and, as the muscles relax, downward pressure is imposed through the other arm.

An upslip may be treated with leg traction. The patient lies supine and the therapist holds the leg in slight internal rotation to protect the hip joint. The action is initially leg shortening (contraction of ipsilateral trunk side flexors) followed by leg traction as the muscles are relaxed.

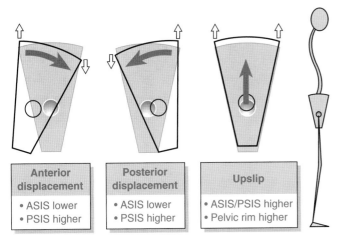

Anterior displacement	Posterior displacement	Upslip
• ASIS lower	• ASIS lower	• ASIS/PSIS higher
• PSIS higher	• PSIS higher	• Pelvic rim higher

Figure 14.24 Positional faults affecting the sacroiliac joint.

Assessment of SIJ stability

The SIJ is stabilized both passively (form closure) and actively (force closure). Failure of the stabilizing mechanisms may be assessed using the active straight leg raise (ASLR) test (Mens et al., 1997). The test first identifies SIJ stability, but, importantly, can also be used to highlight the most appropriate way to stabilize the joint and provides a valuable tool for the reassessment of the treatment intervention. It is therefore the assessment of choice for functional rehabilitation of SIJ dysfunction.

Keypoint

The active straight leg raise (ASLR) test is the assessment of choice for functional rehabilitation of SIJ dysfunction.

The patient is asked to actively lift the leg by 5 cm, keeping it straight, by engaging the hip flexor muscles. Weakness and/or pain on this movement on one side of the body indicates poor dynamic stability of the SIJ (force closure). The test is then performed again while the therapist assists form closure by: (i) compressing the pelvic rims, and (ii) using minimal posterior pelvic tilt (innominate rotation) on the ipsilateral side. Where these techniques reduce pain and increase strength, a SIJ belt should be used initially until force closure has been enhanced. To assess force closure the ASLR test is repeated while engaging the muscle–fascial systems shown in Figure 14.20. For the inner system the transversus abdominis is contracted (abdominal hollowing), for the posterior oblique system the latissimus dorsi is engaged (resisted shoulder adduction).

The ASLR test has been demonstrated radiographically to alter alignment of the pelvic ring using pubic malalignment as a measure. ASLR of the normal limb shows no step deformity across the pubic ramus, but with the symptomatic limb, step deformity of 5 mm together with anterior innominate rotation has been recorded (Mens et al., 1997). In addition, the same study demonstrated that over 70% of symptomatic patients showed less strength in the ASLR and 80% of these showed strength improvement with a SIJ belt. In addition,

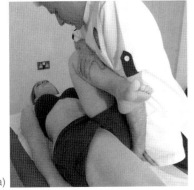

(a)

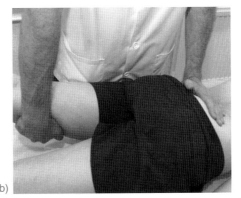

(b)

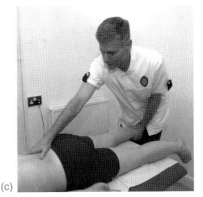

(c)

Figure 14.25 Muscle energy techniques (MET) for the sacroiliac joint. (a) Anterior innominate. (b) Posterior innominate. (c) Upslip.

in all but one patient the ASLR was more powerful with posterior rotation pressure over the ipsilateral ASIS.

SPONDYLOLYSIS

Spondylolysis is a defect in the neural arch (pars interarticularis), in 90% of cases between the lamina and pedicle of the fifth lumbar vertebra (Fig. 14.26). It is a fracture of the pars without slippage, and by the age of 7 years is present in 5% of the population (Reid, 1992). In athletes, however, the incidence may be as high as 20%, and it is often associated with other lumbar anomalies (Hoshina, 1980).

Where symptoms are present but no deformity is detectable on X-ray or bone scan, a pars interarticularis stress reaction has occurred (Weber and Woodall, 1991). At one stage a congenital defect was thought to be present. However, the condition is not present from birth and increases in incidence with age. Furthermore, the ossification centres of the vertebra do not correspond to the position of the defect. Familial tendencies do exist, and racial differences have been described (Colcher and Hursh, 1952).

The most important consideration from the point of view of sport is that of trauma. Direct trauma may result in a non-union of the area or, more likely, a stress fracture forms over a prolonged period, especially as a result of repeated flexion overload, hyperextension, or shearing stress to the lumbar spine. Athletes with hypolordosis in the lumbar spine are at risk from flexion overload whereas those demonstrating hyperlordosis may suffer the condition as a result of forced rotation causing torsion overload (Farfan, Osteria and Lamy, 1976). The pars interarticularis is positioned as a pivot between the disc and facet joints, and so is subjected to considerable stress. The condition has been described in weightlifters and oarsmen (Kotanis et al., 1971), hockey players (Letts et al., 1985), gymnasts (Jackson et al., 1981; Weber and Woodall, 1991), and fast bowlers (Williams and Sperryn, 1976).

> **Keypoint**
>
> Spondylolysis can form over a prolonged period, usually as a result of repeated flexion, hyperextension, or shearing stresses imposed on the lumbar spine.

Repeated stress can lead to microfractures, especially if overtraining has occurred. As these heal they produce an elongated appearance of the bone. Lumbar pain is apparent; this may be unilateral or bilateral but is rarely associated with nerve root compression. Pain is experienced first with hyperextension, such as walk-over movements in gymnastics, and increases in intensity. Pain is aggravated by hyperextension or rotation, and may present with paraspinal muscle spasm. Unilateral pain may be reproduced if the athlete performs hyperextension in single-leg standing. It is thought that this movement causes compression on the pars interarticularis (Weber and Woodall, 1991). Flexion is normally painless

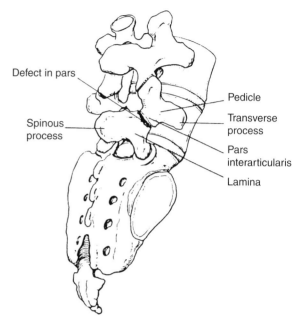

Figure 14.26   Site of defect in spondylolysis. From Gould (1990), with permission.

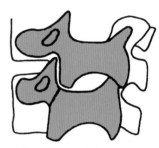

Figure 14.27   An oblique X-ray of the lumbar spine, which has the appearance of a terrier dog. In the lower segment a spondylolysis through the pars interarticularis appears as a collar around the dog's neck. From Corrigan and Maitland (1983), with permission.

although pain may occur as the athlete returns to standing. Oblique X-rays give the classic 'terrier dog' appearance (Fig. 14.27) with the dog's collar represented by the pars interarticularis defect, which is bridged by fibrous tissue rather than bone. A negative X-ray does not rule out spondylogenic conditions, and bone scan may be required (Ciullo and Jackson, 1985).

SPONDYLOLISTHESIS

Spondylolisthesis is an anterior shift of one vertebra on the other, usually L5 on S1. In sport, the condition is usually a progression from spondylolysis, but it may also occur in the elderly as a result of degeneration, or congenitally in association with spina bifida. The first degree injury involves slippage to a distance of one quarter the vertebral diameter, but further movement may occur up to a fourth degree injury which involves a full diameter displacement (Corrigan and Maitland, 1983). The major symptom is of back pain referred to the buttocks which is aggravated by exercise. Sciatica may be present as the condition is associated with disc protrusion in 5% of cases (Williams and Sperryn, 1976). The alteration in spinal alignment causes dimpling of the skin and extra skin folds above the level of injury. A step deformity to the spinous process at the lower level is normally apparent to palpation. The lordosis is usually increased, and severe spasm of the erector spinae may be present. Lumbar extension is often severely limited, and passive intervertebral pressure over the spinous process at the affected level is painful.

MANAGEMENT OF SPONDYLOGENIC DISORDERS

Treatment aims mainly to eliminate the symptoms of the condition rather than to obtain bony union. Initially, rest is required. This varies from 'active rest' by avoiding painful movements with mild conditions to total bed rest with very severe lesions. Occasionally, braces and casts are used to protect the spine until the acute pain subsides, but the most important component of management is closely supervised exercise therapy. Thorough functional assessment is carried out to investigate strength and flexibility. In addition to absolute values in comparison to norms for a particular athlete population, muscle imbalance is important. Transmission of ground forces to the spine is governed to a large extent by hip and spine musculature, and weakness or asymmetry here must be corrected. Anterior shear forces are compensated by an extension moment created by the abdominal muscles (especially the internal obliques and transversus) and the latissimus dorsi pulling on the thoracolumbar fascia. In addition, the paraspinals counteract shear forces in the lumbar spine (Farfan, Osteria and Lamy, 1976).

The use of a stability programme based on motor control (see p. 320) has been shown to be effective in the management of this disorder (O'Sullivan et al., 1997). A 10-week specific stability programme was shown to be more effective than conventional exercise programmes involving gym work, sit-up and swimming using measures of pain intensity, pain description and functional ability. In addition, the benefits of specific stabilization training was maintained at a 30-month follow-up.

SPINAL STABILITY

When the lumbar spine demonstrates instability, there is an alteration of both the quality and quantity of movement available within a vertebral segment. The unstable segment shows decreased stiffness (resistance to bending) and as a consequence movement is increased even under minor loads. Clinical assessment may reveal a number of physical signs as outlined in Table 14.8.

To maintain spinal stability, three inter-related systems have been proposed (Fig. 14.28). Passive support is provided by inert tissues, while active support is from the contractile tissues. Sensory feedback from both systems provides coordination via the neural control centres (Panjabi, 1992).

Table 14.8 Physical signs of instability

Step deformity (spondylolisthesis) or rotation deformity (spondylolysis) on standing which reduces on lying
Transverse band of muscle spasm which reduces on lying
Localized muscle twitching while shifting weight from one leg to the other
Juddering or shaking during forward bending
Alteration to passive intervertebral motion testing, suggesting excessive mobility in the sagittal plane

From Paris, S.V. (1985) Physical signs of instability. *Spine*, 10(3), 272–279 and Maitland (1986), with permission.

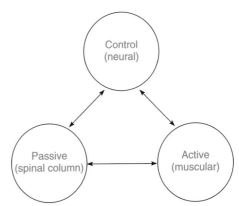

Figure 14.28 The spinal stabilizing system consists of three interrelating subsystems. From Panjabi, M.M. (1992) The stabilizing system of the spine. Part 1. Function, dysfunction, adaptation and enhancement. *Journal of Spinal Disorders*, 5(4), 383–389. With permission.

Importantly, where the stability provided by one system reduces, the other systems may compensate. Thus the proportion of load taken by the active system may increase to minimize stress on the passive system through load-sharing (Tropp, Alaranta and Renstrom, 1993). When this happens, we can view stability as a continuously varying process (Bergmark, 1989). This process is dynamic and quite different to the traditional view of clinical stability being a static mechanical state (stable or unstable).

Keypoint

Instability of the lumbar spine occurs when there is a decreased stiffness (resistance to bending) of a spinal segment. As a result, excessive movement occurs, even under minor loads.

The concept of a dynamic interrelating system gives the physiotherapist the opportunity to reduce pain and improve function by rehabilitating active or functional lumbar stabilization. Such improvement may be accomplished by augmenting both the active and neural control systems. Simply developing muscle strength is insufficient. Moreover, many popular strength exercises for the trunk actually increase mobility in this region to dangerously high levels (Norris, 1993; 1994a). Rather than improving stability, exercises of this type may reduce it and could therefore increase symptoms, especially those associated with inflammation.

Exercise programme to develop active lumbar stability

The lumbar stabilization (back stability) programme (Richardson and Jull, 1994; Norris, 1995; Norris, 2000) is divided into three overlapping stages (Table 14.9), which parallel to a certain degree the three stages of motor learning. In stage I the therapist helps the patient to gain voluntary control of the stabilizing muscles, and then helps to build up their holding capacity. In stage II, dynamic work augments the static activities begun with stage I, and controlled movements are used within mid-range only. In stage III, the speed of muscle contraction is enhanced (through proprioceptive training) in an attempt to redevelop the automatic nature of stabilization.

Phase I (muscle re-education)

The initial aim of the programme is to gain voluntary control over the stabilizing muscles. The stabilizers of the lumbopelvic region are the deep abdominals, the gluteals and the intersegmental muscles of the spine, especially multifidus. These muscles often function poorly after injury, and

may be incorrectly recruited as a result of intense training activities, which lead to muscle imbalance. When this happens the mobilizer muscles of the lumbopelvic region (rectus abdominis, hip flexors and hamstrings) often dominate movements with the stabilizers being poorly recruited. The focus of the back stability programme, therefore, is to reduce the dominance of the mobilizer muscles and enhance the function of the stabilizers.

The process starts with the abdominal hollowing exercise described on page 131. The patient begins traditionally in a prone kneeling position with the spine in its neutral (midrange) position (slight lordosis). The action is to pull the abdominal wall in, and hold the position for 2 seconds initially, building to 5, 10 and eventually 30 seconds, breathing normally. Although initially the action may demand high levels of muscle work to facilitate learning, the eventual aim is to use minimal muscle activity. A useful teaching point is to contract the abdominal muscles as hard as possible and then to relax by half (50% MVC) and then half again (25% MVC). The therapist should monitor the ribcage to ensure that is does not move substantially, and the feeling should be one of the umbilicus drawing inwards and slightly upwards rather than of bulging (doming) or spinal flexion.

Once this has been achieved, the holding capacity of these muscles is built up until the patient can maintain the contraction for 10 repetitions, each held for 10 seconds (Richardson, 1992). Several other starting positions may be used (see Treatment note 14.1) and the most suitable position is chosen for the particular patient being treated.

Table 14.9 Lumbar stabilization

Stage	Method
Muscle re-education	
Single, isolated movements	Perform abdominal hollowing
Slow and precise	4 point kneeling, standing, prone
Focus attention on body part	lying or supine lying
Use visualization and cueing	Build holding time until athlete able to maintain contraction for 20–30 seconds breathing normally, or to perform 10 reps holding each for 10 seconds
Building stability control	
Limb movements	Supine lying – heel slide, bent knee
Maintain neutral position	fall out
Frontal, sagital and transverse plane motions	Prone lying – leg raise
	4 point kneeling – leg and arm movements
	Standing – single leg flexion or abduction
Reduced attention	
Perform secondary movements while maintaining stability	Throwing/catching
	Machine weight activities
Functional actions	Free weight activites
Bending, lifting, sport specific	Balance board, Swiss gym ball
Balance actions	

Phase II (building stability control)

The second phase aims to use the now stable base for movements of the arm and legs. Following abdominal hollowing in crook lying, the next exercise would be the heel slide (Fig. 14.29a). The patient performs the hollowing action, and while maintaining the neutral lumbar position, one leg is straightened, sliding the heel along the ground. The action of the hip flexors in this case tries to tilt the pelvis forwards (iliacus) and increase the lordosis (psoas). The abdominal muscles must work hard to stabilize the pelvis and lumbar spine against this pull. A number of other movements may be used including the bent knee fallout (Fig. 14.29b), which works for rotary stability, and bridging actions (Fig. 14.29c, d and e), which combine abdominal work with gluteal actions.

During stage II, dynamic movements of the spine are also used. Now the aim is to maintain both static (neutral position) and dynamic (lumbopelvic rhythm) alignment. Actions such as the trunk curl and hip hinge are useful, as are more traditional lumbar exercises involving rotation. A variety of additional movements may be used with the aim in each case of maintaining correct alignment of the spine and building holding capacity.

Side support movements (Fig. 14.29f) work the quadratus lumborum and trunk side flexors which are important stabilizers in single handed carrying tasks especially.

Treatment note 14.1   Lumbar stabilization starting positions

Muscle isolation

The lumbar stability programme begins with *muscle isolation*. The aim is to teach the correct abdominal hollowing (AH) action, avoiding substitution strategies such as breath holding, rectus abdominis and external oblique dominance, and obvious ribcage movement. Four starting positions may be used, and the one which is most suitable for the patient forms the basis of the programme progression (Table 14.10).

Table 14.10   Starting positions for abdominal hollowing. From Norris, C.M. (2000) *Back Stability*. Human Kinetics, Champaign, Illinois. With permission.

Starting position	Advantage	Disadvantage
Kneeling (4 point)	Abdominal wall placed on stretch to facilitate AH action Unfamiliar pattern to athletes so avoids 'situp' motor programme Comfortable for LBP patient and during pregnancy	Stress on wrists and knees Difficult for obese subject
Prone lying	Easier to avoid spine movement Good cueing to pull abdominal wall away from table AH can be measured using pressure biofeedback	Inappropriate for obese or pregnant subject due to abdominal compression
Supine lying	Good for self palpation Surface EMG (sEMG) and pressure biofeedback used easily Link to PF contraction easier as patients often lean PF work in this position	Position may lead to situp muscle strategies in athletes (rectus dominance)
Standing (wall support)	Cueing to pull abdominal wall away from waistband of trousers useful for home exercise Appropriate for obese and pregnant patients Functional for daily activities	Weight bearing may not be suitable for disc patients Those with extreme postural abnormalities may find position uncomfortable
	AH = abdominal hollowing LBP = low back pain PF = pelvic floor	

The four point (prone) kneeling position has the advantage that it is comfortable on the spine and is particularly suitable after low back pain or following/during childbirth. In addition, as it is an unfamiliar position for abdominal exercises, the position will not encourage a 'sit-up motor programme' – that is, dominance of the rectus abdominis. This makes the position suitable for use with athletes where the aim is to reduce the reliance on the rectus. As abdominal hollowing is performed the abdominal wall is pulled upwards and a belt may be used to cue this movement, enabling the patient to pull away from the belt. This action is likely to be difficult for obese individuals simply because they have a greater tissue mass to lift, so another starting position may be more appropriate.

Prone lying (lying on the front) supports the back completely and avoids the 'rocking' action which some patients find difficult to control in kneeling. In addition, as the abdominal wall is pulled away from the floor, cueing is provided, and a pressure biofeedback unit (pp. 131–132) may be used to monitor the effect. Again the starting position may not be suitable for an obese subject as tissue mass makes movement initiation difficult.

Supine lying (lying on the back) enables the subject to self-palpate and the use of sEMG also adds to self-measurement. In addition, supine lying is the position often used for retraining pelvic floor (PF) muscle action and linking abdominal hollowing to PF muscle work is a useful method of initiating deep abdominal action. In athletes, however, close supervision will be required as there is a tendency to recruit the rectus abdominis and even to lift the head in this position.

Standing against a wall is most suitable for obese subjects as they can pull the abdominal wall away from a belt (or waistband of the trousers) with minimal muscle work which becomes very motivating. In addition, for those unfamiliar with exercise, standing activities are often better tolerated. Because the position is weight bearing, however, those with acute low back pain may not be able to tolerate prolonged standing and a lying starting position may be more suitable for them.

Phase III (reduced attention)

Once stability has been obtained, the athlete is required to maintain or adopt the stable position only when it is required, relaxing at times when the spine is not under stress. For this to occur, muscle reaction time must be reduced through proprioceptive training. The aim here is to move the spine out of alignment and impose stress upon it so that the stabilizing muscles react quickly to realign the spine and protect it from excessive stress, in a similar approch to that used for the ankle and knee.

More complex activities can now be used which draw the subject's attention away from the spine and into the environment. The aim now is to use proprioception to monitor the position and stability of the spine so that stability becomes more automatic and less attention demanding.

Resistance training appropriate to individual sporting requirements may also be used (Fig. 14.30). The correct relationship between lumbar alignment and pelvic alignment must be rigorously maintained. A convex contour of the abdominal wall (doming or bow-stringing) indicates that the deep abdominals are failing to maintain stability against the pull of rectus abdominis. A maximally flexed or extended lumbar spine indicates that mid-range (active) stability has been lost and joint approximation and inert tissue stretch are providing passive stability only.

The speed and complexity of movements is increased so that the athlete is forced to maintain stability automatically. The athlete's attention is fully taken up by focusing on the complexity of the exercise task (see information processing bottleneck). Spinal alignment must be maintained in sports-related actions such as cycling, jogging, throwing and plyometric actions. Use of a balance board or balance shoes and Swiss gym ball (Fig. 14.29g) is useful (Irion, 1992; Lester, 1992; Lester and Posner-Mayer, 1993).

MID-SECTION TRAINING IN SPORTS

Training the abdominal region is fraught with danger for the lumbar spine, so close analysis of exercises for this region is useful.

Function of the abdominal muscles

The rectus abdominis and lateral fibres of external oblique may be considered as the prime movers of trunk flexion, while the internal oblique and transversus abdominis are the major stabilizers (see Ch. 6). The rectus and external oblique are superficial muscles which often dominate trunk actions, while the transversus and internal oblique are more deeply placed and patients often show an inability to contract them voluntarily.

The rectus abdominis will flex the trunk by approximating the pelvis and rib cage. EMG investigation has shown the supra-umbilical portion to be emphasized by trunk flexion, while activity in the infra-umbilical portion is greater in positions where a posterior pelvic tilt is held (Lipetz and Gutin, 1970; Guimaraes et al., 1991). Some authors however, have questioned these findings, claiming that the differences between the two portions of rectus represent measurement errors rather than muscle function (Lehman and McGill, 2001). Internal oblique and transversus are activated by abdominal hollowing actions (Richardson et al., 1990), and

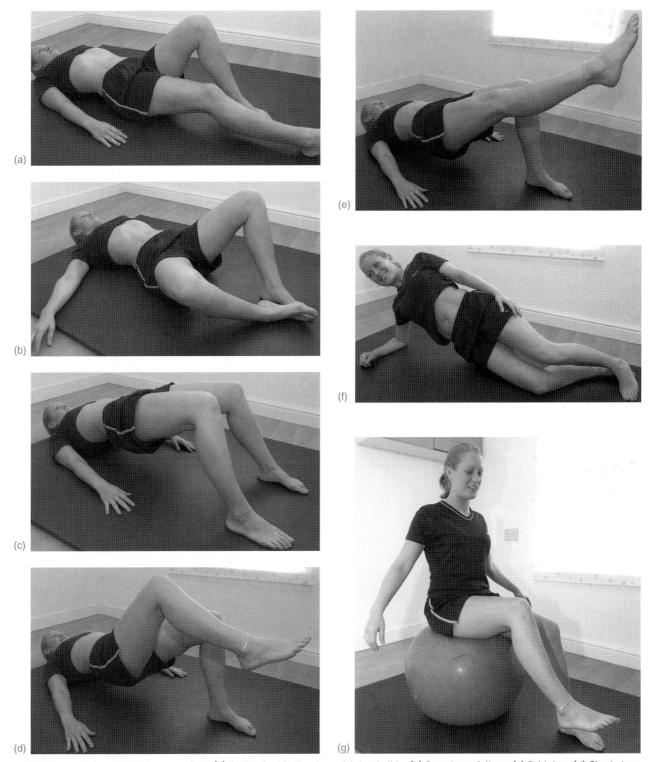

Figure 14.29   Lumbar stabilization exercises. (a) Abdominal hollowing with heel slide. (b) Bent knee fallout. (c) Bridging. (d) Single leg bridge. (e) Single leg bridge with leg straightening. (f) Side support. (g) Gym ball.

the transversus acts at the initiation of movement to stabilize the trunk in overhead and lower limb actions (Hodges, Richardson and Jull, 1996).

In sport, the abdominal muscles essentially function to stabilize the trunk and provide a firm base of support for the arms and legs to work against. If stability is poor (in relation to total power of the athlete), limb actions will cause unwanted displacement of the pelvis and trunk. If we take an overhead pressing movement as an example (Fig. 14.31), where core stability is poor, the neutral position of the spine (p. 137) is lost and the spine is forced into potentially dangerous hyperextension.

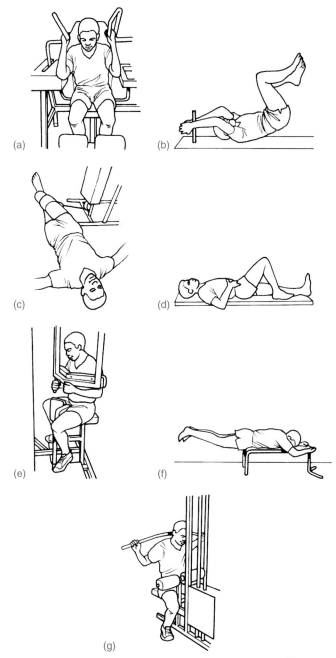

Figure 14.30 Examples of resistance exercises. Stage II (a) sitting abdominal curl, (b) reverse crunch, (c) lying cable trunk rotation, (d) heel slide, (e) sitting trunk rotation, (f) prone leg extension, (g) lateral pull-down. From Norris, C.M. (2000) *Back Stability*. Human Kinetics, Champaign, Illinois. With permission.

Analysis of conventional exercises

Two exercises underlie most abdominal training, the *sit-up* and the *leg-raise*, and we will look at these movements to determine their usefulness.

The sit-up

The sit-up is essentially an action where an athlete comes from a supine lying to a long sitting position by performing

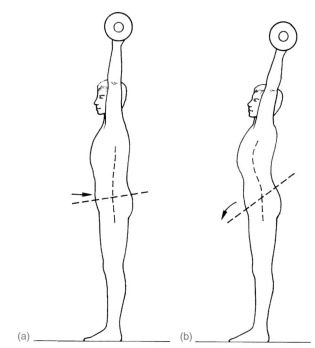

Figure 14.31 Trunk stability in overhead pressing actions. (a) Abdominals pulled in tight, pelvis level. Trunk actively stable, reducing stress on lumbar tissues. (b) Abdominals lax, pelvis tilted. Trunk passively stable, increasing stress on lumbar tissues.

hip flexion, usually with trunk flexion. There are several modifications of this action which will be dealt with below.

In a classic sit-up, as soon as the head lifts, activity is seen in the rectus abdominis, and as a consequence the rib cage is depressed anteriorly. This initial period of flexion emphasizes the supra-umbilical portion of the rectus, the infra-umbilical portion and the internal oblique contracting later (Kendall and McCreary, 1993). As the internal oblique contracts, it pulls on the lower ribs, causing the ribs to flare out and so increase the infra-sternal angle.

Abdominal 'doming' and pelvic fixation   One of the problems that poorly toned individuals face is bow-stringing or 'doming' of the abdominals, which is often seen at the initiation of the sit-up action. For the superficial abdominals (rectus abdominus and external oblique) to pull flat, the deep abdominals (transversus abdominus and internal oblique) must be strong enough to perform an abdominal hollowing action and act as stabilizers, holding the rectus sheath down. Where the deep abdominals are weak and the superficial abdominals are lengthened, the abdominal wall will be seen to dome and the athlete may lift the trunk with the lumbar spine extended or flat rather than flexed (Fig. 14.32).

Definition
Abdominal doming is said to occur when the abdominal wall bulges rather than flattens during a trunk exercise.

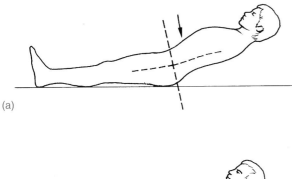

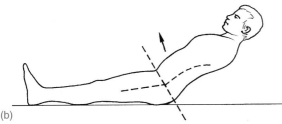

Figure 14.32 Trunk alignment during a sit-up exercise. (a) Deep abdominals pull abdominal wall flat. (b) Deep abdominals allow abdominal wall to 'dome', lengthened superficial abdominals allow anterior pelvic tilt, and hollow back.

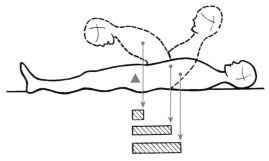

Figure 14.33 Changing leverage of the trunk. As the trunk flexes, the centre of gravity of the upper body moves closer to the hip, reducing the leverage effect. From Norris (1994a), with permission.

Definition

A flexor synergy occurs when several flexor muscles work together to perform an action, in this case anterior motion of the lower limb.

Fixation of the pelvis is provided by the hip flexors, especially iliacus through its attachment to the pelvic rim. The strong pull of the hip flexors is partially counteracted by the pull of the lateral fibres of external oblique and the infra-umbilical portion of the rectus abdominis, which tend to tilt the pelvis posteriorly. Action of the external oblique, if powerful enough, will compress the ribs and reduce the infra-sternal angle once more (Kendall, McCreary and Provance, 1993).

Effects of foot fixation   If the sit-up action is attempted from the supine lying position without allowing trunk flexion, there is a tendency for the legs to lift up from the supporting surface. This occurs because the legs constitute roughly one third of the body weight and the trunk two-thirds.

As the abdominal muscles flex the spine, the centre of gravity of the upper body is moved caudally. Movement of the centre of gravity in this fashion reduces the lever arm of the trunk enabling the subject to sit up without the legs lifting (Fig. 14.33).

In cases where the abdominal muscles are weak, maximum spinal flexion will not occur and so the lever arm of the trunk remains long. Now, the greater weight and lever arm of the trunk causes it to remain on the floor and the legs are seen to lift.

If the feet are fixed, the hip flexors can now pull powerfully without causing the legs to lift. In addition, the act of foot fixation itself may facilitate the iliopsoas (Janda and Schmid, 1980). Foot fixation requires the subject to pull against the fixation point by active dorsiflexion. This process stimulates the gait pattern at heel contact, increasing activity in the tibialis anterior, quadriceps and iliopsoas (flexor synergy).

Modifications of the sit-up
The bent knee sit-up and trunk curl   The bent knee sit-up is performed from the crook-lying starting position, with the knees flexed to 90° and hips flexed to 45°. The action is one of trunk flexion followed by, or performed with, hip flexion. The trunk curl is performed from the same starting position, but no hip flexion occurs, the lumbar spine remaining in contact with the supporting surface. The bench-curl is performed from a starting position of 90° hip flexion, the shin being supported on a bench or chair.

Bending the knees and hips to alter the starting position of the sit-up will affect both the passive and active actions of the hip flexors, and the biomechanics of the lumbar spine. In supine lying, the iliopsoas is on stretch, and aligned with the horizontal (Fig. 14.34). In this position, vertebral compression is at its greatest as the muscle contracts, and trunk lifting is at a mechanical disadvantage. The ratio of lifting to compression is therefore approximately 1:10 (Watson, 1983). As the knees are flexed, the iliopsoas is pulled more vertically and so the ratio of trunk lifting to vertebral compression is reduced to 2:5 in crook lying and 1:1 in bench lying.

With 45° hip flexion, tension development in the iliopsoas has been shown to be 70–80% of its maximum, while with the hips and knees flexed to 90° this figure reduces to between 40 and 50% (Johnson and Reid, 1991).

However, passive tension developed by the iliopsoas due to elastic recoil must also be considered. If the hips are flexed, the iliopsoas will not be fully stretched, and will not be able to passively limit the posterior tilt of the pelvis. Instead, to fix the pelvis and provide a stable base for the abdominals to pull on, the hip flexors will contract earlier in the sit-up action. This contraction, although occurring earlier, is of reduced intensity (Walters and Partridge, 1957) due to the length–tension relationship of the muscle.

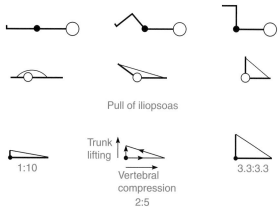

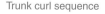

Trunk curl sequence

1. Pelvic tilt
2. Hollowing
3. Fingers to heels

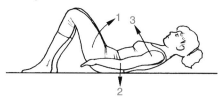

Figure 14.35 Trunk curl sequence.

Figure 14.34 Mechanical advantage of iliopsoas during the sit-up. As the hip is flexed, the moment arm of the iliopsoas is lengthened. The muscle can therefore complete the sit-up action by using less force, and so vertebral compression is reduced. From Norris (1994a), with permission.

With the legs straight in the traditional sit-up position, the iliopsoas is stretched, and can passively limit posterior tilting of the pelvis. However, in this stretched position, the iliopsoas is capable of exerting greater force during hip flexion. If the abdominal muscles are too weak to maintain the position of the pelvis, the stronger hip flexors will hyperextend the lumbar spine and cause the pelvis to tilt forwards, lengthening the abdominals, and hyperextending the lumbar spine. This type of action is, therefore, unsuitable for postural re-education if the aim is to shorten posturally lengthened abdominal muscles.

Correction of posturally lengthened abdominals If the subject has lengthened abdominals, these are shortened by performing an inner range holding movement. This action is a modification of the trunk curl to combine three actions (Norris, 1994a, 1994b). The subject posteriorly tilts the pelvis, performs abdominal hollowing, and depresses the rib cage while exhaling (Fig. 14.35). Maximum trunk flexion is attempted, providing this is not contraindicated by lumbar pathology. If abdominal lengthening has occurred, the subject will show a greater passive range of motion than active range of motion to lumbar flexion.

Keypoint

If abdominal lengthening has occurred, athletes will show a greater passive than active range of motion to lumbar flexion. This is corrected using inner range training and eccentric muscle work.

To correct this, an eccentric action is used. The subject uses his or her finger tips on the outside of the knees to pull the body into full passive lumbar flexion. They set the abdominal muscles and attempt to hold this position as they let the hand grip relax. Initially, they will only be able to decelerate the lowering action using an eccentric contraction of the target muscles. As muscle adaptation occurs, the movement will become more controlled and slower. Eventually an isometric hold will become possible and finally a concentric action. Once this is achieved, full range exercise is begun, using slow movements building up to a total repetition time of 10–30 seconds.

Straight-leg raising

The bilateral straight leg raise has been shown to create only slight activity in the upper rectus, although the lower rectus contributes a greater proportion of the total abdominal work than with the sit-up (Lipetz and Gutin, 1970). The rectus works isometrically to fix the pelvis against the strong pull of iliopsoas (Silvermetz, 1990). The force of contraction of the iliopsoas is at its maximum when the lever arm of the leg is greatest, near the horizontal, and reduces as the leg is lifted towards the vertical.

In subjects with weaker abdominals, the pelvis will tilt and the lumbar spine will hyperextend. This forced hyperextension will dramatically increase stress on the facet joints particularly in the lumbar spine. The movement is likely to be limited by impaction of the inferior articular processes on the laminae of the vertebrae below, or in some cases by contact between the spinous processes (Twomey and Taylor, 1987). Where this action occurs rapidly, damage may result to the facet joint structures. Once contact has occurred between the facet and lamina, further loading will cause axial rotation of the superior vertebra (Yang and King, 1984). The superior vertebra pivots, causing the inferior articular process to move backwards overstretching the joint capsule.

Modification of straight-leg raising As none of the abdominal muscles actually cross the hip, they are not prime movers of the straight-leg raising movement. However, the action is an important one as it emphasizes the pelvic stabilizing function of the infra-umbilical portion of the rectus abdominis, and lateral external oblique.

A number of exercises serve as modifications of the bilateral straight leg raise to reduce the stress on the lumbar spine. The first action is the *heel slide* (Fig. 14.36a). From a crook-lying starting position an abdominal hollowing action is performed to stabilize the spine (p. 000). From this position,

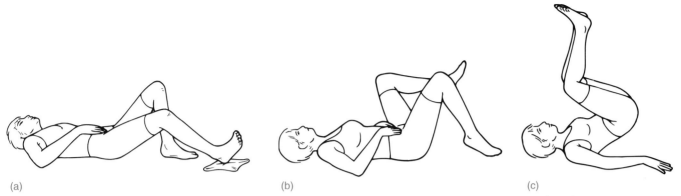

Figure 14.36   Modifications of the straight-leg raise. (a) Heelslide. (b) Leg lowering. (c) Pelvic raise. From Norris (2001), with permission.

one leg is straightened while keeping the heel on the ground and sliding the leg into extension.

The second movement is *leg lowering* (Fig. 14.36b). For this exercise the subject lies supine with the knees and hips bent to 90°. From this position, the lumbar spine is gently flattened into the mat and one leg is lowered by eccentric action of the hip flexors while maintaining the flat contour of the abdomen (avoiding doming) and not allowing any pelvic tilt.

The third exercise uses leg and *pelvic motion* on a fixed trunk to increase the emphasis on the lower abdominals. The subject begins the action in crook lying and draws the knees right up onto the chest (Fig. 14.36c). The action is then a posterior pelvic tilt combined with abdominal hollowing to flex the lower lumbar spine and raise the sacrum off the supporting surface. Again the repetition time is gradually increased to 10–30 seconds. Because both of these exercises flex the lumbar spine, a passive extension action, such as extension in lying and anterior pelvic tilting, should be performed at the end of the exercise bout to compensate for flexion stresses.

References

Adams, M.A. and Hutton, W.C. (1982) Prolapsed intervertebral disc: a hyperflexion injury. *Spine*, **8**, (3) 327

Adams, M.A. and Hutton, W.C. (1983) The mechanical function of the lumbar apophyseal joints. *Spine*, **8**, 327–330

Adams, M.A., Hutton, W.C. and Stott, J.R.R. (1980) The resistance to flexion of the lumbar intervertebral joint. *Spine*, **5**, 245–253

Beattie, P.F., Brooks, W.M. and Rothstein, J.M. (1994) Effect of lordosis on the position of the nucleus pulposus in supine subjects: a study using MRI. *Spine*, **19**, (18) 2096–2102

Bergmark, A. (1989) Stability of the lumbar spine. *Acta Orthopaedica Scandinavica Supplementum*, **230**, (60) 3–54

Bernhardt, M., White, A.A., Panjabi, M.M. and McGowan, D.P. (1992) Lumbar spine instability. In *The Lumbar Spine and Back Pain* (ed. M.I.V. Jayson), 4th edn, Churchill Livingstone, Edinburgh

Bogduk, N. and Engel, R. (1984) The menisci of the lumbar zygapophyseal joints: a review of their anatomy and clinical significance. *Spine*, **9**, 454–460

Bogduk, N. and Jull, G. (1985) The theoretical pathology of acute locked back: a basis for manipulative therapy. *Manual Medicine*, **1**, 78–82

Bogduk, N. and Twomey, L.T. (1987) *Clinical Anatomy of the Lumbar Spine*, Churchill Livingstone, Edinburgh

Bogduk, N. and Twomey, L.T. (1991) *Clinical Anatomy of the Lumbar Spine*, 2nd edn, Churchill Livingstone, Edinburgh

Butler, D.S. (1991) *Mobilisation of the Nervous System*, Churchill Livingstone, Edinburgh

Cappozzo, A., Felici, F., Figura, F. and Gazzani, F. (1985) Lumbar spine loading during half-squat exercises. *Medicine and Science in Sports and Exercise*, **17**, (5) 613–620

Ciullo, J.V. and Jackson, D.W. (1985) Pars interarticularis stress reaction, spondylolysis, and spondylolisthesis in gymnasts. *Clinics in Sports Medicine*, **4**, 95–110

Colcher, A.E. and Hursh, A.M.W. (1952) Pre-employment low back X-ray survey: a review of 1500 cases. *Industrial Medicine and Surgery*, **21**, 319

Corrigan, B. and Maitland, G.D. (1983) *Practical Orthopaedic Medicine*, Butterworth, London

Crock, H.V. and Yoshizawa, H. (1976) The blood supply of the lumbar vertebral column. *Clinical Orthopaedics*, **115**, 6–21

Clinical Standards Advisory Group (CSAG) (1994) *Reports on Back Pain*, HMSO, London

Cyriax, J. (1982) *Textbook of Orthopaedic Medicine*, 8th edn, Baillière Tindall, London, vol. 1

Cyriax, J.H. and Cyriax, P.J. (1983) *Illustrated Manual of Orthopaedic Medicine*, Butterworth, London

Don Tigny, R.L. (1985) Function and pathomechanics of the sacroiliac joint. *Physical Therapy*, **65**, 35–44

Dreyfuss, P., Dreyer, S., Griffin, J., Hoffman, J. and Walsh, N. (1992) Positive sacroiliac screening tests in asymptomatic adults. *Proceedings of the First Interdisciplinary World Congress on Low Back Pain and its Relation to the Sacroiliac Joint*. San Diego, CA

Edmondston, S.J., Song, S. and Bricknell, R.V. (2000) MRI evaluation of lumbar spine flexion and extension in asymptomatic individuals. *Manual Therapy*, **5**, (3) 158–164

Farfan, H.F., Cossette, J.W., Robertson, G.H., Wells, R.V. and Kraus, H. (1970) The effects of torsion on the lumbar intervertebral joints: the role of torsion in the production of disc degeneration. *Journal of Bone and Joint Surgery*, **52A**, 468

Farfan, H.F., Osteria, V. and Lamy, C. (1976) The mechanical etiology of spondylolysis and spondylolisthesis. *Clinical Orthopaedics and Related Research*, **117**, 40–55

Fennell, A.J., Jones, A.P. and Hukins, D.W.L. (1996) Migration of the nucleus pulposus within the intervertebral disc during flexion and extension of the spine. *Spine*, **21**, (23) 2753–2757

Frigerio, N.A., Stowe, R.R. and Howe, J.W. (1974) Movement of the sacro-iliac joint. *Clinical Orthopaedic and Related Research*, **100**, 370

Fryomoyer, J.W. and Cats-Baril, W.L. (1991) An overview of the incidences and costs of low back pain. *Orthopaedic Clinics of North America*, **22**, 263

Gould (1990) *Orthopedic and Sports Physical Therapy*, C.V. Mosby, St. Louis

Grieve, G.P. (1970) Sciatica and the straight leg raising test in manipulative treatment. *Physiotherapy*, **56**, 337

Grieve, G.P. (1976) The sacro-iliac joint. *Physiotherapy*, **62**, (12) 384–400

Guimaraes, A.C.S., Vaz, M.A., De Campos, M.I.A. and Marantes, R. (1991) The contribution of the rectus abdominus and rectus femoris in 12 selected abdominal exercises. *Journal of Sports Medicine and Physical Fitness*, **31**, 222–230

Harreby, M., Hesseloe, G., Kier, J. and Neergaard, K. (1997) Low back pain and physical exercise in leisure time in 38 year old men and women. *European Spinal Journal*, **6**, 181–186

Hirsch, C. and Nachemson, A. (1954) New observations on mechanical behaviour of lumbar discs. *Acta Orthopaedica Scandinavica*, **22**, 184–189

Hirsch, C. and Schajowicz, F. (1952) Studies on structural changes in the lumbar annulus fibrosis. *Acta Orthopaedica Scandinavica*, **22**, 184–189

Hirsch, C., Ingelmark, V.E. and Miller, N. (1963) The anatomic basis for low back pain: studies on the presence of sensory endings in ligamentous capsular and intervertebral disc structures in the human lumbar spine. *Acta Orthopaedica Scandinavica*, **33**, 1–17

Hodges, P., Richardson, C. and Jull, G. (1996). Evaluation of the relationship between laboratory and clinical tests of transverses abdominus function. *Physiotherapy Research International*, **1**, 30–40

Holm, S., Maroudas, A., Urban, J.P.G., Selstam, G. and Nachemson, A. (1981) Nutrition of the intervertebral disc: solute transport and metabolism. *Connective Tissue Research*, **8**, 101–119

Hoshina, H. (1980) Spondylolysis in young athletes. *Physician and Sports Medicine*, **8**, 75–79

Hukins, D.W.L. (1987) Properties of spinal materials. In *The Lumbar Spine and Back Pain* (ed. M.I.V. Jayson), Churchill Livingstone, London

Irion, J.M. (1992) Use of the gym ball in rehabilitation of spinal dysfunction. *Orthopaedic Physical Therapy Clinics of North America*, **23**, 375–398

Janda, V. and Schmid, H.J.A. (1980) Muscles as a pathogenic factor in back pain. *Proceedings of the International Federation of Orthopaedic Manipulative Therapists, 4th Conference*, 17–18, New Zealand

Johnson, C. and Reid, J.G. (1991) Lumbar compressive and shear forces during various curl up exercises. *Clinical Biomechanics*, **6**, 97–104

Kapandji, I. (1974) *The Physiology of Joints*, vol. 3, *The Spine*, Churchill Livingstone, London

Kendall, F.P., McCreary, E.K. and Provance, P.G. (1993) *Muscles: Testing and Function*, 4th edn, Williams and Wilkins, Baltimore

Kesson, M. and Atkins, E. (1998) *Orthopaedic Medicine*, Butterworth-Heinemann, Oxford

Klein, J.A. and Hukins, D.W.L. (1981) Functional differentiation in the spinal column. *Engineering in Medicine*, **12**, (2) 83

Klein, J.A. and Hukins, D.W.L. (1983) Relocation of the bending axis during flexion–extension of the lumbar intervertebral discs and its implications for prolapse. *Spine*, **8**, 659–664

Kotanis, P.T., Ichikawa, N., Wakabayashi, W., Yoshii, T. and Koshimune, M. (1971) Studies of spondylolysis found among weight lifters. *British Journal of Sports Medicine*, **6**, 4

Kraemer, J., Kolditz, D. and Gowin, R. (1985) Water and electrolyte content of human intervertebral discs under variable load. *Spine*, **10**, 69–71

Laslett, M. (1997) Pain provocation sacroiliac joint tests. In *Movement Stability and Low Back Pain* (eds A. Vleeming, V. Mooney, T. Dorman, C. Snijders and R. Stoeckart), Churchill Livingstone, Edinburgh

Laslett, M. and Williams, M. (1994) The reliability of selected pain provocation tests for sacroiliac pathology. *Spine*, **19**, 1243–1249

Leatt, P., Reilly, T. and Troup, J.G.D. (1986) Spinal loading during circuit weight-training and running. *British Journal of Sports Medicine*, **20**, (3) 119–124

Lee, D.G. (1994) Clinical manifestations of pelvic girdle dysfunction. In *Grieve's Modern Manual Therapy*, 2nd edn (eds J.D. Boyling and N. Palastanga), Churchill Livingstone, Edinburgh

Lehman, G.J. and McGill, S.M. (2001) Quantification of the differences in electromyographic activity magnitude between the upper and lower portions of the rectus abdominis muscle during selected trunk exercises. *Physical Therapy*, **81**, (5) 1096–1101

Lester, M.N. (1992) Spinal stabilization and compliance utilizing the therapeutic ball. *Proceeding of the International Federation of Orthopaedic Manipulative Therapists*, Vail, Colorado

Lester, M.N. and Posner-Mayer, J. (1993) *Spinal Stabilization: Utilizing the Swiss Ball* (video), Ball Dynamics, Denver

Letts, M., Smallman, T., Afanasiev, R. and Gouw, G. (1985) Fracture of the pars interarticularis in adolescent athletes: a clinical-biomechanical analysis. *Journal of Paediatric Orthopaedics*, **6**, 40–46

Lipetz, S. and Gutin, B. (1970) An electromyographic study of four abdominal exercises. *Medicine and Science in Sports and Exercise*, **2**, 35–38

McKenzie, R.A. (1981) *The Lumbar Spine: Mechanical Diagnosis and Therapy*, Spinal Publications New Zealand, Waikanae

McKenzie, R.A. (1990) *The Cervical and Thoracic Spine: Mechanical Diagnosis and Therapy*, Spinal Publications New Zealand, Waikanae

McKenzie, R. and May, S. (2003) *The Lumbar Spine: Mechanical Diagnosis and Therapy*, Spinal Publications New Zealand, Waikanae

Magee, D.J. (2002) *Orthopedic Physical Assessment*, 4th edn, Saunders, Philadelphia

Maitland, G.D. (1986) *Vertebral Manipulation*, 5th edn, Butterworth, London

Markolf, K.L. and Morris, J.M. (1974) The structural components of the intervertebral disc. *Journal of Bone and Joint Surgery*, **56A**, 675

Mens, J.M.A., Vleeming, A., Snijders, C.J. and Stam, H.J. (1997) Active straight leg raising test: a clinical approach to the load transfer function of the pelvic girdle. In *Movement Stability and Low Back Pain* (eds A. Vleeming, V. Mooney and T. Dorman), Churchill Livingstone, Edinburgh

Mooney, V. and Robertson, J. (1976) The facet syndrome. *Clinical Orthopaedics*, **115**, 149–156

Mulligan, B.R. (1989) *Manual Therapy – Nags, Snags, and PRPs etc.*, Plane View Services, Wellington, New Zealand

Nachemson, A. (1976) The lumbar spine: an orthopaedic challenge. *Spine*, **1**, 59–71

Nachemson, A. (1987) Lumbar intradiscal pressure. In *The Lumbar Spine and Back Pain* (ed. M.I.V. Jayson), Churchill Livingstone, London

Nachemson, A. and Evans, J. (1968) Some mechanical properties of the third lumbar inter-laminar ligament (ligamentum flavum). *Journal of Biomechanics*, **1**, 211

Nelson, M.A., Allen, P., Clamp, S.E. and De Dombal, F.T. (1979) Reliability and reproducibility of clinical findings in low back pain. *Spine*, **4**, 97–101

Norkin, C.C. and Levangie, P.K. (1992) *Joint Structure and Function: A Comprehensive Analysis*, 2nd edn, F.A. Davis, Philadelphia

Norris, C.M. (1993) Abdominal muscle training in sport. *British Journal of Sports Medicine*, **27**, (1) 19–27

Norris, C.M. (1994a) Abdominal training: dangers and exercise modifications. *Physiotherapy in Sport*, **14**, (5) 10–14

Norris, C.M. (1994b) A flat stomach – the right way. *Exercise Magazine*, November

Norris, C.M. (1995) Spinal stabilisation 2. Limiting factors to end-range motion in the lumbar spine. *Physiotherapy*, **81**, (2) 4–12

Norris, C.M. (2000) *Back Stability*, Human Kinetics, Champaign, Illinois, USA

Norris (2001) *Acupuncture: Treatment of Musculoskeletal Conditions*, Butterworth-Heinemann, Oxford

O'Sullivan, P.B. (2000) Lumbar segmental instability. *Manual Therapy*, **5**, (1) 2–12

O'Sullivan, P.B., Twomey, L.T. and Allison, G.T. (1997) Evaluation of specific stabilizing exercise in the treatment of chronic low back pain with radiologic diagnosis of spondylolysis or spondylolisthesis. *Spine*, **22**, 2959–2967

Oliver, J. and Middleditch, A. (1991) *Functional Anatomy of the Spine*, Butterworth-Heinemann, Oxford

Palastanga, N., Field, D. and Soames, R. (1989) Anatomy and Human Movement, Butterworth-Heinemann, Oxford

Panjabi, M.M. (1992) The stabilizing system of the spine. Part 1. Function, dysfunction, adaptation, and enhancement. *Journal of Spinal Disorders*, **5**, (4) 383–389

Panjabi, M.M., Hult, J.E. and White, A.A. (1987) Biomechanical studies in cadaveric spines. In *The Lumbar Spine and Back Pain* (ed. M.I.V. Jayson), Churchill Livingstone, London

Panjabi, M.M., Jorneus, L. and Greenstein, G. (1984) *Lumbar Spine Ligaments: An In Vitro Biomechanical Study*, ORS Transactions

Paris, S.V. (1985) Physical signs of instability. *Spine*, **10**, (3) 277–279

Pearcy, P., Portek, I. and Shepherd, J. (1984) Three dimensional X-ray analysis of normal movement in the lumbar spine. *Spine*, **9**, 294–297

Potter, N.A. and Rothstein, J.M. (1985) Intertester reliability for selected clinical tests of the sacroiliac joint. *Physical Therapy*, **65**, 1671–1675

Reid, D.C. (1992) *Sports Injury Assessment and Rehabilitation*, Churchill Livingstone, London

Richardson, C., Toppenberg, R. and Jull, G. (1990) An initial evaluation of eight abdominal exercises for their ability to provide stabilization for the lumbar spine. *Australian Journal of Physiotherapy*, **36**, 6–11

Richardson, C.A. (1992) Muscle imbalance: principles of treatment and assessment. *Proceedings of the New Zealand Society of Physiotherapists Challenges Conference*, Christchurch, New Zealand

Richardson, C.A. and Jull, G.A. (1994) Concepts of assessment and rehabilitation for active lumbar stability. In *Grieve's Modern Manual Therapy* (eds J.D. Boyling and N. Palastanga), 2nd edn, Churchill Livingstone, Edinburgh

Roaf, R. (1960) A study of the mechanics of spinal injuries. *Journal of Bone and Joint Surgery (Br)*, **42B**, 810–823

Rockoff, S.F., Sweet, E. and Bleustein, J. (1969) The relative contribution of trabecular and cortical bone to the strength of human lumbar vertebrae. *Calcified Tissue Research*, **3**, 163–175

Silvermetz, M.A. (1990) Pathokinesiology of supine double leg lifts as an abdominal strengthener and suggested alternative exercises. *Athletic Training*, **25**, 17–22

Spitzer, W.O., LeBlanc, F.E. and Dupuis, M. (1987) Scientific approach to the assessment and management of activity related spinal disorders: a monograph for clinicians. Report of the Quebec Task Force on Spinal Disorders. *Spine*, **12**, 7s

Taylor, J.R. and Twomey, L.T. (1986) Age changes in lumbar zygapophyseal joints. *Spine*, **11**, 739–745

Taylor, J.R. and Twomey, L.T. (1994) The lumbar spine from infancy to old age. In *Physical Therapy of the Low Back*, 2nd edn (eds L.T. Twomey and J.R. Taylor), Churchill Livingstone, Edinburgh

Thompson, B. (2002) How should athletes with chronic low back pain be managed in primary care? In *Evidence Based Sports Medicine* (eds D. MacAuley and T. Best), BMJ Books, London

Tkaczuk, H. (1968) Tensile properties of human lumbar longitudinal ligaments. *Acta Orthopaedica Scandinavica*, **115** (Suppl.)

Tropp, H., Alaranta, H. and Renstrom, P.A.F.H. (1993) Proprioception and coordination training in injury prevention. In *Sports Injuries: Basic Principles of Prevention and Care* (ed. P.A.F.H. Renstrom), IOC Medical Commission Publication, Blackwell Scientific, London

Turner, H. (2002) *The Sacro Iliac Joint*, Course notes, Manchester, UK

Twomey, L.T. and Taylor, J.R. (1987) Lumbar posture, movement and mechanics. In *Physical Therapy of the Low Back* (ed. L.T. Twomey), Churchill Livingstone, New York

Tyrrell, A.R., Reilly, T. and Troup, J.D.G. (1985) Circadian variation in stature and the effects of spinal loading. *Spine*, **10**, 161–164

Urban, L.M. (1986) The straight-leg raising test: a review. In *Modern Manual Therapy of the Vertebral Column* (ed. G.P. Grieve), Churchill Livingstone, London

Van Duersen, L.L., Patijn, J., Ockhuysen, A.L. and Vortman, B.J. (1990) The value of some clinical tests of the sacroiliac joint. *Manual Medicine*, **5**, 96–99.

Van Tulder, M., Malmivaara, A., Esmail, R. and Koes, B. (2000) Exercise therapy for low back pain: a systematic review within the framework of the Cochrane Collaboration Back Review Group. *Spine*, **25**, 2784–2796

Vernon-Roberts, B. (1987) Pathology of intervertebral discs and apophyseal joints. In *The Lumbar Spine and Back Pain* (ed. M.I.V. Jayson), Churchill Livingstone, London

Vleeming, A., Mooney, V., Dorman, T. and Snijders, C. (1997) *Movement Stability and Low Back Pain*, Churchill Livingstone, Edinburgh

Vleeming, A., Pool-Goudzwaard, A.L., Stoeckart, R., Wingerden, J.P. and Snijders, C.J. (1995) The posterior layer of the thoracolumbar fascia: its function in load transfer from spine to legs. *Spine*, **20**, 753–758

Waddell, G., Feder, G. and Lewis, M. (1997) Systematic reviews of bed rest and advice to stay active for acute low back pain. *British Journal of General Practice*, **47**, 647–652

Walters, C. and Partridge, M. (1957) Electromyographic study of the differential abdominal muscles during exercise. *American Journal of Physical Medicine*, **36**, 259–268

Watson, J. (1983) *An Introduction for Mechanics of Human Movement*, MTP Press, Lancaster, UK

Weber, M.D. and Woodall, W.R. (1991) Spondylogenic disorders in gymnasts. *Journal of Orthopaedic and Sports Physical Therapy*, **14**, (1) 6–13

Wells, P. (1986) The examination of the pelvic joints. In *Modern Manual Therapy of the Vertebral Column* (ed. G.P. Grieve), Churchill Livingstone, London

Williams, J.G.P. and Sperryn, P.N. (1976) *Sports Medicine*, Edward Arnold, London

Wyke, B. (1972) Articular neurology: a review. *Physiotherapy*, **58**, 94

Yang, K.H. and King, A.I. (1984) Mechanism of facet load transmission as a hypothesis for low-back pain. *Spine*, **9**, 557–565

Chapter 15

The thorax and thoracic spine

CHAPTER CONTENTS

THORACIC SPINE

The unique feature of the vertebrae in the thoracic region is the presence of facets, both on the sides of the vertebral bodies and the transverse processes. These are for articulation with the ribs, forming the costovertebral and costotransverse joints (Fig. 15.1). Most of the ribs articulate with two adjacent vertebral bodies and one transverse process. The facets on the head of the ribs articulate in turn with demifacets on the upper and lower borders of the vertebrae, and the crest on the rib head butts onto the intervertebral disc. The joint capsule is loose and strengthened anteriorly to form the three portions of the radiate ligament. The costovertebral joint cavity is divided into two by the intraarticular ligament, except for ribs one, ten, eleven and twelve which articulate with a single vertebra and have a single joint cavity.

The costotransverse joints are formed only with the upper ten ribs. The joint is made between the articular facet of the transverse process and the oval facet on the rib tubercle. The thin joint capsule is strengthened by the costotransverse ligaments.

Definition

The costovertebral joint is formed between the rib and the vertebral body, the costotransverse joint is formed between the rib and the transverse process of the vertebra.

STERNAL ARTICULATIONS

The sternocostal joints are formed between the medial end of the costal cartilages of ribs one to seven. The joint between the first rib and the sternum is cartilaginous, but all the others are synovial. Each is surrounded by a capsule and supported by radiate ligaments. The fibres of these ligaments fan out and intertwine with those of the ligaments above and below, and also with those of the opposite sternocostal joints. In addition, the radiate ligament fibres fuse with the

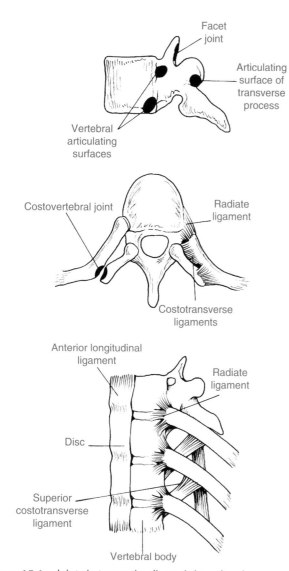

Figure 15.1   Joints between the ribs and thoracic spine.

tendinous fibres of the pectoralis major. The eighth, ninth, and tenth ribs form interchondral joints between their costal cartilages.

The costochondral joints are formed between the end of the rib and the lateral edge of the costal cartilage. The joint formed is cartilaginous, its perichondrium being continuous with the periosteum of the rib itself. Only slight bending and twisting actions are possible at this joint. The manubriosternal articulation is that between the upper part of the sternum and the manubrium. The joint is cartilaginous, with a hollow disc in its centre, and is strengthened by the sternocostal ligaments and longitudinal fibrous bands. About 7° of movement occurs at the joint in association with breathing.

RIB MOVEMENTS

Movement of the diaphragm, ribs and sternum increases the volume within the thorax with inspiration. Each rib acts as a lever, with one axis travelling through the costovertebral and sternocostal joints, and another through the costovertebral and costotransverse joints. The two axes permit two types of motion, known as 'pump handle' and 'bucket handle'. In the pump handle action the upper ribs and sternum are raised, increasing the anteroposterior diameter of the thorax. With bucket handle motion the lower ribs move both up and out, widening the infrasternal angle and increasing the transverse diameter or the thorax. The variation in movement between the upper and lower ribs is due, in part, to the differing structure of their respective costotransverse joints. The upper joints are cup-shaped permitting mainly rotation (pump handle), while those lower down are flat permitting both rotation and gliding movements (bucket handle).

> **Keypoint**
>
> The ribs can move forwards and upwards, increasing the anteroposterior diameter of the thorax (pump handle), and outwards, increasing the lateral diameter of the thorax (bucket handle).

In addition to respiratory motion, the ribs also move in association with the thoracic spine. With flexion of the spine the ribs move closer together and with extension they are pulled further apart, flattening the rib cage. This latter action in the upper ribs is important for the correct movement of the scapulothoracic joint. Lateral flexion causes the ribs on the concave side to move together and those on the convex side to move apart. Rotation gives horizontal gliding of one rib relative to another.

Rib cage shape at rest

The general shape of the ribcage will change as a result of thoracic mobility, with an increased thoracic kyphosis causing a general flattening of the ribcage. In addition, congenital abnormalities occur. A *pigeon chest* is seen when the sternum is orientated downwards and the ribcage becomes pointed because the anteroposterior (AP) diameter is increased. *Funnel chest* occurs when the sternum is pushed backwards in relation to the ribcage, often due to an overgrowth of the ribs (Magee, 2002). On inspiration the depression of the sternum may become more noticeable. Finally, a *barrel chest* deformity occurs when the sternum is orientated forwards and upwards, increasing the AP diameter. This deformity is seen in some pathological lung conditions.

The ribcage will also alter shape in cases of scoliosis. The vertebral bodies rotate towards the convexity of the curve, dragging the ribs with them. The ribs on the convex side of the curve are pushed backwards creating a 'hump' and those on the concave side of the curve move anteriorly causing a 'hollow' (Fig. 15.2). Rotation of the vertebral body causes the

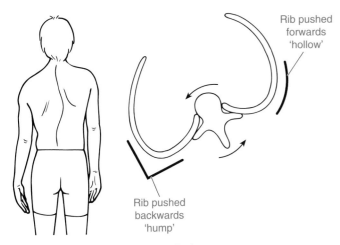

Rib pushed
forwards
'hollow'

Rib pushed
backwards
'hump'

Figure 15.2   Ribcage shape in scoliosis.

spinous processes to move away from the mid-line, in the opposite direction to the scoliosis. Right rotation of the vertebra therefore sees the spinous process deviating to the left.

Definition

Scoliosis is a deformity of the spine where a single or multiple lateral curvature is seen. The scoliosis is named according to the convexity (sharp point) of the curve.

MOVEMENT OF THE THORACIC SPINE

The relative thinness of the discs in the thoracic region, coupled with the presence of the ribs, makes movement here more limited than in other spinal areas. Extension is limited to about 30° with slightly more flexion being possible – roughly 40°. Flexion is freer in the lower thoracic region but still restricted by the ribs. Extension is limited by approximation of the facets and spinous processes as well as tissue tension, and causes the thoracic cage to become flatter. Lateral flexion is limited to roughly 25° to each side, a greater range being available in the lower region. Lateral flexion is accompanied by the same amount of rotation, which occurs contralaterally. For example, right lateral flexion is accompanied by right axial rotation, causing the tip of the spinous process to rest to the left of the mid-line. Rib movements accompany lateral flexion, with the ribs on the concave side compressing and those on the side of the convexity being pulled apart.

The range of rotation is larger than other movements, with 35° being possible to either side. However, when the spine is extended, both lateral flexion and rotation are dramatically reduced. As rotation occurs, the inferior facets of the upper vertebra slide laterally with respect to the lower vertebra, towards the direction of the rotation. Movement of the vertebra is accompanied by distortion of the ribs. The

rib cage becomes more rounded on the side to which the rotation is occurring, and flattens on the opposite side.

Rotation of the thoracic spine is an important constituent of locomotion. In walking, when the right leg swings forward, the lower trunk and the pelvis rotate to the left about the fixed left leg. To keep the head facing forwards the upper spine must rotate to the right, pulling the shoulders back into a forward facing direction. As the upper and lower parts of the spine are rotating in opposite directions, there is a point at which the two movements cancel each other out. This point is the intervertebral disc between T7 and T8 which is not subjected to any rotation, while those vertebra immediately above and below rotate maximally, but in opposite directions.

Keypoint

During walking and running the pelvis rotates to one direction and the shoulders and trunk to the other. The two movements cancel each other out at the T7/8 spinal disc where no rotation occurs at all.

EXAMINATION

The screening examination is essentially similar to that of the lumbar spine, except that rotation is the movement most likely to be revealing as this normally has the greatest range. Rotation is performed in a sitting position, with overpressure being given through the shoulders. Resisted flexion and extension may be performed in a lying or a sitting position. Resisted lateral flexion is tested in a standing position with the therapist initially at the patient's side. The patient's near wrist of the straight arm is gripped, as is the far shoulder. Stability is improved if the therapist widens his or her base of support by placing the near foot between those of the patient (Fig. 1.12, p. 13).

As rotation and lateral flexion accompany each other in the thoracic spine, it is often revealing to combine these movements at examination. Thoracic rotation is performed, and is followed by lateral flexion, first in one direction and then the other.

Palpation takes in the vertebrae, rib joints and ribs themselves, and is carried out with the patient in a prone position with the arms over the couch side to move the scapulae apart. Alternatively, posteroanterior (PA) pressures may be used with the thoracic spine extended using the elbow support prone-lying starting position. In a prone-lying position the spinous processes of the thoracic vertebrae are angled downwards like the scales of a fish. The thoracic vertebrae may be considered in threes, with the transverse processes being found relative to the spinous processes as shown in Table 15.1.

As an approximate guide to levels, the AC joint is normally aligned with the C7–T1 interspace, the spine of the scapula at T3 and the inferior scapular angle at T7.

Table 15.1   Palpation of the thoracic vertebrae

T1, 2, 3	At the same level as spinous process
T4, 5, 6	Between two successive levels
T7, 8, 9	Level with spinous process of vertebra below
T10	Level with vertebra below
T11	Between two successive levels
T12	At same level

Table 15.2   Rib palpation

Rib structure	Region of palpation
1st rib	Above clavicle, within supraclavicular fossa
2nd	End level with manubriosternal joint (angle of Louis)
4th	Lies on nipple line
7th	End level with xiphisternal joint
11th	Tip lies in mid-axillary line
12th	Tip level with L1
Rib angle	3–4 cm lateral to end of transverse process
Costochondral (CC) joint	3 cm lateral to parasternal line at 2nd rib, 12 cm lateral at 7th rib, 18 cm lateral at 10th rib
Costotransverse (CT) joint	Depression between transverse process and rib

The rib angles gradually spread out from the spine with the eighth rib being furthest (about 6 cm) from the mid-line. The rib angles can be palpated at the same levels as the transverse processes down to the T8/T9, by pushing the soft tissue to one side. The facet joints lie in the paravertebral sulci, and the transverse processes, which overlie the costotransverse joints, are found 3–4 cm from the mid-line. Guidelines for rib palpation are shown in Table 15.2.

Modifications to the slump test for the thoracic spine

The slump test was described on page 307. A variation of this test for the cervical and thoracic spine is to perform it in the long sitting position (Fig. 15.3a). From this position thoracic and lumbar flexion are added followed by cervical flexion (Fig. 15.3b). Altering the order of movement will change the neurodynamic demands (Butler and Slater, 1994), enabling the practitioner to refine the test. For example, performing cervical flexion before lumbar and thoracic flexion will challenge the cervical neural tissues more. The test can be further refined to place emphasis on the sympathetic trunk (Slater, Butler and Shacklock, 1994). This is especially relevant in the presence of sympathetic signs in conditions such as T4 syndrome, thoracic outlet syndrome and Raynaud's syndrome, and in cases where cervicothoracic conditions mimic cardiac disease. Sympathetic testing is achieved by adding components of lateral flexion and rotation of the thoracic spine and lateral flexion of the

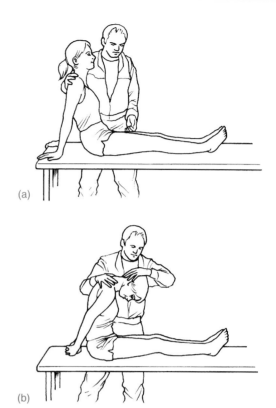

(a)

(b)

Figure 15.3   The slump test (long sitting). (a) Start. (b) Finish. From Butler (1991) with permission.

cervical spine. Additional stress may be imposed by adding a minimal straight leg raise (SLR).

> **Keypoint**
>
> Where sympathetic signs (skin changes, sweating, swelling) are present in conditions such as thoracic outlet syndrome (TOS) and Raynaud's syndrome, modify the slump test to emphasize the sympathetic trunk. Add thoracic lateral flexion and rotation, and cervical lateral flexion to the standard slump test.

INJURY TO THE RIB CAGE

Direct trauma to the rib cage can result in damage to the ribs, intercostal muscles or, indirectly, to the rib joints. Deep breathing will usually reproduce the pain of rib or intercostal injury, and palpation can be used to reveal the exact site of injury as these structures are superficial. Trunk extension will open the rib cage and cause pain, and intercostal muscle tearing will generally give pain to resisted trunk flexion. Rib springing at a distance from the point of injury usually produces pain from a rib fracture.

With rib fracture, it is the tearing of the intercostal muscles which gives the pain rather than the fracture itself (Cyriax, 1982). The acute pain may be relieved by local strapping.

Pre-stretched elastic adhesive strapping is applied across the area to restrict rib cage expansion and give the athlete a feeling of support. In the subacute phase active mobilization is required. If scar tissue formation is excessive and the source of pain, transverse frictions to the intercostal muscles along the line of the ribs are helpful. In addition, holding the rib down with the fingertips and practising deep inspiration will help to stretch the injured area. Exercises to expand the rib cage, such as deep inspiration and overhead reaching, or trunk lateral flexion to the contralateral side with or without rotation is also helpful to stretch the area.

> **Keypoint**
>
> Following rib injury, intercostal muscle stretching is useful. Deep breathing exercises coupled with manual therapy to isolate the movement to a single pair of ribs may also be used.

The sternocostal joints may be sprained giving local swelling and tenderness, as may the costochondral joints (Tietze's syndrome). Pressure on the sternum, or applied to the lateral aspect of the thorax, reproduces the pain, and palpation localizes the lesion. The injury can occur when performing exercises which force the arms into extension and abduction. Weight-training movements such as bench pressing and gymnastic exercises such as dips on parallel bars may both cause problems. Both the costovertebral and costotransverse joints may be subject to sprain, with pain occurring to rib movements and local palpation.

First rib

The first is the shortest and roundest of the ribs. It slopes downwards and forwards from its attachment to the first thoracic vertebra. It forms attachment for the scalene muscles, serratus anterior, and subclavius. Its superior surface bears a deep groove for the subclavian artery (posterior) and the subclavian vein (anterior). The arterial groove is the weakest part of the rib (Gurtler, Pavlov and Torg, 1985).

Fractures of the first rib may either be traumatic or the result of overuse. Overuse injuries have been reported as a result of repeated arm movements, such as heavy lifting and pitching (Bailey, 1985; Lankenner and Micheli, 1985; Gurtler, Pavlov and Torg, 1985). Symptoms are of pain associated with deep breathing, tenderness in the root of the neck, posterior aspect of the shoulder or axilla. Often the patient hears or feels a snap in the shoulder as when performing a sudden violent movement. Range of shoulder movement will usually be full but painful, especially to extension. Accurate diagnosis by radiographs in traumatic lesions is essential because of the proximity of the major vessels, nerves and lung. Bailey (1985) recommended serial radiographs for up to 6 months after stress fracture.

> **Keypoint**
>
> 1st rib injury gives pain on deep breathing. Tenderness is common at the root of the neck, posterior aspect of the shoulder or axilla. Shoulder extension may also cause pain.

Management is by rest from the causal action, with shoulder support in a sling if pain is limiting. Gentle isometric shoulder exercises are used, and the condition usually resolves within 4–6 weeks.

Rib displacement

Respiratory movements of the ribs may be used to assess anteroposterior position, by comparing one side of the body to the other. If a rib on one side stops moving before the rib on the other side during inhalation, the rib is said to be *depressed*. Inhalation involves an upward movement of the rib, so if the rib stops moving, it has been held down. Similarly, if the rib stops moving during exhalation (downward movement) it is said to be *elevated*, because it is being held in an upward position.

Movement may also be forward or backward. An *anterior displacement* may occur with a subluxation of the costovertebral joint, and the rib is sheared forwards. The rib will appear more prominent than its neighbour. This can occur in sport due to a blow to the back, typically when a knee hits the player on the back of the chest in rugby. A *posterior displacement* is more common and presents as a prominence of the rib angle. This is normally due to a blow to the chest, again from a tackle or through seatbelt or steering-wheel trauma in a road traffic accident (RTA). Management of rib displacement is by the use of muscle energy techniques (MET) and rib joint mobilization (see Treatment note 15.1).

MANUAL THERAPY

Joint mobilization

A variety of procedures may be used for the thoracic spine (see Fig. 15.3). Posteroanterior central vertebral pressure (PAVP) is the technique normally used first, in the presence of both unilateral and bilateral symptoms (Maitland, 1986). In the thoracic spine the spinous processes are larger than those of the cervical spine, and so the therapist may use the thumbs either side by side or one in front of the other. For the upper thoracic spine the therapist stands at the patient's head, and for the lower regions at the patient's side. An oscillatory motion is given with the range of movement being particularly great in the middle and lower thoracic areas, but somewhat limited between T1 and T2.

The *costovertebral* and *costotransverse* joints are mobilized by springing the rib. The therapist places his or her thumbs, or the ulnar border of the hand and little finger, along the line of the rib to be mobilized to give a broad (and more comfortable) area of contact. The mobilization must take the

Treatment note 15.1   Manual therapy techniques for rib displacement

Manual therapy techniques encourage correct rib movement during respiration. Essentially they force the rib into the opposite direction to the one in which they are being held. The rib may be bound down by scar tissue, requiring continuous stretching, or through muscle tightness/shortness, requiring PNF stretching. The intercostal muscles (forced expiration), oblique abdominals (trunk rotation), serratus anterior (scapular protraction), latissimus dorsi (arm adduction), scalenes (1st rib, neck sideflexion), and quadratus lumborum (12th rib, trunk sideflexion), should all be considered.

Elevation

An elevated rib does not move down far enough during expiration. The aim is to encourage this movement and draw the rib down as the patient breathes out. For the 1st rib pressure is placed over the rib with the knuckle (key grip) (Fig. 15.4). The head is sideflexed to relax the anterior scalene and the rib is pressed downwards with expiration. The 2nd rib is gripped within the axilla and pulled downwards as the patient exhales powerfully (Fig. 15.5). The remaining ribs may be gripped with the fingertips or pushed downwards using the knife edge of the hand (Fig. 15.6).

Depresssion

The depressed rib is bound down and stops moving upwards during inspiration. The aim is therefore to encourage further upward movement as the patient breathes in. For the 1st rib, stretch of the anterior scalenes is used (sideflex the neck to

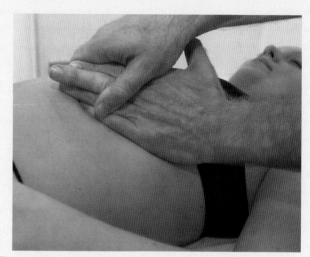

Figure 15.6   General rib mobilization for elevation.

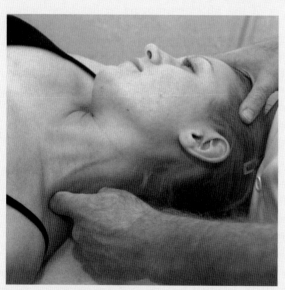

Figure 15.4   Mobilization of an elevated first rib.

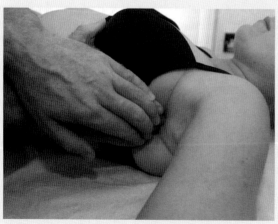

Figure 15.5   Mobilization of an elevated second rib.

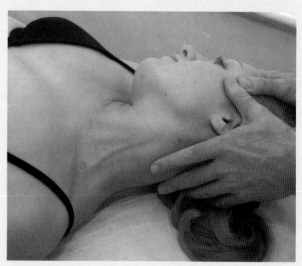

Figure 15.7   Treatment for a depressed first rib using anterior scalene stretch.

the opposite side) to pull the rib upwards (Fig. 15.7). For the 2nd rib the finger or thumb pads press on the rib within the axilla (Fig. 15.8), and for the remaining ribs the thumb pad or pisiform presses on the rib undersurface within the intercostal space (Fig. 15.9).

Anterior displacement

Where the rib lies further forward than the rib on the other side of the body, the aim is to open the rib cage and pull the rib backwards. For an anterior rib on the right, the patient sits at the end of the couch with the therapist to the left. The patient folds the arms across the chest. The therapist hooks his or her fingers over the anterior rib and sidebends the

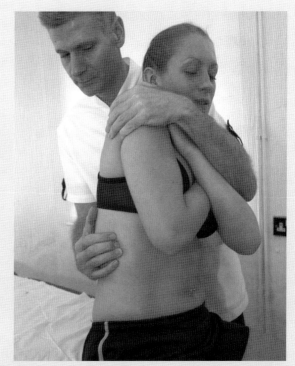

Figure 15.10   Treatment of anterior rib displacement using sidebending.

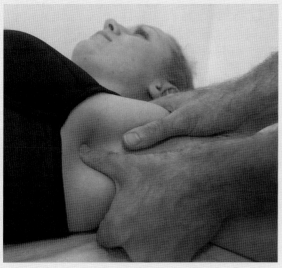

Figure 15.8   Treatment of a depressed second rib using thumb pressure.

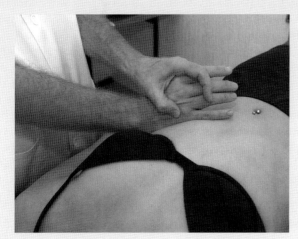

Figure 15.9   Treatment for general rib depression using pisiform grip.

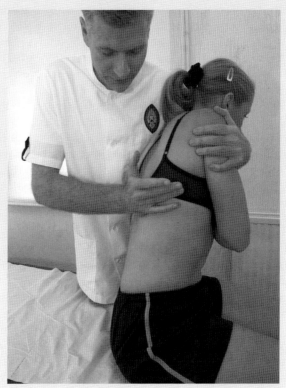

Figure 15.11   Treatment of posterior rib displacement using sideflexion.

patient to the left to open the ribcage, and rotates to the right to encourage the rib to move back (Fig. 15.10).

Posterior displacement
For a posterior rib, the contact area is with the heel of the hand over the rib angle. For a right posterior displacement the action is to sidebend to the left to open the ribcage and rotate to the left to draw the rib forwards (Fig. 15.11). An alternative approach is to perform a posteroanterior mobilization on the rib angle while the patient is prone. The pisiform of one hand performs the action while the pisiform of the other presses over the transverse process of the vertebra on the opposite side to prevent the vertebra from rotating as the rib is mobilized (Fig. 15.12).

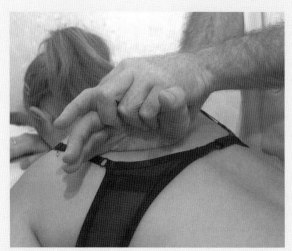

Figure 15.12   Treatment of a posterior rib in prone lying.

patient's respiratory movements into account, pressure for higher grade movements coinciding with expiration.

Anteroposterior movements may be performed on any of the *costal joints* (costochondral, interchondral, sternocostal). The therapist's thumbs are placed over the joint to be mobilized with the fingers fanning out over the patient's chest. The movement may be directed towards the patient's head or feet to reproduce the symptoms, and then continued in this direction at a lesser grade.

Intervertebral rotations may be applied both locally and generally. Local rotation may be carried out using pressure over the *transverse processes*. The thenar eminence of one hand is placed on the transverse process of one vertebra with the fingers pointing towards the patient's head. The hypothenar eminence of the other hand is placed on the transverse process on the opposing side of the spine either of the same vertebra or that of the vertebra below, with the fingers towards the patient's feet. A number of techniques are used. Rotation may be applied by using alternating pressure from one hand and then the other with the hands over the same spinal level (McKenzie, 1990), or a high velocity low amplitude thrust may be applied as the patient breathes out, with the hands over the transverse processes of two levels (Bourdillon, 1982).

General rotation may be performed with the patient seated over the couch end, with the arms folded and the hands gripping the shoulders. The therapist stands to the side of the patient. The patient rotates as far as is possible away from the therapist, who reaches across the patient's chest and grasps the patient's far shoulder. Overpressure is applied as the therapist pulls the far shoulder towards him- or herself and presses the far scapula away with the flat of the hand. Slight traction may be applied by gripping the far elbow rather than the shoulder. The therapist bends his or her knees before applying the grip and then straightens them as he or she pulls up and round. This technique may be used for mobilization or contract-relax stretching.

The close proximity of structures within this area makes it difficult to assess precisely whether a patient's symptoms are coming from the intervertebral joint, the costotransverse joint, the costovertebral joints or a combination of all three. For this reason many of the mobilizations affect all of these joints.

Keypoint

Mobilization techniques for the thoracic spine affect several joints simultaneously.

TRUNK MUSCLES

The trunk muscles are open to injury in the same way as any other muscle in the body, but muscle conditions are often overlooked in the search for signs of more complex injuries involving the intervertebral joints. Injury to the intercostal muscles has already been mentioned, but the abdominal muscles and erector spinae may also give pain from injury or muscle soreness.

The abdominal muscles are tested isometrically to eliminate involvement of the spine. A crook-lying position is preferred, as this partially relaxes the iliopsoas. Straight flexion taxes the rectus abdominis while flexion–rotation works the oblique abdominals. Pure rotation is tested in a sitting position, while lateral flexion is tested either in a sitting or standing position.

The upper (supra-umbilical) portion of the *rectus abdominis* is assessed from a sit-up position, while the lower (infra-umbilical) portion is assessed by lowering the straight legs from 90° hip flexion to work the muscle in a reverse origin to insertion fashion. Comparison is made between the right and left sides of the rectus by palpation, and watching the displacement of the umbilicus which will be pulled to the side of the stronger muscle (Lacote et al., 1987).

The *oblique abdominals* are worked by performing a sit-up motion with rotation, for example reaching the right arm towards the left knee. Rotation to the left works the right external oblique and left internal oblique and vice versa. The transversus abdominis acts to support the viscera and is active in forced expiration. It may be tested with the patient in a prone-kneeling position. From this position the subject breathes out against a resistance (balloon or spirometer) and pulls the abdominal wall in.

The *erector spinae* are tested in a prone-lying position, the subject being asked to extend the trunk and lift the chest from the couch. Isometric contraction is assessed by having the patient (in a prone-lying position) maintain a horizontal position of the trunk with only the legs supported. Alternatively, the patient should rest the chest over the couch end and attempt to straighten the legs to a horizontal position. The *quadratus lumborum* is tested with the subject prone, leg extended and slightly abducted, to elevate the pelvis laterally. Traction is placed through the elevated leg to oppose the pull of quadratus lumborum (Kendall and McCreary, 1983). Abdominal training in sport is covered on pages 323–327.

HERNIA

A hernia is a protrusion of the contents of a cavity through the cavity wall. Most usually an organ or peritoneum is forced through the muscular layer of the abdominal wall at sites of natural weakness where nerves and blood vessels leave the abdomen. The most common types are femoral, inguinal and incisional. Less common types include umbilical, epigastric and hiatus herniae.

Inguinal herniae occur as a result of damage or malformation of the structures forming the inguinal canal (see below). The hernia may be either direct or indirect, and is far more common in men than women. As the testis descends during fetal life, it drags with it a tube-like covering of peritoneum, the processus vaginalis which is usually obliterated. If this tube remains, it constitutes a weakness which may lead to an indirect inguinal hernia. This usually occurs in males and on the right side of the body. Direct inguinal herniae are more common in older men, and rupture through the weak abdominal wall. They are precipitated by obesity, persistent coughing, and straining.

Symptoms of an inguinal hernia are of a dragging sensation in the groin, especially when straining. A swelling may be noticeable over the external ring of the inguinal canal above and medial to the pubic tubercle, the point of attachment of adductor longus. In the case of an indirect hernia, the bulge may be in the upper scrotum. A bulge may be palpated over the hernia when the patient coughs. It is sometimes possible to pass the little finger through the skin of the upper scrotum to the external ring of the inguinal canal, following the line of the spermatic cord. The patient is supine, and the examining finger is directed upwards, backwards and laterally. Again, coughing will produce a bulge when hernia is present.

A *femoral hernia* is a protrusion of abdominal contents through the femoral ring, which is the point below the inguinal ligament where the blood vessels enter the leg. The condition is more common in women than men. The features are essentially similar to that of the inguinal hernia, except that the femoral hernia is generally smaller and more difficult to detect. An *epigastric hernia* travels through the linea alba. A small bulge (usually of fat) is found between the two recti above the umbilicus. An *umbilical hernia* is due to failure of the umbilical ring to close completely. Later in life this may dilate as a result of a rapid increase in intra-abdominal pressure. These hernias may be very large. *Incisional hernias* occur after abdominal surgery through the weak area created by the incision. A hiatus hernia is a rupture of a portion of the stomach through the oesophageal hiatus in the diaphragm. This type of hernia generally gives no symptoms in itself, but may, in turn, cause reflux and oesophagitis, giving heartburn. In addition, reflux of bitter irritating fluid into the pharynx and mouth may occur. Antacids are used to neutralize gastric contents, and weight loss and dietary modification (small frequent meals, avoidance of foods inducing symptoms) are used initially.

Initial management of hernias is conservative, and involves instruction on actions to avoid increasing intra-abdominal pressure. When symptoms persist, surgery is required.

Sportsman's hernia

Sportsman's hernia or groin disruption is a condition which may mimic inguinal hernia in many ways (Gilmore, 1995). To understand the condition we need to look at the structure of the region.

The inguinal canal (Fig. 15.13) is approximately 4 cm long, and transports the spermatic cord in the male, the round ligament in the female, and in both sexes the ilioinguinal nerve. Its anterior wall is formed from the aponeurosis (tendon sheet) of the external oblique supported by the internal oblique muscle at its lateral third. The posterior wall is from the transversalis fascia reinforced by the conjoint tendon at its medial third. The roof of the canal is formed by the internal oblique and transversus abdominis as they merge to form the conjoint tendon running from the

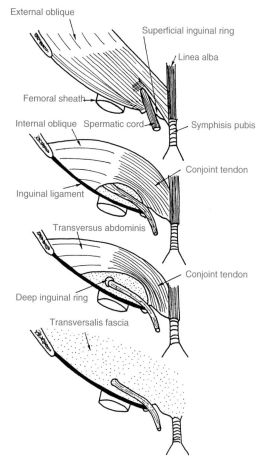

External oblique

Superficial inguinal ring

Linea alba

Femoral sheath

Internal oblique   Spermatic cord

Symphisis pubis

Conjoint tendon

Inguinal ligament

Transversus abdominis

Conjoint tendon

Deep inguinal ring

Transversalis fascia

Figure 15.13   Formation of the inguinal canal. From Palastanga, Field and Soames (1994), with permission.

pubic crest to the pectineal line of the pelvis. The deep inguinal ring is about 1.5 cm above the mid-point of the inguinal ligament and is an opening in the transversalis fascia. The superficial inguinal ring is a hole in the external oblique aponeurosis and lies at the medial end of the tendon above the pubic tubercle.

Definition

The *transversalis fascia* is part of a membranous bag lining the abdomen; (i) it lies on the deep surface of the transversus abdominis muscle, (ii) its thick lower portion is attached to the inguinal ligament, (iii) the femoral vessels drag the fascia with them as they travel into the leg forming the *femoral sheath*.

Sportsman's hernia is a tearing of the external oblique aponeurosis and the conjoint tendon, causing the superficial inguinal ring to dilate. There is a dehiscence (separation) between the conjoint tendon and the inguinal ligament but no hernial sac (Gilmore, 1995). The transversalis fascia may weaken and separate from the conjoint tendon

(Hackney, 1993) and the external oblique has been said to tear at the site of emergence of the anterior ramus of the iliohypogastric nerve (Williams and Foster, 1995).

The condition was originally described in soccer players but may occur in other sports. As many as 28% of soccer players may experience the condition (Kemp and Batt, 1998), and 50% of male athletes presenting with groin pain lasting longer than 8 weeks have been found during surgery to have sports herniae (Lovell, 1995).

There is a gradual onset of pain with one-third of the patients reporting a specific injury which may have resulted in tearing. Pain (in the inguinal, adductor or perineal region) is exacerbated by kicking actions and sudden changes in movement direction. The superficial inguinal ring is often dilated to palpation. Tenderness to palpation over the conjoint tendon and inguinal canal is increased by a resisted sit-up action. It is usually for several pathologies to coexist, with sportman's hernia occurring alongside adductor tendinitis. In a study of athletes with groin pain for more than 3 months, 19 out of 21 were found to have two or more separate pathologies (Ekberg, Persson and Abrahamson, 1988), and in general 25–30% of athletes with this condition can be expected to have a secondary diagnosis (Lovell, 1995).

Keypoint

A *sportsman's hernia* is a separation of the external oblique aponeurosis from the inguinal ligament. It is a muscle attachment injury rather than a true hernia and no protrusion (hernial sac) is present.

Treatment is surgical, with repair of the torn conjoint tendon and approximation of the tendon to the inguinal ligament. The external oblique is repaired and the inguinal ring reconstituted. Surgical success rates have been reported between 63 and 93% (Kemp and Batt, 1998), possibly reflecting the presence of additional pathologies.

Both prevention (Gilmore, 1995; Norris, 1995) and successful rehabilitation of this condition rely heavily on correct abdominal training. One of the factors in the development of this condition may be a muscle imbalance which is created in the athlete by sit-up exercises. Tightness in the hip flexors, combined with preferential recruitment of the rectus abdominis and poor recruitment of the deep abdominals, leaves the lower abdominal area open to injury. Increasing the training emphasis on abdominal hollowing actions and reducing the emphasis on lumbar flexion actions is a key factor which should be combined with stretching of the tight hip flexors.

In addition, dominance of the adductor muscles in certain sports such as soccer should be considered. Stretching the tight adductors and working the abductors proportionally should be considered. It has been suggested that repeated adductor actions create a shearing force across the

Table 15.3 Muscle balance exercises for sports hernia

Hip adductor stretch – straighten and slightly hollow the back by tilting the pelvis forwards. Press the knees downwards and hold the position for 30 s. Repeat 5 times.	
Hip flexor stretch – tighten abdominal muscles to stabilize pelvis and avoid low back extension. Lunge forwards forcing the hip into extension. Hold for 30 s and repeat 5 times.	
Hip abductor inner range work – lift bent knee upwards and outwards (abduction and lateral rotation) avoiding movement of the pelvis or spine. Hold the outer position for 10 s and repeat 10 times.	
Hip extensor (gluteal) inner range work – tighten abdominal muscles to prevent pelvic tilt, and lift bent leg. Maintain position for 10 s and then release.	
Isolation and re-education of the deep abdominals (core stabilizers) – maintain the neutral position of the spine. Draw the abdominal wall inwards in a hollowing action, hold for 10 s (breathing normally). Repeat 10 times.	
Building endurance of the core stabilizers – perform an abdominal hollowing action and maintain the neutral position of the spine. Allow one leg to slide out straight, avoiding pelvic tilt. Perform 5 times on each leg.	

pubic symphysis that places stress on the posterior inguinal wall (Simonet, Saylor and Sim, 1995). In support of this hypothesis, it is common clinically to find athletes who have coexisting osteitis pubis and/or adductor tendinitis. Muscle balance exercises relevant to the prevention and rehabilitation of this condition are shown in Table 15.3.

Keypoint

Muscle balance assessment is essential in the management of sports hernia. Tight hip flexors and hip adductors, together with dominance of the superficial abdominals over the core stabilizers, is often found.

THORACIC OUTLET SYNDROME

Thoracic outlet syndrome (Fig. 15.14) is a compression of the brachial plexus rather than the nerve roots, and so symptoms appear in the arm instead of the neck. The lower trunk (C8/T1) is most commonly affected, with bilateral tingling appearing over the median or ulnar distributions into the forearm and hand. The anatomy of the region favours compression. The nervous structures travel through the costo-clavicular space, formed by the inner clavicle, first rib and insertions of the scalene muscles. The lower trunk of the brachial plexus and the subclavian artery travel through the outlet formed between the scalenus anterior and scalenus medius to rest on the first rib. Symptoms from vascular compression are less common than those from neurological

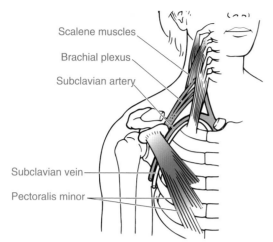

Figure 15.14 Thoracic outlet syndrome.

Table 15.4 Postural presentation in thoracic outlet syndrome

Descended scapulae, compressing the subclavian artery and lower
  trunk of the brachial plexus over the first rib
Possible complication of cervical rib seen on X-ray
Soft tissue contracture limiting range of motion at shoulder joint
  and girdle
Reduced movement in upper/mid-thoracic region (dowager's hump)
Tenderness to palpation of upper/mid-thoracic segments and
  costal joints
Head protraction

Adapted from Grieve (1986) with permission.

involvement, but alteration in blood flow may be used as a test for the condition (see below).

The more oblique slope of the first rib in the female changes the costoscalene angle (Grieve, 1986) and may account for the increased incidence of the condition in females. Lower down, the neurovascular structures pass into the axilla beneath the coracoid process and the tendon of pectoralis minor.

In the non-athlete, middle-aged women are most commonly affected, with the typical clinical picture consisting of a round shouldered posture displaying a 'dowager's hump' between C7 and T1. The thoracic kyphosis is usually stiff, showing tight pectoral tissues and limited shoulder movements. The thoracic segments and rib angles are often exquisitely tender. The pectoral girdle muscles may have weakened through prolonged disuse, and a 'poking chin' head position is common. This postural complex is summarized in Table 15.4.

In the athletic population, postural changes due to the nature of a sport will make the condition more likely. Excessive shoulder depression or overdevelopment of the trapezius and neck musculature in sports such as American football, rugby and throwing sports will put the athlete at risk. Tightness in the pectoralis minor (see p. 136) may occur in swimmers. In tennis players, asymetrical development with excessive scapular depression has been described (Zachazewski, Magee and Quillen, 1996). Athletes complain of pain and difficulty in gripping.

Carrying heavy objects or wearing a heavy coat exacerbates the problem, and simply allowing the arm to hang freely by the side can cause aching. The condition is seen commonly as an occupational injury, with the subject often noticing increased pain when reaching overhead. Typically, this pattern also occurs when a middle-aged woman takes up exercise in a keep-fit class. When severe, vascular signs such as coldness, blueing or whiteness of the skin may occur if the subclavian artery is affected. Equally, the patient may be woken at night with pain, or can experience numbness first thing in the morning.

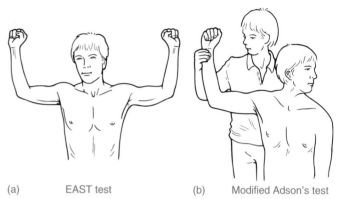

(a) EAST test (b) Modified Adson's test

Figure 15.15 Provocative tests for thoracic outlet syndrome. (a) EAST test. (b) Modified Adson's test.

Provocative tests

Various provocative tests are available which aim to reproduce the patient's symptoms. Sustained scapular elevation, or simply holding the arms overhead may increase the signs. The *Adson test* examines the radial pulse while the patient breathes in deeply and holds the breath, at the same time extending the neck and rotating it either towards or away from the affected side. Abduction of the shoulder to 90° with full external rotation, combined with vigorous hand movements, may give rise to symptoms if compression is significant. This is sometimes called the elevated arm stress test (*EAST*) or abduction-external rotation (AER) position test (Fig. 15.15). In addition, exaggerating the military posture and at the same time placing longitudinal traction through the arms may limit the costoclavicular space and reproduce symptoms (Grieve, 1986).

Examination of the thoracic spine should also be made to differentiate the condition from T4 syndrome (see below), and the long-sitting slump test and upper limb tension tests should be performed.

Treatment

Conservative management is to elevate the scapulae in the first instance. Simply strengthening the trapezius may have little effect, first because the trapezius, as an anti-gravity muscle, is usually very strong, and secondly because the stronger muscle may still not be used correctly. Postural re-education is more successful (Cyriax, 1982), teaching a less depressed shoulder girdle resting position. Enhancment of scapular stability with scapular repositioning exercises (p. 000), and modification of sport technique will also be required.

Tightness of the scalenes and pectoral muscles demands gentle PNF stretching techniques, and trigger point deactivation. Mobilization procedures of the thoracic spine are also helpful. Where neural tension tests are positive, mobilization of the neural tissues is required.

T4 SYNDROME

The T4 syndrome (Maitland, 1986; McGuckin, 1986) produces vague widespread symptoms of pain and paraesthesia in the upper limbs and head, possibly with autonomic involvement. Any region between T2 and T7 may be affected, but the focus is normally around T4. The distribution of symptoms in the hand is glove-like in contrast to that of thoracic outlet syndrome, but many subjects have sensations extending from the wrist and forearm. Head symptoms appear in a 'skull cap' distribution, and the patient is commonly woken with pain. Onset may be due to unaccustomed activities or trauma (road traffic accident), but in many cases there is no specific history of injury. As with thoracic outlet syndrome, a predisposing factor is postural. Head protraction, shoulder girdle protraction and accentuated thoracic kyphosis are common, and place a stretch on the thoracic tissues.

> **Keypoint**
>
> *Thoracic outlet syndrome* gives bilateral tingling over the median or ulnar nerve distributions into the forearm and hand, but generally no head symptoms. *T4 syndrome* gives glove-like symptoms affecting the whole hand, and altered sensation in a skull cap distribution over the head.

On examination, movements can be localized by performing rotations and flexion/extension from a slumped sitting starting position. Palpation is carried out with the patient prone, head in mid-position, with the therapist standing at the patient's head. The patient's forearms hang over the couch side and the upper arms are abducted to 90° to widen the interscapular space. Signs of joint localization include pain, resistance to passive movement and guarding muscle spasm. Common findings include alteration of the alignment of one spinous process in comparison with its neighbours, with local pain to palpation. Examination must take in the cervical spine and first rib. The first rib is palpated above the centre of the clavicle, with the direction of pressure aimed towards the patient's lower scapula.

Mobilization is used for any joints which exhibited signs at examination, and may be carried out with the patient in a supine position, arms folded across the chest and hands placed over the anterior aspect of the shoulders. The therapist places one hand beneath the patient's thoracic spine with the side of his or her thumb or hand in contact with the area to be mobilized. Downward pressure is exerted through the patient's arms onto the therapist's hand. Postural correction may be carried out as with thoracic outlet syndrome.

SCHEUERMANN'S DISEASE

Scheuermann's disease is a condition predominantly affecting the thoracic spine around T9, although the lumbar levels may be involved (Greene, Hensinger and Hunter, 1985). The condition is more common in males, and occurs in about 6% of the adolescent population in the 12–18 age group (Corrigan and Maitland, 1983). There is a disturbance of the normal ossification of the vertebrae. The vertebrae ossify from three centres, one at the centre of the vertebral body and two secondary centres (the ring epiphyses) in the cartilage end plates. In Scheuermanns's disease there is an alteration of the normal development of the ring epiphyses, but avascular necrosis does not occur (Gartland, 1987) in contrast to true osteochondrosis. Penetration of discal material is often seen through the cartilage end plate of the disc and into the vertebral body (Schmorl's nodes). The changes are largely developmental, but trauma may play a part in exacerbating the condition. In contrast, when the central bony nucleus is affected Calve's vertebral osteochondritis is present, a much less common condition affecting a single vertebra.

The changes in Scheuermann's disease are primarily to the anterior margins of the thoracic vertebra as these bear greater weight. The disc narrows anteriorly, and deficient growth of the vertebral body occurs as a result of epiphyseal malformation. The vertebra gradually takes on a wedged formation. Normally, several vertebrae are affected in the thoracic spine. The athlete is usually a skeletally immature adolescent, with a 'rounded back' posture. In the active stage of the condition there may be localized pain, often provoked by repeated thoracic flexion as occurs in certain swimming strokes (butterflier's back) and aerobic dance classes. Deep notches are visible over the anterior corners of the vertebrae on X-ray, and these appear sclerotic rather than rarefied (Fig. 15.16). The ring epiphyses are irregular, but the erythrocyte sedimentation rate (ESR) is normal.

> **Keypoint**
>
> In *Scheuermann's disease* several thoracic vertebrae take on a wedged formation giving a rounded back posture. Pain is exacerbated by repeated thoracic flexion.

The condition is self-limiting, but in the active stage rest is required. In more severe cases, especially those affecting a number of thoracic segments where kyphosis exceeds 30°, a spinal brace (Milwaukee brace) may be required to prevent

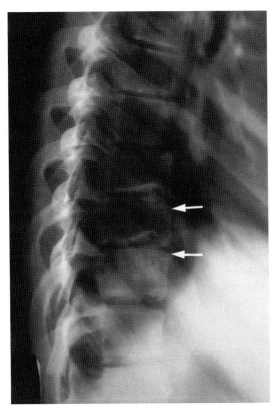

Figure 15.16 Radiographic appearance of Scheuermann's disease. From Read (2000) with permission.

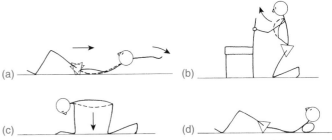

Figure 15.17 Exercise therapy for thoracic extension. (a) Overhead reach. (b) Sternal lift. (c) Chest thrust. (d) Thoracic extension.

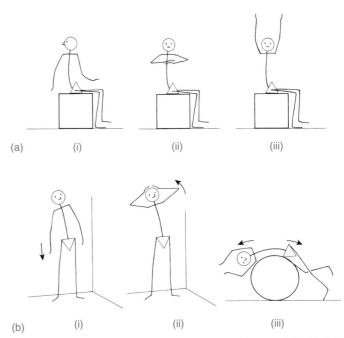

Figure 15.18 (a) Thoracic mobility exercises: (i) upper, (ii) mid, (iii) lower. (b) Thoracic side flexion: (i) lower region, (ii) upper region, (iii) side flexor stretch.

gross deformity. An exercise programme to prevent further deformity is essential. This normally involves strengthening in extension and patient education to avoid repeated flexion during activities and prolonged flexion in sitting and lying. In addition, increasing the lumbar lordosis and stretching the hamstrings has been recommended (Corrigan and Maitland, 1983).

EXERCISE THERAPY FOR THE THORACIC SPINE

As well as restoring fitness components to this body area (such as mobility and strength) following injury, posture is a prime consideration. As was seen on page 139, one of the common postural faults in this region is an increase in kyphosis. The increased thoracic curve often begins with scapular abduction which moves the centre of gravity of the upper body forwards. In time, the thoracic spine flexes further as a result of the change in equilibrium. The increased curvature has a direct effect on scapulohumeral rhythm by limiting scapulothoracic motion and preventing the final degrees of abduction and extension of the glenohumeral joint. Reversing this trend requires a reduction in thoracic curvature to move the centre of gravity posteriorly, shortening of the shoulder retractors, and often restoration of correct shoulder depressor action. Exercises to restore muscle balance for scapulohumeral rhythm are covered on page 373. In the following section, examples are given of exercises to

correct thoracic curvature by increasing extension. General examples of mobility exercises are also given for use in the restoration phase of injury.

Thoracic extension can be performed in a lying position. The pelvis is posteriorly tilted to flatten and block the lumbar spine, and the arms are lifted to the side and eventually overhead (Fig. 15.17a). Lifting the sternum to extend the thoracic spine without expanding the rib cage (Fig. 15.17b) is also a useful exercise and may be practised in a sitting, high kneeling or standing position. In elbow support prone kneeling (Fig. 15.17c) thoracic extension is performed by pressing (thrusting) the chest towards the floor. Passive extension may be performed by lying over a rolled towel, with the towel positioned at the apex of the thoracic curve (Fig. 15.17d). If the head does not rest on the mat, a thin pillow is used to prevent a protracted head position.

Thoracic mobility to rotation and lateral flexion may be localized to various segmental levels (Fig. 15.18). Mobility to rotation is performed in a sitting position, and may be

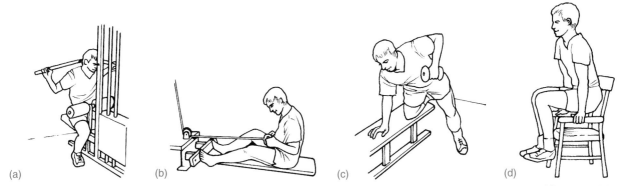

(a)   (b)   (c)   (d)

Figure 15.19   Resistance exercises for the thorax. (a) Lateral pull down. (b) Seated rowing. (c) One arm dumb-bell row. (d) Modified dip.

localized by changing the position of the arms. Leaving the arms at the sides and leading the movement with the head (looking around to the direction of movement) will focus movement to the upper thoracic spine. Holding the elbows horizontally stresses the mid-thoracic spine, which when reaching overhead pulls through the thoracolumbar fascia to stress the lower thoracic spine. Side (lateral) flexion may be mobilized by side-bending against a wall to prevent flexion/extension. With the hands by the sides (reach for the side of the knee) the lower thoracic region is stressed. Placing the hands behind the head and reaching up with the elbow transfers the centre of rotation higher up. Side-lying over a cushion or roll with the upper arm reaching overhead will stretch the muscles of side flexion as well as mobilizing the thoracic spine.

Examples of strength exercises for the thoracic spine musculature include single- or double-handed rowing actions, pull-downs and modified dips (Fig. 15.19).

References

Bailey, P. (1985) Surfer's rib: isolated first rib fracture secondary to indirect trauma. *Annals of Emergency Medicine*, **14**, 346–349

Bourdillon, J.F. (1982) *Spinal Manipulation*, Butterworth-Heinemann, Oxford

Butler, D.S. (1991) *Mobilization of the Nervous System*, Churchill Livingstone, Edinburgh

Butler, D.S. and Slater, H. (1994) Neural injury in the thoracic spine: a conceptual basis for manual therapy. In *Physical Therapy of the Cervical and Thoracic Spine*, 2nd edn (ed. R. Grant), Churchill Livingstone, Edinburgh

Corrigan, B. and Maitland, G.D. (1983) *Practical Orthopaedic Medicine*, Butterworth, London

Cyriax, J. (1982) *Textbook of Orthopaedic Medicine*, 8th edn, Baillière Tindall, London, vol. 1

Ekberg, O., Persson, N.H. and Abrahamson, P. (1988) Longstanding groin pain in athletes: a multidisciplinary approach. *Sports Medicine*, **6**, (1) 56–61

Gartland, J.J. (1987) *Fundamentals of Orthopaedics*, 4th edn, W.B. Saunders, Philadelphia

Gilmore, O.J.A. (1995) personnal communication

Greene, T.L., Hensinger, R.N. and Hunter, L.Y. (1985) Back pain and vertebral changes simulating Scheuermann's disease. *Journal of Pediatric Orthopaedics*, **5**, 1–7

Grieve, G.P. (1986) *Modern Manual Therapy of the Vertebral Column*, Churchill Livingstone, London

Gurtler, R., Pavlov, H. and Torg, J.S. (1985) Stress fracture of the ipsilateral first rib in a pitcher. *American Journal of Sports Medicine*, **13**, 277–279

Hackney, R.G. (1993) The sports hernia: a cause of groin pain. *British Journal of Sports Medicine*, **27**, (1) 58–62

Kemp, S. and Batt, M.E. (1998) The sports hernia: a common cause of groin pain. *Physician and Sportsmedicine*, **26**, (1) 1–6

Kendall, F.P. and McCreary, E.K. (1983) *Muscles Testing and Function*, 3rd edn, Williams and Wilkins, Baltimore

Lacote, M., Chevalier, A.M., Miranda, A., Bleton, J.P. and Stevenin, P. (1987) *Clinical Evaluation of Muscle Function*, Churchill Livingstone, Edinburgh

Lankenner, P.A. and Micheli, L.J. (1985) Stress fracture of the first rib: a case report. *Journal of Bone and Joint Surgery*, **67A**, 159–160

Lovell, G. (1995) The diagnosis of chronic groin pain in athletes. *Australian Journal of Science and Medicine in Sport*, **27**, (3) 76–79

McGuckin, N. (1986) The T4 syndrome. In *Modern Manual Therapy of the Vertebral Column* (ed. G.P. Grieve), Churchill Livingstone, Edinburgh

McKenzie, R.A. (1990) *The Cervical and Thoracic Spine: Mechanical Diagnosis and Therapy*, Spinal Publications, New Zealand

Magee, D.J. (2002) *Orthopedic Physical Assessment*, 4th edn, Saunders, Philadelphia

Maitland, G.D. (1986) *Vertebral Manipulation*, 5th edn, Butterworth, London

Norris, C.M. (1995) *Postural Considerations in Training, Presentation to the Football Association Medical Committee*, Lilleshall, England

Palastanga, N., Field, D. and Soames, R. (1994) *Anatomy and Human Movement*, 2nd edn, Butterworth-Heinemann, Oxford

Read, M.T. (2000) *A Practical Guide to Sports Injuries*, Butterworth-Heinemann, Oxford

Simonet, W.T., Saylor, H.L. and Sim, L. (1995) Abdominal wall muscle tears in hockey players. *International Journal of Sports Medicine*, **16**, (2) 126–128

Slater, H., Butler, D.S. and Shacklock, M.O. (1994) The dynamic central nervous system: examination and assessment using tension tests. In *Grieve's Modern Manual Therapy*, 2nd edn (eds J.D. Boyling and N. Palastanga), Churchill Livingstone, Edinburgh

Williams, P. and Foster, M.E. (1995) Gilmores groin – or is it? *British Journal of Sports Medicine*, **29**, (3) 206–208

Zachazewski, J.E., Magee, D.J. and Quillen, W.S. (1996) *Athletic Injuries and Rehabilitation*, Saunders, Philadelphia

Chapter 16

The cervical spine

CHAPTER CONTENTS

The cervical spine consists of eight mobile segments generally categorized into two functional units. The first comprises the occiput, C1 and C2 (the suboccipital region) and the second the segments from C2 to T1 (the lower cervical region)(see Fig. 6.40, p. 145).

Within the suboccipital region, an important distinction is made between the atlanto-occipital (A/O) and atlantoaxial (A/A) joints. The atlanto-occipital joint, formed between the occipital condyle and lateral masses of C1, allows no rotation but free flexion/extension and some lateral flexion. There are three atlantoaxial joints. The median joint is formed between the odontoid peg of the axis and the anterior arch and transverse ligament of the atlas. The lateral two joints are between the lateral articular processes of the atlas and axis. The atlantoaxial joint allows free rotation to about 35°, and only minimal flexion/extension. As rotation occurs, the head is depressed vertically by about 1 mm, causing ligamentous slackening and increasing the available range of motion.

> **Keypoint**
>
> The atlanto-occipital joint (C0–C1) allows no rotation, but free flexion/extension. The atlantoaxial joint (C1–C2) allows free rotation but only limited flexion/extension.

The discs of the lower cervical region are fairly thick, allowing free movement in all planes. Flexion and extension combined has a range of about 110°, with only 25° being flexion, and the least movement occurring between C7 and T1. With flexion, the upper vertebra of a pair slides anteriorly, pulling its inferior facet up and forwards, thus widening the facet joint space posteriorly. With extension the situation is reversed, the upper vertebra tilting and sliding posteriorly, gapping the facet joint anteriorly but narrowing the intervertebral foramen. Lateral flexion has a range of about 40° to each side. This is not a pure movement, but is combined with rotation and slight extension. Rotation occurs in the lower cervical region in either direction to

Figure 16.1 Structure of the vertebral artery. (a) Anterior and lateral view. (i) Branch from subclavian artery to C6. (ii) Vertical track through foramen transversaria. (iii) Horizontal section from C1. (iv) Entry to foramen magnum to join neighbour. (b) Effect of rotation is to stretch artery forwards. After Grant (1994a), with permission.

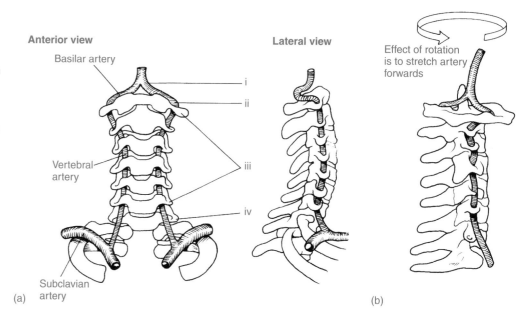

Anterior view

Basilar artery

i

ii

Vertebral artery

iii

iv

Subclavian artery

(a)

Lateral view

Effect of rotation is to stretch artery forwards

(b)

about 50°, and is limited by grinding of the facets and torsion stress on the discs and facet capsules. The function size of the intervertebral foramen is increased on the opposite side to the rotation, but reduced on the same side. Thus, manual therapy to the cervical spine for unilateral pain often involves contralateral rotation to relieve root pressure.

The lateral edge of each vertebra in the cervical region is lipped to form an uncovertebral joint, lying anteriorly to the intervertebral foramen. Each joint is surrounded by a capsule which blends medially with the disc. The joints help to stabilize the neck and control its movements.

Within the total range of any cervical movement some regions move more than others. The upper cervical segments allow more rotation than the lower, but less lateral flexion. With head retraction the upper segments flex while the lower ones extend. In fact, with this movement a greater range of upper cervical flexion is obtained than with neck flexion itself (McKenzie, 1990). As flexion occurs, the spinal canal lengthens, stretching the cord and nerve roots. Extension reverses this effect relaxing the spinal structures.

VERTEBRAL ARTERIES

One important difference between the cervical and other spinal areas is the presence of the vertebral arteries. These branch from the subclavian artery (Fig. 16.1a (i)) and pass through the foramina transversaria of each cervical vertebra from C6 and above (Fig. 16.1a (ii)). When the artery reaches the atlas, it runs almost horizontally (Fig. 16.1a (iii)) and then enters the foramen magnum to join with its neighbour and form the basilar artery (Fig. 16.1a (iv)). The vertebral arteries supply about 11% of the cerebral blood flow, the carotid system supplying 89% (Grant, 1994a).

Variations in the diameter of the vertebral arteries are common, and in some cases the basilar artery is supplied

Table 16.1 Symptoms of vertebrobasilar insufficiency (VBI)

Dizziness (in over 60% of cases)
Visual disturbances
– spots before the eyes
– blurred vision
– hallucination
– field defects
Diplopia
Ataxia
Drop attacks
Visceral/vasomotor disturbances
– nausea
– faintness
– light-headedness
Tingling around lips (perioral dysaesthesia)
Nystagmus
Hemi-anaesthesia
Hemiplegia

From Grant (1994b), with permission.

almost entirely by one dominant vertebral artery (Bogduk, 1986). During its course, the artery is in close relation to a number of structures, including the scalenus anterior and longus colli muscles, the uninate processes, the superior surface of the facet joint, and of course the transverse process itself.

Vertebrobasilar insufficiency (VBI) may occur with occlusion, in which case the predominant symptom is dizziness, although other symptoms may be seen (Table 16.1). Occlusion may be either intrinsic or extrinsic. Intrinsic causes include atherosclerosis blocking the artery, causing either focal narrowing, or more extensive constriction over the whole length of the artery. Extrinsic causes of occlusion occur by compression to the vessel wall. This is most commonly caused during rotation of the neck if an anomaly of the artery exists. Three such anomalies have been described in the lower part of the artery (Bogduk, 1986). First, an irregularity in the origin of the artery from the subclavian, secondly, bands of deep cervical fascia crossing the artery which tighten on rotation, and thirdly squeezing of the artery within the fascicles of either longus colli or scalenus anterior.

The major vertical portion of the artery (Fig. 16.1a) is most commonly affected by osteophytes and adhesive scar tissue, with neck rotation compromising the ipsilateral vessel. In the upper region (Fig. 16.1b), the artery may be occluded should the atlas move on the axis, through trauma, rheumatoid arthritis or abnormalities of the odontoid. Passive rotation of the neck can shut the contralateral artery by stretching it (Brown and Tatlow, 1963). Extension reduces cerebral blood flow less than rotation, but combined rotation—extension in the presence of traction increases the rate of occlusion significantly (Brown and Tatlow, 1963).

> **Keypoint**
>
> Abnormalities of the vertebral artery are common, with some patients having only one fully functioning artery.

Vertebrobasilar insufficiency is a potential danger of any manual therapy to the neck, particularly rotation, with some 60 cases of stroke being reported following neck manipulation (Bogduk, 1986). Twenty six cases reported in one series were subjected to X-ray following the incident. Of these, 23 were reported as normal or showing only minor degenerative changes (Grant, 1994b). In addition, major vascular complications occur predominantly in young (35–40 years) adults, suggesting that bony degenerative changes are not responsible for VBI. Trauma following manipulation occurs predominantly in the atlantoaxial component of the artery, which is stretched forwards during rotation. The more mobile neck of a younger adult will allow a greater range of rotatory motion and therefore greater stretch. Mechanical stress to the vertebral artery may lead to spasm (transient or persistent), subintimal tearing, perivascular haemorrhage or embolus formation leading to brainstem ischaemia. Repeated rotatory manipulation is especially dangerous as it builds on trauma which may already have occurred.

PRE-MANIPULATIVE TESTING OF THE CERVICAL SPINE

Testing for VBI should be carried out for all patients undergoing cervical manipulation (APA, 1989; Grant, 1994a, 1994b). Aspects of these tests (especially subjective history) will be relevant for all manual therapy procedures. Initially, subjective examination is used to determine the presence of dizziness or other symptoms suggesting VBI. The frequency of these symptoms and aggravating and alleviating factors are noted, especially with relevance to the neck. Any

Table 16.2 Physical examination for vertebrobasilar insufficiency (VBI)

No history of VBI	History of VBI (dizziness)
Sustained extension	Sustained extension
Sustained rotation (left and right)	Sustained rotation (left and right)
Sustained rotation with extension (left and right)	Sustained rotation with extension (left and right)
Simulated manipulation position	Test position or movement which provokes dizziness
	Rapid movement of relevant head position within available range

After Grant (1994b), with permission.

previous treatment (particularly multiple rotatory manipulation or manipulation under strong axial traction) is noted.

Physical examination includes sustained movements (10 s or less if symptoms are provoked) of extension, rotation, and combined extension/rotation (Table 16.2). Where there is no history of VBI, the patient is positioned in a simulated manipulation position which is again sustained. If the subjective examination suggests dizziness, the position which provokes this symptom is used in a sustained fashion. In addition, rapid head movement is used to distinguish between dizziness due to VBI and that due to vestibular origin. This is especially relevant where the patient describes rapid movement as a precipitating factor in the subjective examination. The therapist holds the patient's head (but not covering the ears) and body rotation is performed (for example in a swivel chair, or trunk twisting in standing) to both sides and held for 10 seconds. As the head itself is not moving, any symptoms are due to cervical rotation rather than vestibular disturbance.

Measurement of vertebral artery blood flow using ultrasound can also be a useful clinical tool (Johnson et al., 2000). Reliability is high when testing the vertebral artery at C5–C6 level singly (volume flow rate) and using a mean of three tests at C1–C2 (peak velocity).

The production of VBI symptoms is an obvious bar to full range rotation manipulation. However, even if the test is negative, a small risk still remains, so the patient should be continually questioned about dizziness throughout any treatment involving rotation techniques.

NATURE OF CERVICAL INJURY IN SPORT

The most common mechanism of severe cervical injury is axial loading (Torg et al., 1985). This may be caused as a player hits another by using his or her head as a battering ram (spearing), or if the athlete falls on to his or her head or runs into an object head-first. In this situation, the neck is slightly flexed, flattening the cervical lordosis. Now, the cervical spine absorbs considerably less energy than it would in its normal state as a flexible column. Initially, maximal discal compression occurs, and then the spine rapidly buckles and fails in flexion, resulting in fracture, subluxation or dislocation.

An illustration of the importance of this mechanism and its preventive possibilities is found in American football. The incidence of cervical quadriplegia in this sport dropped dramatically from a peak of 34 cases per year to 5 since head-first tackling and blocking were forbidden (Torg et al., 1985).

A similar mechanism has been described in rugby football. Cord injuries have occurred in scrum, ruck and maul situations when a player was attempting to pick the ball up from the ground (Silver and Gill, 1988), and as two forwards engage (Taylor and Coolican, 1987). The vertex of the head is restrained, either against another player or the ground, and the trunk continues to move forwards forcing the cervical spine into flexion and dislocation (McCoy, Piggott and Macafee, 1984).

In ice hockey, axial loading is again the culprit, when a player hits the boards or an opponent with his helmeted head while the neck is slightly flexed (Tator and Edmonds, 1986).

Where significant axial loading has occurred, permanent abnormalities exist within the cervical spine (Torg et al., 1993). These may include interspace narrowing at C5–C6 with deformity of the C5 end plate due to Schmorl's node formation. In addition, reversal of the cervical spine lordosis with fixation from C2 to C6 may be seen. Where these changes are present, they should preclude an athlete from participation in sports involving collision activities.

Definition

A *Schmorl's node* is a herniation of the nucleus pulposus of the spinal disc through the disc end plate and into the vertebral body.

In all full-body contact sports such as rugby, American football and ice hockey it is essential that players are taught that the initial point of contact in a tackle or block should be the shoulders or chest and not the head. In addition, strengthening the neck musculature may reduce the intensity of injury (Torg, 1982).

Less severe trauma may occur to the neck with indirect impact or a sudden mistimed movement. A type of whiplash injury may occur in a rear impact where one player runs into another. Hyperextension of the neck can result, with varying degrees of tissue damage.

Diving into a shallow swimming pool or lake is also a common cause of injury, with fracture dislocation occurring as the neck is forced into flexion (or extension in some cases) when the head strikes the pool bottom. The condition may occur if a swimming pool is too shallow, especially if left unsupervised or without depth markings. In addition, this tragic injury is common in lakes and rivers with youngsters under the influence of alcohol or drugs.

In gymnastics the most usual mechanism of injury is flexion of the cervical spine, with injury occurring most commonly at C4 and C7 levels (Silver, Silver and Godfrey, 1986). Again, there is an axial loading, with the gymnast landing on his or her head. Of note is the potential for abuse of the trampette by young athletes. This piece of equipment enables the young athlete to gain both height and speed in an inverted body position – a potentially lethal combination.

SCREENING EXAMINATION

The subjective assessment will give the practitioner an indication of the depth of examination required objectively. A great number of tests and procedures exist, but not all will be used with every patient. Following the subjective assessment, a screening examination is used to indicate where further tests, including palpation, should concentrate.

Initial objective examination includes posture and head position in both sitting and standing. Muscle tension and both active and passive motions are examined. Flexion/extension, rotation and lateral flexion are examined for range and end-feel. Movements are isolated by eliminating unwanted shoulder elevation or trunk rotation. Resisted movements may be similarly tested, and the shoulder range to abduction and flexion/abduction assessed to determine if there is an associated shoulder or arm pathology. Pain referral and any sensation loss is mapped, and upper limb muscle power and reflexes assessed if the history suggests neurological involvement.

Two further movements and their adaptations are important with reference to mechanical therapy, these are head protrusion (protraction) and retraction. As with other tests, the location and intensity of symptoms is established prior to testing. Head protrusion is performed in a sitting position, with the patient instructed to slide the head forwards horizontally as far as possible by 'poking the chin out'. This is performed singly and to repetition. Head retraction is the opposite action, sliding the head back and 'pulling the chin in'. Again, overpressure may be used to assess end-feel and symptoms. Where postural pain is suspected, the movements are performed statically and maintained to load the structures and cause tissue deformation. The capsular pattern of the cervical spine is an equal limitation of all movements except flexion, which is usually of greater range. Asymmetrical limitation of movement suggests a noncapsular lesion such as disc displacement (Cyriax and Cyriax, 1983).

Classification of disc displacement by pain pattern and presence of deformity is similar to that of the lumbar spine (McKenzie, 1990). Derangements one and two give pain travelling as far as the shoulder, three and four give pain referred into the arm but no further than the elbow. Derangements five and six can refer pain down to the wrist. Derangements one, three, and five do not show deformity, whereas derangement two may show cervical kyphosis, and derangements four and six may show torticollis.

Special tests

Further detail in cervical examination is gained by palpation to test accessory movements, and special tests such as the quadrant position and the upper limb tension test (ULTT). These two latter procedures are useful where the clinical picture is not clear, and to confirm or refute involvement of the cervical spine.

Quadrant test

The quadrant test combines extension, lateral flexion and rotation to the same side. For the *lower cervical spine*, the neck is taken back into extension and lateral flexion towards the painful side, and then rotated, again towards the pain. Testing the *upper cervical spine* is performed by extension with pressure to localize the movement to the upper cervical segments. When full extension has been gained, rotation is added towards the pain, and then followed by lateral flexion. Various sequences of combined movements may produce the patient's symptoms, and it is important that the same sequence of movements be used when making comparisons between both sides, or assessing prior to and following treatment.

Adding compression to these test positions (*foraminal compression test*) can also be clinically revealing in cases where patients have intermittent symptoms not present at the time of examination. Initially, the head and neck are compressed (using a straight vertical force) with the head in neutral. If this fails to reproduce the patient's symptoms compression is used in extension and finally in extension/rotation. In the latter case the movement is to the unaffected side first; if symptoms are not reproduced, the affected side is then used. Where symptoms are present at the time of examination, a distraction test may be used in the neutral position with the aim of alleviating symptoms (*foraminal distraction test*).

Upper limb tension test

The upper limb tension test (ULTT) or brachial plexus provocation test (BPPT) (Elvey's test) may be thought of as the 'straight leg raise of the upper limb'. It develops tension in the cervical nerve roots and their sheaths and dura, and places greatest stress to the C5 and C6 structures. Four variations are used to place greater or lesser stress on particular nerves (ULTT1, ULTT2a, ULTT2b, ULTT3).

For ULTT1 (Fig. 16.2) the patient is supine with the therapist facing the patient and standing at his or her side. The patient's shoulder girdle is depressed by caudal pressure from the therapist's hand. The forearm is supinated and the wrist and fingers extended, and then the shoulder is laterally rotated and the elbow extended. Finally, cervical

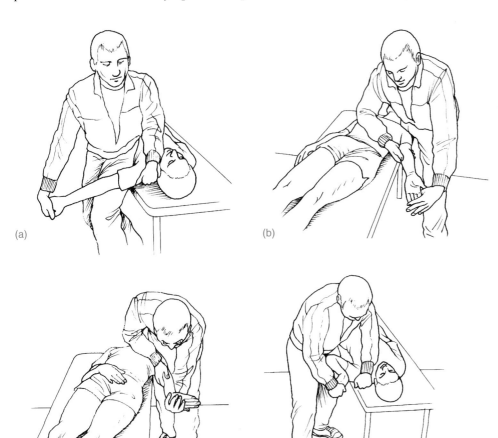

(a)

(b)

(c)

(d)

Figure 16.2 The upper limb tension test (ULTT). Finishing positions are shown. (a) ULTT 1: Median nerve. Shoulder abduction. (b) ULTT 2a: Median nerve. Shoulder girdle depression and external rotation of shoulder. (c) ULTT 2b: Radial nerve. Shoulder girdle depression and internal rotation of shoulder. (d) ULTT 3: Ulnar nerve. Shoulder abduction and elbow flexion. From Butler (1991), with permission.

lateral flexion (but not rotation) is added away from the tested arm. The instruction to 'keep looking at the ceiling but take your ear away' is helpful.

Pain from two-joint muscle stretch over the shoulder is eliminated by altering the head or finger position (which will not affect the shoulder muscles but will alter the nerve tension) to establish if this affects the pain. In normal subjects an ache is usually felt in the cubital fossa, and some sensation on the radial side of the forearm and hand is common. The test is only positive if symptoms other than these, and similar to the patient's complaint, are produced.

ULTT2a is used to place bias on the median nerve. The test is performed by depressing the patient's shoulder girdle and extending the elbow. The shoulder is laterally rotated and the wrist, fingers and thumb are then extended. Slight abduction of the shoulder may be added to sensitize the test. ULTT2b places bias on the radial nerve. From the previous position, the shoulder is medially rotated and the forearm pronated. The wrist is then flexed, and ulnar deviation of the wrist further sensitizes the nerve.

ULTT3 is used to test the ulnar nerve. The patient's wrist is extended and forearm supinated, and then the elbow is flexed. The shoulder girdle is depressed, and the glenohumeral joint abducted as though trying to place the patient's hand over his or her ear.

The ULTT is useful in patients with shoulder girdle or upper limb involvement where the origin of the symptoms is unclear, or where other tests do not reproduce the symptoms (Magarey, 1986). For a test to be positive, it must reproduce the patient's symptoms and be different from the uninjured side of the body. Furthermore, the test responses should be altered by movement of the distal body parts (forearm, wrist and fingers).

Brachial plexus injury in sport

In sport, traction injury of the brachial plexus can occur, in a position similar to that of the ULTT. With blocking or tackling in rugby or American football, the shoulder may be forcibly depressed while the cervical spine is simultaneously laterally flexed to the contralateral side. The upper trunk of the brachial plexus may suffer a neurapraxia as a result. Nerve function is temporarily disturbed and a burning sensation is felt in the upper limb. The condition is often referred to as a 'stinger' or 'burner' by players, and recovery is usually full in a matter of minutes.

The stinger may also be associated with extension compression, and during this mechanism the athlete with cervical spine stenosis is more at risk. The presence of such stenosis also makes the likelihood of developing a stinger three times greater (Meyer et al., 1994). Decreased canal diameter is associated with a narrow intervertebral foramen, and it is this structure which is likely to cause compression of the nerve root.

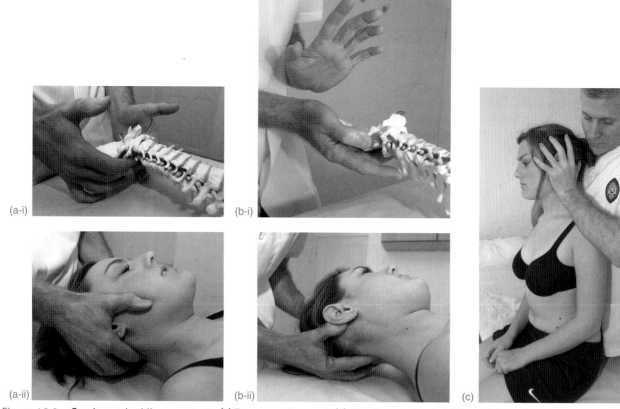

Figure 16.3   Craniovertebral ligament tests. (a) Transverse ligament. (b) Alar ligament test. (c) Tectorial membrane test.

MOTION TESTS FOR THE CERVICAL SPINE

Following traumatic injury such as occurs in sport or a road traffic accident (RTA), ligamentous tearing within the upper cervical spine (craniovertebral ligaments) can create structural instability. Testing the motion of the atlanto-occipital (C0–C1) and atlantoaxial (C1–C2) joints can therefore be revealing. The aim of the tests is to assess not specifically range of motion, but the reproduction of cord signs as the test is performed. Several tests are available (Pettman, 1994) with movement of the skull on C1, or the skull and C1 on C2, forming the basis of each.

In the first test the patient lies supine and the therapist sits at the patient's head. The transverse processes of C1 are palpated with the index fingers and the other fingers curl around the occiput. The action is for C2 to remain relatively fixed through bodyweight and for the therapist to lift the skull and C1 vertically away from the couch (Fig. 16.3a). Normally this movement is restricted by the *transverse ligament*, but if it is ruptured excessive motion will occur giving symptoms.

The second test begins in the same starting position but this time the therapist palpates the spinous process of C2. The action now is to compress the top of the head (vertex) to lock the atlanto-occipital joint and then to side bend the neck (Fig. 16.3b). As this occurs, the spinous process of C2 should move in the opposite direction (right sidebending giving left rotation) due to tightness in the *alar ligament*. If this ligament is ruptured, severe muscle spasm will be seen with cord signs.

For the third test, minimal distraction is used to test the *tectorial membrane*. The patient is sitting and the therapist stands behind. The side of the head is gripped and a distraction force imparted firstly in neutral and then in cervical flexion (Fig. 16.3c). Cord signs indicate a positive test.

> ### Definition
>
> The *transverse ligament* runs between the tubercles of the atlas (C1), the *alar ligament* runs from the sides of the odontoid peg of the axis (C2) to the base of the skull (occiput). The *tectorial membrane* is an extension of the posterior longitudinal ligament. It attaches to the vertebral body of atlas and onto the occiput (Fig. 16.4).

MANUAL THERAPY FOR THE CERVICAL SPINE

Physiological joint movements

One of the most useful mobilization techniques for the cervical spine in the presence of unilateral symptoms is rotation, usually performed in a direction away from the patient's pain (Maitland, 1986). The patient lies supine on the treatment couch with the head extending over the couch end. The therapist grasps the patient's occiput and chin (or side of the head), and rotates the head away from the painful side. The upper cervical (suboccipital) spine is better mobilized with the head and neck in line. With the lower cervical area, the neck is flexed further the lower down the spine the lesion is. The movement can be refined to rotate the atlantoaxial joint by flexing the cervical spine maximally and adding slight compression through the vertex (Fig. 16.5).

> ### Keypoint
>
> The upper cervical spine is mobilized with the head and neck in line (neutral). For the lower cervical area, the neck is flexed further the lower down the spine the lesion is.

Where pain is intense, or if the patient is particularly nervous, longitudinal oscillations are useful. The same grip may be used as with rotation movements, and the longitudinal motion is imparted by the therapist pulling through his or her arms. Stronger manual traction is also of use (Cyriax, 1980). This may be applied with the patient's shoulders stabilized by an assistant, couch horns, or body weight with heavier patients. Traction is applied through straight arms by the therapist leaning back. The use of a belt

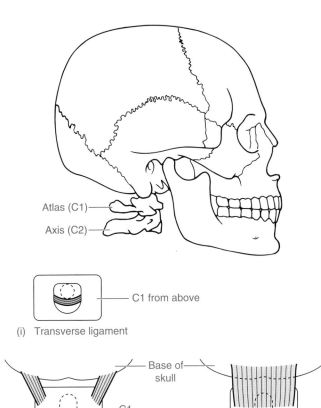

Atlas (C1)

Axis (C2)

(i) Transverse ligament — C1 from above

(ii) Alar ligaments

(iii) Tectorial membrane

Base of skull

C1

C2

Figure 16.4 Diagrammatic representation of craniovertebral ligaments.

or harness can reduce the strain on the therapist considerably (see Treatment note 16.1).

Rotation mobilizations and manipulations may also be applied during traction. Some authors claim that this procedure makes cervical manipulation safer by ensuring that any displaced fragment will move centrally (Cyriax and Cyriax, 1983). Others dispute this claim, arguing that the mechanics of the vertebral arteries makes injury more likely with this technique (Grieve, 1986; Grant, 1994a).

Lateral flexion movements are useful for muscle stretching (especially the upper trapezius) as well as joint mobilization (p. 000). For the lower cervical spine the whole head moves, the nose tracing the path of an arc. For the mid-cervical spine the head tips, the nose remaining still and representing the pivot point. For the suboccipital region (in particular C0–C1), the head and neck are side glided and lateral flexion is then imposed. Side gliding to the right is performed with lateral flexion (tipping) to the left (Fig. 16.6).

Accessory movements

Accessory intervertebral movements are normally performed with the patient in a prone lying position with the hands beneath the forehead. The chin is tucked in slightly to reduce the cervical lordosis. The tips or pads of the therapist's thumbs are used to impart the mobilization. Power for the movement comes from the shoulders and is transmitted through the arms and hands, so that the thumbs deliver rather than create the force.

Posteroanterior central vertebral pressures are performed with the therapist's thumbs in contact with the patient's spinous process. More pressure is required to feel movement in the mid-cervical region than in the suboccipital or lower cervical areas. The atlas has no spinous process, but rather a posterior tubercle, and pressure here is through the overlying muscles and ligaments. The spinous process of C2 overhangs that of C3, so palpation is aided in this region by asking the patient to tuck the chin in further and so increase cervical flexion. The oscillation is repeated two or three times each second, and the direction of travel may be angled towards the patient's head or feet depending on comfort. Posteroanterior central pressures are very useful where symptoms are central, or evenly distributed to either side (Fig. 16.7).

> **Keypoint**
>
> For the suboccipital region, asking the patient to tuck the chin in (upper cervical flexion) flattens the cervical curve and aids PA mobilizations.

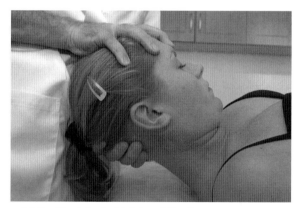

Figure 16.5   Physiological joint mobilization.

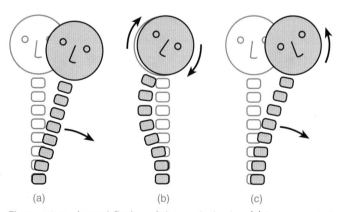

(a)   (b)   (c)

Figure 16.6   Lateral flexion of the cervical spine. (a) Lower cervical spine (C4–C7). (b) Upper cervical spine (C2–C4). (c) Atlanto-occipital joint (C0–C1).

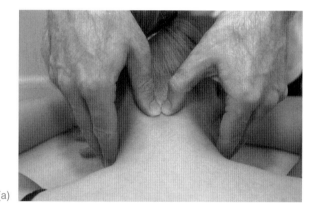

(a)

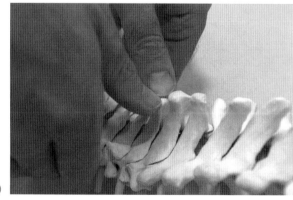

(b)

Figure 16.7   Accessory joint mobilization. (a) Surface palpation. (b) Position on skeleton.

Treatment note 16.1   Seatbelt techniques for cervical traction

Cervical traction is a technique used widely in the treatment of cervical conditions, with recommended poundages being quite high in some cases (Cyriax, 1982). Although mechanical traction may be used, it does not give the precision or variability that manual techniques can produce. However, to provide strong manual traction or repeated longitudinal mobilizations can be stressful to the practitioner's hands. The use of a seatbelt provides the advantages of manual techniques while reducing practitioner stress.

Starting position and grip

Counter-traction is provided by the patient's bodyweight and so they may be treated either with the couch flat, or in inclined sitting. Traction may be localized further down the cervical spine by adding flexion. The head may either be gripped with one hand cupped beneath the chin (ensure that the fingers are away from the trachea) and the other cradling the occiput (Fig. 16.8), or by both hands over the side of the head and fingertips folded beneath the angle of the jaw (Fig. 16.9). The later position is not as strong, but has the advantage that the patient can speak throughout the treatment.

A stride standing position is taken up so that the therapist can transfer bodyweight from the front foot to the back foot to provide the force for the action. Make sure that a balanced gait is maintained throughout the action so that the therapist does not risk slipping.

Belt position

The belt is fastened and measured from the therapist's shoulder to his or her outstretched hand (Fig. 16.10). The belt then passes around the hips, on the outside of the forearms and the backs of the hands. The elbows are held out slightly to hold the belt away from the side of the head

(Fig. 16.11). Once the belt is positioned, a powerful grip is not required from the therapist. As a measure the therapist should be able to comfortably move the fingers while traction is on.

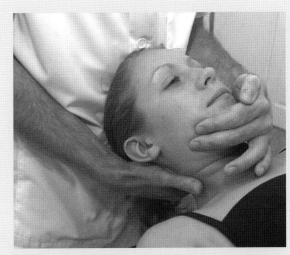

Figure 16.9   Hand grip using chin and occiput.

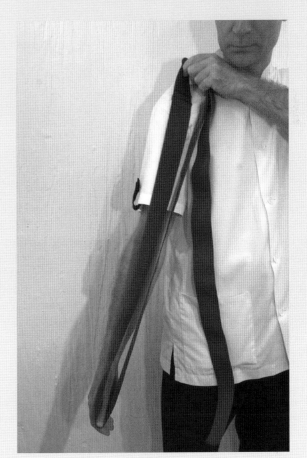

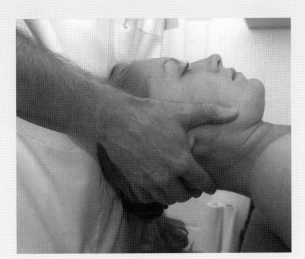

Figure 16.8   Hand grip on side of head.

Figure 16.10   Measuring the belt.

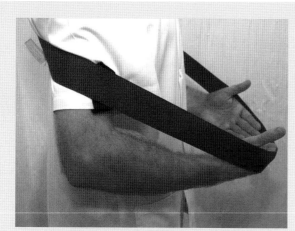

Figure 16.11   Belt position.

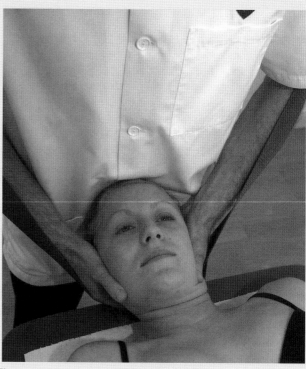

Figure 16.13   Lateral glide using belt.

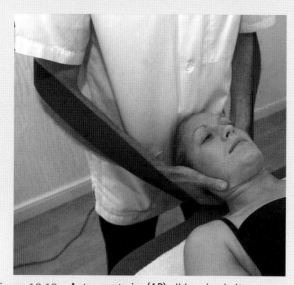

Figure 16.12   Anteroposterior (AP) glide using belt.

Variations

Several mobilization techniques may be given while traction is maintained. A gross AP glide may be given by bending and straightening the knees (Fig. 16.12) and a lateral glide may be performed by tucking the elbows into the sides of the body and shifting the pelvis from side to side (Fig. 16.13).

Posteroanterior unilateral pressures are similarly performed, but this time the therapist's thumbs are in contact with the patient's articular processes, and angled towards the mid-line. The technique is used for unilateral symptoms over the painful side. Transverse vertebral pressures are given against the side of a single spinous process with one thumb reinforcing the other. This technique is used mostly where there are unilateral symptoms which are well localized to the vertebrae. The movement is usually performed from the painless side pressing towards the pain.

MECHANICAL THERAPY

The same rules apply for the assessment of mechanical lesions as for the lumbar spine. The postural syndrome is managed largely by correcting sitting posture with the slouch overcorrect exercise. This time, however, the elimination of head protrusion is an important aim.

Extension dysfunction occurs more commonly in the lower cervical spine, making it impossible for the patient to sit correctly. Retraction is performed initially in sitting or standing, followed by extension. Overpressure is most easily given with the patient in a prone lying position. From this position the patient props him or herself up on the elbows, and places the fingers beneath the chin, pushing the head into further extension. Alternatively, a supine lying position may be used with the head over the couch end. The patient allows the head to slowly move back into full extension (traction being applied by the weight of the head). Small rotation movements may be used at end-range to complete the movement. This latter procedure is really only suitable for younger patients, and even then caution should be exercised with consideration to the vertebral arteries.

Rotation and flexion movements may also be performed with overpressure. The patient gently presses on his or her chin or pulls the back of the head down, respectively.

NAGS and SNAGS

NAGS (natural apophyseal glides) are mid-range oscillatory mobilizations applied to the facet joints between C2 and T3 in an anterosuperior direction (Mulligan, 1989). They are used with the patient seated, placing the cervical spine in a functional weight-bearing position.

Assuming the therapist is using the right hand, he or she stands to the right of the patient, blocking any unwanted shoulder movement with his or her own lower trunk. The patient's head is held in the therapist's cupped right hand, with the little finger hooked below the spinous process at the level to be treated. The therapist's left thenar eminence reinforces the pressure of the right little finger. The mobilization is applied through the hand and little finger at an angle of 45° to the cervical spine, and repeated 6–10 times.

Varying degrees of flexion, and traction may be applied until a movement is found which reduces the patient's symptoms. The cradled head position is particularly useful in that it gives confidence to the especially nervous patient.

SNAGS (sustained natural apophyseal glides) are sustained motions applied at end range. The therapist places the side of his or her thumb over the level to be treated, and presses upwards along the plane of the facet joint as the patient rotates or laterally flexes the head. The thumb follows the motion as the neck moves. Similar SNAGS may be used where flexion or extension is limited, and to C2 in the case of headaches. In this case the direction of movement is horizontal, again in line with the facet joint plane.

SOFT TISSUE TECHNIQUES

Several muscles in the area can develop painful trigger points and shorten, requiring release. Direct pressure (ischaemic pressure) massage and muscle stripping (pp. 77–78), and dry needling are all useful. On the posterior aspect, many of the muscles run to the base of the skull (Fig. 16.14) and so massage must be extended right up onto the occipital rim. The suboccipital muscles may be massaged and stretched in the supine-lying position, and several trigger points may be identified. The therapist places his or her supinated forearms beneath the patient's head, and grips the suboccipital structures with the pads of the flexed fingers. Gently gripping and relaxing the fingers imparts the massage. The muscles are stretched by retracting and flexing the neck, and then applying gentle overpressure. Transverse frictions may be given in prone lying or lean support sitting, using the thumb and forefinger, or forefinger supported by the middle finger (Fig. 16.15).

Four muscle layers are present (Table 16.3) and palpation will often identify trigger points at the muscle attachments or within their bellies. The main muscle to consider on the posterior aspect is the trapezius (see Treatment note 5.1, p. 104). Laterally, the sternomastoid may give pain as well as the scalenes. Trigger points (TrPs) for the sternomastoid

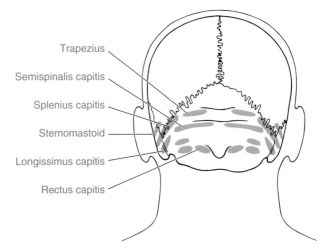

Figure 16.14　Muscles attaching to the base of the skull.

- Trapezius
- Semispinalis capitis
- Splenius capitis
- Sternomastoid
- Longissimus capitis
- Rectus capitis

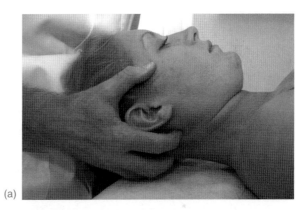

(a)

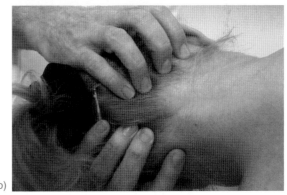

(b)

Figure 16.15　Soft tissue treatment of the suboccipital structure. (a) Whole hand position. (b) Detail of finger position.

may be found within the muscle belly or at the muscle attachment to the mastoid process. The clavicular portion of the muscle may give a TrP close to the clavicular attachment on the superior surface of the medial third of the clavicle (Fig. 16.16). The scalenes may present TrPs close to the transverse processes of the cervical vertebrae. These are best located by drawing the sternomastoid muscle forwards and palpating behind it. The muscles may be stretched by combining neck and shoulder movements. The sternomastoid

Table 16.3 Posterior muscle layers of the neck

Layer	Category	Muscles
First	Superficial extrinsic	Trapezius, latissimus dorsi, levator scapulae, rhomboids
Second	Superficial intrinsic	Splenius capitis, splenius cervicis
Third	Erector spinae group	Longissimus capitis, longissimus cervicis (both part of erector spinae)
Fourth	Deep intrinsic	Semispinalis capitis, multifidus, rotatores

After Gunn (1996), with permission.

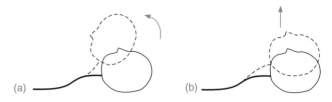

Figure 16.17   Neck flexion test. (a) Normal: cervical lordosis reverses and neck flexes. (b) Abnormal: cervical lordosis increases as chin juts forwards. Upper cervical spine hyperextends.

cervical spine in the suboccipital region, and the head then follows an arc-like movement as flexion continues in the lower cervical region only. This is more apparent when slight resistance is given against the forehead, and sternomastoid is seen to stand out prominently as soon as the movement begins (Janda, 1994).

> **Keypoint**
>
> Muscle imbalance of the cervical region exists when the deep neck flexors are poorly recruited and the superficial flexors are overactive.

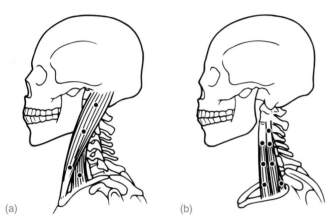

Figure 16.16   Trigger points on the lateral aspect of the neck. (a) Sternocleidomastoid, (b) Scalenes.

by depressing the shoulder then laterally flexing away from the tight side and rotating towards it, and the scalenes by stabilizing the 1st rib then rotating away from the tight side and flexing towards it.

STABILIZATION TECHNIQUES FOR THE CERVICAL SPINE

Restoration of cervical function using exercise therapy begins with spinal stabilization. This topic was covered for the lumbar spine in Chapter 14, and the principles are broadly similar for the cervical spine. The stabilizers of the cervical spine are the deep neck flexors (longus coli, rectus capitis, longus capitis). These have a tendency to be poorly recruited following injury, while the superficial neck flexors (sternomastoid and scalenes) tend to be overactive. Retraining cervical stabilization depends on increasing the work of the deep neck flexors while reducing that of the superficial muscles.

Imbalance of the cervical region is usefully assessed by a screening test in a supine lying position. The patient is instructed to flex the neck ('look at your toes'). If the deep neck flexors are overpowered by the superficial neck flexors, the chin juts forwards at the beginning of the movement (Fig. 16.17). This leads to hyperextension of the

Re-education of deep neck flexor activity begins in a supine-lying starting position. The head rests on the couch or small pad so that its weight does not act as a resistance to the movement. A pressure biofeedback unit is used to monitor head/neck movement. The cuff of the unit is folded and placed behind the upper cervical spine. The aim is to achieve suboccipital rather than lower cervical flexion. The action is a minimal flexion or 'nodding' action of the head alone (dropping the chin to the throat), avoiding forceful actions or lifting the head from the couch. The cuff is inflated sufficiently to fill the space between the cervical spine and couch, which is usually about 20 mmHg. The action is to slowly draw the chin back (chin tuck) to increase the pressure by 6–10 mmHg. If the pressure reduces, the head is being lifted by the sternomastoid and scalenes, so the exercise is restarted. The holding time of the movement is built up until the patient can maintain 10 repetitions each of 10 seconds duration.

CERVICAL STRENGTHENING IN SPORT

Following the restoration of appropriate stabilization and segmental control, many sports require general muscle strengthening. This may be achieved by resisted movements (partner or elastic band) through range and static muscle work in bridging. Several exercise examples are given in Figure 16.18. In each case it is essential to maintain cervical alignment. Once good alignment is lost the exercise should be stopped.

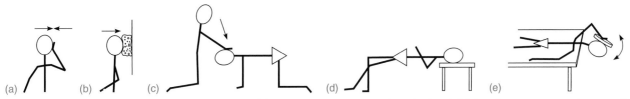

Figure 16.18 Examples of neck strengthening exercises. (a) Isometric resistance against the hand. (b) Pressing a sponge against a wall. (c) Resistance provided by a partner. (d) Neck bridge on a bench. (e) Resistance provided by a weight disc.

References

Australian Physiotherapy Association (APA) (1989) Testing of the cervical spine prior to manipulation. *Physiotherapy Practice*, **5**, 207–211

Bogduk, N. (1986) Cervical causes of headache and dizziness. In *Modern Manual Therapy of the Vertebral Column* (ed. G.P. Grieve), Churchill Livingstone, Edinburgh

Brown, B. St J. and Tatlow, W.F.T. (1963) Radiographic studies of the vertebral arteries in cadavers. *Radiology*, **81**, 80–88

Butler, D.S. (1991) *Mobilisation of the Nervous System*, Churchill Livingstone, Edinburgh

Cyriax, J. (1980) *Textbook of Orthopaedic Medicine*, vol. 2, 10th edn, *Treatment by Manipulation Massage and Injection*, Baillière Tindall, London

Cyriax, J. (1982) *Textbook of Orthopaedic Medicine*, 8th edn, Baillière Tindall, London

Cyriax, J.H. and Cyriax, P.J. (1983) *Illustrated Manual of Orthopaedic Medicine*, Butterworth, London

Grant, R. (1994a) Vertebral artery concerns: pre-manipulative testing of the cervical spine. In *Physical Therapy of the Cervical and Thoracic Spine*, 2nd edn (ed. R. Grant), Churchill Livingstone, Edinburgh

Grant, R. (1994b) Vertebral artery insufficiency: a clinical protocol for pre-manipulative testing of the cervical spine. In *Grieve's Modern Manual Therapy*, 2nd edn (eds J.D. Boyling and N. Palastanga), Churchill Livingstone, Edinburgh

Grieve, G.P. (1986) *Modern Manual Therapy of the Vertebral Column*, Churchill Livingstone, Edinburgh

Gunn, C.C. (1996) *Treatment of Chronic Pain*, 2nd, edn, Churchill Livingstone, Edinburgh

Janda, V. (1994) Muscles and motor control in cervicogenic disorders: assessment and management. In *Physical Therapy of the Cervical and Thoracic Spine*, 2nd edn (ed. R. Grant), Churchill Livingstone, Edinburgh

Johnson, C., Grant, R., Dansie, B., Taylor, J. and Spyropolous, P. (2000) Measurement of blood flow in the vertebral artery using colour duplex Doppler ultrasound. *Manual Therapy*, **5**, (1) 21–20

McCoy, G.F., Piggot, J. and Macafee, A.L. (1984) Injuries of the cervical spine in schoolboy rugby football. *Journal of Bone and Joint Surgery*, **66B**, 500–503

McKenzie, R.A. (1990) *The Cervical and Thoracic Spine: Mechanical Diagnosis and Therapy*, Spinal Publications, New Zealand

Magarey, M.E. (1986) Examination and assessment in spinal joint dysfunction. In *Modern Manual Therapy of the Vertebral Column* (ed. G.P. Grieve), Churchill Livingstone, Edinburgh

Maitland, G.D. (1986) *Vertebral Manipulation*, 5th edn, Butterworth, London

Meyer, S.A., Schulte, K.R., Callaghan, J.J. and Albright, J.P. (1994) Cervical spinal stenosis and stingers in collegiate football players. *American Journal of Sports Medicine*, **22**, 158–166

Mulligan, B.R. (1989) *Manual Therapy – Nags, Snags, and PRPs etc*, Plane View Services, New Zealand

Pettman, E. (1994) Stress tests of the craniovertebral joints. In *Grieve's Modern Manual Therapy*, 2nd edn (eds J.D. Boyling and N. Palastanga), Churchill Livingstone, Edinburgh

Silver, J.R. and Gill, S. (1988) Injuries of the spine sustained during rugby. *Sports Medicine*, **5**, 328–334

Silver, J.R., Silver, D.D. and Godfrey, J.J. (1986) Injuries of the spine sustained during gymnastic activities. *British Medical Journal*, **293**, 861–863

Tator, C.H. and Edmonds, V.E. (1986) Sports and recreation are a rising cause of spinal cord injury. *Physician and Sports Medicine*, **14**, 157–167

Taylor, T.K.F. and Coolican, M.R.J. (1987) Spinal-cord injuries in Australian footballers, 1960–1985. *Medical Journal of Australia*, **147**, 112–118

Torg, J.S. (1982) *Athletic Injuries to the Head, Neck and Face*, Lea and Febiger, Philadelphia

Torg, J.S., Sennett, B., Pavlov, H., Leventhal, M.R. and Glasgow, S.G. (1993) Spear tackler's spine: an entity precluding participation in tackle football and collision activities that expose the cervical spine to axial energy inputs. *American Journal of Sports Medicine*, **21**, 640–649

Torg, J.S., Vegso, J.J., Sennett, B. and Das, M. (1985) The national football head and neck injury registry: 14-year report on cervical quadriplegia, 1971 through 1984. *Journal of the American Medical Association*, **254**, 3439–3443

Chapter 17

Facial injury

CHAPTER CONTENTS

OCULAR INJURY

Eye injuries may arise from collisions in which a finger or elbow goes into the eye. Small balls (squash balls, shuttlecock) may cause ocular damage, while larger balls (cricket or hockey) are more likely to cause orbital fractures. Mud, grit or stone chips can enter the eye and cause both irritation and damage. It is interesting to note the speed at which a ball may move. In squash, the ball can travel at 140 m.p.h., in cricket at 110 m.p.h. and in football 35–75 m.p.h. (Reid, 1992). A small object travelling at these speeds obviously creates considerable force and potential for damage. This is borne out by the sad fact that over 10% of eye injuries in sport result in blindness in that eye (Pashby, 1986).

Where a foreign body is in the eye, quantities of water should be used to irrigate the eye and wash the object out (a squeeze bottle is particularly useful). Sit the athlete down and get him or her to look up, right, left and then down as sterile/clean water is poured into the inner corner of the eye. No attempt should be made to probe the eye as this may cause the object to scratch the cornea.

Keypoint

An *eyewash bottle* (sterile water) is an essential item for first aid in sport. With the athlete sitting, pour water into the inner corner of the eye while they look up, right, left, and then down.

In some instances, particularly if the foreign body is an eyelash, the eyelid may be rolled back on itself. This procedure is carried out by first asking the athlete to look down. The practitioner then grasps the lashes of the upper lid, pulling them gently down and out, away from the eye. A cotton swab is placed on the outside of the lid level with the lid crease. The lashes are then folded upwards over the swab to reveal the inside of the eyelid, and the foreign body is washed away. The eyelid goes back to its normal position when the athlete looks up and blinks.

A foreign body is one of the most common eye problems on the sports field. The reaction is usually pain and tear production. If the object is not removed, blinking may cause corneal abrasion and extreme pain for about 48 hours. It is important not to allow the athlete to touch the foreign body as this will simply increase the area of abrasion. If the object cannot be washed out easily, cover the eye with a sterile dressing and take the athlete to hospital. Encourage the athlete to keep the eyes still as movement of the uninjured eye will also move the injured one increasing tissue damage.

Contact lenses can cause problems. Hard lenses may break or become scratched or roughened causing corneal damage. Soft lenses are easily torn. When the eye has been injured or infected, a contact lens should never be reinserted until the eye has healed completely for at least 24 hours.

When contact lenses become dislodged, the wearer, with the aid of a mirror, is often the person most capable of removing them. Hard lenses may be removed with a small suction cup available from an optician, and persistent soft lenses may be dislodged by water from a squeeze bottle, or by gently wiping with a cotton swab.

Following injury, basic vision assessment should be carried out and if any abnormalities are detected the athlete should be referred to an ophthalmologist. A distance chart (placed 6 metres from the subject) and a near vision chart (35 cm from the eyes) should be used. Failure to read the 20/40 line on either chart is a reason for referral (Ellis, 1987). Visual fields are tested in all four quadrants. One eye is covered, and the athlete should look into the examiner's eyes. The examiner moves a finger to the edge of the visual field in both horizontal and vertical directions until the athlete loses sight of it. Decreased visual acuity or loss of the visual field in one area warrants referral (Ellis, 1987).

Pupil reaction may be tested with a small pen torch. Pupil size, shape and speed of reaction are noted. Pupil dilation in reaction to illumination requires immediate referral, as does any irregularity in pupil shape and an inability to clear blurring of vision by blinking. A number of common eye symptoms and possible causes are listed in Table 17.1

Eye protection

Sports trauma accounts for 25% of all serious ocular injuries (Jones, 1989), an even more tragic statistic when we realize that 90% of sports injuries to the eye could be prevented by wearing eye protection (Pashby, 1989). Prevention of ocular trauma comes from two sources, sports practice and eye protection.

Changes in sports practice include rule modification and increasing player awareness. For example, rule changes in

Keypoint

Most sports injuries to the eye could be prevented if athletes wore eye protection.

Table 17.1 Common eye symptoms encountered in sport

Symptoms	Possible cause
Eye itself	
Itching	Dry eyes, fatigue, allergies
Tears	Hypersecretion of tears, blocked drainage, emotional state
Dry eyes	Decreased secretion through ageing, certain medications
Sandy/gritty eyes	Conjunctivitis
Twitching	Fibrillation of orbicularis oculi muscle
Eyelid heaviness	Lid oedema, fatigue
Blinking	Local irritation, facial tic
Eyelids sticking together	Inflammatory conditions of lid or conjunctiva
Sensation of 'something in the eye'	Corneal abrasion, foreign body
Burning	Conjunctivitis
Throbbing/aching	Sinusitis, iritis
Vision	
Spots infront of eyes	Usually no pathology, but if persists consider possible retinal detachment
Flashes	Migraine, retinal detachment
Glare/photophobia	Iritis, consider meningitis
Sudden vision distortion	Macular oedema, retinal detachment
Presence of shadows or dark areas	Retinal haemorrhage, retinal detachment

Adapted from Magee (2002), with permission.

Canadian ice hockey to prevent high sticking have greatly reduced eye injury. Injury in badminton is more frequent at the net, so teaching young players to cover their face with the racquet when receiving a smash at the net would seem sensible.

Individual athletes should also protect themselves. The eye protectors worn must be capable of dissipating force, but should not restrict the field of vision or the player's comfort. In addition, if they are to be acceptable to a player they must be cosmetically attractive and inexpensive.

Each sport will have its own specific requirements. Where the blow is of great intensity, the eye protector must be incorporated into a helmet, and if there is a danger of irritation (chlorine in a swimming pool) the material used must be chemically resistant. Goggles for skiing must filter out ultraviolet light, while those for shooting may have to be suitable for low light conditions or capable of screening out glare.

For general protection in racquet sports, polycarbonate lenses mounted in plastic rather than wire frames are the choice. The nasal bridge and sides of such a protector should be broad and strong to deflect or absorb force.

DENTAL INJURY

The simplest form of tooth injury is a concussion in which the anterior teeth are knocked against something. This may occur from a head butt, a punch, or someone running into a piece of apparatus. There is only minor soft tissue damage and the teeth and mouth are sore. The front teeth may be painful on eating, so the athlete should avoid eating hard foods until the pain subsides.

Tooth subluxation occurs when a tooth becomes mobile after a direct injury, but is not displaced. On examination, the tooth may be loose and tender, and there may be some gum damage. It is usual for the teeth to tighten up and heal within a week, but the athlete should see his or her dentist. A subluxed tooth may have damaged its dental artery or vein. When this happens the venous blood can stagnate in the tooth and the haemoglobin seeps into the dentine turning the tooth dull yellow and eventually grey.

Displacement of a tooth is more common when a gum shield is not worn. The displaced tooth should be washed in tepid water and replaced in the socket, taking care to put the tooth back the right way round. The athlete may hold the tooth in place by biting on a cloth or handkerchief until specialist advice can be sought. In children, a displaced tooth may be soaked in whole milk (Mackie and Warren, 1988) until help is available. The tooth should be handled by the crown to avoid further damage to the cells at its root. Good results may be expected if reimplantation is carried out within 30 minutes of trauma, but after 2 hours the prognosis is poor.

Examination of the tooth after an impact injury initially is by a pressure test. The biting edge of the tooth is gently pressed inwards towards the tongue and then outwards towards the lips. If the tooth is painless (but not numb) and moves only as much as its neighbours, injury is normally restricted to the gums alone. If the tooth is numb, painful, mobile, or depressed below the level of the other teeth, the athlete requires dental referral.

Keypoint

After an impact injury affecting the teeth, tooth numbness, excessive mobility or depression below the level of the other teeth indicate the need for dental referral.

A number of tooth fractures may occur (Fig. 17.1). A small corner of the tooth may be chipped off, leaving a sharp edge which may cut into the tongue. Larger chips can expose the tooth dentine, causing pain when the athlete sucks air into the mouth, or the tooth pulp, which can be seen by looking

up into the mouth. This latter injury is a dental emergency, as are complete tooth fractures of the root apex or at gum level.

Mouth guards

Custom-made mouth guards (gum shields) have been shown to reduce the incidence of dental injuries by as much as 90% (Jennings, 1990). In addition, they stop the teeth from cutting into the lips and cheeks. When the jaw is hit from below, the bottom teeth will impact into the guard, absorbing some of the impact force. A mouth guard will also modify the transmission of force through the temporomandibular joints. The combination of altered force transmission and shock absorption can reduce the likelihood of concussion and mandibular fracture (Chapman, 1990). Any guard must cover the surfaces of the upper teeth, be comfortable to wear, and allow unhindered breathing and speech. Furthermore, it must show good properties of retention in the mouth, and give proper inter-maxillary positioning.

Mouth guards were originally worn in boxing, when they were simply curved pieces of rubber gripped between the teeth. Progress has been made in their design, and nowadays three types are available, custom-made, mouth-formed and ready moulded. Most protection is given to the upper front teeth, these being the ones most susceptible to injury.

For custom-made gum shields the first step is to take an impression of the upper teeth using a material such as alginate. Dental stone is poured into the impression to create a positive model of the teeth. Polyvinyl acetate-polyethelene (PVAc-PE) is vacuum formed over the model, and the mouth guard is trimmed and smoothed off (Kerr, 1986).

Self-moulded guards come in two types. The first is soaked in hot water to soften it and moulded over the upper teeth ('boil and bite'). The second type consists of a preformed outer shell into which a plasticized acrylic gel or silicone rubber is added. The outer shell and fluid gel are placed over the teeth and pressed into position until the gel sets.

The dentally fitted type of mouth protector is better in terms of both safety and effectiveness. The model made from the impression of the athlete's mouth can be reused to form a number of mouth shields.

The ready moulded kind are available off the shelf in many sports shops. They do not fit well, and have to be held in place by gritting the teeth. They should not be recommended to athletes as they are easily dislodged and may block the airway.

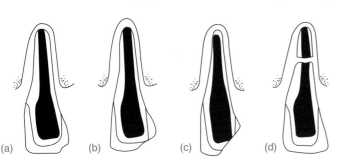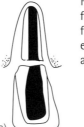

Figure 17.1 Tooth fractures. (a) Small corner fracture involving enamel only. (b) Larger corner fracture with dentine exposure. (c) Nerve root pulp exposed. (d) Fracture close to root apex. (e) Fracture at gum level. From Reid (1992) with permission.

(a)   (b)   (c)   (d)   (e)

> **Keypoint**
>
> Ready moulded mouth guards (gum shields) which are held in place by gritting the teeth are dangerous. They are easily dislodged and may block the airway. Use a self fitted (boil and bite) or dentally fitted unit instead.

AURICULAR INJURY

Cauliflower ear

Auricular haematoma ('cauliflower ear') is normally caused by a direct blow to the ear. Blood and serum accumulate between the perichondrium and external ear cartilage, and secondary infection may arise. First aid treatment involves the use of ice and compression. As soon as possible the haematoma should be aspirated or drained through an incision, and the ear compressed to prevent further fluid accumulation. The injury occurs particularly in contact sports such as wrestling, boxing and rugby, and is very common. Schuller et al. (1989) found 39% of high school and collegiate wrestlers from a group of 537 with one or both of the auricles permanently deformed by injury. Some degree of prevention may be achieved by wearing protective headgear.

Underwater diving injury

Air either side of the tympanic membrane should be at equal pressure. Externally, the air is at atmospheric pressure, and internally the Eustachian tube leads to the nasopharynx. Pressure changes such as those that occur in an aeroplane are equalized by swallowing or yawning, through the Eustachian tube mechanism. If the free exchange of air is impaired, barotrauma may occur. If the outside air pressure rises, such as may occur in diving, and the Eustachian tube mechanism is unable to equalize pressure, pain will result, a condition referred to as 'the squeeze'. Small haemorrhages may occur in the middle ear and the tympanic membrane may burst in depths below 3 m (Sperryn, 1985). With a severe cold, the Eustachian tube may be blocked, so an athlete should not dive (or fly if the condition is severe).

Barotrauma to the inner ear secondary to decompression is less common, but considerably more serious. This type of trauma usually occurs at depths below 35 m. Symptoms may be caused by the formation of gas bubbles in the blood vessels supplying the inner ear (Renon et al., 1986).

The reduction in air volume at increasing depths is responsible for another danger with diving and underwater swimming, the phenomenon of 'mask squeeze'. A relative vacuum is created in a diving mask or swimming goggles as the diver descends. With a mask, this is equalized by breathing out through the nose into the mask, but with swimming goggles this is not possible. A swimming pool may be as deep as 3 or 4 m. Children who dive down for objects at this depth face the very real danger of conjunctival haemorrhage and oedema (Craig, 1984). As the air space within the goggles is not connected to a body cavity, the air pressure will not be equalized. The pressure within the goggles will drop lower than that inside the body causing the ocular vascular system to over-distend and fluid to accumulate in the tissues covered by the goggles.

> **Keypoint**
>
> Conjunctival haemorrhage or oedema (bleeding or swelling of the eye membrane) may occur in children who wear swimming goggles and dive for objects in a deep pool.

Diving with ear plugs in or with an upper respiratory tract infection should also be avoided because of danger to the eardrum (tympanic membrane). Water pressure will press an ear plug further in, compressing the air between the plug and eardrum. This can cause severe pain and may even rupture the drum. During any change in air pressure, the pressure inside the eardrum is equalized through the Eustachian tube mechanism when swallowing or yawning. With upper respiratory tract infections, this tube can become blocked, giving severe pain (middle-ear squeeze) as the eardrum is stretched inwards.

Swimming pool ear

Swimming pool ear (otitis externa) is an irritable condition of the outer ear which can occur in athletes who swim regularly (Eichel, 1986). The symptoms are mainly itching, bordering on pain, but in extreme cases discharge may occur and even partial hearing loss. The ear canal produces its own protective layer of cerumen (wax). With prolonged exposure to chlorinated water especially, the wax may degenerate and the skin of the inner ear can become macerated. This leaves the ear open to bacterial or fungal infection, especially as the skin is damaged by vigorous drying (corner of a towel or cotton swabs) or scratching (finger nail).

Prevention is the key to this condition. Ear wax should not be removed, and nothing inserted into the ear. If ear protection is required, a drop of sterile baby oil placed in the ear will form a protective coating. To limit water contact, rather than using ear plugs a close fitting swimming cap can be used. Where itching is present, anti-bacterial eardrops should be used and the athlete should avoid water contact until the symptoms settle.

MAXILLOFACIAL INJURIES

Sport accounts for about 12% of maxillofacial injuries (Handler, 1991), with fractures of the maxilla and zygomatic bones being more common in contact sports (Fig. 17.2). If the upper jaw has been subjected to a blow, injury should be suspected if the teeth are out of alignment or one half of the cheek feels numb. Direct palpation of these fractures is painful, and pain may be elicited as far back as the

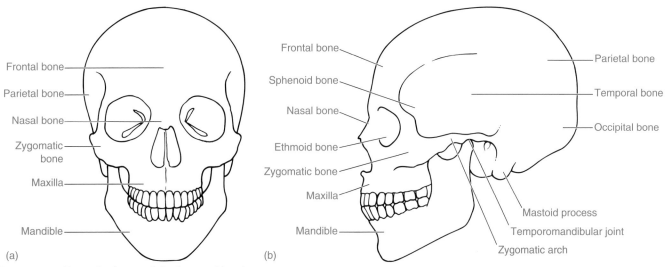

Figure 17.2   The major bones of the face and head.

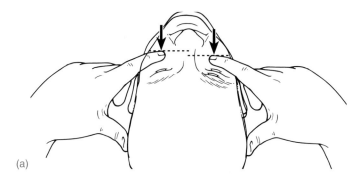

(a)

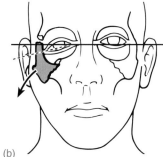

(b)

Figure 17.3   Assessing zygomatic fractures. (a) Checking for bone deformity. (b) Depression of the lateral canthus. After Magee (2002) with permission.

temporomandibular joint if the athlete is asked to bite on a folded cloth or tongue depressor. Chewing will be painful and local swelling may be apparent.

> ### Keypoint
>
> To assess fractures of the maxilla or zygomatic bones, ask the athlete to bite on a folded cloth or tongue depressor and palpate for pain.

Bony deformity of the *zygoma* is often better assessed by looking at both cheekbones from the top of the patient's head (Fig. 17.3a). Gently palpate the zygoma with the flat of the finger and compare finger levels. In addition, with fractures of the zygoma, as the bone drops inferiory it will pull the lateral canthus down with it (Fig. 17.3b).

The *maxilla* may be assessed by stabilizing the head with one hand and reaching up inside the mouth to grip the bone above the upper teeth. Assess for pain and anterior bony displacement. *Mandibular* fracture may occur with a direct blow to the chin, with pain being experienced, as the mouth is opened or closed, in an area in front of the ear. There is malocclusion and abnormal mobility of the mandible.

Most of these fractures extend through the intraoral mucosa and so bleeding is often noticed from the mouth. The primary aim is to ensure a clear airway. Blood, bone and tooth fragments and saliva must be cleared from the mouth. The mobile jaw fragment may be temporarily secured with a bandage around the head and chin.

The local application of ice will ease pain, and direct pressure by the athlete supports the area until hospitalization is achieved.

TEMPOROMANDIBULAR JOINT PAIN

The temporomandibular joint (TMJ) can give rise to facial pain of various types, and although not strictly a sporting injury, will be briefly considered. TMJ pain may be the result of alterations in the way the teeth come together (occlusion), and this in turn is affected by mouth guards used in contact sports.

Structure and function

The TMJ is a synovial condyloid joint found between the mandibular fossa of the temporal bone, and the condyle of the mandible. The two bony surfaces are covered with fibro-cartilage and separated by an articular disc. Movements of the jaw include protraction, retraction, elevation, depression and lateral gliding, all of which are used to some extent when chewing. The three main muscles contributing to TMJ motion are the temporalis, masseter and the pterygoids, and dry needling may be used to treat trigger points within these (see Treatment note 17.1). The temporalis fans out from the temporal fossa to insert into the coronoid process of the mandible. The masseter has both deep and superficial portions, and attaches from the zygomatic arch and maxillary process to the angle of the mandible. The medial pterygoid is similar in position to the masseter, but the lateral pterygoid arises from the sphenoid bone and inserts into the mandibular condyle and articular disc, playing a large part in stabilization of the TMJ.

In the occluded position, the upper teeth are normally in front of the lower ones. As the mouth is opened, the lower inscisors move downwards and forwards, a movement encompassing forward gliding and rotation at the TMJ. Depression of the mandible is controlled by eccentric action of the temporalis, but if resisted, the geniohyoid, mylohyoid and digastric muscles contract. The jaw is closed powerfully by masseter, temporalis and the medial pterygoid. The lateral pterygoid pulls the mandible forwards (protraction) while the temporalis is the main effector of retraction.

Pathology

Dysfunction of the TMJ may present as local muscle tenderness, limited motion and a general dull ache over the side of the face. Clicking may be present, and patients often protrude the mandible as the jaw is opened, or sublux the joint. When chronic, the condition may show reduced range of motion, with contracture of the masticatory muscles. Pain and muscle spasm are common, with the lateral pterygoids most usually affected (Hertling and Kessler, 1990). Emotional stress which presents as teeth clenching is a common factor, as is an alteration in bite pattern and chewing action.

Trauma to the area is common in contact sports, and soft tissue damage and subluxation/dislocation may occur. Whiplash injuries can also give rise to the condition. As the head tips back rapidly, the jaw flies open, stretching the masseter and joint structures. Immediately following this the jaw snaps shut, which may in turn compromise the articular meniscus.

Management

Joint mobilization

With the patient in a side-lying starting position (Fig. 17.4), the head of the mandible may be palpated just in front of the ear canal (external auditory meatus) and felt to move as the mouth is opened and closed. *Anteroposterior* and *posteroanterior* joint mobilization may be performed using one thumb pad as the other thumb monitors movement at the TMJ. By reaching inside the mouth (gloved hand) the thumb may be placed along the medial surface of the mandible (Fig. 17.4b) and can then be used to produce *lateral gliding*. By altering the thumb position slightly and gripping the mandible inside the mouth with the thumb and outside with the fingers, a *longitudinal* mobilization may be performed.

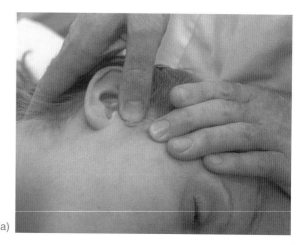

(a)

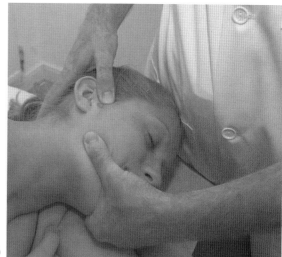

(b)

Figure 17.4 Mobilization techniques for the temporomandibular joint (TMJ). (a) Anteroposterior (AP) mobilization. (b) Lateral glide.

Home exercise/movement techniques

Normal functional opening of the mouth is between 25 and 35 mm depending on body size (Magee, 2002). This may be assessed by asking the patient to place two of their knuckles into their mouth (Fig. 17.5). Inability to do this indicates TMJ hypomobility. Self-stretching begins by asking the patient to simply open and close the mouth, gradually increasing the range until a yawning motion is used. Prolonged static stretch is used by placing a single knuckle and then two knuckles between the teeth. The stretched position is maintained for 5–10 minutes until the muscles relax.

Translation movements occur when the mouth is opened further than about 1 cm. From this position the patient is instructed to protrude and retract the chin, and to use lateral gliding movements (Fig. 17.6).

Mandibular repositioning devices

In persistent cases referral to a dental practitioner is recommended. Bite patterns may be corrected with the use of a

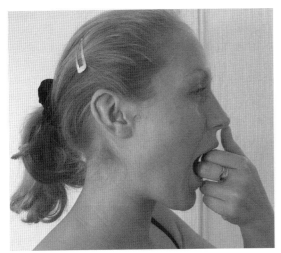

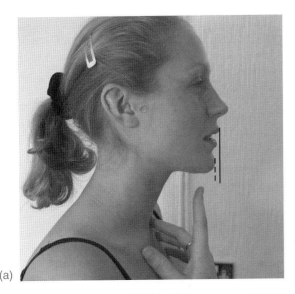

Figure 17.5   Self-stretching procedure for the temporomandibular joint (TMJ).

(a)

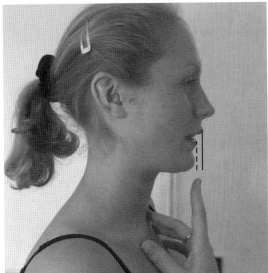

(b)

Figure 17.6   Temporomandibular joint (TMJ) home exercise. (a) Chin protraction. (b) Chin retraction.

Treatment note 17.1   Dry needling in the treatment of TMJ pain

The three muscles giving pain in TMJ conditions are the lateral pterigoid, masseter and the temporalis. All of these muscles may develop painful trigger points (TrP) which can be successfully treated using ischaemic pressure or dry needling. In addition, several traditional acupuncture points are found in this region which may be used in the treatment of TMJ pain and facial pain in general.

Trigger points

The lateral pterygoid muscle is claimed to be the main source of TrP pain to the TMJ (Simons, Travell and Simons, 1999). It can only be effectively palpated through the masseter muscle and then only with the mouth open by 2–3 cm. The muscle lies between the mandibular notch and the zygomatic arch.

TrPs for the temporalis muscle are found 1–2 finger breadths above the zygomatic arch and also towards the anterior aspect of the muscle at its attachment behind the supraorbital ridge. Interestingly this is the precise location of a traditional acupuncture point (extra point) called Taiyang meaning 'supreme yang' regularly used for the relief of frontal headaches. TrPs for the masseter are more easily found with the mouth open. Central TrPs are located on a diagonal bisecting the angle of the mandible and attachment TrPs up towards the zygomatic process (Fig. 17.7).

Traditional acupuncture points

The stomach (ST), small intestine (SI) and gallbladder (GB) acupuncture meridians (channels) all travel on the side of the face and have important points which can be used in the treatment of TMJ pain. The point ST-6 lies within the belly of the masseter muscles and is often tender to palpation. The point GB-8 lies within the temporalis muscle

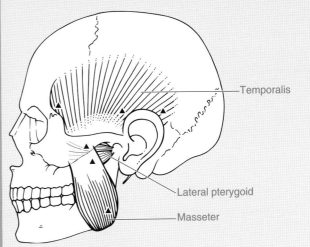

Figure 17.7   Trigger points in relation to the temporomandibular joint (TMJ).

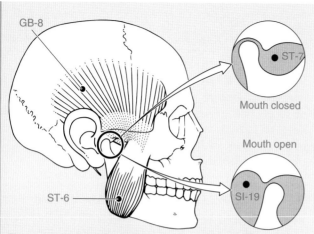

Figure 17.8 Traditional acupuncture points in relation to the temporomandibular joint (TMJ).

and again may be painful. The point SI-19 lies directly behind the TMJ and the point ST-7 lies directly in front. Both may be used in TMJ treatment (Fig. 17.8).

Dry needling technique

The superficial nature of the structures in the face make precise needling essential. The point ST-6 should be needled no deeper than 0.5 cm, if needling perpendicularly, and deeper only if a transverse insertion is used. For this type of insertion a fold of skin is lifted and the needle placed into the skin only.

GB-8 lies 1.5 cm above the apex of the ear, and at this point there is a slight depression. Again needle insertion is superficial – 0.5–1.0 cm, angled transversely. Both SI-19 and ST-7 are located by first palpating the condlye of the mandible just in front of the ear. As the mouth is opened the condyle slides down and forwards and SI-19 is located in the gap behind the condyle. The point is then needled with the mouth slightly *open* to a depth of no more than 1 cm. ST-7 is located in the hollow in front of the condyle when the mouth is *closed* and is then needled to a depth of 0.5–1.0 cm. Importantly, both points are not needled at the same time: palpation will reveal the more tender point which is then chosen.

dental appliance, but the precise value of mandibular orthopaedic repositioning appliances (MORA) is still largely uncertain. Some authors (Laskin and Greene, 1972; Gelb, 1977) have used these devices to optimize the positioning of the condyles and fossa of the TMJ to restore neuromotor function to the joint. It has been suggested (Gelb, 1977) that in addition to TMJ pain, cervical and spinal problems may also benefit, and muscle strength may be enhanced in other body parts (Schwartz and Novich, 1980). The use of a MORA has however been criticized. Burkett and Berstein (1982), and McArdle et al. (1984) found no increase in strength with subjects using a MORA, and Kerr (1986) concluded that physiological improvement by the use of a MORA had not been scientifically proven.

In all cases of TMJ pain, the cervical and thoracic spines must be examined and excluded as a cause or contributory factor of the patient's complaint.

NASAL INJURY

Nasal injuries mainly require treatment for haemorrhage (nose bleed). Direct pressure should be applied to the distal part of the nose with the head held forward. The athlete is able to breathe through the mouth. In cases where bleeding is severe, a cotton-wool ball or compress may be placed inside the nostril providing the pad is large enough not to be inhaled. If bleeding continues, hospitalization may be required to cauterize the ruptured vessels or apply vessel-constricting agents.

Nasal fracture is one of the most common maxillofacial injuries in sport. Often the nasal bones are obviously deviated to one side or depressed. Gently running the finger down the edge or bridge of the nose may reveal a step deformity, but this can easily be disguised when oedema is excessive (frequently the case). Radiographs are useful, but not definitive as many nasal features cannot be identified on X-ray (Handler, 1991). The nasal septum and orbit must be examined at the same time as the nose, as concurrent injures here can often go unnoticed.

Reduction of a displaced fracture should be performed within 7 days, because, after this, fibrosis makes accurate realignment of the bony fragments difficult.

References

Burkett, L.N. and Berstein, A.K. (1982) Strength testing after jaw repositioning with a mandibular orthopaedic appliance. *Physician and Sports Medicine*, **10**, (2) 101–107

Chapman, P.J. (1990) Orofacial injuries and international rugby players' attitudes to mouthguards. *British Journal of Sports Medicine*, **24**, 3

Craig, A.B. (1984) Physics and physiology of swimming goggles. *Physician and Sports Medicine*, **12**, (12) 107

Eichel, B.S. (1986) How I manage external otitis in competitive swimmers. *Physician and Sports Medicine*, **14**, 108

Ellis, G.S. (1987) Sports eye injuries: first aid and prevention. In *Sports Ophthalmology* (eds L.D. Pizzarello and B.G. Haik), Charles C. Thomas, Springfield, Illinois

Gelb, H. (1977) *Clinical Management of Head, Neck and Temporomandibular Joint Pain and Dysfunction*, W.B. Saunders, Philadelphia

Handler, S.D. (1991) Diagnosis and management of maxillofacial injuries. In *Athletic Injuries to the Head, Neck, and Face*, 2nd edn (ed. J.S. Torg), Mosby Year Book, St Louis

Hertling, D. and Kessler, R.M. (1990) *Management of Common Musculoskeletal Disorders*, J.B. Lippincott, Philadelphia

Jennings, D.C. (1990) Injuries sustained by users and non-users of gum shields in local rugby union. *British Journal of Sports Medicine*, **24**, 3

Jones, N.P. (1989) Eye injury in sport. *Sports Medicine*, **7**, 163–181

Kerr, I.L. (1986) Mouth guards for the prevention of injuries in contact sports. *Sports Medicine*, **3**, 415–427

Laskin, D.M. and Greene, G.S. (1972) Splint therapy for the myofacial pain dysfunction (MPD) syndrome in a comparative study. *Journal of the American Dental Association*, **84**, 624–628

Mackie, I.C. and Warren V.N. (1988) Dental trauma: 4. Avulsion of immature incisor teeth. *Dental Update*, December, 406–407

Magee, D.J. (2002) *Orthopedic Physical Assessment*, 4th edn, Saunders, Philadelphia

McArdle, W.D., Goldstein, L.B., Last, F.C., Spena, R. and Lechtman, S. (1984) Temporomandibular joint repositioning and exercise performance: a double blind study. *Medicine and Science in Sports and Exercise*, **16**, (3) 228–233

Pashby, R.C. (1986) Sports injuries to the eye. *Medical Clinics of North America*, **33**, 4672

Pashby, T. (1989) Eye injuries in sports. *Journal of Ophthalmic Nursing and Technology*, **8**, (3) 99–101

Reid, D.C. (1992) *Sports Injuries: Assessment and Rehabilitation*, Churchill Livingstone, Edinburgh

Renon, P., Lory, R., Belliato, R. and Casanova, M. (1986) Inner ear trauma caused by decompression accidents following deep sea diving. *Annals of Otolaryngology (Paris)*, **103**, 259–264

Schuller, D.E., Dankle, S.K., Martin, M. and Strauss, R.H. (1989) Auricular injury and the use of headgear in wrestlers. *Archives of Otolaryngology: Head and Neck Surgery*, **115**, 714–717

Schwartz, R. and Novich, M.M. (1980) The athlete's mouthpiece. *American Journal of Sports Medicine*, **8**, (5) 357–359

Simons, D.G., Travell, J.G. and Simons, L.S. (1999) *Travell and Simons' Myofascial Pain and Dysfunction*, vol. 1, 2nd edn, Lippincott, Williams and Wilkins, Philadelphia

Sperryn, P.N. (1985) *Sport and Medicine*, Butterworth, London

Chapter 18

The shoulder

FUNCTIONAL ANATOMY

The upper limb attaches to the trunk via the shoulder (pectoral) girdle. The shoulder complex in total consists of the scapula and clavicle, articulating with the ribcage and sternum to form four joints, all of which require attention in the management of shoulder pain (Fig. 18.1). The clavicle forms a strut for the shoulder, holding the arm away from the side of the body and allowing a greater range of unencumbered movement. At one end the clavicle joins the sternum through the sternoclavicular joint, while at the other it joins the scapula via the acromioclavicular joint.

Definition

The *acromioclavicular* (A/C) joint is formed between the acromion process of the scapula and the lateral (outer) end of the clavicle. The *sternoclavicular* (S/C) joint is formed between the top of the sternum and the medial (inner) end of the clavicle.

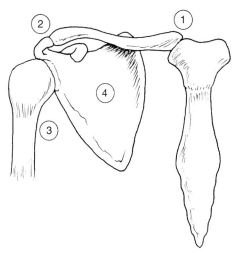

Figure 18.1   Joints of the shoulder complex. 1. Sternoclavicular joint. 2. Acromioclavicular joint. 3. Glenohumeral joint. 4. Scapulothoracic joint.

The scapula rests on the ribcage through muscle tissue alone, an essential point when dealing with stability of the shoulder complex. The glenohumeral joint is the articulation between the head of the humerus and the shallow glenoid fossa of the scapula.

The glenoid fossa is only one third the size of the humeral head, but the fossa is extended by the glenoid labrum attached to its periphery. This fibrocartilage rim is about 4 mm deep with its inner surface lined by, and continuous with, the joint cartilage. The joint itself is surrounded by a loose capsule with a volume twice as large as the humeral head. The anterior capsule is strengthened by the three glenohumeral ligaments. The lower portion of the capsule is lax in the anatomical position, and hangs down in folds. It has two openings, one for the passage of the long head of biceps and the other between the superior and middle glenohumeral ligaments which communicates with the subscapular bursa (between subscapularis and the joint capsule). The capsule is further strengthened by the rotator cuff muscles which act as 'active ligaments' and blend with the lateral capsule. The 'roof' of the joint is formed by the bony coracoid and acromion processes and the coracoacromial ligament which runs between them, the three structures together forming an arch.

Rotator cuff action

Most joints have a high degree of passive stability provided by their capsules and ligaments (see also Table 18.3). The shoulder, however, depends more on the active stability provided by its muscles to maintain joint integrity. In the anatomical position, the weight of the arm is largely supported by the coracohumeral ligament and superior capsule. When the arm moves away from the side of the body, tension in the superior capsule is immediately lost. Now joint stability is provided by the rotator cuff muscles alone.

The fibres of the joint capsule are angled forwards and slightly medially when the arm is hanging by the side of the body. As abduction progresses, tension within these fibres causes the shoulder to passively externally rotate. This movement prevents the humeral head from being pulled closer to the glenoid and facilitates a greater range of movement. Importantly, the external rotation also allows the greater tuberosity to clear the acromion process (see below).

Abduction of the humerus is accomplished by the supraspinatus and deltoid, acting as the prime movers. With the arm dependent, contraction of the deltoid (particularly the middle fibres) merely approximates the joint (upward translation), because the medial muscle fibres run almost parallel with the humerus. Unopposed, this pull would force the head of the humerus into the coracoacromial arch, resulting in impingement. Contraction of the infraspinatus, subscapularis, and teres minor (Fig. 18.2) causes compression and downward translation to offset the upward translation of deltoid (Culham and Peat, 1993). In an overhead throwing or serving action (Fig. 18.3) the subscapularis moves superiorly because the humerus has externally

Figure 18.2 (a) Deltoid pull at 30° and 90° abduction. (b) Muscles counteracting pull of deltoid. (i) Supraspinatus, (ii) infraspinatus and teres minor. (c) Subscapularis. Resolution of muscle force: S, shear; C, compression.

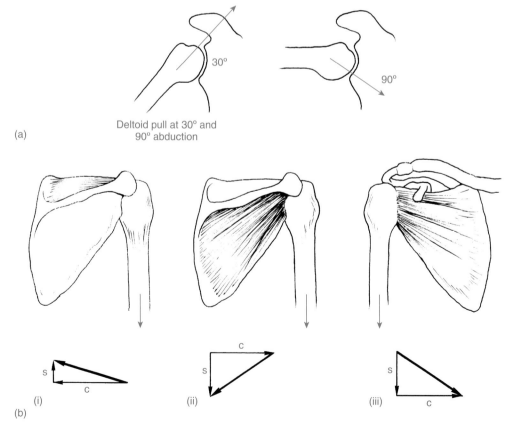

Deltoid pull at 30° and 90° abduction

(a)

(i)   (ii)   (iii)

(b)

rotated and the muscle can no longer effectively control the humeral head. The infraspinatus and to a lesser extent the teres minor stabilize the joint anteriorly in this position (Cain, Mutschler and Fu, 1987). For this reason sEMG addresses this muscle in stabilization programmes targeted at throwing sports (p. 394). By 90° abduction, the pull of the deltoid no longer tends to cause impingement, as shear forces are exceeded by compression, and the humeral head is stabilized into the glenoid (Perry and Glousman, 1995).

The supraspinatus is better placed to produce a rotatory action and therefore initiates abduction for the first 20°. The line of action of supraspinatus is such that less translation is caused, and its contribution to abduction is to reduce the reliance on deltoid and, as a consequence, reduce translation. After 30° of abduction the scapula starts to rotate to alter the glenoid position (see pp. 374–375).

> **Keypoint**
>
> The rotator cuff muscles downwardly translate the humeral head to guard against the risk of impingement caused by upward translation initiated by the deltoid.

Scapulohumeral rhythm

Motion of the shoulder girdle as a whole changes the position of the glenoid fossa, placing it in the most favourable location for the maximum range of humeral movement. When the glenoid cavity moves, it does so in an arc, the diameter of which is the length of the clavicle (Palastanga, Field and Soames, 1989). The medial border of the scapula moves in a similar but smaller arc and as a consequence the positions of the shoulder girdle structures change in relation to each other.

As the scapula moves medially and laterally towards and away from the vertebral column, the curvature of the ribcage forces the scapula to change from a frontal to a more

sagittal position. This, in turn, alters the direction in which the glenoid cavity faces. With elevation, the scapula is accompanied by some rotation, the glenoid cavity gradually pointing further upwards as the scapula gets higher.

With both shoulder abduction and flexion, the clavicle axially rotates. As the scapula twists, the coracoclavicular ligament 'winds up' and tightens, causing the clavicle itself to rotate. As the arm is abducted to 90° (phase I and II, see below) the clavicle elevates by 15° but does not rotate. Above 90° (phase III) further elevation of the clavicle occurs (up to 15°) but marked posterior rotation now occurs to 30–50° (Magee, 2002). For this reason a diminished range of movement at either SC or AC joints which reduces clavicular rotation will also impair scapular and therefore glenohumeral motion.

THE ABDUCTION CYCLE

Movement of the arm into abduction may be divided into three overlapping stages (Table 18.1).

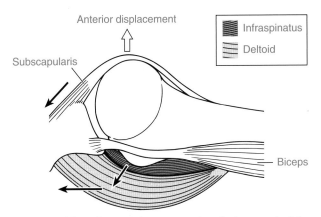

Figure 18.3 Muscular restraints to anterior displacement of the humeral head in an overhead throwing action. Adapted from Reid (1992), with permission.

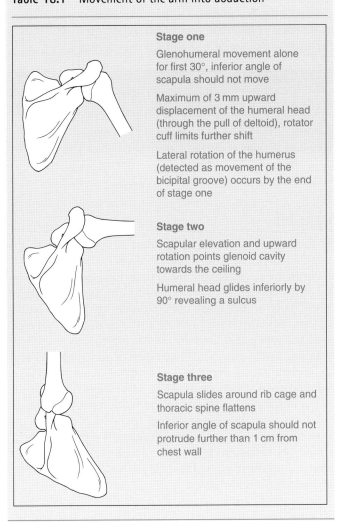

Table 18.1 Movement of the arm into abduction

Stage one

Glenohumeral movement alone for first 30°, inferior angle of scapula should not move

Maximum of 3 mm upward displacement of the humeral head (through the pull of deltoid), rotator cuff limits further shift

Lateral rotation of the humerus (detected as movement of the bicipital groove) occurs by the end of stage one

Stage two

Scapular elevation and upward rotation points glenoid cavity towards the ceiling

Humeral head glides inferiorly by 90° revealing a sulcus

Stage three

Scapula slides around rib cage and thoracic spine flattens

Inferior angle of scapula should not protrude further than 1 cm from chest wall

Stage (I)

In stage (I), no movement of the scapula should occur. The scapular stabilizers (serratus anterior especially) should hold the scapula firmly on the ribcage, providing a stable base for the humerus to move upon. As the arm abducts, lateral rotation of the humerus may be detected by palpation of the bicipital groove (intertubercular sulcus). If the humerus is maintained in a neutral position, abduction in the frontal plane is limited to about 90°. Laterally rotating the humerus increases this range to 120° (Lucas, 1973). When the arm is elevated in the sagittal plane, abduction is accompanied by medial rotation due to tightness in the coracohumeral ligament (Gagey, Bonfait and Gillot, 1987). No rotation is required for elevation in the scapular plane (30–45° anterior to the frontal plane). In this position, the joint capsule does not undergo torsion, and the deltoid and supraspinatus are optimally aligned.

At the beginning of abduction in the frontal plane, slight approximation of the humerus should occur (maximum 3 mm) to overcome the weight of the arm as the fibres of the joint capsule are taken off stretch and no longer support the arm through elastic recoil. No noticeable elevation of the shoulder should occur, unless the upper fibres of trapezius dominate the movement. The instantaneous axis of rotation in stage (I) is near the root of scapular spine, and moves superiorly and laterally as abduction progresses.

> **Keypoint**
>
> Stage (I) of the abduction cycle is the stage of scapular stability. The scapula should remain fixed to the ribcage, and no winging or marked elevation of the scapula should occur.

Stage (II)

By the beginning of stage (II), from 30° of abduction, the scapula should be upwardly rotating to maintain clearance between the acromion and the approaching greater tuberosity of the humerus. Scapular rotation in the beginning of stage (I) occurs as a result of elevation of the clavicle on the SC joint. Between 80 and 140° the instantaneous axis of rotation (IAR) migrates towards the AC joint along the upper central scapular area. Movement then occurs as elevation of the clavicle on the SC joint, and rotation of the scapula on the clavicle at the AC joint. More movement occurs at the glenohumeral joint than at the scapulothoracic joint. Ratios of 2:1 are normally quoted, giving 120° of movement at the glenohumeral joint and 60° at the scapulothoracic joint in a total abduction range of 180°. However, some authors (Lucas, 1973) have argued that the ratio is closer to 5:4 or 3:2 after phase (I) of abduction.

Scapular rotation occurs as a result of force-couples between the various muscles attached to the scapula (Fig. 18.4). Upward (lateral) rotation accompanying shoulder joint abduction or flexion is brought about by contraction of the upper and lower fibres of trapezius and the lower portion of serratus anterior. Serratus anterior is probably the most important of the group. It has two sets of fibres. The fibres of the upper portion run horizontally and slightly upwards, while those of the lower portion are aligned downwards. Both sets pull powerfully on the scapula, anchoring it to the ribcage and causing scapular upward rotation as trapezius lifts the lateral end of the clavicle and acromion process. If serratus anterior and the lower fibres of trapezius are ineffective, the upper trapezius will dominate the movement. In this case, these fibres show increased tone and can be tight. As the abduction moves further into stage (II), the moment arm of lower trapezius is lengthened and this portion of the muscle becomes increasingly active in the movement.

Downward (medial) rotation frequently occurs as a result of eccentric action of the above muscles. However, in activities such as hanging and chinning a beam, active scapular rotation is accomplished by levator scapulae and the rhomboids pulling upwards on the medial side of the

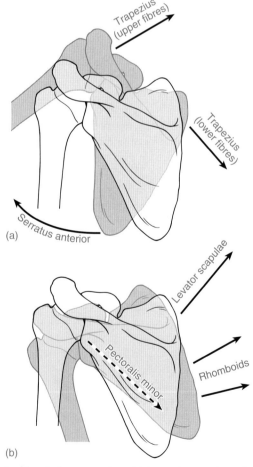

Figure 18.4   Muscle force couples which create scapular rotation. (a) Lateral rotation. (b) Medial rotation. From Palastanga, Field and Soames (1989), with permission.

scapula together with pectoralis minor pulling the coracoid process down. In cases where these muscles are tight or overactive, upward rotation of the scapula will be limited during abduction.

As scapular rotation progresses, lateral rotation of the humerus should be apparent as the cubital fossa and thumb orientate towards the ceiling. Ineffective scapular upward rotators, especially lengthening of the lower fibres of trapezius, will prevent correct orientation of the glenoid and increase the risk of impingement. Tightness in the medial rotators, especially the pectoralis major and sub-scapularis, combined with lengthening and weakness of the lateral rotators, may lead to delayed lateral rotation at the glenohumeral joint, resulting in impingement of the greater tuberosity against the inferior acromion.

During stage (II), as the humerus reaches 90° abduction, its head slides beneath the acromion, and a noticeable dip is formed in the skin. Failure of the shoulder musculature to pull the humerus into this position may result in the head slipping beneath the acromion with a sudden thud as the arm raises above 90° and similarly in this position during descent.

> **Keypoint**
>
> In the first half of stage (II) the scapula is seen to upwardly rotate. At the end of stage (II) the humeral head is pulled beneath the acromion forming a noticeable sulcus.

Stage (III)

During stage (III), as the arm approaches 120° abduction, no further movement is available from the glenohumeral joint. Additional range to reach the arm overhead is achieved by sliding the scapula over the thorax into further upward rotation and abduction. To facilitate this movement, the thor-acic spine must reverse its kyphosis and flatten. A kyphotic posture and inflexibility in the thoracic spine will therefore limit the final degrees of abduction. As a simple test for this, the patient is asked to stand with the back flat against a wall and the pelvis posteriorly tilted to avoid any possibility of hyperextension at the lumbar spine. Both arms are then abducted, keeping them in full contact with the wall. If thor-acic extension is limited, the patient will be unable to per-form pure abduction to full range. Instead, the arm moves through flexion–abduction to bring it in front of the fore-head. In conditions where abduction is limited, therefore, greater range may often be gained by mobilizing the thor-acic spine as well as working on the glenohumeral joint.

As the arm moves into its final overhead position and the scapula rotates maximally, the inferior angle of the scapula juts out through the outer edge of the thorax. However, no more than 1–2 cm of the inferior angle should be visible at

this point. During this final phase the IAR moves to the AC joint. Clavicular elevation is limited by tension in the costo-clavicular ligament. As the coracoid process moves away from the clavicle, tension in this ligament causes dorsal rotation of the clavicle about its long axis.

> **Keypoint**
>
> To reach the arm overhead, the scapula must slide over the thorax. To facilitate this movement, the thoracic spine should reverse its kyphosis and flatten. A kyphotic posture, with an inflexible thoracic spine will therefore limit the final degrees of abduction.

THE BIOMECHANICS OF THROWING

In sport, throwing is to the upper limb what gait is to the lower limb. It is an activity seen in many sports in some form, and there are similarities between all types of throw and with shots in racquet sports. Throwing can be divided into five stages which form a single continuous motion (Fig. 18.5). In the early stages, up to ball release, the body is accelerating the object. By the later stages, following release, the aim is to decelerate and reduce the effect of stress on the body.

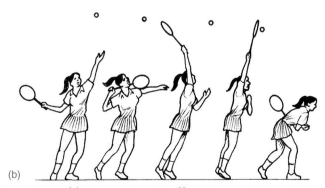

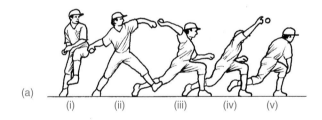

Figure 18.5 (a) Stages of throwing. (i) wind-up – athlete positions him- or herself for the throw; (ii) cocking – lead leg moves forwards, arm moves backwards, stretching body; (iii) acceleration – body drives forwards, leaving arm behind; (iv) deceleration – object released. Elbow continues to extend and shoulder to internally rotate; (v) follow through – trunk and lead leg show eccentric activity to dissipate energy. (b) Similarity to tennis serve. After Fleisig, Dillman and Andrews (1994), with permission.

In the wind-up phase (I) the athlete positions him- or herself in the best position for the throw. A right-handed thrower will plant the back foot on the ground and turn the body perpendicular to the direction of throw (left side of the body forward). The thrower then steps towards the target and begins to move the arms. During the cocking phase (II), the front leg moves forwards and the throwing arm moves backwards, effectively stretching the body out and building elastic energy. The shoulder is abducted to 90° and taken into extension and external rotation. The elbow is flexed to 45°. In the acceleration phase (III) the body moves forwards leaving the arm behind. The elbow begins to extend and the shoulder internally rotates.

The deceleration phase (IV) sees the release of the object being thrown, and the energy built up to throw the object must now be effectively dissipated to reduce stress on the body tissues. The arm continues to extend at the elbow and internally rotate at the shoulder, bringing the knuckles up. The rotator cuffs (external rotators) decelerate the internal rotation motion, and limit distraction to the glenohumeral joint. The elbow flexors similarly decelerate extension and limit hyperextension of the elbow joint. In the final phase, the follow through (V), the trunk is flexed eccentrically and the lead leg is extended pushing into the ground eccentrically to absorb energy. The throwing arm continues to move, giving a longer period over which to dissipate energy, and the hand may end up near the knee of the lead leg. Angular displacement for the shoulder and elbow throughout the throwing action is shown in Fig. 18.6.

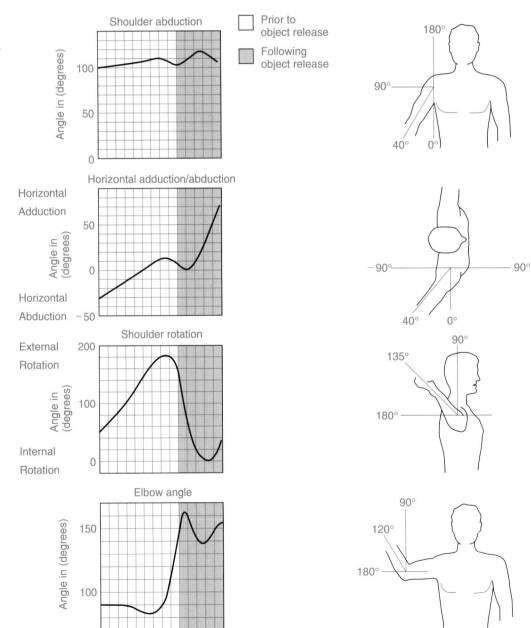

Figure 18.6 Angular displacement of the shoulder during a throwing action. After Fleisig, Dillman and Andrews (1994), with permission.

SCREENING EXAMINATION OF THE SHOULDER COMPLEX

After a subjective history has been taken, a screening examination is performed to enable the examiner to focus more closely on the injured area. The patient's posture and actions are noted while undressing, and the area is inspected for swelling, colour and deformity. A combination of active, resisted and passive movements are used to assess the shoulder complex (Cyriax, 1982). The patient is viewed from behind to note any alteration in scapulohumeral rhythm. It is helpful to have the patient facing a full length mirror, so the anterior aspect of the shoulder and the patient's facial expression may also be assessed. Active abduction and flexion–abduction are performed with overpressure applied at end-range, to assess end-feel. Positional changes of the scapula, either at rest or during movement, warrant closer inspection. Active glenohumeral rotation may be performed by asking the patient to place a hand behind the back (medial rotation) and then behind the head (lateral rotation). Passive lateral rotation is performed with the elbow flexed and upper arm held into the side. This is also the position for resisted lateral and medial rotations. Passive medial rotation is performed with the patient placing a hand into the small of the back. The examiner stabilizes the upper arm, and keeps the patient's elbow tucked into the side of the body. The examiner then gently pulls the patient's forearm away from the body, increasing medial rotation. Any limitation of movement is noted, and the percentages of limitation relative to each other reveal if a capsular pattern exists. The capsular pattern for the glenohumeral joint is gross limitation of abduction with some limitation of lateral rotation and little limitation of medial rotation.

> **Keypoint**
>
> The capsular pattern for the glenohumeral (shoulder) joint is gross limitation of abduction with some limitation of lateral rotation and little limitation of medial rotation.

Resisted abduction and adduction are performed in midrange, the examiner stabilizing the patient's pelvis to prevent any lateral trunk flexion occurring at the same time as the shoulder moves. Elbow flexion, extension and forearm rotation may be assessed at the same time with the elbow flexed and the upper arm held close to the body. The patient's forearm rests on the examiner's when testing the triceps, and resistance is given from above when testing the biceps. Resisted shoulder shrugging tests the trapezius. When a small physiotherapist is examining a large athlete, it is particularly important that resistance is applied from a position which gives maximum mechanical advantage to the therapist.

Referred pain from the neck must always be considered in cases of shoulder pain, and the neck screening examination is performed to establish whether movement is painful or reproduces the patient's shoulder symptoms. This simple but methodical examination should take no more than 2–3 minutes and tells the examiner whether the shoulder is the cause of pain, if a contractile or non-contractile structure is affected, and reveals if a capsular pattern exists to suggest an intracapsular lesion.

Locking test and quadrant test

Should movement apparently be full and painless at the glenohumeral joint, two further procedures are useful to reproduce the patient's symptoms. These are the locking test and the quadrant position (Maitland, 1991). Both tests refer to the position of the greater tuberosity relevant to acromial arch and glenoid (Corrigan and Maitland, 1994). The locking position combines internal rotation, extension and abduction of the shoulder with the scapula fixed. In this position the subacromial space is compressed and will give pain should an impingement syndrome be present. Cadaveric studies have shown that in the locking position the posterosuperior tip of the glenoid is in contact with the humeral head (Mullen, Slade and Briggs, 1989). The quadrant position stresses the anterior and inferior capsule, and combines external rotation, slight flexion and full abduction of the shoulder. Each test should be assessed for pain and end-feel, and compared with the uninjured side.

> **Keypoint**
>
> The locking position compresses the subacromial space and gives pain with an impingement syndrome. The quadrant position stresses the joint capsule and indicates capsular tightening.

To perform the tests, the patient is in a supine position, and the practitioner stands by the patient's side towards the shoulders. To test the locking position, the therapist places the palmar aspect of his or her forearm beneath the patient's shoulder, and grips the trapezius muscle to stop the shoulder shrugging. The therapist holds the patient's elbow, slightly medially rotates the arm, and lifts it into abduction (Fig. 18.7a).

For the quadrant position (Fig. 18.7b) the therapist's forearm still grips the patient's shoulder to prevent shrugging. The action is to hold the elbow and move the patient's arm into abduction, allowing the humerus to move from medial rotation (palm to chest) to lateral rotation (palm to ceiling). The point at which the humerus begins to change from medial to lateral rotation marks the beginning of the quadrant (Petty and Moore, 2001). From this point horizontal extension is examined by pressing the elbow to the floor, releasing it and then moving into further abduction before pressing again. Both the quality and the range of motion are assessed, as well as the occurrence of muscle spasm. The affected shoulder is compared to the unaffected side.

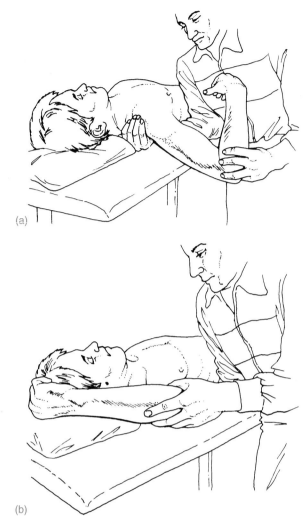

(a)

(b)

Figure 18.7   Locking position and quadrant position.

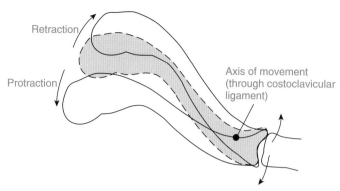

Figure 18.8   Movement of the clavicle. After Palastanga, Field and Soames (1994), with permission.

STERNOCLAVICULAR JOINT

The sternoclavicular (SC) joint provides, via the clavicle, the only structural attachment of the scapula to the rest of the body (Norkin and Levangie, 1992). The joint performs functionally as a ball and socket. The medial end of the clavicle articulates with the clavicular notch of the sternum, and the adjacent edge of the first costal cartilage. The congruity of the joint is enhanced by the presence of an interarticular fibrocartilage disc, which separates the joint cavity into two. In addition to improving the congruity of the joint, the disc also provides cushioning between the two bone ends. Furthermore, it holds the medial end of the clavicle against the sternum, preventing it moving upwards and medially when pushing actions are performed.

The joint is strengthened by a capsule attached to the articular margins, and four ligaments (anterior SC, posterior SC, interclavicular, and costoclavicular). Three degrees of movement are possible at the joint, elevation–depression, protraction–retraction and axial rotation. The axis of rotation for the first two movements (not rotation) is lateral to

the joint itself, passing through the costoclavicular ligament. Consequently, when the lateral end of the clavicle moves in one direction, its medial end moves in the opposite direction (Fig. 18.8), an important consideration with clavicular joint dislocation.

A total of about 60° of elevation and depression is available, elevation being limited by tension in the costoclavicular ligament, and depression by the interclavicular ligament and articular disc. When the lateral end of the clavicle is protracted, the medial end moves backwards, the opposite movement occurring with retraction. The total range of motion here is about 35°. This fact may be used in the emergency situation where posterior SC dislocation is causing asphyxia (blocked oxygen intake). A folded towel is placed on the ground between the athlete's shoulders to act as a fulcrum and the arm on the injured side is pushed firmly backwards to draw the medial aspect of the clavicle forwards and away from the trachea.

Keypoint

When the lateral (outer) end of the clavicle moves forwards in a protraction movement, the medial (inner) end moves back. In retraction the movement is reversed.

Axial rotation is purely a passive action accompanying scapular movements. The range of rotation is small (20–40°), but increases slightly as the lateral end of the clavicle is pulled back.

Injury

Injury to the SC joint is unusual, forming about 3% of all shoulder girdle trauma. Anterior dislocations occur more commonly than posterior dislocations in a ratio of 20:1 (Zachazewski, Magee and Quillen, 1996). Normally, the clavicle will fracture or the acromioclavicular joint will give way before the SC joint is seriously injured. However, when damage does occur, it is frequently the result of direct lateral compression of the shoulder, such as occurs when

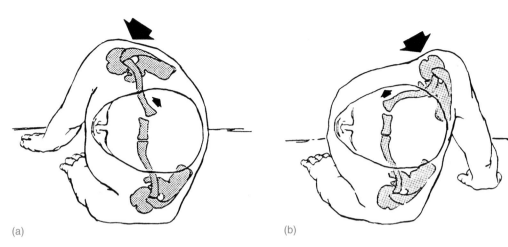

Figure 18.9
Sternoclavicular dislocation.
(a) Anteriorly directed force
causes posterior dislocation.
(b) Posteriorly directed force
causes anterior dislocation.
From Garrick and Webb
(1990), with permission.

(a)

(b)

falling onto the side of the body. The injury is more common in horse-riding and cycling where sufficient force is produced, but is seen in rugby and wrestling.

The SC joint will dislocate in the opposite direction to the applied force (Fig. 18.9), thus an anterior force (falling onto the back) will dislocate the joint backwards. Several important structures lie in close proximity to the joint including the oesophagus, trachea, lungs, pleurae, brachial plexus and major arteries and veins. Posterior dislocation therefore, if it is severe, may be potentially life-threatening. In contrast, anterior dislocation can occur in the absence of trauma, and frequently results only in slight discomfort.

Keypoint

The SC joint can dislocate in a fall onto the side of the body. The joint will move in the opposite direction to the applied force, an anteriorly directed force causing the joint to move backwards. If severe, this may be potentially life-threatening as the trachea may be damaged.

Initial examination (of posterior dislocation) on the field must obviously be aimed at ruling out life-threatening injury. The presence of stridor, dyspnoea, cyanosis, difficulty with speech, pulsating vessels and neurological signs may all necessitate immediate hospitalization.

If these are not present, joint examination may continue. Pain is generally well localized, and may become progressively more limiting over time. Anterior dislocation leaves a visible step deformity, and with posterior dislocation the usual prominence over the medial clavicle is lost. Local swelling is sometimes present, with crepitus and pain to motion, especially horizontal flexion. The shoulder is frequently held protracted.

Radiographic investigation will rule out clavicular fracture, and may enable differentiation between fracture and epiphyseal injury in the young (below 25 years) athlete. Closed reduction is often possible immediately after injury if pain is not too severe and before muscle spasm sets in.

Both anterior and posterior dislocations may be reduced by placing a knee between the scapulae of the seated athlete and gently pulling the shoulders back. The joint often reduces with an audible thud. After reduction the joint is immobilized with a figure-of-eight bandage and ice is used to reduce local swelling.

Posterior dislocations, even if successfully reduced, will still require hospital referral and observation. Posterior dislocations usually stay reduced, but anterior dislocations are apt to recur. Surgical fixation of anterior dislocation is possible, but the number of complications makes the procedure undesirable. Migration of a Steinmann pin or Kirchner wire into the heart or major vessels has been reported (Garrick and Webb, 1990). Rockwood and Odor (1989) reported excellent results following conservative management of atraumatic anterior displacement 8 years after initial treatment. Patients treated surgically (not by these authors) in the same study had complications including scarring, instability, pain and limitation of activity.

Even though the joint is frequently hypermobile, joint mobilizations may be used to relieve pain (Maitland, 1991). Anteroposterior gliding may be performed with the therapist placing his or her thumbs over the sternal end of the clavicle.

ACROMIOCLAVICULAR JOINT

This joint is formed between the oval facet on the lateral end of the clavicle and the similarly shaped area on the acromion process. The lateral end of the clavicle overrides the acromion, slightly. The joint capsule is fairly loose and strengthened above by fibres from trapezius, and by capsular thickenings which make up the superior and inferior acromioclavicular (AC) ligaments. As with the SC joint there is an intra-articular disc, but this time it does not divide the cavity into two. The joint is further stabilized by the coracoclavicular ligament, divided into its conoid and trapezoid parts. The conoid ligament is fan-shaped and resists forward movement of the scapula, while the stronger trapezoid ligament is flat and restricts backward movements.

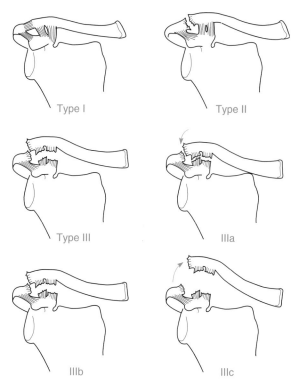

Figure 18.10 Acromioclavicular joint injuries. Type I (sprain), type II (subluxation), type II (dislocation), type IIIa (reduces as weight taken), type IIIb (no change as weight taken), type IIIc (lateral end of clavicle more prominent as weight taken).

As with the SC joints, the AC joint moves only in association with the scapula. Three types of movement are again present, protraction–retraction, elevation-depression and axial rotation.

Injury

The most common conditions affecting the AC joint are sprains and degeneration. AC joint sprains vary in intensity between minor grade I injuries to grade III ruptures representing complete disruption of the coracoclavicular ligament and AC joint dislocation (sprung shoulder) (Fig. 18.10). The injury may be further classified using weight-lifting radiographs. Here, the anterior deltoid is contracted by having the patient hold a weight with the elbow flexed and arm next to the body. If the clavicular attachment of the deltoid is intact, the joint may reduce as weight is taken (IIIa), or there may be no change in the joint appearance (IIIb). However, if the lateral end of the clavicle becomes more prominent, the clavicular attachment of the deltoid may have been stripped off (Dias and Gregg, 1991). Radiographs are also used to differentiate the condition from fractures of the distal clavicle where this is suspected.

Injury is usually the result of a superiorly directed force as occurs with a fall onto the point of the shoulder or being struck from above. The force drives the scapula downwards, an action resisted by the coracoclavicular ligament.

Examination reveals local tenderness over the AC joint, sometimes with a noticeable step deformity. The deformity may occur later, if initial muscle spasm reduces acromioclavicular separation.

Initial treatment aims to reduce the symptoms. Ice and a sling support to take the weight of the arm are recommended. The joint is immobilized in the sling for 2–3 weeks, and then gradually mobilized within pain-free limits. With grade I injuries, some relief may be provided by taping.

Acromioclavicular taping

Stress may be taken off the AC joint by a simple taping designed to press the clavicle down and take some of the weight of the arm away from the distal shoulder structures (Austin, Gwynn-Brett and Marshall, 1994; Macdonald, 1994). The athlete is positioned in sitting at the side of the couch with the elbow flexed to 90° and the shoulder abducted to 30°. The shoulder is slightly elevated and the arm rests on the couch. The shoulder and chest on the injured side of the body should be shaved of long hair. Spray adhesive is applied, making sure that the athlete turns the head away from the spray and covers the eyes with the unaffected hand. Also, the nipple area must be protected with a non-adhesive pad.

A felt pad is placed over the acromion to protect it from abrasion. Two anchors of 7.5 cm elastic adhesive tape are applied. The first runs horizontally from the sternum to the paravertebral area on the side of injury. The second is placed around the mid-humerus with light tension, ensuring that the limb is not excessively compressed (Fig. 18.11a). Two stirrups of 7.5 cm elastic adhesive tape are placed (prestretched) from the front to the back of the chest anchor, passing over the acromion (Fig. 18.11b). These are then reinforced by two strips of 5 cm zinc oxide taping. Two further strips of elastic adhesive tape are placed (pre-stretched) laterally from the arm anchor across the anterior aspect of the shoulder to join the chest stirrups over the acromion, and laterally from the anchor, passing posteriorly over the shoulder to the acromion (Fig. 18.11c). Again, these stirrups are reinforced by 5 cm zinc oxide taping. If the shoulder stirrups have been applied correctly, their tension will tend to lift the arm into abduction slightly. The chest and arm stirrups are closed by reapplying the chest and arm anchors (7.5 cm elastic adhesive tape) to act as fixing strips. Sensation and pulse should be re-tested after tape application.

In the acute phase of injury, the forearm weight may also be taken by a collar and cuff sling. With time, when pain-free

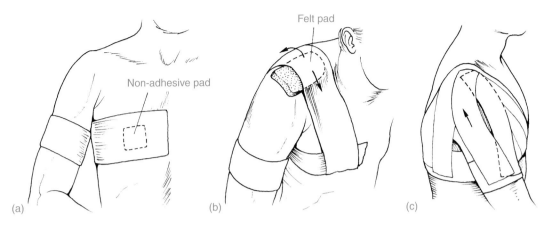

Figure 18.11
Acromioclavicular joint taping. (a) Anchors. (b) Stirrup applied under tension. (c) Arm stirrups.

Non-adhesive pad

Felt pad

(a)   (b)   (c)

arm motion to 90° is available, the humeral portion of the tape may be dispensed with.

Specific exercise therapy

As inflammation subsides, exercise therapy is commenced to restore function. This is used initially to maintain muscle tone in the absence of joint movement. Isometric contractions of the scapular and glenohumeral muscles are used, and the athlete maintains general fitness and lower body strength by exercising with the AC joint taped. When pain subsides and movement commences, gentle scapular actions are used, such as shoulder shrugging and bracing within the limits of pain. These may progress to a scapular stabilization programme. Range of motion exercises for the glenohumeral joint are begun, ensuring that correct scapulohumeral rhythm is maintained.

When full pain-free motion is obtained, the athlete may be seen to have a permanent step deformity, and some joint degeneration may occur in later years. The major problem resulting from this injury is lack of confidence when falling in contact sports. The effects of direct trauma may be limited by placing a felt doughnut pad over the joint. Confidence is built using progressive closed chain exercises and rehearsal of falling actions. These may begin with forward rolls onto the outstretched arm on a mat, initially from a kneeling position, progressing to standing and finally a diving forward roll over a bench. Pressure over the point of the shoulder begins with log rolling on the floor, and builds up to shoulder blows on to a rolled mat or punch bag.

Surgical intervention

There is some controversy concerning the treatment of this condition. Both conservative and surgical approaches restore function to a similar degree (Larsen, Bjerg-Nielsen and Christensen, 1986; Dias et al., 1987; Bannister et al., 1989), and some surgical methods have been shown to give long-term functional detriment. Certainly, removal of the distal end of the clavicle (Gurd, 1941) will disrupt the acromioclavicular ligament, a main stabilizer of the joint

(Fukuda et al., 1986). In the literature, the main argument for surgery has been the development of degenerative changes in the joint as a result of non-operative management. However, degeneration does not occur in all patients, and when it does occur, it is not necessarily a limitation (Dias et al., 1987). In addition, surgery is often as effective if done in the acute or chronic condition, so there is normally no advantage to operating immediately. Importantly, surgery carries with it a high risk of complications (Ejeskar, 1974; Lancaster, Horowitz and Alonso, 1987; Taft, Wilson and Oglesby, 1987).

In a literature review of 11 papers detailing the long-term results of both surgical and conservative management of this injury, Dias and Gregg (1991) found poor results to have occurred in 13 out of 247 patients treated conservatively (5.3%), and 22 out of 233 managed surgically (9.4%). These authors argued that as comparable results were obtained regardless of the method used, conservative management was the treatment of choice for most AC injuries. Looking at strength testing following grade III AC injuries treated conservatively (average 4.5 year follow-up), Tibone, Sellers and Tonino (1992) found no subjective complaints in patients, all of whom were able to participate in sport. Full motion occurred in all subjects, and no significant differences were found in muscle strength of injured and non-injured sides in rotation, abduction/adduction or flexion/extension.

AC joint degeneration

Joint degeneration is common in later years following injury, regardless of the grade of damage which occurred, and particularly after repeated trauma. In addition, some sports, such as weight-lifting, have a higher incidence of degenerative changes in the AC joint, even where no incidents of trauma may have occurred. Cahill (1982) reported 46 cases of osteolysis of the distal clavicle, all but one occurring in weight-lifters. He argued that degeneration occurred as a result of subchondral stress fractures resulting from repeated microtrauma. The condition presents as pain, usually dull and aching in nature, brought on by activities such as lifting and throwing. To examination there is point tenderness

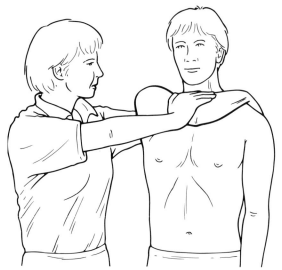

Figure 18.12   The cross body test for acromioclavicular (AC) joint dysfunction (the scarf test).

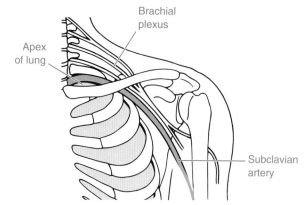

Figure 18.13   Structures close to the clavicle.

over the joint, with pain and crepitus to passive horizontal adduction, taking the hand across the chest and placing on top of the other shoulder (cross body or scarf test) (Fig. 18.12).

Keypoint

Where the AC joint is suspected to be the source of pain, horizontal adduction with overpressure ('cross body' or 'scarf' test) can be used as a confirmatory test.

Where the diagnosis is uncertain, radiographs will frequently reveal degeneration, and injection of local anaesthetic into the joint is helpful to establish if the degeneration is the cause of the patient's symptoms.

Movements which stress the joint (for example, press-ups, weight training or throwing) should be avoided. Initially, immobilization in a sling may be required in the very acute lesion. Later, joint mobilization provides good results. Anteroposterior gliding may be performed with the patient in a sitting position. The therapist grasps the distal end of the clavicle with his or her thumb and forefingers of one hand, and the acromion process in a similar fashion with the other hand. The hands are worked against each other to glide the joint. Injection of corticosteroid may give many months of relief, a technique made easier if the shoulder is laterally rotated to distract the AC joint.

FRACTURES OF THE CLAVICLE

The most common mechanism of injury is a fall onto the outstretched arm, and occasionally direct trauma to the shoulder. Although common, these injuries should not be taken too lightly, as it must be remembered that the subclavian vessels and the medial cord of the brachial plexus lie in close proximity, as does the upper lobe of the lung (Fig. 18.13). Neurovascular and pulmonary examination may therefore be required.

There is usually a cracking sensation at the time of injury, with immediate pain over the fracture sight and rapid swelling. Signs of injury to vital structures are rare, but include dyspnoea and paraesthesia and obviously warrant immediate hospitalization. Laceration of the subclavian artery presents as a readily expanding pulsating haematoma. Deformity is common, as is crepitus.

Fractures of the proximal and middle thirds of the clavicle make up the largest proportion (80%) of such injuries. If not displaced these should be immobilized with the shoulders retracted in a figure-of-eight bandage for 6 weeks. With young athletes the risk of non-union may make it necessary to curtail activity for up to 3 months after injury. Figure-of-eight bandages must not be applied so tightly as to constrict the blood or nerve supply to the arm. When little displacement is present, support in a sling may be all that is required. Some step deformity usually occurs as complete immobilization of athletes (other than in a cast) is difficult. This type of deformity is usually cosmetic rather than functional.

Distal fractures tend to be displaced by retraction immobilization, and are better wired. Internal fixation of the proximal clavicle carries with it similar complications to that of the sternoclavicular (SC) joint. Fractures to the extreme proximal end of the clavicle may be misdiagnosed as SC dislocations, and in the younger individual epiphyseal injury should be considered in this region. It should be noted that the sternoclavicular epiphysis may remain open until the age of 25 (Zachazewski, Magee and Quillen, 1996), so radiological examination must be accurate.

WINGED SCAPULA

During normal scapulohumeral rhythm, the scapula slides over the ribcage, and is held in place by the serratus anterior. If weakness or paralysis of the serratus anterior occurs, the scapula will stand prominent from the ribcage when the arm is protracted against resistance. In addition to muscular weakness, there are a number of other causes including damage to the long thoracic nerve, brachial plexus injury, conditions affecting the fifth, sixth and seventh cervical nerve roots, and certain types of muscular dystrophy (Apley and Solomon, 1989).

Where weakness is due to nerve palsy, spontaneous recovery is to be expected. Re-education of scapulohumeral movement is required as habitual alteration of scapulohumeral rhythm is often seen. Strengthening the shoulder musculature in general, and especially serratus anterior, is also useful.

Occasionally, a congenitally undescended scapula (Sprengel's shoulder) is seen, sometimes associated with marked thoracic kyphosis. Normally, the scapulae descend completely by the third month of fetal life. However, if undescended, the scapula appears slightly smaller, higher, and more prominent. Scapulohumeral rhythm is affected and abduction is limited as a consequence. Minor cases respond to rehabilitation although marked deformity may require surgery.

Apparent winging may occur when the scapulae abduct through lengthening of the scapular retractors and tightening of the protractors. As the scapulae move away from the mid-line, they roll around the ribcage, lifting their medial border. This is not true winging, however, because the condition is present at rest and during muscle contraction.

IMPINGEMENT SYNDROME

The subacromial space (Fig. 18.14) lies beneath the coracoacromial arch formed by the coracoacromial ligament together with the coracoid and acromion the so-called 'roof of the joint'. The coracoacromial arch is covered by the deltoid, and inferiorly its fascia is continuous with that of the supraspinatus. The arch prevents upward dislocation of the glenohumeral joint. The supraspinatus passes beneath the arch, being separated from it by the subacromial bursa. The subacromial distance (space between the inferior acromion and the head of the humerus) is normally about 1 cm (Petersson and Redlund-Johnell, 1984). If the supraspinatus tendon has ruptured, or the muscle is no longer active, this space will reduce by as much as 50% due to the unopposed pull of the deltoid.

> ### Keypoint
>
> The subacromial space may reduce by as much as 50% if the supraspinatus muscle is dysfunctional.

During elevation and internal rotation, the greater tuberosity, with the supraspinatus riding on top, may press against the anterior edge of the underside of the acromion (or a spur from a degenerating AC joint) causing impingement

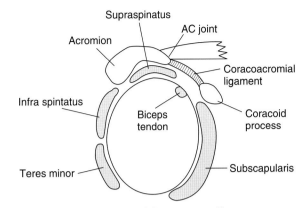

Figure 18.14 Impingement of the rotator cuff.

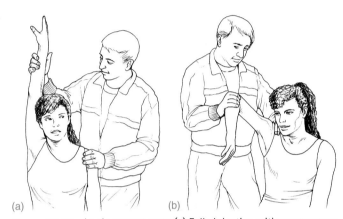

Figure 18.15 Impingement tests. (a) Full abduction with overpressure to the internally rotated shoulder. (b) Hawkin's sign. Flexion and internal rotation. Overpressure to internal rotation and abduction or horizontal flexion.

pain. During flexion, impingement may also involve the long head of biceps (Peat and Culham, 1994).

The action of abduction involves a complex series of movements, as described on page 374. At the point where the greater tuberosity comes close to the acromion (70–120° abduction), a number of structures may be pinched between the involved bones or the tuberosity and the coracoclavicular ligament. Normally, the structures affected are the supra sinatus tendon, the long head of biceps and the sub acromial bursa.

Examination

Following the screening examination described on page 000, two further tests are useful. In test one (Fig. 18.15a) the arm is fully abducted and overpressure is put onto the internally rotated (thumb forwards) shoulder. For the second test (Fig. 18.15b), the glenohumeral joint is flexed and internally rotated (Hawkins test). Overpressure is then added to internal rotation and abduction or horizontal flexion. Resisting flexion by placing pressure over the elbow may also bring on the athlete's pain (Hawkins and Hobeika, 1983; Reid, 1992).

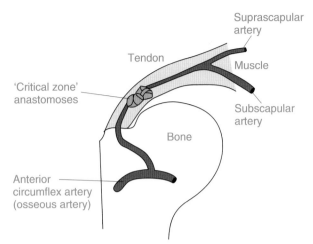

Figure 18.16 Vascularity of the critical zone. From Keirns (1994) with permission.

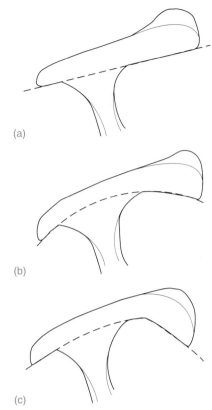

Figure 18.17 Acromion types. (a) Type I, flat. (b) Type II, curved. (c) Type III, hooked. After Ticker and Bigliani (1994).

In addition to a purely mechanical impingement, changes in the microvascular supply to the area have been noted. Pressure exerted by the humeral head on the supraspinatus tendon, has the effect of 'wringing out' the tendon vessels and creating an avascular zone (Rathbun and Macnab, 1970). This area, known as the critical zone (Fig. 18.16), is an anastomosis between the osseous vessels and the tendinous vessels (Moseley and Goldie, 1963). Furthermore, repeated microtrauma results in local oedema within the tendon and an increase in tissue volume. This in turn makes the structures more susceptible to impingement by reducing the subacromial space and so perpetuates the problem.

A reduction in the subacromial space may be the result of individual variation in the anatomical architecture of this region, with some individuals more prone to impingement than others (Ticker and Bigliani, 1994). Cadaveric studies of 140 specimens have identified three types of acromion associated with full thickness tears of the rotator cuff (Bigliani, Morrison and April, 1986). The flat (type I) acromion occurred in 17% of subjects, the curved (type II) acromion was seen in 43%, and the hooked (type III) type in 39% (Fig. 18.17). The hooked acromion was present in 70% of rotator cuff tears whereas the flat type was only seen in 3%. By assessing the supraspinatus outlet view X-ray, Morrison and Bigliani (1987) showed 80% of those with positive arthrograms to have a hooked acromion. The same authors showed that 66% of patients who underwent open subacromial decompression had a hooked acromion.

Impingement is not simply the result of a lack of subacromial space, however. Weakness in the rotator cuff (or pain inhibition) can cause instability (see below) and allow the humeral head to ride up through deltoid contraction, making examination of rotator cuff strength and order of muscle contraction vital with this condition. The interaction between biomechanics, physiology and pathology creates a painful progressive condition which ultimately may cause mechanical failure, as detailed in Fig. 18.18.

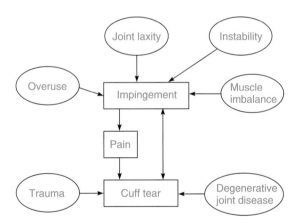

Figure 18.18 Interrelation between pain, impingement and cuff tear. After Reid (1992) with permission.

Stages of impingement

Three stages of impingement have been described (Neer, 1972). Stage I is a self-limiting overuse syndrome. It presents as a dull ache occurring after repeated overhead activity. The most significant sign is a painful arc of movement. Here, as abduction is commenced, no pain is felt. As the tuberosity moves closer to the glenoid, structures are compressed and pain occurs between 70 and 120°. As abduction goes further, the tuberosity moves away from the acromion and pain subsides as the arm is taken overhead (Fig. 18.19).

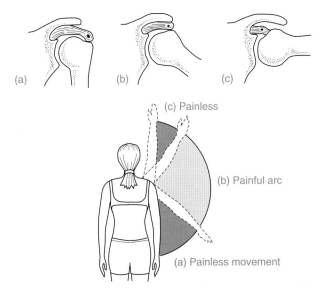

Figure 18.19 The painful arc. (a) No impingement, painless. (b) Tuberosity pinches painful structure. (c) Tuberosity moves beneath acromion, pain disappears.

In addition to a painful arc, palpable pain may be found over the anterior edge of the acromion in some cases. Resisted movements may or may not be painful depending on whether a contractile structure is impinged. If the supraspinatus is affected, the painful arc exists in combination with pain to resisted lateral rotation and sometimes initiation of abduction. However, the situation is far from being clear-cut because pain is frequently caused when a resisted movement approximates the joint, pulling the humerus onto the acromion. In addition, pain in this condition may be so acute that resisted actions appear weak. The weakness, however, is due to the pain itself rather than neurological involvement. Involvement of the biceps tendon gives pain along the intertubercular sulcus with resisted shoulder and elbow flexion in combination with resisted forearm supination.

The stage I lesion is basically inflammatory in nature and so reversible. Treatment aims to reduce pain and swelling, and to remove the cause of impingement by resting the impinged structures through training modification. If modalities are used, the position of the athlete for treatment must be considered. The standard resting position of adduction and neutral rotation causes the blood vessels within the region to be tractioned and compressed (McNab, 1973). A better resting position during treatment is to have the athlete sit at the side of the couch with the arm abducted to 30–70° and the forearm supported (Lovinger, Mangus and Ingersoll, 1991). There should be neutral rotation of the glenohumeral joint and slight extension.

Stage II lesions involve the development of thickening and fibrosis. They generally give more intense pain, at night as well as with activity, and are not so readily reversed. Movement becomes increasingly limited as fibrosis and scarring occur in the subacromial space. Pain relief and reduction of inflammation are as for a stage I condition, but now stretching exercises become more important to limit loss of range through fibrosis. The stage III lesion involves chronic bony changes and is more usually seen in the older athlete (Thein, 1989). Prolonged mechanical impingement gives rise to sclerosis and osteophyte formation of the acromion and tuberosity, and occasionally calcification of the supraspinatus tendon. Active movements are more limited than passive, with weakness and rotator cuff atrophy being commonly seen. Treatment aims are essentially to restore limited function, and frequently require surgical intervention. Both decompression and anterior acromioplasty are used.

> **Keypoint**
>
> Stage I lesions are inflammatory, stage II see the development of fibrosis and adhesion. In stage III lesions chronic bony changes, including sclerosis and osteophyte formation, may be present.

Internal rotation of the shoulder is one biomechanical factor which predisposes to impingement (Halbach and Tank, 1990), and should be limited in patients with this condition. While external rotation helps the greater tuberosity clear the acromion, internal rotation has the reverse effect, compressing the two structures. Exercise therapy aims to redevelop scapular stability and to restore the normal internal/external rotation, ratio of the glenohumeral joint to 3:2 (Baechle, 1994). As the supraspinatus is affected, external rotation range and strength is normally greatly reduced in these athletes. External rotation exercises, beginning with the arm held to the side and eventually in 90° abduction, are therefore used. Combinations of abduction, extension and external rotation may be performed on a pulley or with elastic tubing, within the pain-free range.

The structures affected by impingement may also be injured in isolation. So, either the supraspinatus or biceps tendons may be subjected to tendinitis, and the subacromial bursa inflamed without muscular involvement.

TENDON INJURIES

Rotator cuff

Tendinitis of the rotator cuff muscles is common both as a result of overuse and through trauma. Common examples of overuse include excessive repetitions on a single weight-training exercise, while trauma may result from an ill-timed 'wrenching' action which combines rotation with abduction.

The most commonly affected tendon in the shoulder is that of the supraspinatus. Pain is elicited with resisted external rotation and initiation of abduction. More specifically, pain occurs with the arms abducted to 90°, brought forwards into 30° flexion and internally rotated so that the thumbs point towards the floor (Reid, 1992).

Palpation to the muscle insertion is performed with the injured arm medially rotated (hand behind the back) to bring the greater tuberosity forwards and make the tendon more superficial (Fig. 18.20a). This is also the most convenient position for transverse frictions, the area of scarring being found by palpating about one finger's width below the anterior tip of the acromion. The musculotendinous junction is more conveniently palpated with the injured arm abducted to 90° and supported (Cyriax and Cyriax, 1983). The palpating finger is directed at the space between the posterior aspect of the lateral clavicle and the scapular spine. Again, this is the most convenient starting position for transverse frictional massage (Fig. 18.20b).

Pain on resisted lateral rotation but not abduction implicates the infraspinatus. Local pain may be found by palpation to the posterior aspect of the greater tuberosity with the patient's shoulder flexed, slightly adducted and laterally rotated. The most convenient position for this is elbow support in a prone-lying position, with the patient leaning forwards and outward over the injured shoulder (Fig. 18.20c).

If resisted medial rotation alone gives pain, the subscapularis is most likely affected, at its insertion into the lesser tuberosity. This structure may be palpated and treated along the inner edge of the intertubercular sulcus. The patient is in a long sitting position, and the therapist grasps the hand on the affected side. A transverse frictional mobilization is carried out by medial and lateral rotation of the patient's shoulder against the palpating finger of the therapist (Fig. 18.20d).

Pain in combination with resisted adduction implicates the muscles (pectoralis major, latissimus dorsi and teres major) attaching within the intertubercular sulcus. These muscles are usually tight and they show tendinitis less commonly than muscle tearing.

Calcification of the supraspinatus (or rarely the other rotator cuff tendons) may develop following chronic tendinitis within the critical zone (Moseley and Goldie, 1963),

Figure 18.20 Palpation and treatment of rotator cuff tendon injury. (a) Supraspinatus: tendon. (b) Supraspinatus: musculotendinous junction. (c) Infraspinatus. (d) Subscapularis. After Cyriax and Cyriax (1983), with permission.

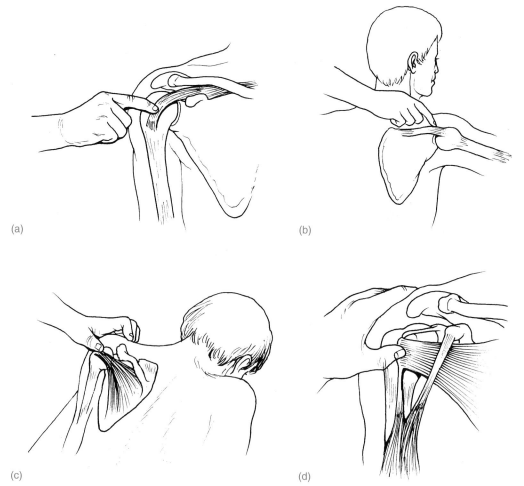

an area susceptible to injury due to reduced vascularity (Rothman and Parkes, 1965). This area, near the attachment of the supraspinatus (see Fig. 18.16), tends to be wrung out when the arm is held in its resting position of adduction and neutral rotation. Compression of the tendon vessels and microtrauma leads to repetitive hypoxia, and is especially common in activities which involve repeated internal rotation at 90° shoulder abduction. Fibrocytes within the tendon are transformed to chondrocytes, and collagen disintegration, coupled with the accumulation of mucopolysaccharides, begins. Hydroxyapatite mineral deposit deposition is then initiated (Lemak, 1994).

During the acute and subacute phase the deposit is of toothpaste-like consistency (and will escape into the subacromial bursa if punctured during an injection procedure). Conservative management is usually successful if the

---

Treatment note 18.1   Rotator cuff trigger points

Trigger points (TrPs) within the rotator cuff muscles can give pain in shoulder conditions such as impingement where there is a painful arc, and adhesive capsulitis where movement is severely limited. TrPs in these cases are often secondary to other pathologies, but may, in some instances, actually be the primary cause of pain (Simons, Travell and Simons, 1999; Gunn, 1996).

Supraspinatus
The supraspinatus may refer pain into the point of the shoulder and as far down the arm as the lateral epicondyle. TrPs may be found in the muscle bulk, which are usually very painful to palpation as the muscle is more superficial here (Fig. 18.21). As the muscle travels across the head of the humerus it is covered by the deltoid and so less painful to palpation, but at its insertion onto the superior aspect of the greater tuberosity again it may be tender. TrPs may be treated by ischaemic compression and dry needling. When needling over the scapula the possibility of incomplete ossification of the scapula surface must be considered and deep needling (greater than 1.0 cm) should be used with caution.

Infraspinatus
TrPs from the infraspinatus refer to the shoulder and arm in much the same way as the supraspinatus. Differentiation is through palpation and pain to abduction (supraspinatus). In addition, the larger origin of the infraspinatus can refer pain between the scapulae into the rhomboid region. TrPs may be in the belly of the muscle, normally located just below the medial third of the scapular spine, and occasionally right onto the medial border of the scapula (Fig. 18.22). To facilitate palpation ask the patient to place the arm across the chest to grasp the opposite shoulder and place the muscle on slight stretch.

Teres minor
The teres minor has the same action as infraspinatus but a different innervation (teres minor the axillary nerve, infraspinatus the suprascapular nerve). TrPs are often secondary to those of infraspinatus and lie within the muscle belly. They are located at the lateral edge of the scapula between the infraspinatus above and the teres major below.

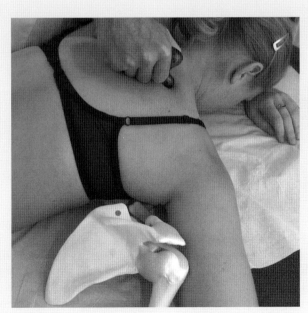

Figure 18.21   Supraspinatus.

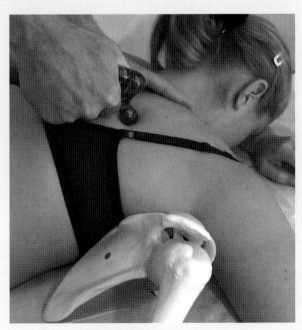

Figure 18.22   Infraspinatus.

Subscapularis

TrPs in this muscle have been described as 'the key to frozen shoulder' (Simons, Travell and Simons, 1999) and this claim certainly coincides with the pathological changes found within the rotator interval in adhesive capsulitis (see Fig. 18.34). Referred pain is to the posterior aspect of the shoulder and can extend down the posterior aspect of the arm. TrPs are mostly beneath the scapula and only accessible by placing the patient supine with the arm abducted to 45°. The therapist then places traction through the arm to draw the scapula laterally and locates the lateral edge of the scapula beneath the medial to the latissimus dorsi. A pincer grip is used between the thumb and forefinger (Fig. 18.23).

East meets West

Many traditional acupuncture points correspond to TrPs. SI-12 (Small Intestine 12) lies directly within the belly of the supraspinatus, while SI-10 lies on the belly of infraspinatus, and SI-9 within teres minor. The Small Intestine acupuncture channel (meridian) is often used in cases of posterior shoulder pain (Fig. 18.24).

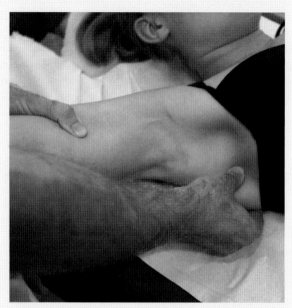

Figure 18.23   Subscapularis, anterior approach.

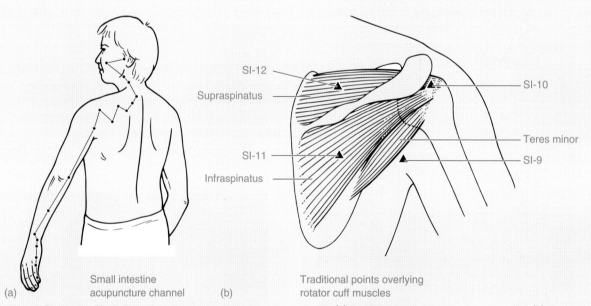

(a) Small intestine acupuncture channel

(b) Traditional points overlying rotator cuff muscles

SI-12
Supraspinatus
SI-11
Infraspinatus
SI-10
Teres minor
SI-9

Figure 18.24   Rotator cuff trigger points in relation to acupuncture points. (a) Small intestine acupuncture channel. (b) Traditional points overlying rotator cuff muscles.

condition is caught early enough. Active rest and exercise are called for. The repetitive forces causing hypoxia must be removed by correcting impingement. Exercise therapy is then used to enhance the blood supply of the tendon, and healing is good. High repetitions are performed in the pain-free range (Torstensen, Meen and Stiris, 1994) avoiding both the resting position (adduction and neutral rotation) and

internal rotation. All other sporting activities which cause pain are curtailed.

In the chronic phase the deposit is gritty and sand-like. This later stage is more painful and may require surgical intervention. Arthroscopy is normally performed to debride the calcific portion of the tendon and remove any necrotic tissue. The tendon should then heal well.

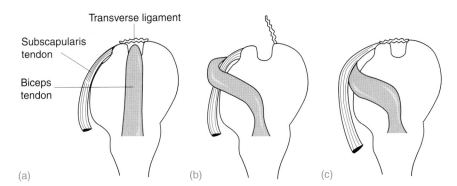

Figure 18.25 Biceps tendon subluxation. (a) Normal alignment. (b) Transverse ligament tears, biceps tendon rides over subscapularis. (c) Transverse ligament intact, biceps tendon slides beneath subscapularis. After Reid (1992), with permission.

Biceps

The long head of biceps originates at the supraglenoid tubercle and passes intracapsularly into the bicipital groove (intertubercular sulcus). The tendon is round at its origin, flattens as it passes over the shoulder joint and narrows within the intertubercular sulcus (Mariani and Cofield, 1988). As the humerus moves, the tendon slides within its groove by as much as 3–4 cm. The tendon is held in the groove by both the transverse ligament and the coracohumeral ligament (the latter attaching from the lateral edge of the coracoid to the lesser and greater tuberosities). Cadaveric studies have shown that the biceps tendon will not displace when the transverse ligament is cut, if the coracohumeral ligament remains intact (Slatis and Alato, 1979). The tendency for subluxation or dislocation of the tendon from the bicipital groove is dependent on a number of factors including the depth of the groove, and angle of the medial wall of the groove and the presence of a supratubercular ridge. Normally, the medial wall of the bicipital groove forms an angle of 60–70°, and angles of less than 30° when combined with a shallow groove have been shown to be associated with tendon subluxation (O'Donoghue, 1973). A supratubercular ridge is present in 55% of the population, and well developed in 18% (Reid, 1992). It is a proximal extension of the medial wall of the bicipital groove, and may force the biceps tendon against the transverse ligament thus increasing tension. When the tendon subluxes, it does so in one of two ways, both normally associated with trauma to the humerus or rotator cuff (Petersson, 1986). The tendon usually moves medially and will lie superficial to the subscapularis if the transverse ligament ruptures. If the subscapularis remains attached to the transverse ligament, the biceps tendon may end up deep to the subscapularis tendon itself (Fig. 18.25).

Biceps tendon dislocation typically occurs after a violent overhead action, with the athlete feeling pain on the anterior aspect of the shoulder. The shoulder will feel weak or 'dead' and often the athlete describes feeling 'something going out' or 'snapping'. On examination there is tenderness to palpation over the tendon, and medial and lateral rotation may elicit a palpable click. This may be further investigated using Yergason's sign (Yergason, 1931) or Speed's test. For Yergason's test the patient attempts to supinate the flexed elbow while externally rotating the shoulder. Speed's test involves shoulder flexion from a position of extension with the forearm supinated. Management of the condition is usually surgical followed by intensive rehabilitation to restore correct scapulothoracic and glenohumeral function.

> **Keypoint**
>
> Both Yergason's test and Speed's test attempt to reproduce biceps tendon dislocation using resisted shoulder and elbow movements.

Tendinitis of the long head of biceps presents as pain to resisted shoulder and elbow flexion and resisted forearm supination. Yergason's sign and Speed's test may again be used. The teno-osseous junction of the muscle at the supraglenoid tubercle and adjacent glenoid labrum is difficult to palpate directly, but the tendon itself within the intertubercular sulcus is easier. A painful arc is only present with these conditions if the inflamed area of tendon is within a pinchable position in mid-range abduction, in which case impingement tests will be positive.

Overuse is the predominant causal factor with alteration in the biomechanics of overhead actions often being present. The synovial sheath of the tendon may become swollen and inflamed, with thickening and haemorrhaging frequently seen. Adhesions are often present. If the locking position and quadrant test reproduce pain, posteroanterior (PA) gliding should be assessed. If limited, PA pressures against the humeral head (see below) should be used.

Rupture of the biceps brachii occurs more commonly at the insertion of the long head into the supraglenoid tubercle, but tears to the short head, distal attachment or belly may occur (Fig. 18.26c). The rupture more frequently follows subacromial impingement and tendon degeneration (Reid, 1992). The mechanism of injury for proximal tendon injuries is normally a forced extension while the muscle is contracting. This can result from an arm tackle or block, where the arm is held abducted and then pushed back behind trunk level. Distal tendon injuries may occur as a result of heavy lifting with the elbow flexed to 90°.

> **Keypoint**
>
> The biceps ruptures more commonly at its long head attaching into the supraglenoid tubercle. The injury normally occurs with forced arm extension as the muscle is contracting.

On examination, pain is elicited to resisted elbow flexion and supination (which may be combined with shoulder flexion), and passive end-range extension. A visible defect may be noted in the muscle, with retraction of the tendon. In the case of the long head, the tendon may no longer be palpable in the intertubercular sulcus, and as the muscle is contracted the belly of the long head is seen to bunch up into a ball-shaped mass. Local swelling and bruising are noted, and lead to an increased arm girth measurement.

Both surgical and conservative management have been recommended in the literature (Friedman, 1963; Morrey et al., 1985; Bandy, Lovelace-Chandler and Holt, 1991). Surgical management is normally favoured (in the young especially) because conservative treatment has been said to give a loss of supination power (Baker and Bierwagen, 1985; Morrey et al., 1985). However, the reason for this deficit may be the lack of adequate rehabilitation following conservative management (Bandy, Lovelace-Chandler and Holt, 1991).

Conservative management consists of the RICE protocol to minimize inflammation, with gentle mobility exercises to the elbow within the pain-free range. Exercise therapy is used to maintain shoulder function. Multi-angle isometric training begins as soon as possible to reduce muscle atrophy, the deciding factor for starting this being pain. As pain to resisted movement reduces, dynamic exercise is begun against manual, and later isokinetic, resistance. PNF techniques combining shoulder flexion/adduction/medial rotation with elbow flexion/supination are used, as well as static stretching to elbow and shoulder extension. The resistance training programme is progressed with power actions, and functional sporting activities are introduced. The long-term prognosis is good in terms of restoration of function, but a palpable defect will usually remain in the muscle.

Surgery for distal tendon injuries includes re-inserting the tendon into the radial tuberosity, or the use of a fascia lata graft, where surgery has been delayed and the tendon has retracted. The long head may be re-inserted into the supraglenoid tubercle in the case of an avulsion or, in some instances, to the wall of the bicipital groove.

Pectoralis major

Rupture of the pectoralis major is unusual, but when it does occur, the muscle is usually already under tension when further force is imposed on it (Fig. 18.26a). The most common example of this scenario is the bench press exercise in weight-training. The injury normally occurs during the eccentric phase of the exercise as the bar is being lowered. During the last 30° of humeral extension of this action the inferior fibres of the muscle have been shown to lengthen disproportionately (Wolfe, Wickiewicz and Cavanaugh, 1992). In addition, with fatigue, the athlete may move the whole body in an attempt to lift the weight, and so bring accessory muscle groups into action enabling the athlete to exceed his or her safe limit. When lowering this excessive weight, the athlete loses control and the injury occurs.

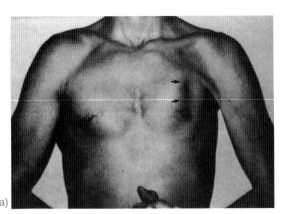
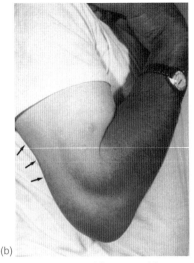
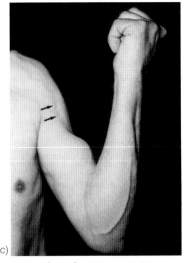

(a)   (b)   (c)

Figure 18.26 Ruptures to muscles in the shoulder region. (a) Pectoralis major. (b) Triceps. (c) Biceps. After Reid (1992) with permission.

A tearing sensation is felt, and a large haematoma is apparent over the anterior axilla. Weakness and pain to resisted adduction and medial rotation is noted to manual muscle testing. No defect may be seen at rest, but if the muscle is contracted isometrically by asking the athlete to press the hands together as if clapping, a defect may be apparent. Following injury, the muscle does not retract very far, perhaps due to its varied fibre direction and wide origin. The insertion into the humerus (just lateral to the intertubercular sulcus) of the non-dominant arm is more normally affected (Kretzler and Richardson, 1989).

Non-surgical treatment can be successful for partial tears (Roi, Respizzi and Dworzak, 1990), and in the non-athletic individual (Delport and Piper, 1982). However, surgical management is more generally recommended (Kretzler and Richardson, 1989; Reut, Bach and Johnson, 1991). At operation the deltoid is retracted and the tendon is reattached either via drill holes in the humerus or by suturing the tendon to the remnant of tissue insertion.

The arm is immobilized in a sling and isometric contractions started as soon as the pain stabilizes. Assisted movements are begun 1 week after surgery, and thereafter the rehabilitation programme aims to restore strength, mobility and function. As strength training progresses, eccentric movements must be used to prepare the muscle for its action of decelerating the bar in the bench press exercise. In addition, pectoral muscle stretches and retraction work must be used to avoid a protracted shoulder posture.

Triceps

In addition to the more common elbow site for triceps injury, occasionally the muscle may avulse from its glenoid attachment (O'Donoghue, 1976), especially in throwing athletes (Fig. 18.26b). Pain occurs to triceps stretching, often palpable at the inferior rim of the glenoid. With rest, a fibrous union will normally fix the fragment back in place, but surgery to remove the avulsed fragment and re-suture the tendon may be required where the injury recurs. When the muscle belly itself is injured, it is usually the medial head which is involved and the treatment of choice is conservative (Kunichi and Torisu, 1984).

It is important to note that the normal tendon is capable of sustaining considerable force before it will rupture, making avulsion fracture the more usual injury. Where tendon rupture occurs, an underlying pathology may be present.

High dosage oral steroids may weaken the tendons (Hunter, Shybut and Nuber, 1986), a situation especially important with athletes using heavy resistance exercise or power movements. Conditions such as rheumatoid arthritis, systemic lupus erythematosus and hormone disorders may also predispose to tendon rupture (Reid and Kushner, 1989).

BURSITIS

Gray's Anatomy (Warwick and Williams, 1973) lists some eight bursae around the shoulder joint, but the one most commonly affected in sport is the subacromial (subdeltoid) bursa. This lies between the deltoid and the joint capsule and stretches beneath the acromion process and coracoacromial ligament. The bursa extends over the supraspinatus tendon (Fig. 18.27), and does not usually communicate with the joint capsule except in the case of a supraspinatus tear, where the bursa may be damaged as well. Acute subacromial bursitis is unusual and occurs with sudden onset. The whole bursa is inflamed, and this severely limits abduction, but not in the capsular pattern. Pain is acute and often referred as far down as the wrist in extreme cases. Resisted movements are largely painless, and a painful arc only appears in a subacute case as initially no abduction at all is possible. Treatment in this acute stage is aimed at reducing the intense pain. The arm is supported in a sling to limit all glenohumeral movement, and anti-inflammatory modalities used.

Chronic subacromial bursitis occurs when the bursal sac becomes thickened and adherent, but in one part only. The condition is not a progression of acute bursitis but a separate clinical entity (Cyriax, 1982). The onset is gradual and a painful arc is present, but movements are largely of full range. Injecting the bursa with a local anaesthetic to inflate it is surprisingly effective, and may act mechanically by simply pushing the walls of the bursal sac apart.

In all cases of bursitis, shoulder mechanics should be closely examined to detect any abnormality which may give rise to microtrauma. Typically, postural changes around the

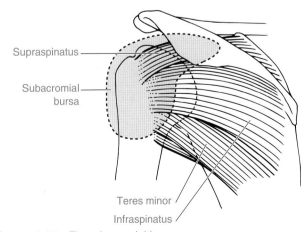

Figure 18.27 The subacromial bursa.

chest and shoulder can alter the mechanics of glenohumeral movement. This may predispose the athlete to impingement leading eventually to bursitis.

SHOULDER INSTABILITY

The stability of the glenohumeral joint lies very much on a continuum. At one end there is the stable, fully functional joint and at the other the dislocated joint requiring surgery. In many cases, there is a progression which begins with a reduction of stability through alteration in static, dynamic or proprioceptive factors. Individual differences in bony or soft tissue configuration can give some athletes a greater risk of instability, and training activities can alter the subtle muscle balance that exists around the joint. Trauma will cause both mechanical changes to stabilizing structures and alteration in proprioception. Any or all of these factors may coexist to push the athlete from a position of stability to one of instability of some degree. The progression from minor instability to major instability may then occur with time, unless there is treatment intervention of some type.

Instability may be classified using the TUBS/AMBRI acronyms (Matsen, Harryman and Sidles, 1991). These acronyms represent two ends of the spectrum (Table 18.2) from instability through trauma to instability through congenital factors. The patient with a TUBS lesion will have suffered trauma instability in one direction only (unidirectional). The glenoid labrum will have been detached from the anterior rim of the glenoid (Bankart lesion) and surgery will probably be required, although rehabilitation should be tried first as this can be successful with minor degrees of injury. The AMBRI patient has an atraumatic aetiology causing multidirectional instability in both shoulders (bilateral). Usually this patient responds well to intensive rehabilitation, but if surgery is required, an inferior capsular shift is normally the treatment of choice.

Shoulder stability is supplied by both static and dynamic factors. Static stability is provided by the glenoid labrum, joint capsule and ligaments, while dynamic stability comes from muscle action (Table 18.3). As the arm hangs by the side of the body, the pull of gravity is resisted by the superior capsule and the coracohumeral ligament. If the arm is loaded, when carrying a bag for example, the greater force is resisted by the supraspinatus which shares a common distal attachment with the two previous structures and has a line of action which is virtually identical to them (Norkin and Levangie, 1992).

The middle glenohumeral ligament lies directly under the tendon of subscapularis and is attached to it (Fig. 18.28). The ligament varies tremendously between subjects. In some it may be 2 cm wide, while in others it may be completely absent (Peat and Culham, 1994). Both the subscapularis and middle glenohumeral ligament limit external rotation and are important anterior stabilizers in the lower and middle ranges of abduction.

The inferior glenohumeral ligament (the thickest position of the glenohumeral ligament in total) is the most

Table 18.3   Stability of the glenohumeral joint

Dependent position	Coracohumeral ligament
	Superior glenohumeral ligament
	Supraspinatus muscle
Elevation	
Lower range (0–45°)	Anterior capsule
	Superior glenohumeral ligament
	Coracohumeral ligament
	Middle glenohumeral ligament
	Subscapularis, infraspinatus, and teres minor muscles
Middle range (45–75°)	Middle glenohumeral ligament
	Supscapularis muscle (decreasing importance)
	Infraspinatus and teres minor muscles
	Inferior glenohumeral ligament (superior band)
Upper range (>75°)	Inferior glenohumeral ligament (axillary pouch)
Throughout elevation	Dynamic activity of rotator cuff

From Peat and Culham (1994), with permission.

Table 18.2   Classification of shoulder instability

TUBS Born loose ⟷	AMBRI Torn loose
T – Traumatic aetiology	A – Atraumatic aetiology
U – Unidirectional instability	M – Multidirectional instability
B – Bankart lesion	B – Bilateral condition
S – Surgical repair	R – Rehabilitation normally successful
	I – Inferior capsular shift if rehabilitation fails

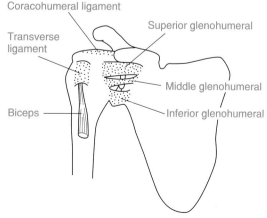

Figure 18.28   Anterior ligaments of the glenohumeral joint.

important passive stabilizing structure in overhead actions. The ligament is divided into three bands with the inferior portion forming the axillary pouch. The anterior band wraps around the humeral head at 90° abduction with external rotation and prevents anterior head migration (O'Brian et al., 1990). It is therefore the anterior band of the inferior glenohumeral ligament which is most significant in stabilizing the arm in overhead throwing sports. As this ligament tightens, abduction is limited and the humerus must laterally rotate and move towards the scapular plane.

The glenohumeral and coracohumeral ligaments form a 'Z' shape on the anterior aspect of the shoulder, with the middle glenohumeral ligament providing the crossbar of the Z. Above and below the crossbar are spaces which create areas of potential weakness. Superiorly (foramen of Weitbrecht) the opening allows the subscapularis bursa to communicate with the joint cavity. Inferiorly, a smaller bursa is sometimes present (Ferrari, 1990). In some subjects, if the Z crossbar (middle glenohumeral ligament) is missing, the anterior defect formed may contribute to anterior instability.

Active stability is provided by the rotator cuff muscles (Fig. 18.29). As previously stated the pull of the deltoid is almost vertical and it tends to cause upward translation of the humeral head. This is counteracted by the rotator cuff muscles, which tend to downwardly translate the head. The combination of the two sets of muscle translation forces stabilize the head of the humerus in the glenoid. These compressor forces are at their maximum between 60 and 80° and are minimal after 120° (Comtet, Herberg and Naasan, 1989). Where a massive tear of the rotator cuff muscles occurs, stability of the joint can still be maintained by the middle deltoid alone compressing the humeral head into the glenoid (Gagey and Hue, 2000).

Assessing instability

Static instability may be assessed clinically by a number of drawer and apprehension tests. Anterior and posterior instability is initially tested with the athlete in a sitting position. The therapist grasps the athlete's upper arm over the humeral head and applies forward and backward pressure while stabilizing the scapula (Fig. 18.30). The injured and uninjured sides are compared for range and end-feel. Excessive anterior glide leaves a posterior hollow, and the movement can be graded as mild (less than one third of the head coming off the glenoid), moderate (head riding on the edge of the glenoid, but spontaneously reduces when released) or severe (complete dislocation of the head). Posterior subluxation is considered abnormal when more than 50% of the humeral head comes off the glenoid.

The apprehension test is again performed in a sitting position. The athlete's arm is taken into 90° abduction and externally rotated. At the same time an anterior pressure is exerted on the proximal humerus (Fig. 18.31a). The test is

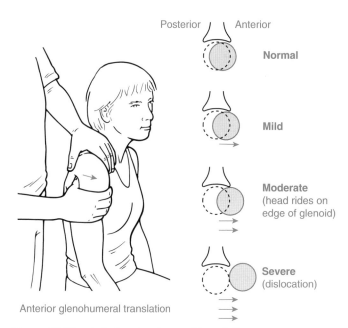

Figure 18.30   Anterior glenohumeral translation.

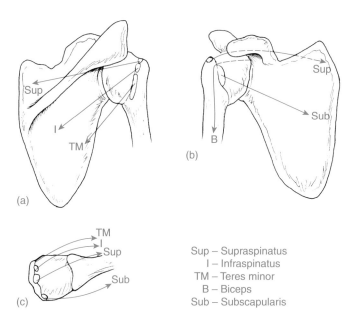

Figure 18.29   Active stabilizers of the glenohumeral joint. (a) Posterior. (b) Anterior. (c) Superior.

Sup – Supraspinatus
I – Infraspinatus
TM – Teres minor
B – Biceps
Sub – Subscapularis

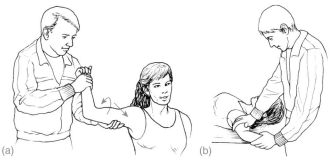

Figure 18.31   (a) Apprehension test – pain/apprehension increases as an anteriorly directed force is applied. (b) Modified apprehension test – pain reduces with posterior pressure.

positive in the presence of spasm or a feeling of impending (or actual) subluxation. A more rigorous procedure is to position the athlete in a supine-lying position, with the injured shoulder over the table edge. The arm is abducted to 90° and externally rotated. From this position the examiner applies an anteriorly directed pressure to increase pain and a posteriorly directed pressure to reduce pain (Fig. 18.31b).

EXERCISE THERAPY

In an overhead motion the arm externally rotates, causing the humeral head to move superiorly. In this position the subscapularis is not able to control the humeral head any longer and the tendency to anterior translation is therefore increased. The joint must depend on the inferior glenohumeral ligament for passive stability, the only effective active control coming from the infraspinatus. If the ligamentous control is failing, enhancement of infraspinatus action can effectively control the humeral head (Reid, 1992).

> **Keypoint**
>
> When the arm is overhead and ligamentous stability of the humeral head is inadequate, the infraspinatus muscle can provide active stability.

As with all shoulder rehabilitation, the cornerstone of exercise therapy is scapular stabilization. Proximal stability must be obtained before distal mobility and function are attempted. In cases of anterior instability of the glenohumeral joint, single channel sEMG is an extremely useful rehabilitation tool. The sEMG electrode is placed over the bulk of the infraspinatus below the scapular spine avoiding the posterior deltoid. The shoulder is flexed to activate the sEMG signal and the athlete is instructed to maintain the audible or visual signal from the machine by tightening the rotator cuff muscles. Isometric rotator cuff tightening is performed for multiple repetitions (10 sets of 10 repetitions), and then holding time is built (up to a 10-second hold) before active glenohumeral movements are commenced. Short lever shoulder flexion (in neutral rotation) is performed between 70 and 90° as the patient tries to push the sEMG signal up as high as possible. If pain or apprehension occur, the exercise is regressed to isometric holding alone. As sEMG signals can be maintained with active shoulder flexion, further exercises are added in a progression (Table 18.4). When painless and confident full-range motion has been obtained, general shoulder rehabilitation is begun.

Although anterior instability is by far the most common type, posterior or inferior instability is seen. Rehabilitation follows similar guidelines, building scapular stability and

Table 18.4 Use of surface EMG in rehabilitation of anterior instability of the shoulder

1	Forward flexion with a straight elbow
2	Forward flexion with increasing external rotation
3	Abduction with flexion, progressing to elbow extension
4	Abduction with elbow extension with increasing external rotation
5	Abduction from flexion
6	Abduction from flexion with increasing external rotation
7	Reaching for objects behind the back or overhead

From Reid (1992), with permission.

then emphasizing general rotator cuff control while avoiding movements which stress the pathological joint.

TAPING AND MOBILIZATION WITH MOVEMENT

When assessing static alignment of the glenohumeral joint, no more than one third of the head of the humerus should lie anterior to the acromion. In cases where the head of the humerus lies further forward (normally with impingement or instability symptoms), mobilization with movement and taping may be of help. Mobilization with movement (MWM) is a technique where a sustained mobilization is applied to a joint, normally at 90° to the plane of movement, to correct joint tracking (Mulligan, 1989).

The mobilization is applied at the same time as the patient performs a painful action with the affected joint. In the case of the shoulder, the painful action is abduction. The therapist stands behind the patient with one hand cupped over the anterior aspect of the shoulder, and the other braced against the scapula. A posterior gliding force is applied over the head of the humerus as the patient performs a previously painful abduction movement. The aim of the MWM is to allow the patient to perform the action painlessly to repetition. Eventually, the posterior glide is released, and the patient should still be able to perform the action with less (or no) pain.

If this technique is successful, a proprioceptive taping, which gives the patient the feeling of posterior glide and scapular depression, is often helpful (McConnell, 1992). The taping consists of the strips of 5 cm zinc oxide taping placed over adhesive net tape (Fig. 18.32). The first strip passes from the anterior aspect of the shoulder around the lateral aspect of the joint and down to the inferior angle of the scapula. The second strip passes from the anterior aspect of the shoulder, over the middle fibres of trapezius and again down to the inferior angle of the scapula. The adhesive net tape is placed on the shoulder in a relaxed state, but the zinc oxide tape pulls the skin to give the patient the sensation of posterior gliding (strip one) and scapula depression (strip two). The gap between the two pieces of tape should correspond to the sulcus which appears at the tip of the acromion at 90° abduction. As with the MWM, the taping should reduce the pain of abduction to re-test.

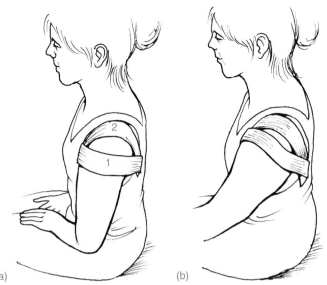

Figure 18.32 Proprioceptive taping of the shoulder. (a) Strip 1 passes from the anterior shoulder to the inferior angle of the scapula. Strip 2 passes over the middle trapezius. (b) Gap between the two strips corresponds to the humeral sulcus at 90° abduction.

> **Keypoint**
>
> With impingement syndrome, if the humeral head is anteriorly displaced, joint tracking may be improved using as sustained posterior glide during movement. Proprioceptive taping to reinforce both posterior glide and scapular stabilization may be used between treatment sessions.

GLENOHUMERAL DISLOCATION

Dislocation (often a progression of instability) is a commonly seen shoulder injury, with anterior displacement being encountered more often than posterior. Forced movements involving rotation and abduction are common mechanisms, and a fall onto the outstretched arm is also a frequent aetiology. Acute anterior dislocation gives considerable pain. The arm is usually held slightly abducted and externally rotated, and the normal rounded contour of the shoulder is lost. Close inspection shows the acromion process to be more prominent than usual, and a hollow is visible below it. The displaced humeral head can usually be felt on the anterior aspect of the shoulder.

The question of whether to reduce an acute injury is one of debate. On the positive side, early reduction of an uncomplicated injury may be achieved without anaesthetic and with little discomfort. If left, muscle spasm sets in, making reduction under anaesthetic necessary. The main problem is the likelihood of further injury by reduction without X-ray by inexperienced staff. Fracture of the head or neck of the humerus may have occurred at the time of injury and epiphyseal displacement is seen with adolescents. Displaced bone

fragments may easily be pulled onto the circumflex or radial nerves causing injury, and vascular damage may also occur.

Where an area of numbness is present over the deltoid, injury to the axillary nerve should be suspected, and swelling in the hand and fingers together with a loss of pulse suggests arterial damage as a result of humeral fracture (Reid, 1992). For these reasons, an acute injury occurring for the first time is better referred to an orthopaedic consultant.

> **Keypoint**
>
> Following shoulder dislocation, the presence of numbness over the shoulder, swelling in the fingers or a loss of pulse suggest complications requiring urgent medical attention.

Recurrent anterior dislocation may be reduced more easily. The forces required to dislocate the shoulder in the first place are considerably less than with the acute injury, and so the chance of associated fracture is minimal. Spontaneous reduction may occur, and frequently the athlete has learnt to reduce the dislocation him- or herself, and the joint is fairly lax. For assisted reduction a number of techniques are available:

With the patient in a supine position on the ground, the therapist sits on the patient's injured side. The therapist places his or her stockinged foot just below the ipsilateral axilla, while holding the patient's arm. The therapist then simply leans back to provide traction, and may gently rotate the arm to facilitate reduction.

The simplest self-reduction procedure is for the athlete to bend the ipsilateral leg and grasp the knee with both hands, keeping the arms locked straight. Slowly leaning back produces in-line traction which usually allows the shoulder to reduce. It must be emphasized that these procedures should only be performed in the absence of pain and spasm. The traction is applied gently, brute force or 'yanking' the arm by another athlete being obviously contraindicated.

As an alternative the patient may lie prone on a couch or gym bench with the arm hanging over the edge of the couch (hand off the floor). The weight of the arm will usually provide sufficient traction to initiate spontaneous reduction. Holding a weight in the hand (small dumbell) will assist the traction force. If the recurrently dislocated shoulder does not reduce readily, referral is still necessary.

Acute posterior dislocation is not as obvious as anterior. Pain is still intense, with the arm held adducted and internally rotated. Any attempt to move the arm is resisted by intense muscle spasm. In thin individuals the coracoid process is more visible than usual, and fullness is often apparent posteriorly. Heavy musculature in an athlete will, however, obscure these signs. Posterior dislocations require referral and reduction under sedation. Gentle in-line traction is applied to the adducted/internally rotated arm with gentle pressure over the humeral head.

Table 18.5 Guidelines for rehabilitation following anterior glenohumeral dislocation

Initial post-reduction period
Rest and ice
Immobilization

0–3 weeks
Isometrics twice daily
Minimal abduction for axillary hygiene only
Limited flexion and extension
Avoid external rotation
Gentle pendular swinging in transverse and sagittal planes
Scapular stability work

3–6 weeks
Resisted internal rotation
External rotation to neutral only
Abduction limited to 45°
Re-education of scapulohumeral rhythm
Extension/adduction/medial rotation pattern on pulley
Limited range resisted adduction
Pendular swinging giving way to automobilization techniques
Proprioceptive work including static joint repositioning

6–8 weeks
Abduction increased to 90°
External rotation gradually increased
Flexion/abduction/lateral rotation pattern on pulley
Full resistance training below shoulder height
Introduce fast throwing and catching below head height
Closed chain work on balance board and trampette (two hands)

Final rehabilitation
Full range motion resisted
Ensure muscle balance (internal rotation:external rotation ratio)
Closed chain work (single arm)
Push up with clap
Fast reaction work – throwing/catching/blocking
Re-education of falling – forward roll/handstand/fall back

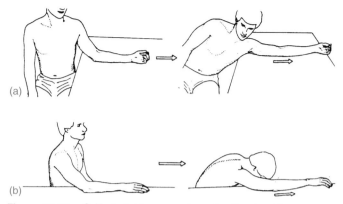

Figure 18.33 Self-stretching procedures for the shoulder.

Rehabilitation following anterior dislocation

Following reduction, rest and ice are used to limit inflammation. The arm is immobilized, and the initial period of immobilization is an important determinant of recurrence. Normally the recurrence rate for young (20–30 years) athletes may be as high as 85% (Halbach and Tank, 1990). However, this may be reduced considerably, with one study of 50 individuals showing a recurrence rate of 20% after 6 weeks immobilization (Reid, 1992). Exercise therapy is divided into four phases (Table 18.5).

In phase one (0–3 weeks), isometric exercises are used. These are performed twice daily with only minimal active abduction allowed to facilitate axillary hygiene. Limited flexion and extension are allowed, but external rotation is avoided. Gentle pendular swinging actions are used in transverse and sagittal planes. In phase two (3–6 weeks), active resisted internal rotation is used, and external rotation to

neutral using elastic tubing. Abduction is limited to 45° and exercise for the rest of the body is progressed. Strengthening concentrates on medial rotation, to strengthen the subscapularis and support the anterior joint, and limited range adduction to work latissimus dorsi, teres major, the pectorals and coracobrachialis to resist abduction forces.

After 6–8 weeks (phase three), abduction increases to 90° and limited external rotation is used to reduce stiffness. Only when strength has increased to 75% of the uninjured shoulder should full-range motion be attempted. To reduce stiffness, self-stretches such as 'finger walking' along a table top or up a wall, and limited joint distractions are useful (Fig. 18.33). Autotherapy distractions may be performed in a prone kneeling position, holding the couch end.

Slow velocity (<90°/s) isokinetics may be used, with the velocity gradually increasing to functional sporting levels as the athlete is able to control the movement. Pool exercises are used to incorporate faster actions against the resistance of a paddle, and range of motion exercise using flotation to take the weight of the arm. PNF techniques involving extension/adduction/medial rotation are used initially against manual resistance and subsequently with a weight and pulley system. Later, flexion/abduction/lateral rotation is used with caution. Restoration of kinaesthetic awareness is important after anterior dislocation (Smith and Brunolli, 1989) and is described on page 148.

FROZEN SHOULDER

Frozen shoulder or 'adhesive capsulitis' is an increasingly common pathology found in sport. As the number of elderly people involved in sport continues to rise, this condition is likely to be seen even more frequently. Between 2 and 3% of the adult population between the ages of 40 and 70 develop the problem and the condition is more common in women. It presents as a gradual loss of shoulder movement, with or without pain. The initial loss of movement may go unnoticed until function is limited. Patients complain that activities of everyday living become increasingly difficult. Combing the hair at the back of the head and fastening a bra strap are frequent sources of complaint. Active sports persons frequently notice the onset of the condition earlier than sedentary individuals. Elderly athletes often complain that their golf swing is affected, or overhead badminton shots are painful for example.

The term 'frozen shoulder' (Codman, 1934) is not an accurate diagnosis, but rather a description of the major symptom, which is lack of movement. 'Adhesive capsulitis' (Neviaser, 1945) describes the finding of capsular thickening, contraction and adhesions. The condition may appear as a primary (insidious) or secondary (traumatic) adhesive capsulitis. Secondary types can be associated with a number of soft tissue and medical pathologies including rotator cuff injuries, impingement syndrome, traumatic arthritis, osteoarthritis, shoulder joint immobilization, autoimmune disease, diabetes and thyroid dysfunction (Boissonnault and Janos, 1989; Hertling and Kessler, 1990; Ott, Clancy and Wilk, 1994).

The joint capsule seems to be a major source of movement limitation in this condition. The capsule is thickened and may adhere to the humeral head, with the axillary pouch frequently being obliterated. A reduction in joint volume has been noted on arthrogram (Reeves, 1966), and a loss of bone mineral content can be seen on X-ray (Lundberg and Nilsson, 1968). An increase in vascularity and thickening has been noted in the subacromial bursa and rotator cuff (Simmonds, 1949), and a contracture of the coracohumeral ligament (Ozaki et al., 1989). Many studies, subsequent to Neviaser, have noted an absence of adhesions and degenerative changes (Ha'eri and Maitland, 1981; Uitvlugt, Detrisac and Johnson, 1988). Changes to the subscapular bursa, rotator cuff, and biceps tendon (Uitvlugt, Detrisac and Johnson, 1988; Wiley, 1991) indicate that these structures may be key factors in the initiation of the condition. Arthroscopic examination has revealed fibrous contracture of the rotator interval and coracohumeral ligament which primarily limits lateral rotation (Bunker, 1997). Histological evaluation of the fibrous tissue has shown it to be similar to that found in Dupuytren's contracture (Cleland and Durall, 2002).

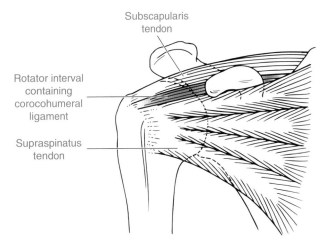

Figure 18.34 The rotator interval.

pain is the dominant feature, which almost completely prevents movement. With stage II conditions, painful limitation is again a feature. This time, however, some movement is present, and when the joint is stretched the pain increases. Stage III lesions have restricted range but very little pain.

Management

Management of adhesive capsulitis includes physiotherapy, medication and surgery. Physiotherapy tends to use joint mobilization, acupuncture/dry needling and exercises. Surgical intervention is mainly by manipulation under anaesthesia (MUA) and arthrsocopic dissection. Medication on the whole includes corticosteroid injection and the use of non-specific anti-inflammatory drugs (NSAIDs) or analgesics. Corticosteroid injection has been shown to be effective in the short term but to have little long term (6–18 months) benefit (Van der Windt and Koes, 2002). Patients treated with MUA have been shown to achieve a 50 point functional improvement score while those treated with physiotherapy gained a 78 point score (Melzer et al., 1995). However, physiotherapy for adhesive capsulitis can be protracted with studies reporting 12–29 treatment sessions on average (Cleland and Durall, 2002). Following an active physiotherapy programme which includes home exercise, 90% of patients have reported a satisfactory result (Griggs, Ahn and Green, 2000) and patients rated their shoulder function improvement as excellent (57%) or good (29%) (Vermeulen et al., 2000). Although spontaneous recovery may occur, as many as 50% of patients can still have symptoms up to 7 years later if not treated (Shaffer, Tibone and Kerlan, 1992).

Manual therapy

Pain may be greatly reduced by posteroanterior (PA) oscillations (Maitland, 1991), and scapulothoracic mobilization,

---

Definition

The *rotator interval* is the space between the anterior border of the supraspinatus tendon and the superior border of the subscapularis tendon (Fig. 18.34). The space is filled by the coracohumeral ligament which limits inferior translation and lateral rotation.

On examination, movement is usually limited in a capsular pattern (subacute) or by muscle guarding (acute), but resisted movements are normally pain free. Accessory movements are limited, particularly inferior and anterior gliding, and the quadrant position is limited and painful when compared to the uninvolved side. Three stages of the condition have been described (Maitland, 1991). In stage I, and these are the manual treatments of choice for the stage I lesion. For PA mobilization, the patient lies in a supine position with the arm supported in a pain-free position. The elbow is flexed with a folded towel placed under the arm. The patient's forearm rests on the trunk. This position limits adduction, extension and excessive medial rotation. The therapist kneels on the floor and directs his or her thumbs to the posterior aspect of the humeral head. The oscillations are produced by the therapist's arms rather than the finger flexors. For scapulothoracic mobilization the patient lies on the side with the injured arm uppermost. The arm should be in a pain-free position supported by towels. The therapist grasps the medial edge of the scapula with his or her fingertips in an attempt to release the scapula from the ribcage first, and secondly to abduct it, easing it away from the spine.

With the stage II condition, the pain is limited first, and then stiffness is addressed. As pain is reduced, the starting position is changed to use the patient's upper arm as a lever. The therapist grips the patient's upper arm in his or her cupped hands, high into the axilla. Initially, the arm is by the patient's side (Fig. 18.35a). From this position the slack is taken up in the joint by lifting it anteriorly, and then the arm is lifted and lowered to perform the PA glide. As pain lessens and movement returns, the same action is performed with the arm held abducted to 45° (Fig. 18.35b), and then in full flexion overhead (Fig. 18.35c).

Inferior gliding, if limited, may be regained with the patient's shoulder flexed to 90° and the patient's hand on the trapezius (central fibres). The therapist stabilizes the patient's elbow against his or her own shoulder and grips the upper arm in cupped hands. The gliding motion pulls the humeral head inferiorly. As pain reduces, a similar movement may be performed with the patient's arm abducted and supported. The therapist pushes down on the humeral head with the web of his or her free hand (Fig. 18.36).

The final range of movement may be regained using the quadrant position (see above) as a mobilization to stretch the anterior capsule. This is only used when pain is minimal and stiffness is the predominant symptom (late stage II and stage III lesions). The therapist stands at the head of the couch with his or her knee resting on the couch top (Fig. 18.37a). The arm is then oscillated through approximately 30° to facilitate a grade II mobilization. A grade IV movement may be used by placing the therapist's nearside arm under the patient's upper rib angles; a small 5° oscillation is all that is required (Fig. 18.37b).

Exercise therapy

In stage (I), the primary aim is to reduce pain and ensure that the joint is not irritated to increase the inflammatory reaction of the involved soft tissues (Table 18.6). Pendular swinging actions may be used to great effect. The patient leans over a table with the unaffected hand supporting

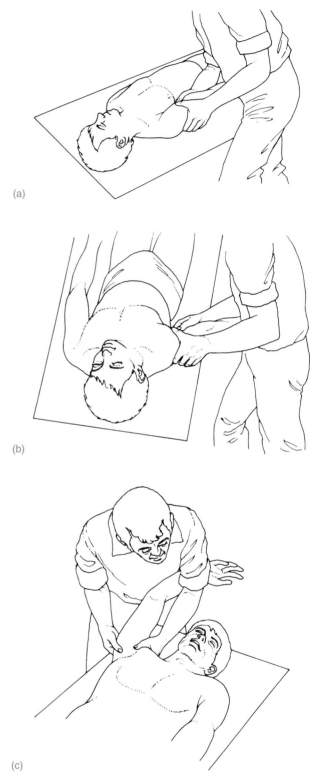

(a)

(b)

(c)

Figure 18.35 Posteroanterior glenohumeral joint movement. (a) Patient's arm by his or her side. (b) 45° abduction. (c) Maximal flexion–abduction.

them. The affected arm is allowed to relax and 'go heavy', allowing arm weight to slightly traction the joint in its flexed–abducted position. The action is to sway the body and impart a gentle circling movement on the straight arm

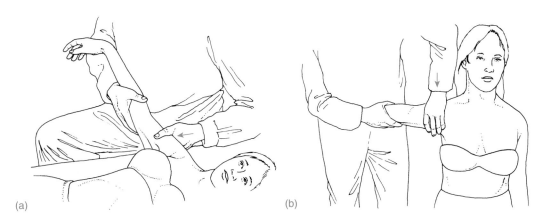

Figure 18.36 Inferior gliding, glenohumeral joint. Patient in (a) supine, or (b) sitting position. The arm is grasped near the elbow to stabilize it in 90° abduction. The web of the other hand contacts the head of the humerus. The head of the humerus is then depressed inferiorly.

(a) (b)

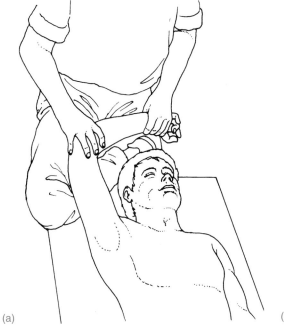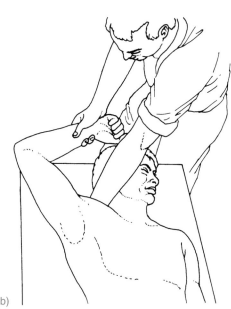

Figure 18.37 Glenohumeral mobilizations in the quadrant position to regain final degrees of movement.

(a) (b)

Table 18.6 Movement therapy for adhesive capsulitis

Stage	Pathology and signs	Exercise therapy
(I) 'Freezing'	Scar tissue forming and maturing. External rotation of shoulder markedly reduced, abduction less limited. Spasm end feel	Active range of motion exercise Joint mobilization for pain relief, not increased range Pendular swinging
(II) 'Frozen'	Scarring mature. Glenohumeral joint lost mobility. Patient unable to lie on affected side at night. Elastic end-feel	More aggressive joint mobilizations providing joint is not irritated Stretching Strengthening within pain-free ranges
(III) 'Thawing'	Arm pain dominates, shoulder pain less intense. Gross reverse scapulohumeral rhythm. Hard leathery end-feel	Scapular stability Aggressive glenohumeral joint mobilization. End range stretching Movement re-education

which is transmitted to the glenohumeral joint (Fig. 18.38a). It must be emphasized that shoulder muscle action should not create the movement, but rather bodysway. The action should be performed in both clockwise and anticlockwise directions and repeated every 2 hours throughout the waking day.

In stage (II), pendular swinging may be continued for pain relief, but stretching and strengthening should begin.

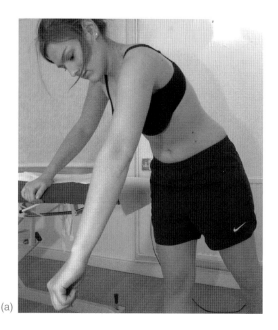

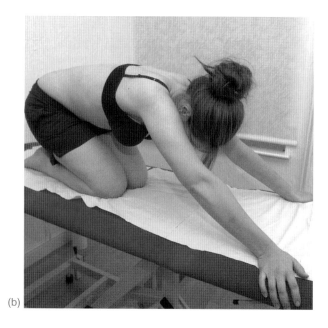

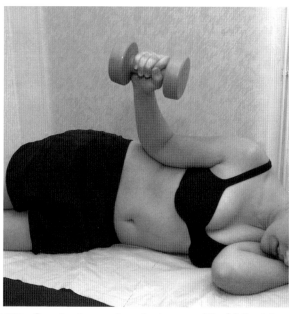

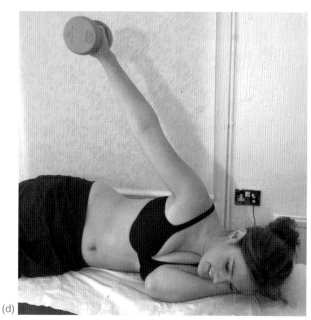

Figure 18.38 Exercise therapy for adhesive capsulitis. (a) Pendulum swinging. (b) Flexion–abduction with traction. (c) Resisted lateral rotation. (d) Initial range of abduction.

Flexion–abduction with traction may be used in kneeling, holding onto an object or simply gripping the floor with the fingertips and moving the bodyweight backwards to sit on the heels (Fig. 18.38b). The aim is to encourage movement rather than force it. Resisted lateral rotation may be used in side lying with the weight of the arm initially and a light dumbell as pain allows (Fig. 18.38c). Abduction within the pain-free range should be used in side lying (Fig. 18.38d) rather than standing at this stage. In standing, the increased leverage as the arm reaches the horizontal position encourages shoulder shrugging and reverse scapulohumeral rhythm.

Scapular stability work should begin and as abduction and lateral rotation range increases, all three movements

Definition
Normally in arm abduction there is more glenohumeral movement than scapulothoracic movement (ratio 2:1). With reverse scapulohumeral rhythm, glenohumeral movement is reduced and scapulothoracic movement increased to compensate.

should be combined in sitting (Fig. 18.39). The patient begins the action by drawing the scapula down gently. While maintaining this position, the bent arm is laterally rotated and the elbow lifted from the couch. The distance

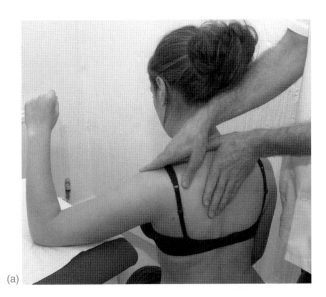

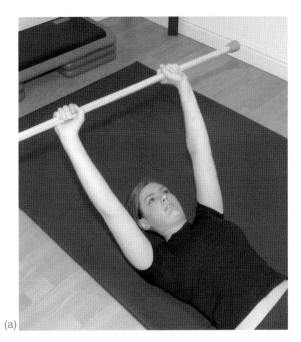

(a)

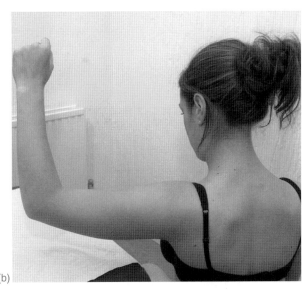

(b)

Figure 18.39   Combining shoulder lateral rotation and abduction with scapular stability. (a) Scapular repositioning. (b) Arm lifting.

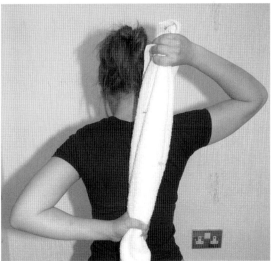

(b)

Figure 18.40   Full range stretching exercises for the shoulder.

between the ear and the shoulder should be maintained as shoulder shrugging is avoided.

In stage (III) end-range stretching and further strengthening is used. The sit to heels exercise and sitting abduction-lateral rotation may be continued with the aim of increasing range of motion in each. Passive abduction and lateral rotation using a stick or towel in lying (Fig. 18.40a) is useful as the leverage involved assists in obtaining the final few degrees of movement. Both medial and lateral rotation may be gained using a hand behind neck (HBN) and hand behind back (HBB) action (Fig. 18.40b). Several weight training exercises may be used to regain should strength and improve range of motion, including shoulder press, lateral pull-downs, and pulley abduction movements (Fig. 18.41).

SNAPPING SCAPULAE

This unusual condition occurs especially in adolescent females just after skeletal maturity, and in both sexes following surgery. Patients experience a snapping sensation, which is sometimes audible, near the vertebral border of the scapula. Pain is often localized to the rhomboids and levator scapulae over the medial scapular border or the trapezius over the medial aspect of the scapular spine. One possibility is that tendinitis occurs to the muscles, another that the bursa located beneath the medial border of the scapula becomes inflamed.

The condition occurs through microtrauma from excessive shearing forces beneath the scapula due to abnormal scapulothoracic rhythm. Management relies on the restoration of a

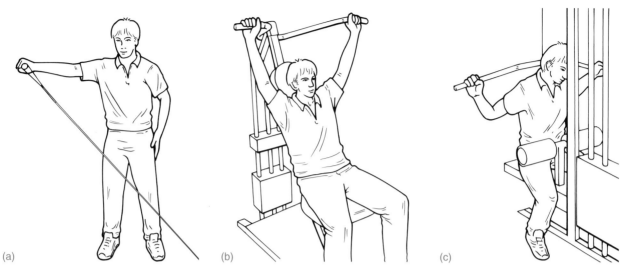

Figure 18.41   Weight training actions for the shoulder. (a) Cable lateral raise. (b) Shoulder press. (c) Lateral pull-down. From Norris, C.M. (1996). *Weight Training*. CD-ROM Package. Exercise Association, London. With permission

more normal scapulothoracic rhythm (Percy, Birbrager and Pitt, 1988).

NERVE ENTRAPMENT SYNDROMES

Two relatively uncommon nerve entrapments are seen around the shoulder, quadrilateral space syndrome and entrapment of the suprascapular nerve.

The quadrilateral (quadrangular) space lies between the teres minor and the subscapularis above and the teres major below. The long head of triceps forms its medial wall and the surgical neck of the humerus lies laterally (Fig. 18.42a). Entrapment by tethering can occur to both the axillary nerve and circumflex humeral artery (Cahill and Palmer, 1983). The patient, frequently a throwing athlete, is usually young (22–35 years) and complains of shoulder pain of insidious onset. Muscle fatigue and loss of abduction power are apparent and tenderness may be elicited to palpation over the involved quadrilateral space. Arteriograph frequently shows posterior circumflex artery occlusion. Most patients respond to alteration of throwing technique but some may go on to surgical decompression.

The suprascapular nerve (Fig. 18.42b) may be trapped as it passes through the suprascapular notch beneath the suprascapular ligament, or as it winds around the lateral edge of the scapular spine. Direct blows in contact sports are one cause as the nerve is superficial, and occult ganglions pressing on the shoulder have been described (Fritz et al., 1992; Gerscovich and Greenspan, 1993). Entrapment can affect the motor response of both the supraspinatus and infraspinatus, either together or in isolation (Black and Lombardo, 1990). The patient presents with visible muscular atrophy and weakness is often noticed to backhand shots or in serving. Vague pain occurs deep in the posterior aspect of the shoulder. Treatment involves decompression of the nerve at the suprascapular notch and scapular nerve block.

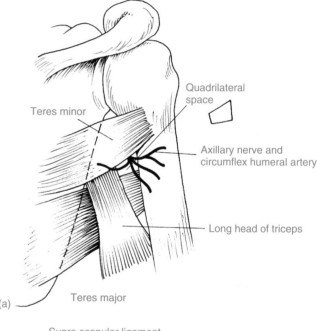

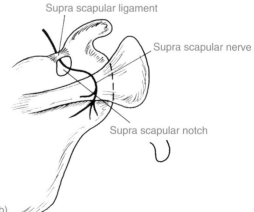

Figure 18.42   Entrapment neuropathy in the shoulder. (a) Quadrilateral space. (b) Suprascapular notch.

SHOULDER REHABILITATION

Shoulder rehabilitation begins with an assessment of scapulohumeral rhythm and then localized scapula stability exercises as detailed in Chapter. It is essential that provision of a stable base is made before further shoulder work is begun. Rehabilitation must start at the base of the kinetic chain and progress outward into the extremity (Kibler, 1991).

GLENOHUMERAL STABILITY

The glenohumeral joint must then be restored and a balanced action of all the rotator cuff muscles obtained. Glenohumeral stability has been described as a circle concept (Dempster, 1965; Wilk and Arrigo, 1993). Translational movement of the humeral head is related to laxity of both the anterior and posterior structures. For example, anterior translation may be caused by tightness in the anterior structures, but will only be noticeable if the posterior structures are lax. Active stability is achieved through co-contraction of the rotator cuff muscles compressing the humeral head into the glenoid. Rehabilitation must involve work for the entire rotator cuff, rather than simply the supraspinatus, which has a contributory role only (Wilk and Arrigo, 1993).

> **Keypoint**
>
> For the glenohumeral joint to be unstable there must be both anterior and posterior laxity. To regain stability the same process applies, with work on both the anterior and posterior muscles being required.

A differentiation must be made between joint laxity and functional instability. Shoulder laxity is present when the humeral head can be passively translated on the glenoid. Functional instability, on the other hand, exists when unwanted humeral head motion compromises the comfort and function of a movement (Matsen, Harryman and Sidles, 1991). The difference is the patient's ability to control the translational motion of the humeral head. Three interrelating systems exist to contribute to glenohumeral stability. The first is an increase in joint compression brought about by a force couple between the deltoid and rotator cuff. Secondly, dynamic stability is provided by the rotator cuff tendons with the shoulder capsule. Muscular contraction directly tensions the joint ligaments, therefore creating 'dynamic ligament tension' (Cleland, 1866). The third method of stabilization is via neuromuscular control. Proprioceptive rehabilitation (movement awareness drills) has been shown to reduce muscle reaction speed in a number of joints and has been used successfully for shoulder rehabilitation (Smith and Brunolli, 1989; Lephart et al., 1994).

Exercises begin in starting positions which place minimal stress on the shoulder joint capsule. Initially, the arm is held

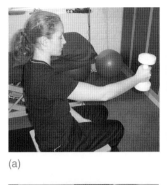
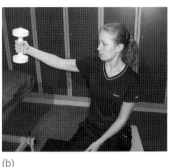

(a) (b)

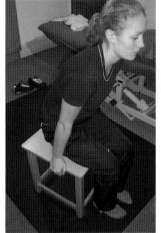
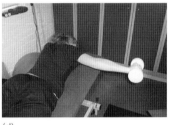

(d)

(c)

Figure 18.43 Glenohumeral exercises. (a) Elevation and lateral rotation in the sagittal plane. (b) Elevation and lateral rotation in the scapular plane. (c) Sitting press-up. (d) Horizontal abduction in lateral rotation.

by the side with the elbow flexed to 90°. The patient is instructed to hold the arm inactive against alternating manual pressure (medial and lateral rotation) from the therapist to apply rhythmic stabilization. The movement then progresses to 45° and finally 90° of shoulder abduction.

A variety of weight-training exercises may be performed to re-strengthen the shoulder musculature. Fig. 18.43 illustrates four movements which work both the glenohumeral and scapulothoracic muscles in both open and closed chain. The movements minimize the risk of impingement by combining lateral rotation movements with abduction in the scapular plane.

In overhead motions, the cocking phase provides an eccentric pre-stretch to the muscles (adductors and internal rotators) closely followed by an explosive acceleration phase. Concentric-eccentric coupling of this type requires plyometric rehabilitation. Plyometrics involve a pre-stretch (eccentric) and short amortization phase where the movement direction is reversed, and finally a rapid facilitated concentric action. Activities include overhead soccer throws, basketball chest passes, single arm tennis ball throws, use of exercise tubing in PNF patterns and use of small medicine balls (Wilk et al., 1993).

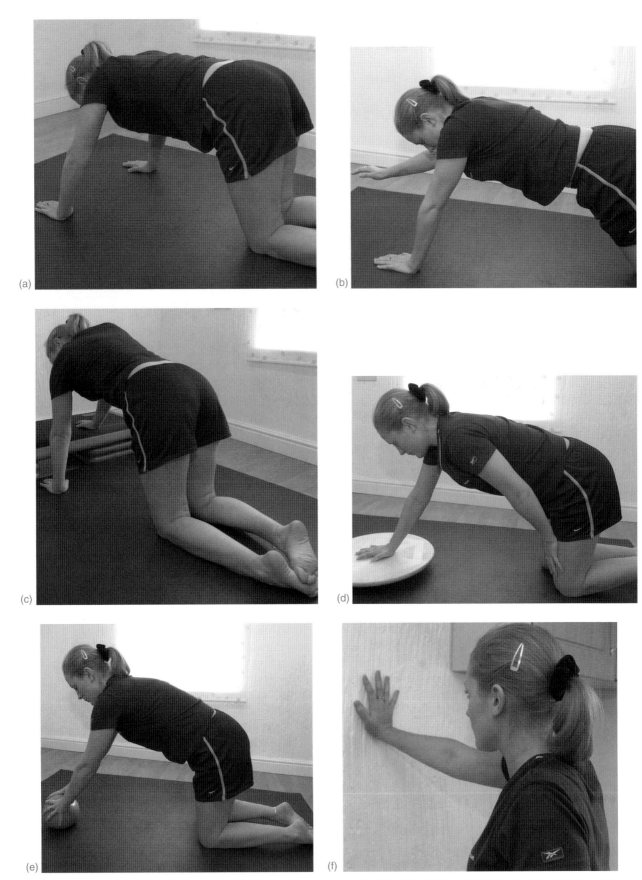

Figure 18.44   Closed chain shoulder rehabilitation. (a) Knee push-up. (b) Hand walking flat. (c) Stool. (d) Wobble board. (e) Gym ball. (f) Single arm wall lean.

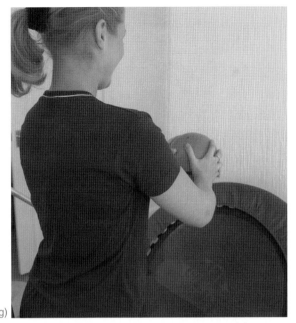

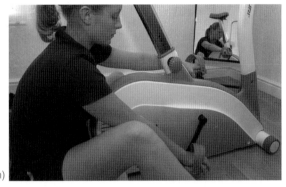

Figure 18.44 (cont.)   (g) Throw and catch on trampette. (h) Hand work on static cycle.

CLOSED KINETIC CHAIN ACTIVITIES

The concept of kinetic chain activity was introduced on page 19. Essentially, closed kinetic chain activity involves movement of the proximal body segment on a fixed distal segment. This is common in the lower limb, during the stance phase of gait for example. In the upper limb the majority of daily actions occur in open chain format, with the distal segment (arm) moving on a fixed proximal base (thorax). However, the upper limb must be able to work in a closed kinetic chain pattern for 'fall' and 'push' actions. In many sports, the athlete is likely to fall onto the hand or elbow, and in some sports, such as gymnastics, complex closed kinetic chain actions are involved (handstand/ vault). During a closed chain action, such as falling onto the outstretched arm, gravity assists in closing the chain of movement, approximating the joint surfaces. The muscle action is primarily eccentric to control the deceleration of movement and provide a protective role. As concentric action begins to accelerate the body segment, the joint surfaces are still approximated (push-up) whereas during open chain actions, the joint surfaces are under traction (throwing).

> **Keypoint**
>
> In closed kinetic chain exercises the muscle action is mainly eccentric to control excessive movement and protect the joint.

Traditional closed chain exercises include body weight (push-ups, dips) resistance and weights (bench and shoulder presses). Additional movements include the push-up with a press, and the sitting push-up. Hand walking activities are useful and may be performed on a wall, floor, treadmill, stepper, static cycling or on steps, either from a kneeling or prone falling position. Use of a rocker board for double-handed activities and a balance board for single handed activities is also useful for closed kinetic chain rehabilitation and is challenging to proprioception. The same would apply to activities on the Swiss ball and slide trainer (Fig. 18.44).

References

Apley, A.G. and Solomon, L. (1989) *Concise System of Orthopaedics and Fractures*, Butterworth, London

Austin, K.A., Gwynn-Brett, K.A. and Marshall, S.C. (1994) *Illustrated Guide to Taping Techniques*, C.V. Mosby, St Louis

Baechle, T.R. (1994) *Essentials of Strength Training and Conditioning*, Human Kinetics, Champaign, Illinois

Baker, B.E. and Bierwagen, D. (1985) Rupture of the distal tendon of the biceps brachii: operative versus non-operative treatment. *Journal of Bone and Joint Surgery*, **67A**, 414–417

Bandy, W.D., Lovelace-Chandler, V. and Holt, A. (1991) Rehabilitation of the ruptured biceps brachii muscle of an athlete. *Journal of Orthopaedic and Sports Physical Therapy*, **13**, (4) 184–190

Bannister, G.C., Wallace, W.A., Stableforth, P.G. and Hutson, M.A. (1989) The management of acute acromioclavicular dislocation: a randomised prospective controlled trial. *Journal of Bone and Joint Surgery*, **71B**, 848–850

Bigliani, L.U., Morrison, D.S. and April, E.W. (1986) The morphology of the acromion and its relationship to rotator cuff tears. *Orthopaedic Transactions*, **10**, 228

Black, K. and Lombardo, J. (1990) Suprascapular nerve injuries with isolated paralysis of the infraspinatus. *American Journal of Sports Medicine*, **18**, (3) 225–228

Boissonnault, W.G. and Janos, S.C. (1989) Dysfunction, evaluation, and treatment of the shoulder. In *Orthopaedic Physical Therapy* (eds R. Donatelli and M.J. Wooden), Churchill Livingstone, Edinburgh

Bunker, T.D. (1997) Frozen shoulder: unravelling the enigma. *Annals of the Royal College of Surgeons of England*, **79**, 210–213

Cahill, B.R. (1982) Osteolysis of distal part of clavicle in male athletes. *Journal of Bone and Joint Surgery*, **64A**, 1053–1058

Cahill, B.R. and Palmer, R.E. (1983) Quadrilateral space syndrome. *Journal of Hand Surgery*, **8**, 65

Cain, P.R., Mutschler, T.A. and Fu, F.H. (1987) Anterior stability of the glenohumeral joint: a dynamic model. *American Journal of Sports Medicine*, **15**, 144

Cleland, J. (1866) On the actions of muscles passing over more than one joint. *Journal of Anatomy and Physiology*, **1**, 85–93

Cleland, J. and Durall, J. C. (2002) Physical therapy for adhesive capsulitis: systematic review. *Physiotherapy*, **88**, (8) 450–457

Codman, E.A. (1934) *The Shoulder*, Thomas Todd, Boston

Comtet, J.J., Herberg, G. and Naasan, I.A. (1989) Biomechanical basis of transfers for shoulder paralysis. *Hand Clinics*, **5**, 1

Corrigan, B. and Maitland, G.D. (1994) *Musculoskeletal and Sports Injuries*, Butterworth-Heinemann, Oxford

Culham, E. and Peat, M. (1993) Functional anatomy of the shoulder complex. *Journal of Orthopedic and Sports Physical Therapy*, **18**, (1) 342–350

Cyriax, J. (1982) *Textbook of Orthopaedic Medicine*, 8th edn, Baillière Tindall, London, vol. 1

Cyriax, J.H. and Cyriax, P.J. (1983) *Illustrated Manual of Orthopaedic Medicine*, Butterworth, London

Delport, H.P. and Piper, M.S. (1982) Pectoralis major rupture in athletes. *Archives of Orthopaedic and Traumatic Surgery*, **100**, 135–137

Dempster, W.T. (1965) Mechanisms of shoulder movement. *Archives of Physics in Medicine and Rehabilitation*, **46**, 49–70

Dias, J.J. and Gregg, P.J. (1991) Acromioclavicular joint injuries in sport. *Sports Medicine*, **11**, 125–132

Dias, J.J., Steingold, R.F., Richardson, R.A., Tesfayohannes, B. and Gregg, P.J. (1987) The conservative treatment of acromioclavicular dislocation: review after five years. *Journal of Bone and Joint Surgery*, **69B**, 719–722

Ejeskar, A. (1974) Coracoclavicular wiring for acromioclavicular joint dislocation: a ten year follow-up study. *Acta Orthopaedica Scandinavica*, **45**, 652–661

Ferrari, D.A. (1990) Capsular ligaments of the shoulder: anatomical and functional study of the anterior superior capsule. *American Journal of Sports Medicine*, **18**, 20

Fleisig, G.S., Dillman, C.J. and Andrews, J.R. (1994) Biomechanics of the shoulder during throwing. In *The Athlete's Shoulder* (eds J.R. Andrews and K.E. Wilk), Churchill Livingstone, Edinburgh

Freidman, E. (1963) Rupture of the distal biceps tendon. Report on 13 cases. *Journal of the American Medical Association*, **184**, 60–63

Fritz, R.C., Helms, C.A., Steinbach, L.S. and Genant, H.K. (1992) Suprascapular nerve entrapment: evaluation with MR imaging. *Radiology*, **182**, 437–444

Fukuda, K., Craig, E.V., An, K., Cofield, R.H. and Chao, E.Y.S. (1986) Biomechanical study of the ligamentous system of the acromioclavicular joint. *Journal of Bone and Joint Surgery*, **68A**, 434–439

Gagey, O. and Hue, E. (2000) Mechanics of the deltoid muscle. *Clinical Orthopedics*, **375**, 250–257

Gagey, O., Bonfait, H. and Gillot, C. (1987) Anatomic basis of ligamentous control of elevation of the shoulder. *Surgical and Radiological Anatomy*, **9**, 19

Garrick, J.G. and Webb, D.R. (1990) *Sports Injuries: Diagnosis and Management*, W.B. Saunders, Philadelphia

Gerscovich, E.O. and Greenspan, A. (1993) Magnetic resonance imaging in the diagnosis of suprascapular nerve syndrome. *Canadian Association of Radiologists Journal*, **44**, 307–309

Griggs, S.M., Ahn, A. and Green, A. (2000) Idiopathic adhesive capsulitis: a prospective functional outcome of non-operative treatment. *Journal of Bone and Joint Surgery*, **82**, 1398–1407

Gunn, C.C. (1996) *Treatment of Chronic Pain*, 2nd edn, Churchill Livingstone, Edinburgh

Gurd, F.B. (1941) The treatment of complete dislocation of the outer end of the clavicle: a hitherto undescribed operation. *Annals of Surgery*, **113**, 1041

Ha'eri, G.B. and Maitland, A. (1981) Arthroscopic findings in the frozen shoulder. *Journal of Rheumatology*, **8**, 149

Halbach, J.W. and Tank, R.T. (1990) The shoulder. In *Orthopaedic and Sports Physical Therapy*, 2nd edn (ed. J.A. Gould), C.V. Mosby, St Louis

Hawkins, R.J. and Hobeika, P.E. (1983) Impingement syndrome in the athletic shoulder. *Clinics in Sports Medicine*, **2**, 391

Hertling, D. and Kessler, R.M. (1990) *Management of Common Musculoskeletal Disorders*, J.B. Lippincott, Philadelphia

Hunter, M.B., Shybut, G.T. and Nuber, G. (1986) The effect of anabolic steroid hormones on the mechanical properties of tendons and ligaments. *Transactions of the Orthopaedic Research Society*, **11**, 240

Jobe, F.W., Giangarra, C.E. and Kvitne, R.S. (1991) Anterior capsulolabral reconstruction of the shoulder in athletes in overhand sports. *American Journal of Sports Medicine*, **19**, 428

Keirns, M.A. (1994) Conservative management of shoulder impingement. In *The Athlete's Shoulder* (eds J.R. Andrews and K.E. Wilk). Churchill Livingstone, New York

Kibler, W.B. (1991) Role of the scapula in the overhead throwing motion. *Contemporary Orthopaedics*, **22**, 525–532

Kretzler, H.H. and Richardson, A.B. (1989) Rupture of the pectoralis major muscle. *American Journal of Sports Medicine*, **17**, 453–458

Kunichi, A. and Torisu, T. (1984) Muscle belly tear of the triceps. *American Journal of Sports Medicine*, **12**, (6) 485

Lancaster, S., Horowitz, M. and Alonso, J. (1987) Complete acromioclavicular separations: a comparison of operative methods. *Clinical Orthopaedics and Related Research*, **216**, 80–88

Larsen, E., Bjerg-Nielsen, A. and Christensen, P. (1986) Conservative or surgical treatment of acromioclavicular dislocation: a prospective controlled randomised study. *Journal of Bone and Joint Surgery*, **68A**, 552–555

Lemak, L.J. (1994) Calcifying tendonitis. In *The Athlete's Shoulder* (eds J.R. Andrews and K.E. Wilk), Churchill Livingstone, Edinburgh

Lephart, S.M., Warner, J.P., Borsa, P.A. and Fu, F.H. (1994) Proprioception of the shoulder in normal, unstable, and surgical individuals. *Journal of Shoulder and Elbow Surgery*, **3**, (4) 116–119

Lovinger, A., Mangus, B.C. and Ingersoll, C.D. (1991) Shoulder positioning for optimal treatment effects. *Athletic Training, Journal of the National Athletic Training Association*, **26**, 81–82

Lucas, D.B. (1973) Biomechanics of the shoulder joint. *Archives of Surgery*, **107**, 425–432

Lundberg, B.J. and Nilsson, B.E. (1968) Osteopenia in the frozen shoulder. *Clinical Orthopaedics and Related Research*, **60**, 187

McConnell, J. (1992) *The Challenge of the Problem Shoulder*, Course notes, London

Macdonald, R. (1994) *Taping Techniques: Principles and Practice*, Butterworth-Heinemann, Oxford

McNab, I. (1973) Rotator cuff tendinitis. *Annals of the Royal College of Surgeons of England*, **53**, 271

Magee, D.J. (2002) *Orthopaedic Physical Assessment*, 4th edn, Saunders, Philadelphia

Maitland, G.D. (1991) *Peripheral Manipulation*, 3rd edn, Butterworth-Heinemann, Oxford

Mariani, E.M. and Cofield, R.H. (1988) The tendon of the long head of biceps brachii: instability, tendinitis, and rupture. *Advances in Orthopaedic Surgery*, **11**, 262

Matsen, F.A., Harryman, D.T. and Sidles, J.A. (1991) Mechanics of glenohumeral instability. *Clinical Sports Medicine*, **10**, (4) 783–788

Melzer, C., Wallny, T., Wirth, C.J. and Hoffman S. (1995) Frozen shoulder: treatment and results. *Archives of Orthopaedic Trauma Surgery*, **114**, 87–91

Morrey, B.F., Askew, L.J., An, K.N. and Dobyns, J.H. (1985) Rupture of the distal tendon of the biceps brachii: a biomechanical study. *Journal of Bone and Joint Surgery*, **67A**, 418–421

Morrison, D.S. and Bigliani, L.U. (1987) The clinical significance of variations in acromial morphology. *Orthopaedic Transactions*, **11**, 234

Moseley, H.F. and Goldie, I. (1963) The arterial pattern of the rotator cuff of the shoulder. *Journal of Bone and Joint Surgery*, **45B**, 780

Mullen, F., Slade, S. and Briggs, C. (1989) Bony and capsular determinants of glenohumeral locking and quadrant positions. *Australian Journal of Physiotherapy*, **35**, 202–208

Mulligan, B.R. (1989) *Manual Therapy*, Plane View Services, Wellington, New Zealand

Neer, C. (1972) Anterior acromioplasty for the chronic impingement syndrome in the shoulder. *Journal of Bone and Joint Surgery*, **54A**, 41–50

Neviaser, J.S. (1945) Adhesive capsulitis of the shoulder. *Journal of Bone and Joint Surgery*, **27**, 211

Norkin, C.C. and Levangie, P.K. (1992) *Joint Structure and Function*, 2nd edn, F.A. Davis, Philadelphia

Norris, C.M. (1996) *Weight Training*, CD-ROM Package, Physiotools, Helsinki

O'Brian, S.J., Neves, M.C., Arnoczky, S.P. et al. (1990) The anatomy and histology of the inferior glenohumeral ligament complex of the shoulder. *American Journal of Sports Medicine*, **18**, 451

O'Donoghue, D.H. (1973) Subluxing biceps tendon in the athlete. *Journal of Sports Medicine*, **1**, 20

O'Donoghue, D.H. (1976) *Treatment of Injuries to Athletes*, W.B. Saunders, Philadelphia

Ott, J.W., Clancy, W.G. and Wilk, K.E. (1994) Soft tissue injuries of the shoulder. In *The Athlete's Shoulder* (eds J.R. Andrews and K.E. Wilk), Churchill Livingstone, Edinburgh

Ozaki, J., Nakagawa, Y., Sakurai, G. and Tamia, S. (1989) Recalcitrant chronic adhesive capsulitis of the shoulder. *Journal of Bone and Joint Surgery*, **71A**, 1511

Palastanga, N., Field, D. and Soames, R. (1989) *Anatomy and Human Movement*, Heinemann Medical, Oxford

Palastanga, N., Field, D. and Soames, R. (1994) Anatomy and Human Movement, 2nd edition, Butterworth-Heinemann, Oxford

Peat, M. and Culham, E. (1994) Functional anatomy of the shoulder complex. In *The Athlete's Shoulder* (eds J.R. Andrews and K.E. Wilk), Churchill Livingstone, Edinburgh

Percy, E.C., Birbrager, D. and Pitt, M.J. (1988) Snapping scapula: a review of the literature and presentation of 14 patients. *Canadian Journal of Surgery*, **31**, 248–250

Perry, J. and Glousman, R.E. (1995) Biomechanics of throwing. In *The Upper Extremity in Sports Medicine*, 2nd edn (eds. J.A. Nicholas and E.B. Hershman), C.V. Mosby, St Louis

Petersson, C.J. (1986) Spontaneous medial dislocation of the tendon of the long biceps brachii: an anatomic study of prevalence and pathomechanics. *Clinical Orthopaedica and Related Research*, **211**, 244

Petersson, C.J. and Redlund-Johnell, I. (1984) The subacromial space in normal shoulder radiographs. *Acta Orthopaedica Scandinavica*, **55**, 57

Petty, N.J. and Moore, A.P. (2001) *Neuromusculoskeletal Examination and Assessment*, 2nd edn, Churchill Livingstone, Edinburgh

Rathbun, J. and Macnab, I. (1970) The microvascular pattern of the rotator cuff. *Journal of Bone and Joint Surgery*, **52B**, 540–553

Reeves, B. (1966) Arthrographic changes in frozen shoulder and post traumatic stiff shoulders. *Proceedings of the Royal Society of Medicine*, **59**, 827

Reid, D.C. (1992) *Sports Injury Assessment and Rehabilitation*, Churchill Livingstone, Edinburgh

Reid, D.C. and Kushner, S. (1989) The elbow region. In *Orthopaedic Physical Therapy* (eds R. Donatelli and M.J. Wooden), Churchill Livingstone, Edinburgh

Reut, R.C., Bach, B.R. and Johnson, C. (1991) Pectoralis major rupture: diagnosing and treating a weight-training injury. *Physician and Sports Medicine*, **19**, (3) 89–96

Rockwood, C.A. and Odor, J.M. (1989) Spontaneous atraumatic subluxation of the sternoclavicular joint. *Journal of Bone and Joint Surgery*, **71A**, 1280–1288

Roi, G.S., Respizzi, S. and Dworzak, F. (1990) Partial rupture of the pectoralis major muscle in athletes. *International Journal of Sports Medicine*, **11**, (1) 85–87

Rothman, R.H. and Parkes, W.W. (1965) The vascular anatomy of the rotator cuff. *Clinical Orthopaedics and Related Research*, **41**, 176

Shaffer, B., Tibone, J.E. and Kerlan, R.K. (1992) Frozen shoulder: a long term follow up. *Journal of Bone and Joint Surgery*, **74**, 738–746

Simmonds, F.A. (1949) Shoulder pain with particular reference to the frozen shoulder. *Journal of Bone and Joint Surgery*, **31B**, 426

Simons, D.G., Travell, J.G., and Simons, L.S. (1999) *Travell and Simons' Myofascial Pain and Dysfunction*, vol. 1, 2nd edn, Lippincott, Williams and Wilkins, Philadelphia

Slatis, P. and Alato, K. (1979) Medial dislocation of the tendon of the long head of biceps brachii. *Acta Orthopaedica Scandinavica*, **50**, 73

Smith, R.L. and Brunolli, J. (1989). Shoulder kinesthesia after anterior glenohumeral joint dislocation. *Physical Therapy*, **69**, 106–112

Taft, T.N., Wilson, F.C. and Oglesby, J.W. (1987) Dislocation of the acromioclavicular joint: an end-result study. *Journal of Bone and Joint Surgery*, **69A**, 1045–1051

Thein, L.A. (1989) Impingement syndrome and its conservative management. *Journal of Orthopaedic and Sports Physical Therapy*, **11**, (5) 183–191

Tibone, J., Sellers, R. and Tonino, P. (1992) Strength testing after third degree acromioclavicular dislocations. *American Journal of Sports Medicine*, **20**, 328–331

Ticker, J.B. and Bigliani, L.U. (1994) Impingement pathology of the rotator cuff. In *The Athlete's Shoulder* (eds J.R. Andrews and K.E. Wilk), Churchill Livingstone, Edinburgh

Torstensen, T.A., Meen, H.D. and Stiris, M. (1994) The effect of medical exercise therapy on a patient with chronic supraspinatus tendinitis. Diagnostic ultrasound-tissue regeneration: a case study. *Journal of Orthopaedic and Sports Physical Therapy*, **20**, 319–327

Uitvlugt, G., Detrisac, D.A. and Johnson, L.L. (1988) The pathology of the frozen shoulder: an arthroscopic perspective. *Arthroscopy*, **4**, 137

Van der Windt, D. and Koes, B. (2002) Are corticosteroid injections as effective as physiotherapy for the treatment of a painful shoulder? In *Evidence Based Sports Medicine* (eds D. MacAuley and T. Best), BMJ Books, London

Vermeulen, H.M., Obermann, W.M., Burger, B.J. and Kok, G.J. (2000) End range mobilisation techniques in adhesive capsulitis of the shoulder joint. *Physical Therapy*, **80**, 1204–1213

Warwick, R. and Williams, P.L. (1973) *Gray's Anatomy*, 35th edn, Longman, Harlow

Wiley, A.M. (1991) Arthroscopic appearance of frozen shoulder. *Arthroscopy*, **7**, 138

Wilk, K.E. and Arrigo, C. (1993) Current concepts in the rehabilitation of the athletic shoulder. *Journal of Orthopaedic and Sports Physical Therapy*, **18**, (1) 365–378

Wilk, K.E., Voight, M.L., Keirns, M.A., Gambetta, V., Andrews, J.R. and Dillman, C.J. (1993) Stretch shortening drills for the upper extremities: theory and clinical application. *Journal of Orthopaedic and Sports Physical Therapy*, **17**, (5) 225–239

Wolfe, S.W., Wickiewicz, T.L. and Cavanaugh, J.T. (1992) Ruptures of the pectoralis major muscle: an anatomic and clinical analysis. *American Journal of Sports Medicine*, **20**, 587–593

Yergason, R.M. (1931) Supination sign. *Journal of Bone and Joint Surgery*, **13A**, 160

Zachazewski, J.E., Magee, D.J. and Quillen, W.S. (1996) *Athletic Injuries and Rehabilitation*, W.B.Saunders, Philadelphia

Chapter **19**

The elbow

STRUCTURE AND FUNCTION

The primary purpose of the shoulder is often described as positioning the arm to facilitate hand action. The elbow, in turn, functions to shorten or lengthen the arm, largely to allow the hand to be brought to the mouth. The elbow complex consists of the humeroulnar and humeroradial articulations and the superior radioulnar joint, all of which share the same capsule (Fig. 19.1).

Definition

Joints within the elbow are: *humeroulnar* between the trochlea of the humerus and the trochlea notch of the ulnar; *humeroradial* between the capitulum of the humerus and the superior surface of the head of the radius; *superior radioulnar* between the circumference of the head of the radius and the fibro-osseous ring formed by the radial notch of the ulna and the annular ligament.

When viewed from the side, the distal end of the humerus is larger anteriorly and inferiorly, and sits at an angle of 45° to the longitudinal axis of the bone. Similarly, the trochlear notch of the ulna bulges, making a comparable angle to its axis. This structure postpones contact between the humerus and ulna on flexion, and allows more space between the bones to accommodate soft tissues. The 'nutcracker effect' is therefore reduced as the bones come together.

Bony alignment and joint contact areas

Viewed from the front, the radius and ulna are slanted laterally to the shaft of the humerus, the angulation forming the carrying angle (Fig. 19.2a). This is approximately 10–15° for men, increasing to 20–25° for women. This bony alignment means that normally, as the arm is flexed the hand moves towards the shoulder, and the radius and ulna end up in line with the humerus (Fig. 19.2c). Variations in carrying angle between individuals, mainly due to altered configuration of the trochlear groove, may occur and will alter the resting

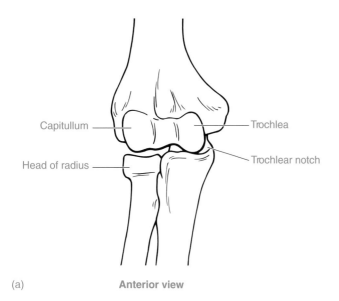

Capitullum — Trochlea

Head of radius — Trochlear notch

(a) **Anterior view**

Humerus —

Head of radius

Olecranon —

Ulna

(b) **Lateral view**

Figure 19.1 Articulations forming the elbow joint. (a) Anterior view. (b) Lateral view.

Figure 19.2 (a) Carrying angle. (b) Lateral orientation. (c) Most common configuration of the trochlear groove. (d) Medial orientation. After Norkin, C.C. and Levangie, P.K. (1992) *Joint Structure and Function*, 2nd edn. Davis, Philadelphia. With permission.

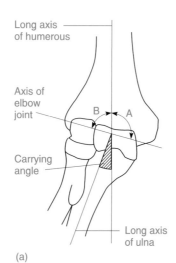

Long axis of humerous

Axis of elbow joint

B A

Carrying angle

Long axis of ulna

(a)

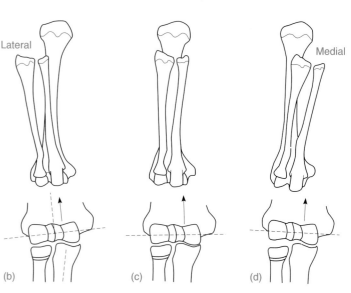

Lateral

Medial

(b) (c) (d)

position of the radius and ulnar at full flexion (Fig. 19.2b,d). Changes in bony alignment may also occur after injury – an important factor in rehabilitation following elbow fractures.

The contact area between the joint surfaces of the elbow complex increases throughout flexion. In full extension the lower medial part of the trochlear notch of the ulna is used, with no contact occurring between the radius and ulna. At 90° the contact area is a diagonal (lower medial to upper lateral) across the trochlear surface, with only slight pressure between the humerus and radial head. In full flexion definite contact occurs between the radius and ulna, and the trochlear contact areas increase (Fig. 19.3). Full flexion is thus required to ensure adequate nutrition of the whole articular cartilage, a situation sometimes not possible in obese or heavily muscled individuals due to the approximation of the flexor soft tissues.

Collateral ligaments

The elbow collateral ligaments are positioned on the ulnar (inner) and radial (outer) aspects of the joint. The ulnar or medial collateral ligament (MCL) spreads out from the medial epicondyle to form two thick anterior and posterior bands, joined by a thinner intermediate (oblique) portion. The radial or lateral collateral ligament (LCL) is a single triangular structure attaching just below the lateral epicondyle and blending with the annular ligament of the radius.

As occurs in the knee, the collateral ligaments of the elbow become taut at different degrees of flexion. The anterior fibres of both the medial and lateral collateral ligaments are taut in extension, whereas the posterior fibres are taut in flexion. Protection is provided against valgus and varus strains throughout the whole range of joint movement as a result.

Flexion is limited by muscle contact and impingement of the radial head on to the radial fossa. In addition, tension occurs in the triceps and posterior joint capsule, and finally, in lean individuals, the shafts of the radius and humerus themselves come into contact (Fig. 19.4a).

In extension, when the muscles are relaxed, valgus stability is provided by the medial collateral ligament, anterior capsule and bony configuration. As the elbow flexes, the anterior capsule relaxes, and its role is taken on by the medial collateral ligament, which provides 31% of joint stability in extension and 54% at 90° flexion (Table 19.1). In contrast, varus stress is resisted in the main by bone contact supplemented by the anterior capsule. The lateral collateral ligament only contributes 14% of the total stability of the joint with the elbow in full extension, and 9% with it flexed to 90° (Morrey and Kai-Nan, 1983). With joint distraction, the main limiting factor in extension is the joint capsule, and

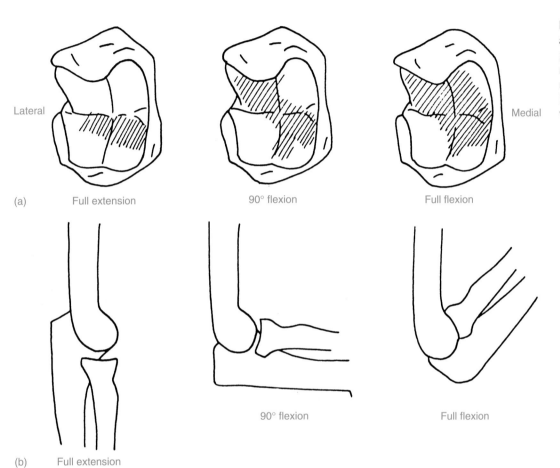

(a)   Full extension   90° flexion   Full flexion

(b)   Full extension   90° flexion   Full flexion

Figure 19.3   Contact areas at different elbow positions. (a) The trochlear notch. (b) The head of the radius. From Palastanga, Field and Soames (1989) with permission.

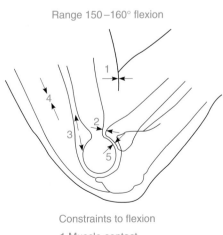

Range 150–160° flexion

Constraints to flexion

1 Muscle contact
2 Radial head impingement
3 Posterior capsule tension
4 Triceps tension
5 Radius–humerus contact

(a)

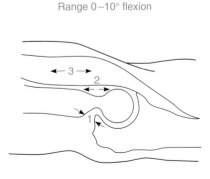

Range 0–10° flexion

Constraints to extension

1 Olecranon impingement
2 Anterior capsule tension
3 Biceps tension

(b)

Figure 19.4   Constraints to (a) flexion and (b) extension. From Reid (1992) with permission.

Table 19.1 Percentage contribution of elbow structures to stability of the joint

Limiting structure	Valgus %		Varus %		Distribution %	
	0°	90°	0°	90°	0°	90°
Medial collateral ligament	31	54	–	–	6	78
Lateral collateral ligament	–	–	14	9	5	10
Joint capsule	38	10	31	13	85	8
Bone contact	31	33	55	75	–	–

After Morrey, B.F. and Kai-Nan, A. (1983) Articular and ligamentous contributions to the stability of the elbow joint. *American Journal of Sports Medicine*, 11, 315–318. With permission.

Table 19.2 General causes of tennis elbow

Radiohumeral bursitis
Periostitis of the common extensor tendon
Tendinitis: extensor carpi radialis brevis, supinator
Microtendinous tears of the common extensor tendon with subtendinous granulation and fibrosis
Myofascitis
Radial head fibrillation/chondromalacia
Calcification
Radial nerve entrapment and subsequent fibrosis
Stenosis of the orbicular ligament
Hyperaemic synovial fringe
Inflammation of the annular ligament
Cervical radiculopathy

From Lee, D.G. (1986) Tennis elbow: a manual therapist's perspective. *Journal of Orthopaedic and Sports Physical Therapy*, 12(2), 81–87. With permission.

with the joint flexed to 90°, the medial collateral ligament. End-range is limited by a combination of the olecranon impinging into the olecranon fossa, and tension in the anterior capsule and biceps (Fig. 19.4b).

Pronation and supination of the forearm involve not just the superior and inferior radioulnar joints, but also the ulnohumeral, radiohumeral and radiocarpal joints. With pronation, the head of the radius twists on the capitulum and swings on the radial notch of the ulna, tightening the quadrate ligament. The radial head tilts, and is pulled into the capitulotrochlear groove, and the ulna moves into slight extension and abduction at the ulnohumeral joint (Lee, 1986). Consequent to this, at the inferior radioulnar joint the ulnar notch of the radius swings medially over the ulnar head. A traumatic injury to the elbow is therefore likely to affect the wrist, and, to be complete, clinical examination should include both joints.

SCREENING EXAMINATION

Following inspection, objective examination begins with flexion and extension, each performed to full range, noting the joint end-feel. The normal end-feel to extension is hard while that to flexion is soft. Pronation and supination are performed with the elbow held to the side of the body and arm flexed to 90°. The end-feel should be springy. Further differentiation may be obtained by combining flexion and extension with abduction and adduction (valgus/varus) stresses, and by assessing gliding motions of the individual component joints of the elbow complex (see Treatment note 19.1). The capsular pattern is of flexion more limited than extension, and rotations relatively free.

The inferior radioulnar joint is stressed by pronation and supination, and may require further examination if pain is produced. Screening examinations of the neck and shoulder are performed if referred pain is suspected, and full neurological examination may be required. The front of the elbow lies within the C5 and C6 dermatomes, while the back of the elbow is in the C7 dermatome. Pain may therefore be referred to the elbow from the cervical nerve roots or the shoulder region.

The contractile structures are examined by resisted movements, performed firstly with the elbow flexed to 90°. One of the therapist's hands supports the elbow to restrict shoulder movement and the other applies resistance to flexion and extension. For pronation and supination, the lower forearm (not the hand) is gripped. The grip must be tight and positioned over the radial styloid to avoid a friction burn to the patient's skin. Resisted wrist flexion and extension are performed with the elbow locked.

Ligamentous instability may be assessed by combining movement of the forearm and upper arm. The MCL is assessed by applying an abduction force to the forearm with the elbow unlocked. At the same time the humerus is laterally rotated. For the LCL the technique is reversed, an adduction force being imposed on the forearm and the humerus pulled into medial rotation. In each case both excessive movement and reproduction of the patient's symptoms indicate a positive test result.

LATERAL PAIN

The term 'tennis elbow' is often used colloquially as a blanket description for any soft tissue pain between the shoulder and wrist, and there has been little agreement in the past as to the exact site of the lesion. The condition was first documented in the late 1800s when it was described as 'lawn tennis arm'. Cyriax (1936) described 26 different lesions to which the condition had been attributed, while Lee (1986) cited 12 more general causes, as shown in Table 19.2. The terms 'lateral' and 'medial tennis elbow' have been used (Nirschl, 1986), but in this book the name tennis elbow is used to describe lateral epicondylitis while 'golfer's elbow' refers to medial epicondylitis. The ratio of lateral to medial epicondylitis encountered clinically has been shown to be 7:1 (Leach and Miller, 1987).

Tennis elbow is a lesion to the common extensor origin (CEO), with the primary site being the tendon of extensor

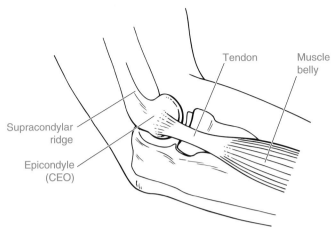

Supracondylar ridge

Tendon   Muscle belly

Epicondyle (CEO)

Figure 19.5   Palpation of tennis elbow.

carpi radialis brevis (ECRB) . Less frequently, the extensor carpi radialis longus (ECRL) is affected at its attachment to the supracondylar ridge, and in some cases the anterior portion of the extensor digitorum. Most commonly, the injury is at the tenoperiosteal junction, but scar tissue may form onto the tendon itself or the musculotendinous junction (Fig. 19.5).

> **Keypoint**
>
> Tennis elbow affects: (i) the tendon of extensor carpi radialis brevis at the epicondyle; (ii) tendon of extensor carpi radialis longus onto the supracondylar ridge.

Repeated activity causes microtrauma, with subsequent granulation tissue formation on the underside of the tendon unit and at the tenoperiosteal junction. The granulation tissue formed appears to contain large numbers of free nerve endings, hence the pain of the condition. The major problem is that the granulation tissue does not progress quickly to a mature form, and so healing fails to take place, almost a type of tendinous 'non-union' (Goldie, 1964; Bernhang, 1979).

Clinical presentation

Tennis elbow usually presents as pain over the region of the lateral epicondyle, extending distally. The pain may build up slowly (overuse) or be the result of a single incident (trauma). Pain is usually increased with resisted wrist extension. Depending on the site of the lesion, pain can be made worse by adding forearm supination (but see radial tunnel syndrome, below), and radial deviation of the wrist (Halle, Franklin and Karalfa, 1986). Performing resisted wrist extension with the elbow fully extended will usually elicit pain, even in mild cases.

The condition is most common with athletes over 30 years of age, and occurs normally when repeated wrist extension is combined with forearm supination. Racquet sports involve this action, but several occupational stresses

can also be causal factors. Hammering, painting and using heavy spanners will all exacerbate the problem, so any training modification which is prescribed must also take into account an athlete's job. Pain usually increases when small objects are gripped, as this hand position places additional stretch on the forearm extensors.

> **Keypoint**
>
> Tennis elbow is exacerbated by activities involving repeated wrist extension while gripping a thin object.

As with most overuse syndromes, the ache may initially subside when the stressful activity is discontinued, but as the condition progresses pain even occurs at rest. Patients complain of a weak grip, and wasting of the affected muscles may be seen in long-standing cases. Close inspection will often reveal slight swelling over the affected area, but this is rarely obvious to the patient.

Treatment

Treatment aims initially to reduce pain and swelling. The RICE protocol is used, and several authors have reported good results by using ultrasound, alone or with hydrocortisone gel (Griffen and Touchstone, 1963; Klienkort and Wood, 1975; Halle, Franklin and Karalfa, 1986). Reducing the stress applied to the tendon is important. Rest from exacerbating activities and the use of counterforce bracing are effective. The counterforce brace consists of a tight strap which is placed around the upper forearm to create a lateral pressure when an object is gripped. The aim is to redirect and disperse overload to healthy tissue or to the band itself, and in so doing reduce painful inhibition and permit a more forceful contraction. Using this technique, grip strength has been shown to improve (Burton, 1985; Wadsworth et al., 1989), and a positive effect has been shown using biomechanical analysis and technique correction of tennis serves and backhand strokes (Groppel and Nirschl, 1986).

As the local swelling adheres and shrinks, inelastic scar tissue is formed. Stretching exercises are therefore of particular value. A useful forearm extensor stretch may be performed with the athlete facing a wall (Fig. 19.6a). The dorsum of the hand is placed flat onto the wall, and the elbow remains locked. By leaning forwards the wrist is forced into 90° flexion, stretching the posterior forearm tissues. Wrist flexion may be combined with a pronation stretch (Fig. 19.6b). Keeping the elbow locked, the forearm is maximally pronated and the wrist flexed. Overpressure is applied with the other hand and a static stretch performed. The scar tissue is more pliable when warm and so the athlete is advised to practise stretching after a hot bath or shower.

Resistance exercises (weight or powerband) are used to re-strengthen the forearm extensors. Wrist extension may be performed holding a small (2 kg) dumb-bell. The forearm

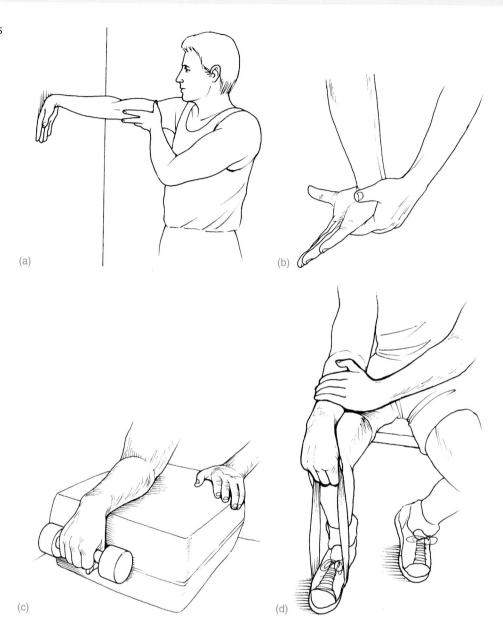

Figure 19.6 Exercise therapy for tennis elbow. (a) Forearm extensor stretch against wall. (b) Combined flexion-pronation of wrist. (c) Resisted forearm extension (dumb-bell). (d) Resisted extension (band).

is supported on a block or over the couch side and full range movement is attempted (Fig. 19.6c). Powerband extension is performed with the athlete sitting. One end of the band is placed beneath the foot and the other end gripped. The forearm is supported along the athlete's thigh (Fig. 19.6d). Initially, eccentric contractions are likely to be less painful than concentric, and the use of ice massage to produce a temporary anaesthesia before exercise is applied (cryokinetics) is often used.

One word of caution: negative transfer effects (see p. 150) have been described by Nirschl (1988) when using high weight, low repetition training following tennis elbow. To avoid this Nirschl (1988) recommended the use of high speed skill training as part of the total rehabilitation programme.

Manual therapy, including local massage to reduce swelling and produce hyperaemia, and transverse frictions

to form a mobile scar are both of use. It is important to locate the exact site of injury for transverse frictions to be effective. The forearm should be pronated and supinated while the area is palpated to find the exact site of the CEO. The lateral epicondyle should be identified as should the supracondylar ridge, and each considered as a possible source of pain. The teno-osseous junction is best frictioned with the forearm in mid-position to let the CEO relax slightly and allow the palpating finger to get right onto the bony surface. The tendon itself is treated on stretch with the elbow and wrist flexed, and forearm pronated (Fig. 19.7a).

Mills manipulation (Mills, 1928), although originally designed to stress the annular ligament, can be performed to stretch the CEO. The patient's arm is held in extension at the shoulder, with the elbow comfortably flexed and wrist and forearm fully flexed and pronated (Fig. 19.7b). A high velocity

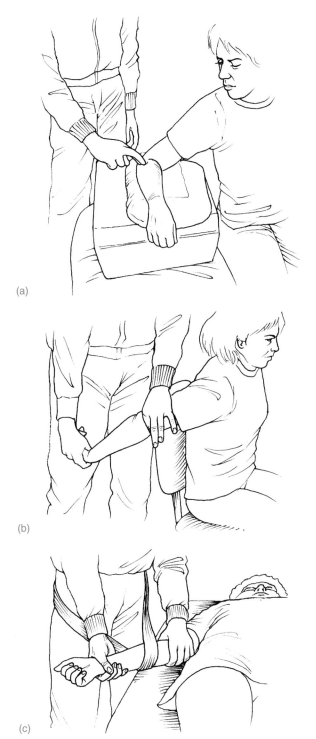

(a)

(b)

(c)

Figure 19.7   Manual therapy for tennis elbow. (a) Deep transverse friction to the common extensor origin. (b) Mills manipulation. (c) Mobilization with movement using belt.

low amplitude thrust is applied to the elbow to fully extend it. Cyriax and Cyriax (1983) claimed this procedure would pull apart the tissue surfaces joined by a painful scar, the fresh tear being replaced by new fibrous tissue under no tension.

Mobilization with movement has been shown to be an effective treatment for this condition (Vicenzino and Wright,

1995). In this technique, a sustained mobilization is applied to a joint, normally at 90° to the plane of movement, to correct joint tracking (Mulligan, 1989). The mobilization is applied at the same time as the patient performs a painful action with the affected joint. In the case of tennis elbow, this action is normally extension of the wrist or fingers (especially the third finger).

With the patient in a supine position, the therapist wraps a belt around his or her own hips and the athlete's forearm. The proximal edge of the belt is level with the elbow joint. The humerus and forearm are stabilized by the therapist's hands. The mobilization (lateral glide of the ulna) is carried out by the therapist gently leaning back (Fig. 19.7c). The aim is to reduce the pain of the finger extension action, initially while the mobilization is applied and eventually during free movement.

Where general elbow stiffness is present as a result of previous inflammation, joint mobilization may be required. Overpressure to either flexion or extension may be combined with adduction and abduction to regain accessory movement. Mobilization of the radial head may also be useful in cases of tennis elbow, and end-range pronation and supination with overpressure may be performed. Direct palpation may be given to the radial head using the therapist's thumbs. For a PA (posteroanterior) glide, the patient's elbow is flexed and the bony contour of the radial head is easily palpable. AP (anteroposterior) glides are performed with the patient's arm extended, and the radial head is palpated through the anterior soft tissues.

Biomechanics

The extensor carpi radialis brevis is under maximum tension when it contracts in a position of forearm pronation, wrist flexion and ulna deviation (Briggs and Elliott, 1985). This is a typical position for a backhand shot in racquet sports, and elements of this anatomical alignment are seen in many repetitive actions in sport. Repeated practice will cause hypertrophy of this muscle and often a resultant loss of flexibility. In addition, an imbalance frequently exists between the forearm flexors and extensors. Normally, the wrist extensors should be at least 50% of the flexors, but in many recreational sports an individual may have considerably weaker wrist extensors in proportion to flexors. The combination of weaker and less flexible wrist extensors placed in a demanding situation of the backhand stroke (or similar occupational action) exceeds the adaptability of the tissues. One action an athlete may take as part of a preventive programme for this condition, therefore, is to maintain the flexibility of the wrist musculature, and build up the strength of the wrist extensors to as much as 75% of the flexor strength (Reid, 1992).

Ergonomics plays an important part in the management of this condition. Enlarging the grip of any object being held, be it a racquet or a spanner, is important in most cases. The correct grip size can be calculated by measuring from the tip

Treatment note 19.1   Trigger points and acupuncture points in the treatment of tennis elbow

Both classical acupuncture points and trigger points (TrPs) are extremely useful in the treatment of tennis elbow, and have been shown to be superior to sham points (Molsberger and Hille, 1994; Fink et al., 2002). TrPs in the extensor carpi radialis longus and brevis may be palpated with the elbow flexed and hand *unsupported*. Begin over the common extensor origin and palpate distally. Central points are located on the ulnar side of the brachioradialis muscle 4–5 cm distal to the elbow crease (at the approximate point of the classical points LI-10, LI-9, and LI-8) while attachment TrPs are located at the common extensor origin. The TrP may be pressed against the radius and flicked transversely to produce a twitch response, causing the patient's wrist to extend and radially deviate.

The TrP may be treated with either dry needling or deep massage. For massage, the therapist's thumbs are used beginning over the patient's supracondylar ridge and epicondyle, extending into the muscle belly. The whole of the area may be treated using a muscle stripping technique pressing in a line from the epicondyle to the thumb. Ischaemic compression may be used over a single active point using a plunger and the patient may be taught self-palpation (Fig. 19.8).

Dry needling uses either an intramuscular technique to a depth of 0.5–1.5 cm depending on muscle bulk, or needling close to the epicondyle with the intention of striking the bone using a periosteal technique. Here, the aim is to stimulate the richly innervated periosteum to give pain relief (Mann, 1992).

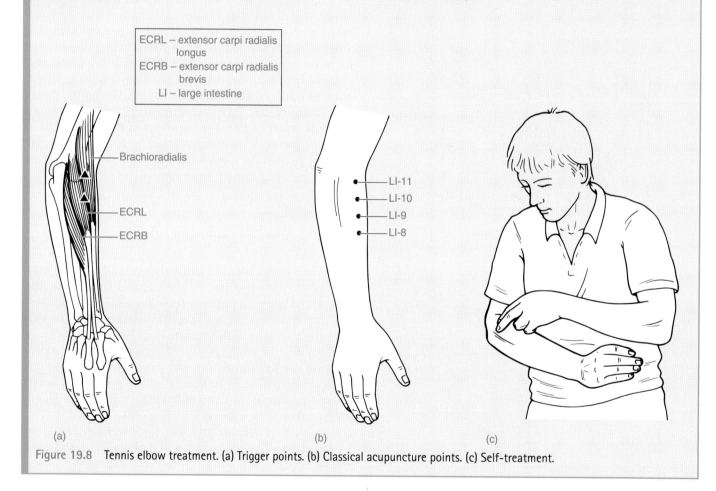

ECRL – extensor carpi radialis longus
ECRB – extensor carpi radialis brevis
LI – large intestine

Brachioradialis

ECRL

ECRB

LI-11
LI-10
LI-9
LI-8

(a)   (b)   (c)

Figure 19.8   Tennis elbow treatment. (a) Trigger points. (b) Classical acupuncture points. (c) Self-treatment.

of the ring finger to the bottom lateral crease of the palm, directly below (Fig. 19.9). The figure obtained represents the circumference of the racquet handle. Placing a thick piece of sponge around a handle is also useful to enlarge the grip and reduce shock travelling from the handle to the hand. In some cases a grip which is too large may also be a problem, so to assess if grip size is a relevant feature, ask the patient to grip a thin object (a pencil) and a large one (a bottle) and find which gives less pain. In general terms, when prolonged grip is applied, the therapist should be able to place one finger between the tips of the athlete's fingers and thumb.

In tennis, higher impact and torsion forces are produced by a wet, heavy ball or a racquet which is too tightly strung. The closer the ball is to the centre of percussion (the

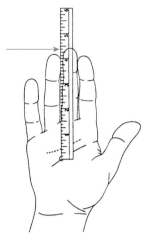

Figure 19.9   Hand measurement to determine proper grip handle size. The distance from the proximal palmar crease to the tip of the middle finger determines the proper size. From Nirschl (1988), with permission.

mathematical point on the racquet face where no torsion will occur on impact), the less strain on the elbow tissues.

Oversize racquets, by increasing the likelihood of keeping the ball away from the frame, may reduce torsion and in turn overload stress on the elbow. In addition, leverage forces may be reduced in these racquets by moving the centre of percussion closer to the racquet handle (Nirschl, 1988). A heavier racquet will have more momentum, and will place a greater strain on the forearm. Nirschl (1988) recommended a mid-sized (90–100 square inch) graphite composite light-weight racquet to give the best protection, and Bullard (1982) recommended fibreglass or graphite as the best materials to absorb vibration.

OSTEOCHONDROSIS

The most common site for osteochondrosis in the elbow is the anterolateral surface of the capitulum (Panner's disease). The aetiology is generally either traumatic or vascular, although some familial tendency may be present. The condition is most commonly related to throwing or racquet sports. In throwing, the angular velocity experienced at the joint may exceed 300°/s (Jobe and Nuber, 1986). This, coupled with a valgus force and an extension stress, causes the radial head to impinge against the capitulum. Ultimately, a breakdown can occur in the capitulum surface and the radial head may hypertrophy.

The vascular supply to the area can be disrupted by this repeated trauma. Up until the age of 5 years the capitulum has a good blood supply, but later the nucleus of the capitulum receives only one or two vessels. These pass into the area posteriorly through soft, compressible cartilage- – a possible site of damage.

The typical patient is an athlete in early adolescence (usually male) who shows limitation of elbow extension with local swelling. Onset is often insidious and the patient may have been experiencing difficulties over a protracted period. If the osteochondrotic fragment is free within the joint, locking or catching may be experienced with certain movements. Radiographs may show blunting of the capitulum with enlargement of the radial head. Often an island of bone is seen surrounded by an area of rarefaction. Premature epiphyseal closure may also be noted to either the humerus or the proximal radius.

In the initial stages of the condition with a young athlete, rest is all that is required, splinting being indicated if the patient fails to heed this advice. If stress has been allowed to continue and bony degeneration has occurred, drilling or grafting of the attached fragment may be required. In late stage conditions loose bodies may need to be removed, and unfortunately the prognosis is sometimes poor.

MEDIAL PAIN

Lesions to the medial side of the joint occur most often with throwing actions. Although different sports demand different throwing techniques, similarities still exist. Initially, the shoulder is abducted and taken into extreme external rotation and extension, while the elbow remains flexed (cocking phase). Then, the shoulder and trunk rapidly move forward, leaving the arm behind (acceleration phase). This action imposes a valgus stress on the joint and stretches the ulnar collateral ligament in particular. The shoulder flexors and internal rotators contract powerfully, flinging the arm forward resulting in stress to the olecranon as the arm extends rapidly to full range (deceleration phase and follow-through).

The throwing action imposes a number of stresses on the elbow (Fig. 19.10). The lateral joint line is subjected to compression forces, in the olecranon fossa there are shearing forces, while the medial joint line experiences tensile forces (Jobe and Nuber, 1986). These forces, if repeated, can give rise to specific injuries and general degeneration reflecting the stress imposed on the elbow structures (Table 19.3).

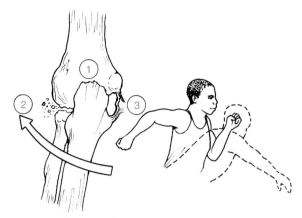

Figure 19.10   Forces on the elbow during throwing. 1. Hypertension—olecranon shear. 2. Valgus—compresses laterally, radial head damage. 3. Valgus—distracts medially, collateral ligament damage.

Table 19.3   Throwing injuries to the elbow

Medial tension	Lateral compression	Posterior shear
Muscular overuse	Osteochondrosis	Muscular strain
Ligamentous injury	Fractured capitulum	Impingement
Capsular injury	Lateral epicondylitis	Olecranon fracture
Ulnar traction spur		Bony hypertrophy
Medial epicondylitis		Loose bodies

MEDIAL EPICONDYLITIS

This is a lesion of the common flexor origin (CFO) on the medial epicondyle, and is commonly called golfer's elbow. The primary site is the origin of pronator teres and flexor carpi radialis on the medial epicondyle. The flexor carpi ulnaris may occasionally be affected. Golfer's elbow is less common than tennis elbow, occurring at a ratio of about 1:15 (Coorad and Hooper, 1973). The injury can be complicated by ulnar nerve involvement, the nerve being compressed at a point distal to the medial epicondyle.

> **Keypoint**
>
> Golfer's elbow (medial epicondylitis) mainly affects the pronator teres and flexor carpi radialis muscle. Flexor carpi ulnaris is affected less often, and ulnar nerve involvement may also occur.

Sensory symptoms are often present and Tinel's sign (tapping the ulnar nerve at the elbow to produce pain or tingling in the ulnar portion of the hand) is positive (Nirschl, 1986). Chronic conditions may see calcium deposits developing within the tendon itself (Leach and Miller, 1987).

Pain is felt more locally than with tennis elbow, and is increased on resisted wrist flexion and sometimes forearm pronation. The condition may be differentiated from chronic medial ligament sprain by applying the valgus stress test which should not give pain or laxity in epicondylitis.

The treatment is for the most part like that for tennis elbow, including soft tissue manipulation and biomechanical changes. Transverse frictions are now performed with the elbow and wrist in extension, with the forearm supinated. Counterforce bracing is again used, but this time the brace extends up to the medial epicondyle to avoid interfering with elbow flexion.

MEDIAL COLLATERAL LIGAMENT (THROWER'S ELBOW)

Repetitive stresses to this ligament are common in throwing athletes, particularly in events such as the javelin. Pain is generally quite localized over the medial joint line, and exacerbated by applying an elbow abduction stress test, forcing a valgus strain on the joint in 20° flexion. With severe injuries, gapping of the joint may be apparent.

Initial treatment is to remove the causal stress and rest from throwing. Operative repair of a ruptured medial collateral ligament is often recommended for athletes and those involved in heavy manual labour. The theory is that instability may produce problems later in life. However, Kuroda and Sakamaki (1986) reported surgical repair in 10 patients and conservative management in three others. Before surgery, valgus instability averaged 14.9°. Those treated surgically later showed average laxity of 5.1° while those managed conservatively had average values of 8.0°. With figures for instability which are so similar, it may be questionable whether surgery offers substantial advantage over conservative management in many cases.

POSTERIOR ELBOW PAIN

Pain at the back of the elbow is common in sports which rapidly extend or hyperextend the joint. These include the throwing sports, punching in martial arts and pressing actions in weight training. Structures involved, either individually or in combination, include the insertion of the triceps, the olecranon bursa and the olecranon itself.

Olecranon bursitis

The olecranon bursa is placed at the bony point of the elbow, over the olecranon process subcutaneously. A deeper bursa is sometimes present between the capsule and triceps. When the elbow is extended, the margins of the olecranon bursa cause a circular ridge of skin about 1.5–2 cm in diameter to be pulled up on the posterior aspect of the elbow.

The bursa can become inflamed by leaning on the elbow for a prolonged period (student's elbow), or from a direct fall onto the point of the elbow. This latter case may induce haemorrhage into the bursal sac itself. Examination of the joint reveals no abnormality, but pain and thickening occur to direct palpation over the bursa. Treatment is to remove the cause, pad the point of the elbow and aspirate the fluid.

Triceps insertion

Triceps tendinitis may occur in throwing athletes (especially javelin) and weight-lifters. Inflammation and microtrauma are usually limited to the olecranon insertion of the muscle. Damage is usually to the musculotendinous or teno-osseous junctions, and cessation of activity and correction of technique, coupled with modalities to reduce local inflammation and pain, are usually curative. Unusually, the medial head of the triceps may sublux over the medial epicondyle during flexion causing a snapping sensation ('snapping elbow syndrome'; Dreyfuss and Kessler, 1978). This must be distinguished from subluxation of the ulnar nerve from its groove, which is common in 16% of the population (Reid, 1992). This is normally due to laxity of the ulnar collateral ligament and/or a shallow ulnar groove.

> **Keypoint**
>
> Laxity of the ulnar collateral ligament and a shallow ulnar groove can allow the ulnar nerve to sublux and causes neurological symptoms into the 4th and 5th fingers.

Rupture of the triceps tendon, either partial or complete, is unusual, and the muscle belly itself is even less frequently injured. When rupture does occur, there is usually a palpable defect in the musculotendinous junction of the muscle, with scarring in the chronic injury. Active extension is lost, and a large haematoma, later developing into bruising, is noted locally. The majority of patients are in their 30s or 40s, and the injury almost always occurs either following a fall onto the outstretched hand or a 'chopping' action. In either case, the stress is one of deceleration imposed on an already contracting muscle.

A small fragment of the olecranon may be avulsed and show up on a lateral radiograph of the elbow, and occasionally radial head fractures are associated with the condition. Conservative management is reserved for partial ruptures (Bach, Warren and Wickiewicz, 1987) distinguished by an ability to partially extend the arm against gravity. Surgical management for avulsion injuries involves drilling the olecranon and suturing the muscle. Postoperatively, the patient is immobilized for 3–4 weeks in a cast or splint at 30–45° elbow flexion.

POSTERIOR IMPINGEMENT

Posterior impingement of the olecranon into its fossa is common in sports where the elbow is 'snapped back'. This is especially the case with rapid weight (circuit) training, and martial arts, where athletes reach upwards as if 'punching

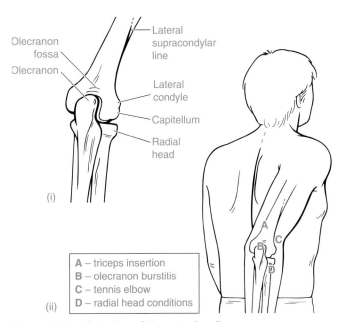

Figure 19.11 Palpation of the posterior elbow.

the air' while performing forms. Throwing events will tend to cause impingement of the medial aspect of the olecranon on the follow-through movement.

Examination usually reveals point tenderness over the posterior or posteromedial aspect of the olecranon (Fig. 19.11). This is made worse by forced extension, and extension/abduction. Chronic injuries may show osteophyte formation posteromedially. Cortical thickening is also usually seen on radiograph, but this is thought to represent adaptation of the bone to repetitive stress (Garrick and Webb, 1990).

Treatment is initially to limit extension and valgus stress by strapping, or if this fails, to rest the elbow completely. The elbow flexors are strengthened (especially eccentrically) to enhance their action as decelerators of elbow extension, and to shorten them and therefore limit hyperextension.

Stress fracture of the olecranon is a rare but often overlooked outcome of posterior impingement, and has been described in javelin throwers (Hulkko, Orava and Nikula, 1968) and baseball pitchers (Nuber and Diment, 1992). Pain usually follows the pattern typical of a stress fracture, eventually limiting performance. Many lesions will respond to rest and splinting, but some require surgery including excision of the olecranon tip and inlaid bone block graft (Torg, 1993).

MUSCULAR INJURY

The biceps, triceps and brachialis may all be injured in sport. The most common injury for the biceps is to its long head, but its lower insertion may also be injured occasionally. Pain is reproduced to resisted elbow flexion and supination, and passive pronation, resisted shoulder flexion may also be added. If resisted flexion is painful but supination is not, the brachialis is indicated. The site of pain is the centre of the front of the arm, often radiating as far as the wrist in severe cases.

The usual site for injury to the triceps is the musculo-tendinous junction, but the belly may be injured. Pain on resisted elbow (and shoulder) extension is the clinical sign, but when this test gives pain in the upper arm felt nearer to the shoulder, referred pain from impingement of a shoulder structure should be considered. In this case the triceps contraction pulls the humerus up into the acromion approximating the joint.

MYOSITIS OSSIFICANS TRAUMATICA

Injury to the brachialis should always be treated with caution, because this muscle shares with the quadriceps the potential for myositis development.

The history is usually that of a direct blow, for example from a knee or head in rugby or a foot in martial arts. Most commonly, a second blow has been experienced to the same area. The typical findings are tenderness persisting for 2–3 weeks after injury, and difficulty in regaining full range motion. On examination, a fibrous mass is often palpable within the muscle over the anterior aspect of the arm.

> **Keypoint**
>
> The possibility of myositis in the brachialis muscle exists when: (i) there is a history of a number of direct blows to the same area; (ii) tenderness has persisted for 2–3 weeks after injury; (iii) full range of motion cannot be regained; (iv) there is a palpable mass over the anterior aspect of the arm when compared to the uninjured side.

Where these findings are present, X-ray is required. Often heterotrophic bone formation is seen, showing a diffuse fluffy callus. As the callus matures it will shrink and its margins become better defined. Bone scan will reveal whether the condition is still active.

Management aims initially to minimize the damage. Local swelling is reduced where possible, and activity limited. Mobility exercise is begun with caution when radiographic evidence shows that the condition is no longer active. Resisted work is the last exercise to be started, and when sport is resumed, the area is protected with padding.

ELBOW DISLOCATIONS

Posterior or posterolateral dislocation of the elbow is seen following a fall onto the outstretched arm, sometimes associated with a fracture to the olecranon or coronoid process. This is common when falling from a horse or bicycle, and from gymnastic accidents. Roller-skating and skateboarding are also prime causes, as the athlete usually falls backwards onto an abducted straight arm. There is often a snap or crack at the time of injury with immediate swelling. On

examination, the arm is held flexed, and a gross deformity is apparent on the posterior aspect of the elbow. The normal triangular alignment of the olecranon and two epicondyles is lost (Fig. 19.12). Radiographic examination is required to assess bony damage, and on no account should reduction on the field be attempted because of the risk of neural complications. Reduction is achieved by downward pressure on the forearm initially to disengage the coronoid from the olecranon fossa and then the forearm is brought forwards. As with the shoulder, reduction, unless immediate, will usually require analgesia. Operative intervention has often been recommended where reduction is unstable due to ligament avulsion. However, Josefsson et al. (1987) compared the results of patients treated by primary surgical repair to those treated by closed reduction. Although the surgery group included those with complete collateral ligament ruptures or avulsions (all patients) and muscle origin tears from the humeral epicondyles (half the patients), the results from the two groups were the same.

If the arm is immobilized for more than a week, the resting position should be in as much extension as possible (Garrick and Webb, 1990). This is important because reduced flexion is far easier to regain during rehabilitation than is extension. With an uncomplicated injury, gentle isometric exercise is begun as pain and swelling settles. After 2–3 days, active mobility exercise is started with caution in the pain-free range, the athlete remaining in a sling between exercise periods for protection.

Early mobilization of this injury is essential. Mehlhoff et al. (1988) described 52 adults with elbow dislocation. Those immobilized for less than 18 days showed significantly better results than those inactive for longer periods, and patients immobilized for more than 4 weeks all showed only fair or poor results. None of the patients redislocated.

Following this injury, there is normally a slight loss of extension. If the elbow has previously hyperextended, this is not usually a problem. However, where the arm remains slightly flexed, weight-bearing activities, such as handstands and cartwheels, will tend to push the arm into flexion. To

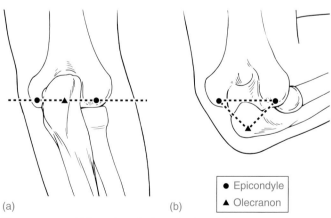

(a) (b)

● Epicondyle
▲ Olecranon

Figure 19.12 Triangular relation of epicondyles and olecranon with elbow flexion.

stabilize the arm and obtain some degree of functional locking, the triceps must be built up extensively.

RADIAL HEAD

Compression fracture of the radial head may occur with a vertical fall onto the outstretched arm, but more commonly the injury which affects the radial head is a dislocation. This is usually seen in children, where the radial head is pulled through the annular ligament, limiting extension. The peak incidence of injury occurs between the ages of 2 and 3 years, this being the age when the annular ligament is thinner and more easily disrupted. The injury is twice as common in girls as in boys (Quan and Marcuse, 1985), and the left elbow is affected more often than the right (Corrigan and Maitland, 1994). The mechanism of injury is a sudden traction applied to an extended and pronated arm as an adult lifts the child while gripping the child's hand.

Reduction, if carried out before muscle spasm sets in, may be performed by holding the elbow flexed to 90° and lightly rotating the forearm. The therapist holds the child's elbow in his or her cupped hand and places the thumb over the radial head. The other hand holds the child's hand, and the manipulation is produced with a high velocity supination of the patient's forearm while maintaining thumb pressure over the radial head. At the same time, the radius and humerus are gently pulled together and the radial head is felt to click back beneath the annular ligament on full supination. Often this condition reduces spontaneously.

NERVE INVOLVEMENT

Ulnar nerve

The ulnar nerve may be involved with medial collateral ligament injuries of the elbow, as outlined above. Friction against this nerve or its sheath may give rise to symptoms, described by Wadsworth and Williams (1973) as the 'cubital tunnel syndrome'. Since the sensory fibres of the ulnar nerve are more superficial than the motor fibres, sensory symptoms are more prevalent, with paraesthesia occurring in the fourth and fifth fingers.

The nerve passes through the groove behind the medial epicondyle and is covered by a fibrous sheath, forming the cubital tunnel (Fig. 19.13a). The roof of the tunnel is the aponeurosis of the two heads of flexor carpi ulnaris. This is taut at 90° flexion, constricting the tunnel, and slack on extension. The floor of the cubital tunnel is formed from the tip of the trochlea and the medial collateral ligament. The ligament bulges with elbow flexion, an additional factor leading to nerve compression, especially with prolonged periods of end-range flexion.

Definition
Cubital tunnel syndrome occurs when there is friction of the ulnar nerve or its sheath. Altered sensation and tingling (paraesthesia) occurs in the 4th and 5th fingers.

Dislocation of the nerve from the ulnar groove can also occur following fracture and is accompanied by a persistent tingling sensation with certain elbow actions. If motor symptoms are present, wasting may be seen in the hypothenar eminence and the first dorsal interosseous space. Tinel's sign (see p. 431) and the elbow flexion test may be positive. This latter test involves maximal flexion of the elbow for 5 minutes to compress the cubital tunnel. Symptoms produced, including pain, altered sensation and numbness, constitute a positive test.

Management depends very much on the severity of the symptoms. Often rest and elbow padding to avoid irritation

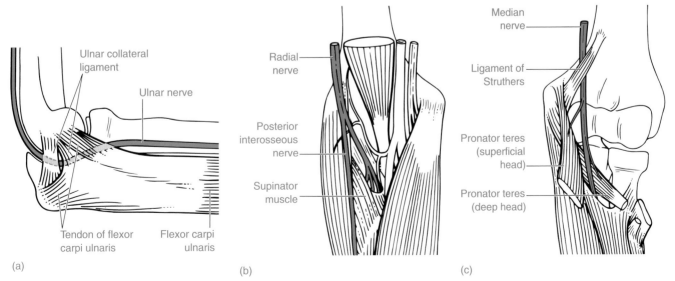

Figure 19.13 Nerve compression in the elbow. (a) Ulnar nerve, cubital tunnel. (b) Radial nerve, arcade of Frohse. (c) Median nerve, pronator teres.

in contact sports may be all that is required for frictional neuritis. Corticosteroid injection along the cubital tunnel may be useful (Corrigan and Maitland, 1994). Surgery, if performed early, can be successful. Nerve transposition combined with excision of a portion of the medial epicondyle and division of the tendinous origin of the flexor carpi ulnaris has been described (Hirsch and Thanki, 1985).

Radial nerve

The radial nerve can be injured in the elbow region. The nerve travels in front of the lateral condyle of the humerus to divide into deep (posterior interosseous) and superficial branches. The superficial branch may be exposed to direct trauma, sometimes being damaged as a complication of fractures to the radial head or neck.

Radial tunnel syndrome (Roles and Maudsley, 1972) occurs when the deep branch of the radial nerve is compressed as it passes under the origin of the extensor carpi radialis brevis and along the fibrous edge of the supinator muscle (arcade of Frohse, Fig. 19.13b). Pain is produced when the arm is fully pronated with the wrist flexed.

Differential diagnosis of radial tunnel syndrome is made by eliciting pain by palpation of the radial head, and pain on resisted supination. True tennis elbow will give pain over the lateral epicondyle (not the radial head), with pain on resisted wrist extension but not supination alone (Lee, 1986). The condition is seen following repeated contraction of the wrist extensors and forearm supinators against resistance, as in racquet sports in a novice sportsperson (Cailliet, 1983).

Treatment by local injection and surgery have both been described (Moss and Switzer, 1983).

Median nerve

In general usage, the medial nerve is most commonly injured by laceration at the wrist, giving an inability to abduct the thumb, a classic 'pointing (index) finger' and sensory loss over the radial 3½ digits. In sport, however, medial nerve compression may occur, although it is unusual. At the elbow, the median nerve passes beneath the ligament of Struthers. This is an anomaly found in about 1% of the general population running from a bony spur on the shaft of the humerus to the medial epicondyle (Fig. 19.13c). Symptoms are generally sensory, with paraesthesia in the forearm and hand. If left, motor symptoms affecting the thumb and forefinger may also occur. Lower down the forearm the medial nerve passes between the two heads of pronator teres, and it may be compressed here. Resisted pronation may be weak, more noticeably if the movement is maintained for 30–60 seconds, and sensory symptoms may be seen as before. The condition usually responds to an alteration in training, but surgical release may be required.

TESTING THE ELBOW FOLLOWING INJURY

A sportsperson must be able to perform actions relevant to his or her sport and to his or her competitive role within that sport (Wright, 1981). Maximal functional work of the biceps may be performed by the subject chinning a bar, and for the triceps dipping between two chairs or performing a push-up with the feet on a chair; both of these actions should be slow and controlled until confidence is built. Faster, more demanding actions include press-ups with a clap in between each repetition, and walking hand to hand while hanging at arm's length from a horizontal ladder.

Racquet sportspeople should mimic their stroke action with a weighted racquet or heavy club, and can assess their resilience to jarring strains by hitting a club or bat against a firm surface (a medicine ball is ideal). The elbow must be able to take repeated traction and approximation strains, and be pain-free when the arm is locked while holding a weight at arm's length.

References

Bach, B.R., Warren, R.F. and Wickiewicz, T.L. (1987) Triceps rupture: a case report and literature review. *American Journal of Sports Medicine*, **15**, (3) 285–289

Bernhang, A.M. (1979) The many causes of tennis elbow. *New York State Journal of Medicine*, **79**, (9) 1363–1366

Briggs, C.A. and Elliott, B.G. (1985) Lateral epicondylitis: a review of structures associated with tennis elbow. *Anatomia Clinica*, **7**, 149

Bullard, J.A.A. (1982) Tennis elbow. *Canadian Family Physician*, **28**, 961–963

Burton, A.K. (1985) Grip strength and forearm straps in tennis elbow. *British Journal of Sports Medicine*, **19**, 37–38

Cailliet, R. (1983) *Soft Tissue Pain and Disability*, F.A. Davis, Philadelphia

Coorad, R.W. and Hooper, W.R. (1973) Tennis elbow: course, natural history, conservative and surgical management. *Journal of Bone and Joint Surgery*, **55A**, 1177

Corrigan, B. and Maitland, G.D. (1994) *Musculoskeletal and Sports Injuries*, Butterworth-Heinemann, Oxford

Cyriax, J. (1936) Pathology and treatment of tennis elbow. *Journal of Bone and Joint Surgery*, **18A**, 921

Cyriax, J.H. and Cyriax, P.J. (1983) *Illustrated Manual of Orthopaedic Medicine*, Butterworth, London

Dreyfuss, U. and Kessler, I. (1978) Snapping elbow due to dislocation of the medial head of triceps. *Journal of Bone and Joint Surgery*, **60B**, 56

Fink, M., Wolkenstein, E., Karst, M. and Gehrke, A. (2002) Acupuncture in chronic epicondylitis. *Rheumatology*, **41**, (2) 205–209

Garrick, J.G. and Webb, D.R. (1990) *Sports Injuries: Diagnosis and Management*, W.B. Saunders, Philadelphia

Goldie, I. (1964) Epicondylitis lateralis humeri: a pathological study. *Acta Chirugica Scandinavica* (Suppl.), **34**, 339

Griffen, J.E. and Touchstone, J.C. (1963) Ultrasonic movement of cortisol into pig tissues. (I). Movement into skeletal muscle. *American Journal of Physical Medicine*, **43**, 77

Groppel, J.L. and Nirschl, R.P. (1986) A mechanical and electromyographical analysis of the effects of various joint counterforce braces on the tennis player. *American Journal of Sports Medicine*, **14**, 195–200

Halle, J.S., Franklin, R.J. and Karalfa, B.L. (1986) Comparison of four treatment approaches for lateral epicondylitis of the elbow. *Journal of Orthopaedic and Sports Physical Therapy*, **8**, (2) 62–69

Hirsch, L.F. and Thanki, A. (1985) Ulnar nerve entrapment at the elbow: tailoring the treatment to the cause. *Postgraduate Medicine*, **77**, 211–215

Hulkko, A., Orava, S. and Nikula, P. (1968) Stress fractures of the olecranon in javelin throwers. *International Journal of Sports Medicine*, **7**, 210

Jobe, F.W. and Nuber, G. (1986) Throwing injuries of the elbow. *Sports Medicine*, **5**, (4) 621–635

Josefsson, P.O., Gentz, C., Johnell, O. and Wendeberg, B. (1987) Surgical versus non-surgical treatment of ligamentous injuries following dislocation of the elbow joint: a prospective randomized study. *Journal of Bone and Joint Surgery*, **69A**, 605–608

Kleinkort, J.B. and Wood, F. (1975) Phonophoresis with 1% versus 10% hydrocortisone. *Physical Therapy*, **55**, 1320

Kuroda, S. and Sakamaki, K. (1986) Ulnar collateral ligament tears of the elbow joint. *Clinical Orthopaedics and Related Research*, **208**, 266–271

Leach, R.E. and Miller, J.K. (1987) Lateral and medial epicondylitis of the elbow. *Clinics in Sports Medicine*, **6**, (2) 259–272

Lee, D.G. (1986) Tennis elbow: a manual therapist's perspective. *Journal of Orthopaedic and Sports Physical Therapy*, **12**, (2) 81–87

Mann, F (1992) *Reinventing Acupuncture*, Butterworth Heinemann, Oxford

Mehlhoff, T.L., Noble, P.C., Bennett, J.B. and Tullos, H.S. (1988) Simple dislocation of the elbow in the adult: results after closed treatment. *Journal of Bone and Joint Surgery*, **70A**, 244–249

Mills, G.P. (1928) Treatment of tennis elbow. *British Medical Journal*, **1**, (12)

Molsberger, A., and Hille, E. (1994) The analgesic effect of acupuncture in chronic tennis elbow pain. *British Journal of Rheumatology*, **33**, (12) 1162–1165

Morrey, B.F. and Kai-Nan, A. (1983) Articular and ligamentous contributions to the stability of the elbow joint. *American Journal of Sports Medicine*, **11**, 315–318

Moss, S.H. and Switzer, H.E. (1983) Radial tunnel syndrome: a spectrum of clinical presentations. *Journal of Hand Surgery*, **8**, 414–420

Mulligan, B.R. (1989) *Manual Therapy*, Plane View Services, Wellington, New Zealand

Nirschl, R.P. (1986) Soft tissue injuries about the elbow. *Clinics in Sports Medicine*, **5**, (4) 637–652

Nirschl, R.P. (1988) Prevention and treatment of elbow and shoulder injuries in the tennis player. *Clinics in Sports Medicine*, **7**, (2) 289–309

Norkin, C.C. and Levangie, P.K. (1992) *Joint Structure and Function: A Comprehensive Analysis*, 2nd edn, F.A. Davis, Philadelphia

Nuber, G.W. and Diment, M.T. (1992) Olecranon stress fractures in throwers: a report of two cases and a review of the literature. *Clinical Orthopaedics and Related Research*, **278**, 58–61

Palastanga, N., Field, D. and Soames, R. (1989) *Anatomy and Human Movement*, Heinemann Medical, Oxford

Quan, L. and Marcuse, E.K. (1985) The epidemiology and treatment of radial head subluxation. *American Journal of Diseases of Children*, **139**, 1194–1197

Reid, D.C. (1992) *Sports Injury Assessment and Rehabilitation*, Churchill Livingstone, Edinburgh

Roles, N.C. and Maudsley, R.H. (1972) Radial tunnel syndrome: resistant tennis elbow as a nerve entrapment. *Journal of Bone and Joint Surgery*, **54B**, 499–508

Torg, J.S. (1993) Comment. *Yearbook of Sports Medicine*, C.V. Mosby, St Louis, p. 72

Vicenzino, B. and Wright, A. (1995) Effects of a novel manipulative physiotherapy technique on tennis elbow: a single case study. *Manual Therapy*, **1**, 30–35

Wadsworth, C.T., Nielsen, D.H., Burns, L.T., Krull, J.D. and Thompson, C.G. (1989) Effect of the counterforce armband on wrist extension and grip strength and pain in subjects with tennis elbow. *Journal of Orthopaedic and Sports Physical Therapy*, **11**, 192–197

Wadsworth, T.G. and Williams, J.R. (1973) Cubital tunnel external compression syndrome. *British Medical Journal*, **1**, 662

Wright, D. (1981) Fitness testing after injury. In *Sports Fitness and Sports Injuries* (ed. T. Reilly), Faber and Faber, London

Chapter 20

The wrist and hand

The wrist area has a series of articulations between the distal end of the radius and the carpal bones (radiocarpal joint), and between the individual carpals themselves (intercarpal joints). The radiocarpal joint is formed between the distal end of the radius and the scaphoid, lunate and triquetral. The end of the radius being covered by a concave articular disc. The eight carpal bones are arranged in two rows, the junction between the rows forming the mid-carpal joint. This joint is convex laterally and concave medially, giving it an 'S' shape (Fig. 20.1).

Definition

The *radiocarpal* joint is formed between the ends of the forearm bones (radius and ulna) and the wrist bones (carpals). The *mid-carpal* joint is between the two rows of carpal bones themselves.

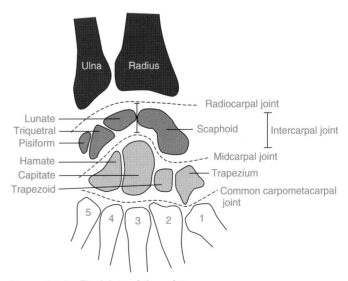

Figure 20.1 The joints of the wrist.

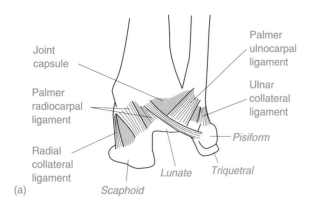

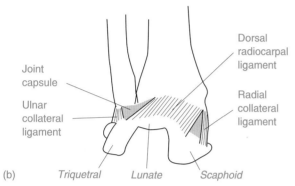

Figure 20.2 The capsular and collateral ligaments of the radiocarpal joint. (a) Anterior. (b) Posterior. After Palastanga, Field and Soames (1994) with permission.

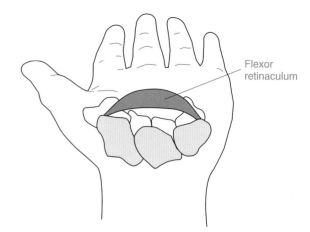

Figure 20.3 Transverse arch of the wrist.

through which runs the tendon of flexor carpi radialis. The space formed beneath the retinaculum is called the 'carpal tunnel', and the tendons of flexor pollicis longus, flexor digitorum profundus, flexor digitorum superficialis and the median nerve pass through it.

On the posterior aspect of the wrist the extensor retinaculum stretches from the radius to the hamate and pisiform bones and extends inferiorly to form six longitudinal compartments for the passage of the extensor tendons.

GRIP

Prehension is an advanced skill in humans, resulting largely from the ability of the thumb to oppose the fingers. Two types of grip may be described, 'precision' involving the thumb and fingers and 'power', involving the whole hand.

With precision grip, the object is usually small and light. The grip is applied with the nails or fingertips (terminal opposition), pads of the fingers (subterminal opposition), or the pad and side of another finger (subterminal-lateral opposition). This action involves rotation of both the carpometacarpal joints of the thumb and fingers involved in the gripping action. The small finger muscles work in combination with the flexor digitorum profundus and superficialis as well as the flexor pollicis longus.

In power grips the long flexors and extensors work to lock the wrist and grip the object. In the palmar grip, the whole hand surrounds the object, and the thumb works against the fingers. The shape taken up by the hand is largely determined by the size of the object, but the grip is strongest when the thumb can still touch the index finger. This is the type of grip used when holding a racquet or javelin. When the fingers are closed firmly, the fourth and fifth metacarpals move over the hamate bone to further tighten the grip and prevent a smooth object from slipping out of the hand. The hook grip is used when lifting something with a handle, such as a suitcase. Now, the object is held between the flexed fingers and palm, the thumb not

The wrist is strengthened by collateral, palmar and dorsal ligaments. The ulnar collateral ligament is a rounded cord stretching from the ulnar styloid to the triquetral and pisiform. The radial collateral ligament passes from the radial styloid to the scaphoid and then to the trapezium. The dorsal radiocarpal ligament runs from the lower aspect of the radius to the scaphoid, lunate and triquetral. On the palmar surface, the radiocarpal and ulnocarpal ligaments attach from the lower ends of the radius and ulna to the proximal carpal bones (Fig. 20.2).

The available range of movement at the wrist is a combination of radiocarpal and mid-carpal movement. Flexion occurs more at the mid-carpal joint, while extension is greater at the radiocarpal joint, but the combined movement is about 85° in each direction. Abduction occurs mostly at the mid-carpal joint and has a range of about 15°, whereas adduction involves more movement of the radiocarpal joint and has a range of 45° (Palastanga, Field and Soames, 1989). The difference in range occurs because the radial styloid comes down further than the ulnar styloid, and so is more limiting to abduction.

The carpal bones form a transverse arch, concave on their palmar aspect (Fig. 20.3). This arch is maintained by the flexor retinaculum, which attaches medially to the pisiform and the hook of hamate. Laterally, the retinaculum binds to the scaphoid tubercle and to the groove of trapezium, being used. Although the grip is quite powerful, the power is in one direction only.

SCREENING EXAMINATION

Initial examination of the wrist utilizes a number of movements to cover all the joints involved in wrist articulation. The superior and inferior radioulnar joints are stressed by passive pronation and supination. The wrist itself is assessed by flexion, extension, abduction and adduction performed both passively and against resistance.

> **Keypoint**
>
> When the wrist is examined, the superior and inferior radioulnar joints should also be assessed, using passive pronation and supination of the forearm.

At the same time as the wrist is examined, the fingers are also assessed as the two areas are intimately linked. Passive and resisted movements are performed at the thumb and finger joints. Again, flexion, extension, abduction and adduction are used. The capsular pattern for the wrist joint is an equal limitation to passive flexion and extension. Painful resisted movement at the wrist indicates that the lesion is not local, but higher up in the muscle bellies, whereas pain to resisted finger movements may give local pain. In addition to pain, crepitus to active movements is an important sign for the long finger tendons.

This examination, described by Cyriax (1982), provides the examiner with enough information to establish whether a lesion is intracapsular or not, and whether contractile tissue is affected. For the physiotherapist, further assessment is usually required to assess and record range of motion and accessory movements. Movements of the individual carpal bones gives more detail about the exact site of the lesion, and the sequence for testing is shown in Table 20.1. In addition, specific tests are used once the initial examination has focused the therapist's attention onto a specific area or series of tissues.

SCAPHOID FRACTURE

The important feature of this fracture is not the frequency with which it occurs, but the number of times it is missed, with pain so often being put down to 'just a sprain'. The usual history is of a fall onto the outstretched arm with the wrist fully extended. When the hand is locked into extension, the athlete is more likely to sustain a scaphoid fracture; this can occur with a vertical fall from gymnastic apparatus for example. When the hand is more relaxed and the force has some horizontal component, as with a fall when running, the distal radius will usually break (Colles' fracture). The scaphoid fracture is common in the young athlete while the Colles' fracture is seen more frequently in the elderly.

Table 20.1   Assessing motion of individual carpal joints

Movements around the capitate
Fixate capitate and move
   1. trapezoid
   2. scaphoid
   3. lunate
Fixate capitate and move
   4. hamate
Movements on the radial side
Fixate scaphoid and move
   5. the two trapezii
Movements of the radiocarpal joint
Fixate radius and move
   6. scaphoid
   7. lunate
Fixate ulna (including the disc) and move
   8. triquetrum (triquetral)
Movements on the ulnar side
Fixate triquetrum and move
   9. hamate
   10. pisiform (position the patient's hand in palmar flexion)

From Kaltenborn, F.M. (1993) *The Spine. Basic Examination and Mobilisation Techniques*, 2nd edn. Olaf Norlis Bokhandel, Oslo, Norway. With permission.

This is partially due to the weakness of the radius with the onset of osteoporosis in the aged.

> **Keypoint**
>
> With a fall onto the outstretched hand, if the wrist is locked a *scaphoid* fracture is common. Where the wrist is more relaxed and some sliding force is present (fall onto the outstretched hand when running) the *distal radius* will more commonly break.

A further cause of injury to the scaphoid is striking an object with the heel of the hand, a mechanism seen in contact sports such as the martial arts or in a collision with another player. In addition, scaphoid fracture can be seen as a punching injury. Horii et al. (1994) described a series of 125 patients with fractured scaphoid, 14% of whom had acquired the injury through punching. Normally it is a bending force within the scaphoid which creates the fracture line when falling onto the outstretched hand. With a punching scaphoid fracture, however, stress force creates the fracture, making displacement and delayed union more likely.

Examination

The major symptom of scaphoid fracture is one of well-localized pain to the base of the thumb, within the 'anatomical snuffbox'. The athlete's hand is pronated and gently stressed into ulnar deviation to make the scaphoid more superficial, as the snuffbox is palpated. Palpation of the scaphoid tuberosity with radial deviation of the wrist may also be painful. In addition, pain is exacerbated by axial (longitudinal) compression of the first metacarpal against the scaphoid by pressing the thumb proximally.

> **Keypoint**
>
> With a fracture of the scaphoid bone there is pain at the base of the thumb within the 'anatomical snuffbox'. Pain is exacerbated by shunting the thumb into itself (longitudinal compression).

Radiographic examination is helpful, but a negative X-ray does not rule out fracture (Garrick and Webb, 1990). Non-displaced fractures are often normal to begin with and only become positive when some bone reabsorption has occurred, the fracture line beginning to show up 2–4 weeks after injury. Plain AP (anteroposterior) views of the wrist may easily miss a scaphoid fracture (Fig. 20.4a), while a specialist scaphoid view which focuses on the bone itself is more reliable (Fig. 20.4b).

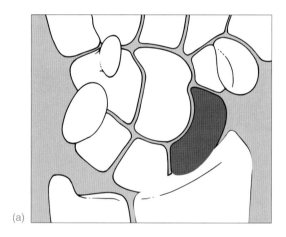

(a)

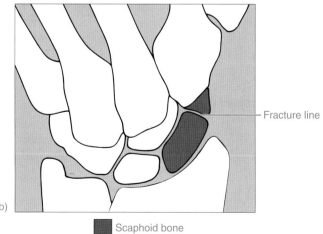

(b)

Fracture line

■ Scaphoid bone

Figure 20.4   The wrist showing the scaphoid bone. (a) Anteroposterior view. (b) Scaphoid view.

The scaphoid is 'nut-shaped' with a narrow waist and two poles (proximal and distal). On the palmar surface of the distal pole there is a tubercle for the attachment of the flexor retinaculum and the tendon of abductor pollicis brevis. The blood supply to the scaphoid enters through the waist (centre) of the bone (Fig. 20.5). Smaller arteries enter from the distal pole and retrograde flow from these supplies the proximal pole, this pole having no separate blood supply itself. This has an important clinical bearing, because fractures to the waist of the bone can sever the communicating vessels, starving the proximal segment of blood (Gutierrez, 1996). This situation makes non-union or malunion more likely.

Classification of injury is important as fractures occurring more proximally tend towards avascular necrosis. In addition, fracture orientation should be noted (see Fig. 20.5) as this will influence stability. Horizontal oblique fractures are generally stable, whereas transverse fractures are inherently unstable.

Management

Scaphoid fracture requires prolonged immobilization of the wrist and thumb. The cast usually extends to the interphalangeal (IP) joint of the thumb to just below the elbow. In some cases an above elbow splint is used to limit pronation and supination. Uncomplicated fractures of the scaphoid tubercle may heal in as little as 4 weeks, but fracture to the proximal part of the bone may take as much as 20 weeks.

Complications to scaphoid fracture have a poor prognosis. Avascular necrosis may require excision of the avascular fragment, or prosthetic replacement of the whole bone. Non-union usually demands bone graft or screw fixation,

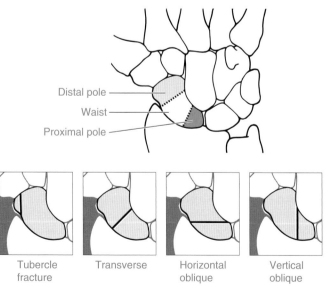

Distal pole
Waist
Proximal pole

| Tubercle fracture | Transverse | Horizontal oblique | Vertical oblique |

Figure 20.5   Classification of scaphoid fracture. From Gutierrez, G. (1996) Office management of scaphoid fractures. *Physician and Sportsmedicine*, 24(8), 1–8. With permission.

but the failure rate can be high. Successful union has, however, been shown in 90% of patients treated with a Herbert differential pitch screw (which is completely buried in the bone) combined with bone grafting (Bunker, McNamee and Scott, 1987). This type of fixation significantly reduces the time to return to active sport. With fixation, return in some athletes is immediate, but on average 4.3 weeks. Athletes treated non-operatively with a playing cast return on average in 11 weeks (Rettig, Weidenbener and Gloyeske, 1994).

Rehabilitation

Immobilization of the wrist can lead to gross movement loss. It is important therefore that athletes perform range of motion exercise of the shoulder and elbow while the cast is still on. Once the cast has been removed, wrist mobilization is essential to regain flexion/extension, abduction/adduction, and pronation/supination. In addition individual carpal joint mobilization will also be required, moving the whole lateral side of the wrist and hand, but particularly focusing on the thumb. Re-strengthening grip and both approximation (push-up) and traction (pull-up on bar) are important if wrist function for sport is not to be limited.

WRIST PAIN

Sprains

A 'sprained wrist' is a common diagnosis, but really only indicates the area of pain, and the fact than soft tissue is the likely structure affected. The most common tissues affected are the intercarpal ligaments, with or without subluxation of a carpal bone. Pain is reproduced to passive wrist flexion and is generally well-localized to the particular tissue injured. Common ligaments affected include the lunate-capitate (Cyriax, 1982) and scapho-lunate (Wilkes, 1989). Transverse frictions to the ligament with the wrist flexed are effective, but manipulation to rupture adhesive scarring is not (Cyriax, 1982).

Sprain to the ulnar or radial collateral ligaments is rare, but if present gives pain to end-range passive abduction and adduction.

Carpal dislocation

Subluxation or dislocation of a carpal bone, rather than a scaphoid fracture, may occur from a fall onto the outstretched hand. The bone most commonly affected is the lunate, although the capitate may also sublux (Cyriax and Cyriax, 1983). Movement is generally limited in one direction only (contrast the capsular pattern). Pain is localized by palpating in a line along the third finger to reach the third metacarpal. In the normal hand the capitate lies in a hollow just proximal to the base of the third metacarpal and the lunate is felt proximal to this, and slightly towards the ulna.

Keypoint

When palpating the dorsum of the wrist the *capitate* bone lies in a hollow just proximal to the base of the third (centre) metacarpal and the *lunate* is felt proximal to this, and slightly towards the ulna (see Fig. 20.1).

When the capitate subluxes, the wrist is held in flexion, and a prominent bump is seen over the dorsum of the wrist as the capitate stands proud of its neighbours. Reduction of a minor subluxation is often spontaneous, but if not, may be achieved during traction by a repeated anterior and posterior glide, with the wrist positioned over the edge of the treatment couch. The wrist is immobilized in a splint until the acute pain subsides, when rehabilitation is begun.

Full dislocation of the lunate may occur with a fall onto the extended wrist. The shape and position of the lunate lying between the lower radius and capitate make it prone to dislocation. On forced wrist extension, the wedge-shaped lunate is squeezed out from between the two bones to lie on the palmar surface of the carpal region (Fig. 20.6) as an apparent 'swelling'. If the athlete is asked to form a fist, the third metacarpal head should normally project above the second and fourth. Where the lunate has dislocated, however, all three metacarpal heads may appear in line (Magee, 2002).

During lunate dislocation, the scaphoid-lunate ligament usually ruptures and the lunate rotates. Radiographs taken with the forearm fully supinated show a separation of the scaphoid-lunate joint of more than 2 mm (Corrigan and Maitland, 1983). The dislocated lunate may impinge on the median nerve, and the flexor tendons may be compressed within the carpal tunnel.

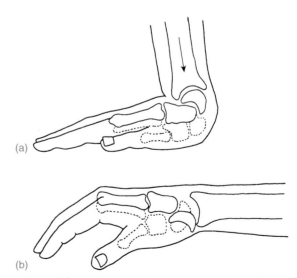

(a)

(b)

Figure 20.6 (a) Lunate dislocation injury occurs when the radius forces the lunate in a palmar direction, (b) resulting in dislocation. From Hertling, D. and Kessler, R.M. (1990) *Management of Common Musculoskeletal Disorders.* J.B. Lippincott, Philadelphia. With permission.

Reduction under anaesthesia is possible if the condition is diagnosed early, with the wrist being immobilized in some degree of flexion initially, and then protected from forced extension when sport is resumed. If left, damage to the median nerve is more likely and open reduction is usually required.

Occasionally, the lunate may stay in place against the radius, and the carpal bones surrounding it dislocate posteriorly to give a perilunar dislocation. This normally occurs in association with a scaphoid fracture, part of the fractured bone remaining with the radius and lunate (O'Donoghue, 1976; Williams and Sperryn, 1976).

WRIST PAIN IN GYMNASTS

Repetitive forced extension causes compression and impaction forces on the wrist. This type of movement is common in gymnastics, and in exercises such as the 'press-up with clap'. In addition, heavy bench press exercises used in training or powerlifting force extension at the wrist. When this occurs, the athlete may experience pain over the dorsum of the wrist, and end-range flexion and extension are painfully limited. The main fault initially may be an impingement of the dorsal wrist structures, resulting in capsular inflammation (Aronen, 1985). If impact forces continue, however, carpal subluxation or fracture may occur in the adult, and epiphyseal damage in the adolescent.

Keypoint

Repetitive forced extension (gymnastics, push-ups, rapid bench press) may cause impingement, inflammation, carpal bone subluxation, and, in children, growth plate injury.

The distal end of the ulna has a fibrocartilage disc which separates it from the lunate. The disc prevents ulnocarpal abutment by cushioning forces between the ulna and lunate. Trauma may cause thinning of the articular disc, and a reduction in shock-absorbing capacity. Cadaver studies have shown that the radius takes 60% of axial loading to the wrist when the articular disc is intact, but this is increased to 95% when the disc is excised (Palmer and Werner, 1981).

Forced extension is of particular concern in the child. Normally, closure of the distal ulnar growth plate should precede that of the radius. However, the structure and function of the distal radial growth plate can be altered by repetitive loading from gymnastics or other sports, and may fuse prematurely giving radial shortening with respect to the normal ulna (Albanese et al., 1989). On posterior-anterior radiographs, the position of the ulna may be compared to that of the radius. If the ulnar is longer, positive ulnar variance exists, if shorter, negative variance is present. As the radial growth plate closes after that of the ulna, negative ulnar variance is the norm. However, gymnasts have been shown to have significant positive ulnar variance when compared to controls (Mandelbaum et al., 1989).

With positive variance, in addition to bone changes, the articular disc between the ulna and lunate may be thinner, and less stable. The combination of reduced shock absorption and stability may lead to a chronic degenerative condition.

In the adolescent, rest from activities involving extension and loading of the wrist is essential. Carter et al. (1988) have demonstrated significant healing of this condition within 3 months following cessation of gymnastics.

KIENBOCK'S DISEASE

This is an aseptic necrosis (osteochondritis) of the lunate. The condition may result from direct trauma, such as a compression fracture (Cetti, Christensen and Reuther, 1982), or following repeated microtrauma from impact stresses. Industrial stresses, such as hammering, and impact forces in sports, such as tennis, karate, volleyball and golf, have been identified as factors (Nakamura et al., 1991). Although the progress of the condition is similar in both sporting and non-sporting populations, athletes develop symptoms more quickly.

The condition is seen from adolescence up to the mid-30s. The lunate atrophies, becomes sclerosed, and later decalcifies, showing flattening and fragmentation on X-ray. The main symptom is wrist pain, with range of motion and grip strength reducing.

Marked deformity of the bone occurs, unless the condition is identified early enough, when pressure on the wrist during sport should be eliminated. If the condition is too advanced to respond to conservative management, surgery is required. As the patients are young, and remodelling of the lunate can be expected, osteotomy is frequently performed rather than carpectomy (Nakamura et al., 1991).

WRIST MOBILIZATION

Mobilization of the various joints of the wrist is useful both for pain reduction and movement enhancement. The inferior radioulnar joint is mobilized by gripping the lower ends of the radius and ulna and working the hands forwards and backwards against each other (Fig. 20.7a). The radiocarpal joint may be mobilized by gripping the athlete's wrist in one hand and hand in the other. The edge of the therapist's hands are aligned with the radiocarpal joint line. Again, the hands are worked against each other to perform transverse mobilizations and anteroposterior movements. Greater purchase may be gained by supporting the athlete's forearm on a low block or on the couch edge (Fig. 20.7b). Pronation and supination at the radiocarpal joint is performed using a 'wringing' action (Fig. 20.7c), and intercarpal

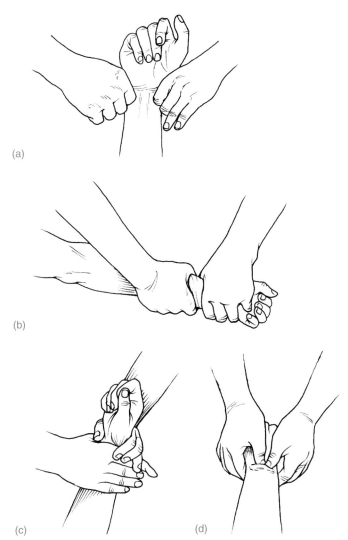

(a)

(b)

(c) (d)

Figure 20.7 Examples of wrist mobilization. From Corrigan and Maitland (1983), with permission.

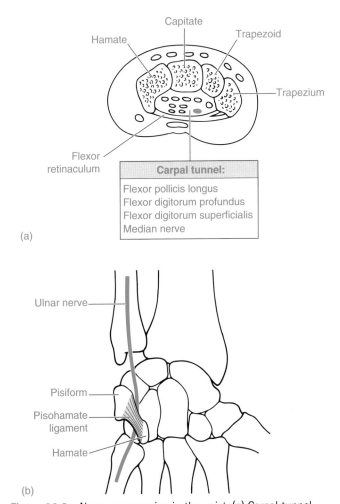

(a)

Carpal tunnel:

Flexor pollicis longus
Flexor digitorum profundus
Flexor digitorum superficialis
Median nerve

(b)

Figure 20.8 Nerve compression in the wrist. (a) Carpal tunnel, (b) Guyon's canal.

movements (see Table 20.1) are performed using the thumb pads (Fig. 20.7d).

COMPRESSION NEUROPATHIES

Carpal tunnel syndrome

Carpal tunnel syndrome is a compression neuropathy of the median nerve as it passes beneath the flexor retinaculum and into the carpal tunnel (Fig. 20.8a). It is more common in women than men, and occurs typically later in life (40–60 years), although it is seen in younger individuals secondary to trauma. Paraesthesia (numbness, burning, tingling) is felt over the first three fingers and the radial half of the fourth. Pain is made worse with repeated movements, and prolonged (1 minute) wrist flexion can reproduce the symptoms (*Phalen's test*). Percussion of the medial nerve (*Tinel's sign*) within the centre of the carpal tunnel with the wrist extended may also be positive.

Keypoint

With carpal tunnel syndrome, numbness, burning and/or tingling are produced with prolonged wrist flexion (Phalen's test) and tapping over the middle of the wrist (Tinel's sign).

A number of factors may contribute to the condition, and these generally fall into one of two categories. First, factors which increase the size of the structures within the carpal tunnel. This could be through swelling of the flexor tendon sheaths (tenosynovitis) as a result of repeated or sustained flexor activity (gymnasts, cyclists, weightlifters). Secondly, factors which reduce the size of the carpal tunnel itself, such as arthritic changes secondary to a Colles' fracture, fluid retention during pregnancy and obesity. The condition must be differentiated from vascular insufficiency which usually gives a glove-like distribution of symptoms, and entrapment of the C6/C7 nerve root, which does not give increased pain to repeated wrist movements.

Management of the condition is initially to rest the wrist in a splint (day and night), as in the neutral position there is less pressure within the carpal tunnel (Hertling and Kessler, 1990). In addition, the flexor retinaculum may be stretched by separating the pisiform and hamate from the trapezium and scaphoid (Maitland, 1991). It is interesting to note that vitamin B_6 may facilitate healing in this condition (Diamond, 1989).

Ulnar nerve compression

Ulnar nerve compression (cyclist's palsy) is an unusual condition. The ulnar nerve passes into the hand through Guyon's canal, a shallow trough formed between the pisiform and the hook of hamate, running beneath the pisohamate ligament (Fig. 20.8b). During cycling, the nerve is stretched by hyperextension and ulnar deviation of the wrist. Stresses taken by the hand in cycling can be greater than the athlete's bodyweight (Haloua, Collin and Coudeyre, 1987), and altered conduction velocity of the distal ulnar nerve has been shown in long-distance cyclists (Wilmarth and Nelson, 1988).

Motor and sensory symptoms may be caused, affecting the fourth and fifth fingers. Weakness and clumsiness of fine finger movements may be seen with a reduction in pinch grip strength. The latter is tested by asking the athlete to pinch a piece of paper between the thumb and radial side of the second finger.

Initial management is by ensuring a correct cycle frame size to prevent the athlete overstretching. Extra padding on the handlebars or in cycling gloves will reduce compression stress, but if symptoms persist, the athlete should refrain from cycling for as long as 4 months to allow recovery of motor function.

> **Keypoint**
>
> Cylist's palsy is: (i) a compression neuropathy of the ulnar nerve as it passes through the wrist and into the hand; (ii) brought on by prolonged hyperextension and ulnar deviation of the wrist; (iii) fine finger movements are eroded, and there is a loss of pinch grip power between the thumb and index finger.

THUMB

Ulnar collateral ligament rupture

Injury to the ulnar collateral ligament (UCL) of the metacarpophalangeal (MCP) joint of the thumb is common in any sport where the thumb is forced into excessive abduction. This may occur in alpine skiing, where the strap of the ski pole pulls the thumb. It has been estimated that around 10% of all alpine skiing injuries involve this ligament, giving a total of between 50000 and 200000 injuries per year

(Peterson and Renstrom, 1986). The injury also occurs less commonly in contact sports when the thumb becomes trapped as a player falls.

Chronic insufficiency of the ligament (gamekeeper's thumb) is distinct from complete rupture (skier's thumb). Complete rupture usually occurs from the distal attachment at the base of the proximal phalanx, and in about 30% of cases an avulsion fracture occurs. The UCL lies beneath the adductor pollicis, and with complete rupture the aponeurosis of this muscle may be trapped between the pieces of torn ligament – a so-called 'Stener lesion' (Stener, 1962). When the ligament is completely ruptured, contraction of the adductor pollicis will tend to sublux the joint rather than give true adduction, and so grip is weakened.

Symptoms are reproduced by passive extension and abduction of the thumb, and the pain is usually well-localized to the ulnar side of the joint. A valgus stress to the MCP joint will stretch the ligament and again gives pain, and this force may also be used to test for ligamentous instability. If the valgus stress is applied with the joint in complete extension (close pack) the joint may appear stable. Unlocking the joint, however, reveals the instability when compared to the non-injured side. In complete rupture, the end-feel of the joint is limp, and a dorsal haematoma may be visible over the thumb interphalangeal joint, indicating that blood has diffused along the extensor pollicis longus (Moutet et al., 1989).

> **Keypoint**
>
> Gamekeeper's or skier's thumb is an injury to the ulnar collateral ligament of the MCP joint of the thumb. Extension and abduction of the thumb causes pain and ligamentous instability may be noted when a valgus stress is imposed on the joint.

Treatment

Treatment of a grade I injury is initially by rest and ice in the acute phase and then the joint is actively mobilized as pain and swelling settle. Grade II injuries require immobilization for as much as 4 weeks in a strapping or splint to limit abduction, and in severe cases a cast may be required. Complete ligamentous ruptures generally require surgery, and about a quarter may be expected to have displaced bone fragments (Moutet et al., 1989) which will require fixation by Kirschner wires.

Following surgical repair, the thumb is immobilized in a cast for 4–6 weeks, and later a full rehabilitation programme is begun.

De Quervain's tenovaginitis

De Quervain's sydrome (also called Hoffman's disease) is an inflammation and thickening of the synovial lining of the

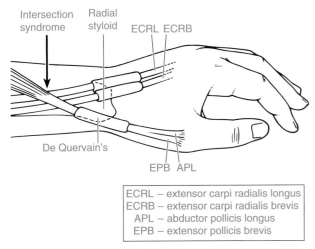

ECRL – extensor carpi radialis longus
ECRB – extensor carpi radialis brevis
APL – abductor pollicis longus
EPB – extensor pollicis brevis

Figure 20.9   Thumb tendinitis.

common sheath of the abductor pollicis longus and extensor pollicis brevis tendons (Fig. 20.9). The thickening occurs particularly at the point where the tendons pass over the distal aspect of the radius (radial styloid or Lister's tubercle). The history is usually of overuse and the condition represents a common occupational injury, but is also seen in rock climbers. There is pain to resisted thumb extension and abduction. In addition, pain is caused by passively ulnar deviating the wrist while keeping the thumb fully flexed (Finkelstein's test), a movement which stretches the tendon and sheath. Local tenderness is found to palpation, again with the tendon on stretch. Crepitus is often present to repeated movements. The condition must be differentiated from arthritis of the carpometacarpal joint of the thumb which will not give pain on resisted movements, or tendon stretch, but will give pain in roughly the same area.

De Quervain's tenovaginitis responds well to frictional massage with the tendon on stretch, and immobilization of the thumb in a splint. Corticosteroid injection into the tendon sheath is reserved for persistent cases.

Importantly, the stressor causing this injury must be identified and removed. Often, the type of grip and repetition of movement are the two deciding factors. Experimenting with alternative grip types and size of grip is useful to increase the variety of stress imposed on the affected tissues.

Intersection syndrome

Intersection syndrome (oarsman's wrist) is a bursitus between the abductor pollicis longus and extensor pollicis brevis (first dorsal compartment of wrist) on one side and the extensor carpi radialis longus and brevis (second compartment) on the other (Fig. 20.9). The two sets of tendons are in separate sheaths which cross each other at a 60° angle about 2–3 finger breadths proximal to the wrist crease, and proximal to the radial styloid (the site of de Quervain's syndrome). The condition is common in rowing and skiing, and

in any activity involving repeated wrist extension and radial deviation. This is often visible swelling along the tendon sheaths and palpable crepitus. Management is by reduction of activity and wrist splinting. Steroid injection into the tendon sheath may be required for persistent cases.

> **Keypoint**
>
> Differentiation of de Quervain's syndrome and intersection syndrome is by palpation. *De Quervain's* gives pain directly over the radial styloid, while *intersection syndrome* gives pain 2–3 cm proximal and medial to this point.

Arthrosis

The capsular pattern at the carpometacarpal joint is a limitation of abduction only. By far the most common intra-articular lesion is osteoarthrosis. The condition is more usual in women and is frequently bilateral, but can also occur secondary to Bennett's fracture. The typical patient seen by the sports physiotherapist is a mature woman who plays casual racquet sports. The pain is made worse with increasing frequency of play, particularly with a sustained grip. Pain is well localized to the base of the thumb and must be distinguished from tenovaginitis (see above). Sudden shooting pains may often cause the patient to drop an object in extreme cases, and accessory movements are limited and painful, particularly axial rotations. Pinch grip power is reduced.

Splinting the joint may allow the acute inflammation to subside. Joint mobilization, including longitudinal oscillations, and abduction/adduction while stabilizing the trapezium are effective for pain relief or increasing motion.

Fracture

The base of the first metacarpal is often fractured from a longitudinally applied force, as occurs from a punch in sports such as boxing and karate. Transverse or oblique fracture lines may occur, and if the fracture line affects the joint surface (Bennett's fracture), secondary osteoarthritis may occur in later years. Oblique fractures are often displaced, with the abductor pollicis longus pulling the shaft of the metacarpal proximally (Fig. 20.10). These injuries require manipulation under anaesthetic to reduce them. Maintenance of reduction is by casting the thumb, wrist and forearm, keeping the first metacarpal in extension. Fixation may be required where the joint surface is involved to improve the alignment of the bone fragments.

Immobilization is usually for a period of about 3 weeks. Active mobility exercises are begun immediately the cast is removed, as stiffness is a severe impairment to normal hand function.

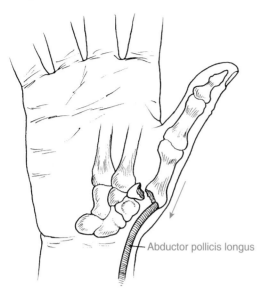

Figure 20.10   Bennett's fracture displaced proximally by the pull of the abductor pollicis longus. From Reid (1992), with permission.

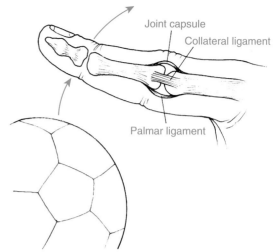

Figure 20.11   Hyperextension injury of the finger. Hyperextension injury (ball hitting finger) may damage the joint capsule and palmar ligament. Greater force creates a dislocation.

THE FINGERS

The fingers are commonly injured in sport by being 'pulled back' when hit by a ball or opponent (Fig. 20.11). In addition, sports which place great strain on the fingers themselves, such as rock climbing and certain martial arts techniques, may also give problems.

Dislocation

Dislocations of the proximal interphalangeal (PIP) joints, especially that of the fifth finger, are the most commonly seen types. These result from a hyperextension force, with posterior dislocation being more common. Radiographic appearance is of the middle phalanx overriding the proximal, a condition which is often associated with detachment of the palmar ligament (volar plate) from the base of the middle phalanx. Once reduced, these injuries should be protected in a splint which prevents hyperextension, but allows early flexion.

Where the force is less severe, dislocation may be avoided, but the palmar ligament and joint capsule may still be disrupted. The anterior aspect of the joint is tender to palpation, and the joint is splinted as for a dislocation.

Fracture dislocation can result when an axially directed force is imposed on a semi-flexed finger. The middle phalanx shears and hits onto the condyle of the proximal phalanx, dislodging a bony fragment. When the fragment involves less than one third of the articular line (Fig. 20.12) the collateral ligament usually remains intact and ensures joint stability. Closed reduction is used, with splinting to prevent the last 15% of extension. Where the joint surface is fragmented the collateral ligament will usually be disrupted, and repeated subluxation is likely to occur. Open reduction with internal fixation is therefore required (Isani, 1990).

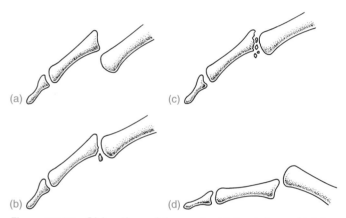

Figure 20.12   Dislocations of the proximal interphalangeal joint. (a) Reducible dislocation. (b) Fracture-dislocation involving less than one third of the articular base. (c) Articular fragmentation involving more than one third of the articular base. (d) Anterior (volar) dislocation.

It is often tempting to reduce finger dislocations straight away, and this is certainly easier than when muscle spasm has set in. As the joint capsule is intact the procedure is usually quite successful. However, the danger of fracture dislocation or the imposition of soft tissue between the bone ends makes it necessary to err on the side of caution. Close examination is needed, and longitudinal traction should be gently applied. The joint may reduce easily, but this should be checked by X-ray (Rimmer, 1981).

Keypoint

Only put back (reduce) a dislocated finger joint after close examination. Do not force the joint, but apply longitudinal traction until the joint reduces spontaneously.

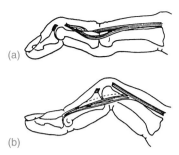

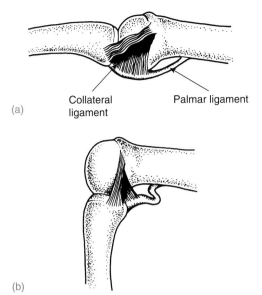

Figure 20.13   Interphalangeal joint of the finger. (a) Extension–collateral ligament lax, palmar ligament tight. (b) Flexion–collateral ligament tight, palmar ligament lax. From Hertling, D. and Kessler, R.M. (1990) *Management of Common Musculoskeletal Disorders.* J.B. Lippincott, Philadelphia. With permission.

Collateral ligament injuries

The MCP and IP joints have loose capsules which are lax in extension. Each joint has obliquely placed collateral ligaments which become increasingly tight with flexion. In addition, the palmar ligaments are fibrocartilage structures attached loosely to the metacarpals but firmly to the bases of the proximal phalanges. Proximally, the palmar ligament thins out to become membranous. During flexion, this thin portion folds like a bellows, but with hyperextension it is stretched and provides the support lacking from the joint capsule (Fig. 20.13). The fibrous flexor sheaths (containing the tendons of flexor digitorum superficialis and flexor digitorum profundus) in turn attach to the palmar ligaments.

Valgus and varus forces directed against the PIP joints will usually result in partial tearing of the collateral ligaments but leave the joint stable. The injuries respond to strapping to the adjacent finger (buddy splinting) to protect the joint and at the same time facilitate early mobility.

Complete ligamentous disruption may warrant surgical intervention, especially where the radial collateral ligament of the index or little finger is affected, as these are subjected to greater stress in normal gripping activities (Isani, 1990). The ligament normally ruptures at the level of the joint line, possibly with avulsion. After suture repair the finger is maintained in 60° flexion for 3 weeks (Rimmer, 1981).

Muscles

The muscles most commonly injured within the hand are the interossei, usually by overstretching the fingers. Pain is highly localized, and increased to abduction (dorsal interossei) or adduction (plantar interossei). As the muscle

Figure 20.14   Results of injury to the extensor tendon mechanism. (a) Mallet deformity. (b) Buttonhole deformity. From Reilly, T. (1981) The concept, measurement and development of flexibility. In *Sports Fitness and Sports Injuries* (ed. T. Reilly). Faber and Faber, London. With permission.

fibres travel parallel to the finger, transverse friction massage is given by the therapist placing his or her finger between those of the athlete and using a rotation action by pronating and supinating his or her own forearm.

Tendon injury

Prolonged gripping with the tips of the fingers, such as may occur in rock climbing, can cause injury to the flexor tendons. The distal IP joint is extended, while the proximal IP is flexed, stressing flexor digitorum profundus. Long-term exposure to this type of stress may also damage the flexor sheath, increasing the bowstringing effect to resisted finger flexion (Bollen, 1988).

Hyperflexion may disrupt the extensor tendon, and avulse it from the base of the distal phalanx (mallet finger) or cause the middle section of the tendon to rupture (boutonniere or 'buttonhole' deformity) (Fig. 20.14). This can occur when the end of the terminal phalanx is struck by a ball for example. When the extensor mechanism is disrupted in this way, the athlete can flex the finger, and while elastic recoil enables the joint to extend slightly, normal extension is impossible.

With mallet finger, tenderness occurs at a point between the nail and the distal IP joint, and the fingertip is held slightly flexed when resting. In a button-hole deformity, tenderness is more proximal, and the finger is hyperextended at the distal interphalangeal joint. Radiographs reveal the avulsed fragment. Treatment is by immobilization in a splint which maintains hyperextension of the distal IP joint, or occasionally surgical intervention. Conservative management has been shown to give a very high satisfaction level. In an evaluation of 26 outcome studies, Geyman, Fink and Sullivan (1998) showed an 83.4% satisfaction level with conservative management and recommended that surgical treatment should be reserved for chronic or recurrent injuries only.

Keypoint

With *mallet finger*, the fingertip is held slightly flexed when resting. In a *button-hole deformity*, the finger is hyperextended at the distal interphalangeal joint.

Inflammation of the extensor tendons (tendinitis), or tendon sheaths (tenosynovitis) may occur with repetitive finger movements. Although more common as an occupational injury (keyboard operators), the condition can occur through excessive training activities. Pain and crepitus occur to repeated movements, with pain localized to the extensor tendon sheaths. Treatment is to remove the stressor and reduce the inflammation with ice and modalities.

REHABILITATION OF WRIST AND HAND INJURIES

There is often a tendency for athletes to play down wrist and finger injuries. Because they can run, and because they largely look normal, athletes may often be found some years later to still have a lack of movement or strength when compared to the uninjured side. This, of course, leads to faults in sports technique in those areas where the hand is used extensively, and lays the foundation for arthritis in later years. Hand rehabilitation is no less important than that of, say, a hamstring or injured collateral ligament of the knee, and this must be stressed over and over again.

For soft tissue injuries, especially those affecting the fingers, mobility following injury is the all-important factor. Where splinting is required, this should be in the 'protective position', which prevents capsular and ligamentous contracture while protecting the joint from further injury. The IP joints are immobilized in extension, the MCP joints in flexion, and the thumb in abduction (Isani, 1990). Movement must be begun as soon as possible after injury. Gentle isometrics and mobility exercise within the pain-free range can usually be begun 1 or 2 days after injury.

Following this, exercise progresses as hand function returns. For convenience, wrist and finger exercises will be dealt with separately, although many of the exercises will be used together.

> ### Keypoint
>
> Early mobilization of finger injuries is vital to prevent long-term stiffness.

Wrist exercise

Three exercises can be used to form a basis for regaining wrist mobility. The first two are performed with the hand flat on a table top. Initially, the hand is placed palm down on the table surface, with the wrist crease at the table edge. The contralateral hand is placed on top of the injured one, and the elbow is moved up and down to produce flexion and extension of the wrist. The leverage of the forearm and bodyweight may be used to actively assist movement at end-range (Fig. 20.15a). The hand is then moved into the centre of the table, so that the whole forearm is supported; again the contralateral hand holds the injured one flat

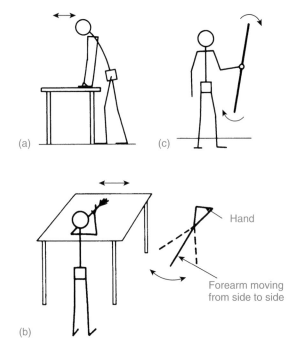

Figure 20.15   Autotherapy wrist mobilizations. (a) Flexion/extension. (b) Abduction/adduction. (c) Pronation/supination with a broom handle.

against the table surface, stopping it moving. The elbow on the injured side is moved from side to side, sliding over the table surface to perform abduction and adduction of the injured wrist (Fig. 20.15b). Finally, the arm is held at 90° flexion with the elbow held close into the side of the body, the injured forearm supported by the cupped contralateral hand. A stick is held in the hand, and pronation and supination performed, aiming to move the stick into a horizontal position (Fig. 20.15c). Range of motion is measured regularly and realistic targets are set for the athlete to achieve.

Strength of the wrist is regained by performing movements against the resistance of a powerband or small weight. Flexion/extension may be performed holding a light dumb-bell, with the forearm supported. The other movements are performed with one weight of the dumb-bell removed (hammerbell), or using a hammer. The forearm is positioned with the side supported, and the hand holds the free end of the dumb-bell. Abduction is performed with the dumb-bell weight above the hand, and adduction with it below; in each case a 'chopping' action is used (Fig. 20.16). Pronation and supination are again executed using the hammerbell. The forearm is supported, and pronated and supinated to perform an arc with the hammerbell weight.

In addition to mobility and strength, compression, distraction and combined movements using functional activities are important. The ability of the wrist to take weight (press-up, bench press), to lock (straight arm actions holding a dumb-bell), and to take tension (chinning a bar) must be redeveloped. Rapid actions such as punching, catching

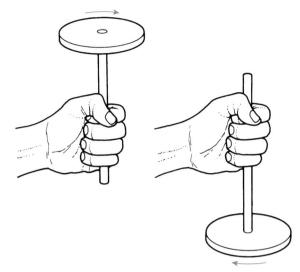

Figure 20.16   Wrist abduction/adduction using a modified dumb-bell.

and throwing all form part of the late stage rehabilitation programme.

> **Keypoint**
>
> Functional wrist exercise includes taking weight (compression) through the wrist, tensioning (traction) the wrist, and locking the wrist at various angles.

Finger exercise

Many finger exercises may be begun using simple pinch grip and power grip actions. Grip and release movements, holding, and lifting may be performed using small objects with two fingers (pinch) or larger objects and all the fingers (power). Mobility may be performed by isolating the movement to the affected joint and simply teaching the athlete to perform autotherapy activities with the other hand. These are easier when the joint is warm and any tight skin is made more flexible, so hot soaking and the use of oil or cream is encouraged.

Isolation exercises for strength may be accomplished using therapeutic putty, rubber bands of varying sizes and small weights. Again, functional activities, the ability to push, pull, and lock, and rapid grip and release actions are important. Simple actions such as screwing and unscrewing varying sized nuts and bolts improve dexterity. Pushing with the finger straight into a thick piece of foam rubber, and pulling using pinch, ring, power and key grips help to restore tension and compression ability. Rapid throwing and catching actions with objects of varying sizes and weight rehabilitate grip and release.

> **Keypoint**
>
> Functional activities for the fingers are vital. Pushing and pulling with the fingers, using the fingers locked (stable) and rapidly gripping and releasing should all be practised.

References

Albanese, S.A., Palmer, A.K., Kerr, D.R., Carpenter, C.W., Lisi, D. and Levinsohn, E.M. (1989) Wrist pain and distal growth plate closure of the radius in gymnasts. *Journal of Pediatric Orthopaedics*, **9**, 23–28

Aronen, J.G. (1985) Problems of the upper extremity in gymnasts. *Clinics in Sports Medicine*, **4**, (1) 61–71

Bollen, S.R. (1988) Soft tissue injury in extreme rock climbers. *British Journal of Sports Medicine*, **22**, (4) 145–147

Bunker, T.D., McNamee, P.B. and Scott, T.D. (1987) The Herbert screw for scaphoid fractures: a multicentre study. *Journal of Bone and Joint Surgery*, **69B**, 631–634

Carter, S.R., Aldridge, M.J., Fitzgerald, R. and Davies, A.M. (1988) Stress changes of the wrist in adolescent gymnasts. *British Journal of Radiology*, **61**, 109–112

Cetti, R., Christensen, S.E. and Reuther, K. (1982) Fracture of the lunate bone. *Hand*, **14**, 80–84

Corrigan, B. and Maitland, G.D. (1983) *Practical Orthopaedic Medicine*, Butterworth, London

Cyriax, J. (1982) *Textbook of Orthopaedic Medicine*, 8th edn, Baillière Tindall, London, vol. 1

Cyriax, J.H. and Cyriax, P.J. (1983) *Illustrated Manual of Orthopaedic Medicine*, Butterworth, London

Diamond, M.R. (1989) Carpal tunnel syndrome: a review. *Chiropractic Sports Medicine*, **3**, (2), 46–53

Garrick, J.G. and Webb, D.R. (1990) *Sports Injuries: Diagnosis and Management*. W.B. Saunders, London

Geyman, J.P., Fink, K. and Sullivan, S.D. (1998) Conservative versus surgical treatment of mallet finger. *Journal of the American Board of Family Practitioners*, **11**, 382–390

Gutierrez, G. (1996) Office management of scaphoid fractures. *Physician and Sportsmedicine*, **24**, (8) 1–8

Haloua, J.P., Collin, J.P. and Coudeyre, L. (1987) Paralysis of the ulnar nerve in cyclists. *Annales de Chirurgie de la Main*, **6**, 282–287

Hertling, D. and Kessler, R.M. (1990) *Management of Common Musculoskeletal Disorders*, J.B. Lippincott, Philadelphia

Horii, E., Nakamura, R., Watanabe, K. and Tsunoda, K. (1994) Scaphoid fracture as a 'Puncher's fracture'. *Journal of Orthopaedic Trauma*, **8**, 107–110

Isani, A. (1990) Prevention and treatment of ligamentous sports injuries to the hand. *Sports Medicine*, **9**, (1) 48–61

Kaltenborg, F.M. (1993) *The Spine. Basic Examination and Mobilisation Techniques*, 2nd edn, Olaf Norlis Bokhandel, Oslo, Norway

Magee, D.J. (2002) *Orthopedic Physical Assessment*, 4th edn, Saunders, Philadelphia

Maitland, G.D. (1991) *Peripheral Manipulation*, 3rd edn, Butterworth-Heinemann, London

Mandelbaum B.R., Bartolozzi, A.R., Davis, C.A., Teurlings, L. and Bragonier, B. (1989) Wrist pain syndrome in the gymnast: pathogenetic, diagnostic and therapeutic considerations. *American Journal of Sports Medicine*, **17**, (3) 305–317

Moutet, F., Guinard, D., Lebrun, C., Bello-Champel, P. and Massart, P. (1989) Metacarpo-phalangeal thumb sprains: based on experience with more than 1000 cases. *Annales de Chirugie de la Main*, **8**, 99–109

Nakamura, R., Imaeda, T., Suzuki, K. and Miura, T. (1991) Sports-related Kienbock's disease. *American Journal of Sports Medicine*, **19**, (1) 88–91

O'Donoghue, D.H. (1976) *Treatment of Injuries to Athletes*, W.B. Saunders, Philadelphia

Palastanga, N., Field, D. and Soames, R. (1989) *Anatomy and Human Movement*, Heinemann Medical, Oxford

Palastanga, N., Field, D. and Soames, R. (1994) *Anatomy and Human Movement*, 2nd edn, Butterworth-Heinemann, Oxford

Palmer, A.K. and Werner, F.W. (1981) The triangular fibrocartilage complex of the wrist: anatomy and function. *Journal of Hand Surgery*, **6**, 153–162

Peterson, L. and Renstrom, P. (1986) *Sports Injuries*, Martin Dunitz, London

Reid, D.C. (1992) *Sports Injury Assessment and Rehabilitation*, Churchill Livingstone, Edinburgh

Reilly, T. (1981) The concept, measurement and development of flexibility. In *Sports Fitness and Sports Injuries* (ed. T. Reilly), Faber and Faber, London

Rettig, A.C., Weidenbener, E.J. and Gloyeske, R. (1994) Alternative management of midthird scaphoid fractures in the athlete. *American Journal of Sports Medicine*, **22**, 711–714

Rimmer, J.N. (1981) Injuries to the hand in sports. In *Sports Fitness and Sports Injuries* (ed. T. Reilly), Faber and Faber, London

Stener, B. (1962) Displacement of the ruptured ulnar collateral ligament of the metacarpophalangeal joint of the thumb: a clinical and anatomical study. *Journal of Bone and Joint Surgery*, **44B**, 869

Wilkes, J.S. (1989) Reconstructive surgery of the wrist and hand. In *Orthopaedic Physical Therapy* (eds R. Donatelli and M.J. Wooden). Churchill Livingstone, Edinburgh

Williams, J.G.P. and Sperryn, P.N. (1976) *Sports Medicine*. Edward Arnold, London

Wilmarth, M.A. and Nelson, S.G. (1988) Distal sensory latencies of the ulnar nerve in long distance bicyclists: pilot study. *Journal of Orthopaedic and Sports Physical Therapy*, **9**, 370–374

Appendix 1

MANUAL MUSCLE TESTS

The upper extremity

The following tests draw largely on the work of Kendall, McCreary and Provance (1993) and Clarkson and Gilewich (1989) to which the reader is referred for further information.

Serratus anterior

The serratus anterior is a scapular abductor and lateral rotator, which works in opposition to the rhomboids. As a screening test, the wall push-up or full push-up is performed and any scapular winging is noted. In both cases winging is more noticeable on eccentric activity. A similar, but less powerful, movement is obtained in a supine-lying position by performing a 'punch with a plus'. Again, weakness is apparent with scapular winging, but it should be noted that pectoralis minor can partially perform the punching action from this starting position by causing the coronoid to pull the scapular into subtle tilt. Resisted shoulder flexion (120°) in sitting is a more accurate test (Fig. A.1). If serratus anterior is weak, the rhomboids are usually found to be tight, due to an inability to abduct the scapulae fully. The rhomboids may be stretched by pulling on the vertebral border of the scapula, or by abducting the scapulae and crossing the arms fully.

Trapezius

The upper trapezius, levator scapulae and the rhomboids all elevate the scapulae. However, the upper trapezius upwardly rotates the scapula while the rhomboids and levator scapulae downwardly rotate it. These latter two muscles may be differentiated through the action of levator scapulae on the cervical spine. Elevation is tested in a sitting position, resisting both elevation of the shoulder and lateral flexion of the cervical spine (Fig. A.2).

The middle fibres of trapezius are tested with the athlete in a prone-lying position with the arm hanging over the couch side initially, and then abducted to 90° (Fig. A.3). The athlete adducts the scapula towards the mid-line. The rhomboids are differentiated from the middle trapezius by their action on scapular rotation. Laterally rotating the humerus, by pointing the thumb to the ceiling, tractions the teres major (a medial rotator of the glenohumeral joint)

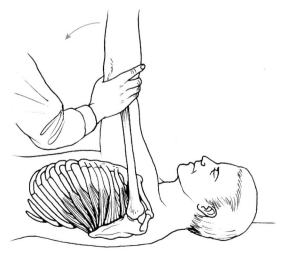

Figure A.1 Serratus anterior.

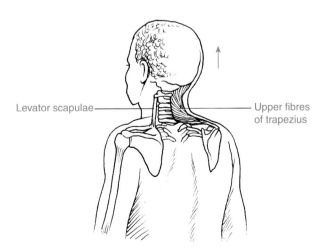

Figure A.2 Levator scapulae and upper trapezius.

Levator scapulae

Upper fibres of trapezius

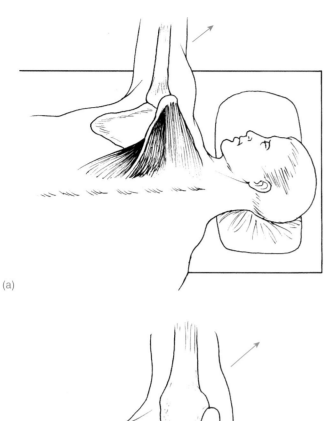

(a)

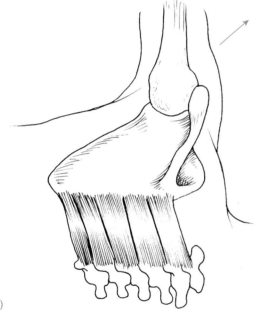

(b)

Figure A.3   (a) Middle trapezius. (b) Rhomboids.

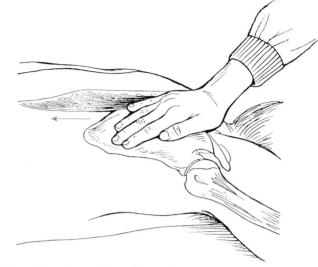

Figure A.4   Lower fibres of trapezius.

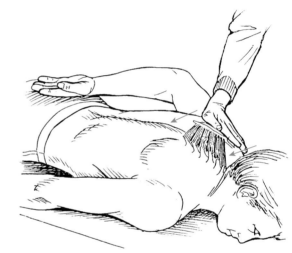

Figure A.5   Rhomboids.

causing it to pull on the axillary border of the scapular sufficiently to draw the scapula into upward rotation. As scapular adduction is begun, movement of the scapula into downward rotation shows the rhomboids to be working with or without the middle trapezius. Medially rotating the humerus (thumb to floor) emphasizes the rhomboids and is an alternative test.

The lower trapezius is again assessed in a prone-lying position. Initially, the scapula is passively depressed and adducted into an optimal position. The arm is held by the side, slightly off the couch and the test assesses the athlete's ability to maintain scapular stabilization against the weight of the arm. Progression is made by lengthening the arm lever while maintaining an optimal scapular position. The

final test position is with the arm held diagonally overhead in line with the lower trapezius fibres (Fig. A.4).

The rhomboids

The rhomboids are tested with the athlete in a prone position (Fig. A.5). The athlete places the dorsum of the hand over the buttock on the non-test side, and attempts to raise the arm away from the back. Resistance is applied over the scapula, not the humerus. Differentiation from the middle trapezius relies on scapular rotation as described above.

Deltoid

Each of the three sets of deltoid fibres are assessed in a sitting position (Fig. A.6). For the anterior fibres, the athlete flexes the shoulder joint to 90° (in slight medial rotation). Where coracobrachialis is tested, the anterior deltoid is placed at a disadvantage by maintaining an externally

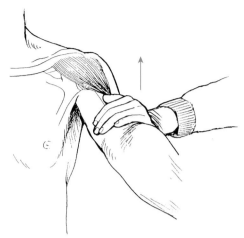

Figure A.6   Anterior deltoid.

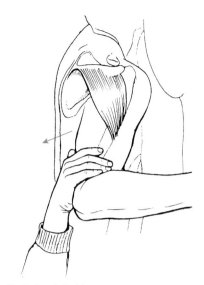

Figure A.8   Posterior deltoid.

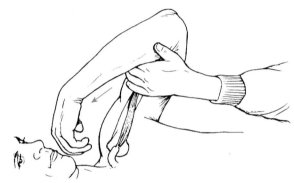

Figure A.7   Coracobrachialis.

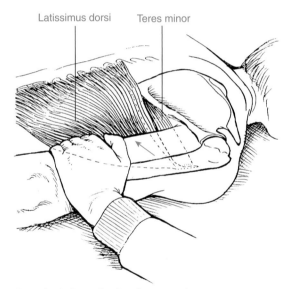

Figure A.9   Latissimus dorsi and teres major.

rotated position. Flexion adduction is used (Fig. A.7). The medial deltoid and supraspinatus are tested with the arm abducted to 90°. Supraspinatus may not be distinguished from the medial deltoid in initiation of abduction, as both muscles are active. However, palpation of supraspinatus and use of surface EMG will indicate if the muscle is contracting. As the muscle is covered by the middle and upper trapezius, the trapezius must remain as relaxed as possible throughout the action. The posterior fibres of the deltoid are assessed using horizontal abduction combined with slight lateral rotation (Fig. A.8).

Latissimus dorsi

The latissimus dorsi and teres major are tested in a prone-lying position with the arm by the athlete's side. The action is to extend the arm while maintaining adduction (Fig. A.9).

Pectoralis major

The pectoralis major is assessed in a supine-lying position. Initially, the whole muscle is tested using horizontal adduction. Any excessive activity in the anterior deltoid is noted. The clavicular and sternal heads of the muscle may be differentiated by aligning the direction of pull with the appropriate

muscle fibres. Both sets of fibres are tested using adduction and slight medial rotation. The clavicular (upper) head is tested from a 70° abducted position, aiming the pull to the sternal end of the clavicle. The sternal head is tested from 135° abduction, pulling towards the opposite iliac crest (Fig. A.10). Pectoralis minor is tested again in supine lying, but the action is a forward thrust with the shoulder region, with no direct movement of the humerus (Fig. A.11). This muscle is commonly short, and an important factor in altered mechanics of the glenohumeral joint.

Internal and external rotation

Rotation is assessed either in a prone-lying position with the shoulder abducted to 90° (upper arm supported) and the elbow flexed, or in a sitting position with the upper arm tucked into the side. Internal rotation tests the subscapularis

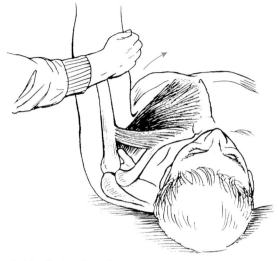

Figure A.10   Pectoralis major.

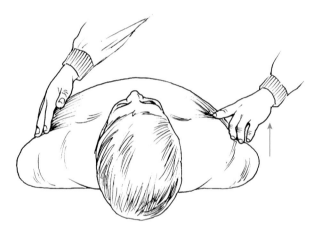

Figure A.11   Pectoralis minor.

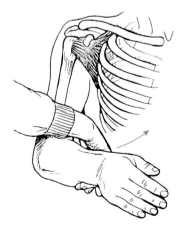

Figure A.12   Internal rotation of subscapularis.

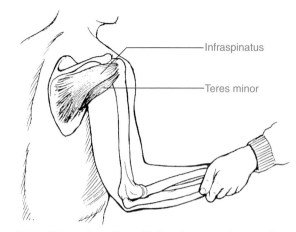

Figure A.13   External rotation of infraspinatus and teres minor.

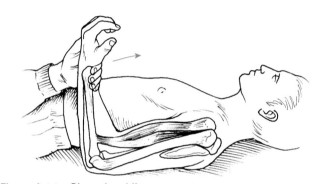

Figure A.14   Biceps brachii.

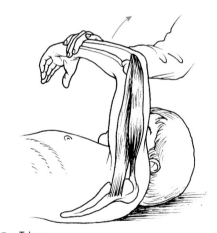

Figure A.15   Triceps.

Elbow flexors

Biceps, brachialis and brachioradialis are all assessed in supine lying with the shoulder adducted. The athlete performs resisted elbow flexion with the forearm supinated for biceps (Fig. A.14), pronated for brachialis and in mid-position for brachioradialis. The effect of biceps on glenohumeral flexion, and radiohumeral supination must also be tested, with the athlete in a sitting position.

with teres major, pectoralis major, latissimus dorsi, and the anterior deltoid acting as assistant movers (Fig. A.12). External rotation tests the infraspinatus and teres minor with the posterior deltoid acting as an assistant (Fig. A.13).

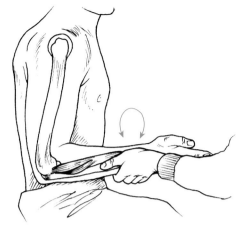

Figure A.16   Supinator.

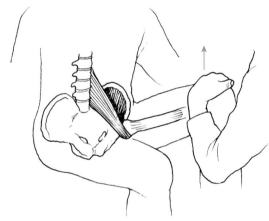

Figure A.17   Iliopsoas.

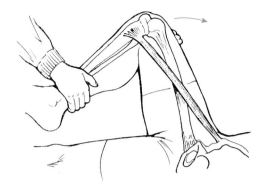

Figure A.18   Sartorius.

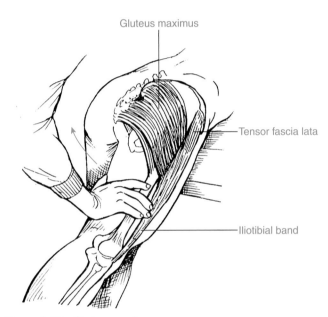

Figure A.19   Gluteus maximus.

Triceps

The athlete may be tested in supine lying, with the shoulder internally rotated and flexed to 90°. Elbow extension is resisted (Fig. A.15). In prone lying, with the shoulder abducted to 90°, elbow extension may be combined with shoulder extension.

Pronation and supination

Both movements are tested with the athlete in a sitting position, with the arm positioned in mid-position (Fig. A.16).

The lower extremity

Iliopsoas

Iliopsoas is tested in a sitting position, with resisted hip flexion, and the knee remaining flexed (Fig. A.17). The muscle is differentiated from rectus femoris by the action of rectus over the knee.

Sartorius

The starting position is supine lying, and hip flexion, abduction and external rotation (FABER) are combined with knee flexion (Fig. A.18).

Gluteus maximus

The athlete is positioned in prone lying, and inner range hip extension is performed with the knee remaining flexed to reduce the activity of the hamstrings. Through range, activity is assessed from four point kneeling, with the athlete's abdomen supported over a stool (Fig. A.19). The movement must be pure extension with no abduction.

Hip abductors

The starting position is side lying. The gluteus minimus and gluteus medius are both tested in side lying (Fig. A.20). Emphasis is placed on the posterior fibres of gluteus medius (postural portion of the muscle) by combining hip abduction with external rotation. Tensor fascia lata is again tested in side lying. It is differentiated from gluteus minimus by the action of tensor fascia lata on hip flexion, knee extension and in tightening the iliotibial band (Fig. A.21).

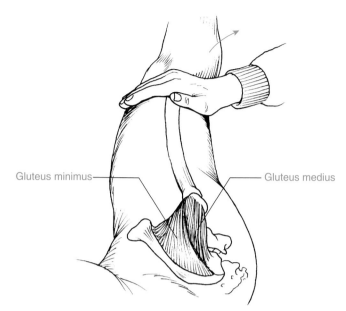

Figure A.20   Gluteus medius.

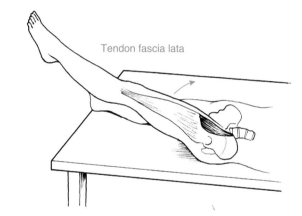

Figure A.21   Tensor fascia lata.

Hip adductors

A side-lying starting position is chosen with the tested leg down (Fig. A.22). Adduction is resisted to test the whole adductor group. Flexing the knee will shorten gracilis and place it at a mechanical disadvantage, thus emphasizing the short adductors. Gracilis should also be tested with the hamstrings by resisted knee flexion. It is differentiated from the hamstrings by its inability to extend the hip. Adductor longus and brevis, together with pectineus, aid in hip flexion, so a tendency for the leg to drift into flexion is an indication that these adductors are dominant and/or that the hip extensors are failing to neutralize the flexion movement.

Hip rotators

A prone-lying starting position may be used with the pelvis stabilized by the therapist. The hip and knee are flexed to 90°, and resisted internal rotation (foot out) and external rotation (foot in) are performed (Fig. A.23).

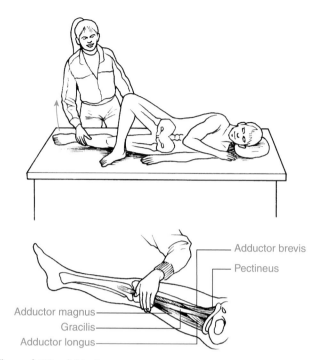

Figure A.22   Adductors.

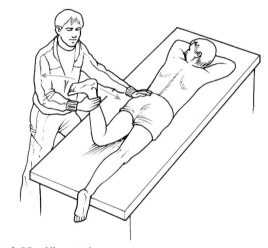

Figure A.23   Hip rotation.

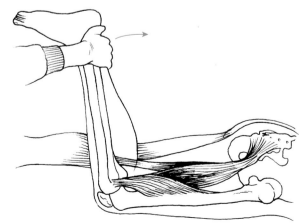

Figure A.24   Hamstrings.

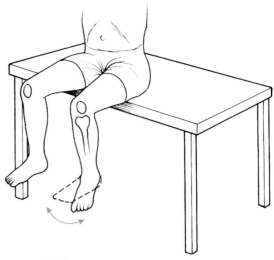

Figure A.26   Popliteus.

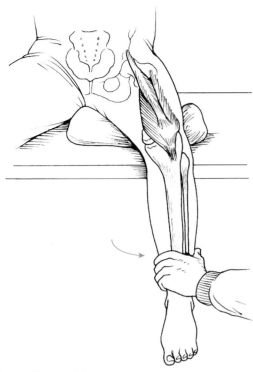

Figure A.25   The quadriceps.

Hamstrings

The starting position is prone lying with the pelvis stabilized. Resisted knee flexion is performed with internal rotation (semimembranosus and semitendinosus) or external rotation (biceps femoris) (Fig. A.24). The action of the hamstrings and gluteus maximus in extending the hip is an important factor to muscle imbalance assessment in this region.

Quadriceps

The quadriceps are tested in a sitting position. Resisted knee extension is performed to assess the vasti, and resisted knee extension and hip flexion are combined to test the rectus femoris (Fig. A.25).

Popliteus

The athlete is tested in a sitting position, and the action is resisted medial rotation of the tibia on the fixed femur. In cases where the lateral hamstrings are dominant over the medial, active medial rotation may be extremely weak. During the test tibial rotation must be differentiated from foot inversion (Fig. A.26).

References

Clarkson, H.M. and Gilewich, G.B. (1989) *Musculoskeletal Assessment*, Williams and Wilkins, Baltimore

Kendall, F.P., McCreary, E. and Provance, P.G. (1993) *Muscles. Testing and Function*, Williams and Wilkins, Baltimore

Appendix 2

Stretching exercises for athletes

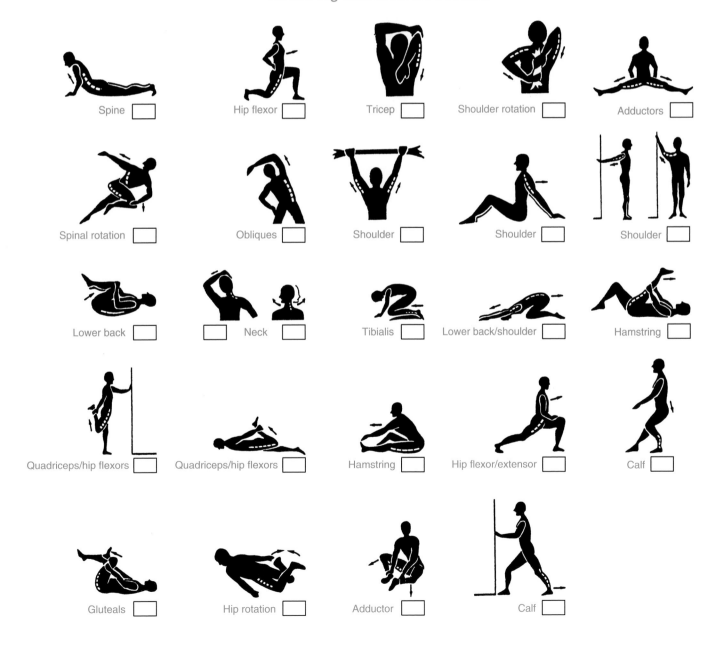

Spine ☐ Hip flexor ☐ Tricep ☐ Shoulder rotation ☐ Adductors ☐

Spinal rotation ☐ Obliques ☐ Shoulder ☐ Shoulder ☐ Shoulder ☐

Lower back ☐ ☐ Neck ☐ Tibialis ☐ Lower back/shoulder ☐ Hamstring ☐

Quadriceps/hip flexors ☐ Quadriceps/hip flexors ☐ Hamstring ☐ Hip flexor/extensor ☐ Calf ☐

Gluteals ☐ Hip rotation ☐ Adductor ☐ Calf ☐

Index

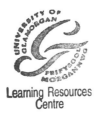